CLEFT PALATE AND CRANIOFACIAL ANOMALIES

Effects on Speech and Resonance

SECOND EDITION

ANN W. KUMMER, PH.D., CCC-SLP, ASHA-F

Professor of Clinical Pediatrics
University of Cincinnati Medical Center

Senior Director of Speech Pathology
Cincinnati Children's Hospital Medical Center

With Contributions

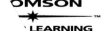
OMSON
LEARNING

Australia • Brazil • Canada • Mexico • Singapore • Spain • United Kingdom • United States

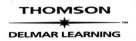

THOMSON

DELMAR LEARNING

Cleft Palate and Craniofacial Anomalies: Effects on Speech and Resonance, Second Edition
By Ann W. Kummer

Vice President, Health Care Business Unit:
William Brottmiller

Director of Learning Solutions:
Matthew Kane

Managing Editor:
Marah Bellegarde

Senior Acquisitions Editor:
Sherry Dickinson

Product Manager:
Natalie Pashoukos

Editorial Assistant:
Angela Doolin

Marketing Director:
Jennifer McAvey

Marketing Channel Manager:
Michele McTighe

Technology Director:
Laurie Davis

Technology Project Manager:
Mary Colleen Liburdi

Production Director:
Carolyn Miller

Content Project Manager:
Katie Wachtl

Senior Art Director:
Jack Pendleton

Library of Congress Cataloging-in-Publication Data
Kummer, Ann W.
Cleft palate and craniofacial anomalies: the effects on speech and resonance/Ann W. Kummer, with contributions.—2nd ed.
   p. ; cm.
   Includes bibliographical references and index.
   ISBN-13: 978-1-4180-1547-3
   ISBN-10: 1-4180-1547-4
   1. Cleft palate—Complications.
   2. Face—Abnormalities—Complications. 3. Skull—Abnormalities—Complications.
   4. Speech disorders. I. Title. [DNLM: 1. Cleft Palate—complications. 2. Cleft Palate—therapy. 3. Craniofacial Abnormalities–complications.
   4. Craniofacial Abnormalities—therapy. 5. Speech Disorders—etiology. 6. Speech Disorders—therapy.
   WV 440 K96c 2008]
   RD763.K86 2008
   617.5'225—dc22
                                    2007022052

Notice to the Reader

DEDICATION

This book is dedicated to the three people who have influenced me most in my life and have helped me to be the best that I can be. Without their love and support, I would never have had a career and certainly would not have had the opportunity to write this book.

The first dedication is to my father, who was a wonderful, caring, and talented otolaryngologist whom I always admired. Dad, I always wanted to be just like you when I grew up.

The next dedication is to my mother, who is the kindest, most thoughtful, and most caring person that I have ever known. Mom, now that I am grown up, I strive to be more like you.

The final dedication is to my husband, who has supported me, encouraged me, and helped me to focus and succeed in my career. John, you have allowed me to spread my wings and fly. For that I will be eternally grateful.

With all my love, Ann

CONTENTS

PART 5

TREATMENT PROCEDURES: SPEECH, RESONANCE, AND VELOPHARYNGEAL DYSFUNCTION...... 507

Legends for Videos

These videos are meant to augment the information that is provided in the text. Videos are organized to specifically go with certain chapters. However, many of the videos can be used to illustrate information provided in other chapters.

The video symbol is used in the text to indicate that at least one video is available to illustrate that point or topic. Viewing additional videos in other chapters will provide multiple examples. Additional videos on a particular topic can be found by going to the main menu of the CD-ROM and clicking on "List of Videos by Topic." The following key words are examples of topics that can be found on the list:

- Adenoid
- Apraxia
- Bubbling of secretions
- Compensatory productions
- Cul-de-sac resonance
- Dysarthria
- Dysphonia
- Epiglottis
- Fistula
- Frequent breaths
- Glottal stops
- Hypernasality
- Hyponasality
- Middorsum palatal stops
- Nasal emission

- Nasal grimace
- Nasalization or nasalized
- Nasal rustle
- Nasopharyngoscopy
- Velopharyngeal closure-Normal
- Obstruction
- Passavant's ridge
- Pharyngeal flap
- Sphincter pharyngoplasty
- Velopharyngeal incompetence
- Velopharyngeal insufficiency
- Velopharyngeal mislearning
- Videofluoroscopy
- Weak consonants

CHAPTER 5

5–01.   Baby feeding with a Haberman bottle.

CHAPTER 7

7–01.   Severe hypernasality. Note that vowels are hypernasal and there is nasalization of oral consonants, resulting in a predominance of /m/ and /n/ sounds.

7–02.   Severe hypernasality and nasal emission. Articulation placement is fairly good, but oral consonants are nasalized. See Video 7–03 for this child's postoperative voice sample.

7–03.   Hyponasality as noted on nasal sounds. This child had airway obstruction following a pharyngeal flap. See Video 7–02 for a preoperative comparison of the same child.

7–04.   Cul-de-sac resonance. This child has a large scar band on the back of the pharynx, just below the base of the tongue. As a result, sound is resonating in the oropharynx. This sounds similar to hyponasality. However, notice how clearly the nasal sounds are produced.

7–05.   Nasal emission. This girl has consistent nasal emission on all sounds, but it is most noticeable on sibilants, particularly /s/. Her articulation is normal, but she has weak consonants.

7–06.   Nasal emission. This woman has excellent articulation. However, she has consistent nasal emission on all sounds, most noticeably on sibilants. She has to take an extra breath when counting, which causes short utterance length. She also demonstrates a nasal grimace during speech.

7–07.   Nasal emission. This young man has a submucous cleft and velopharyngeal insufficiency. There is consistent nasal emission on pressure-sensitive sounds. He also has a frontal lisp on /s/ and /z/.

7–08.   Severe nasal emission. This patient has a history of cerebral palsy and velopharyngeal incompetence. Because of a large velopharyngeal opening, there is significant nasal emission and loss of oral pressure. This causes the consonants to be very weak in intensity and pressure. Notice the fact that she takes frequent breaths while counting to compensate for the loss of air through the nose. This causes short utterance length in connected speech. There is also a nasal grimace, reflecting the effort required for trying to achieve velopharyngeal closure.

7–09.   Severe nasal emission. This patient has a history of myasthenia gravis, with velopharyngeal incompetence and vocal-fold paralysis. As a result, the voice is breathy and there is significant nasal emission, weak oral consonants, and short utterance length. The effort required for producing speech is apparent in this sample.

7–10.   Nasal emission and glottal stops. There is obvious nasal emission on voiceless phonemes. On voiced plosives, this child coarticulates glottal stops with nasal sounds. This is the same child as in Video 7–11.

7–11.   Glottal stops and nasal emission. This is the same child as in Video 7–10 but this video shows connected speech.

7–12.   Glottal stops. There is nasal emission and a nasal grimace on sibilants at the beginning of this segment. However, this child's speech is primarily characterized by glottal stops. Phonation is characterized by mild dysphonia secondary to right vocal-cord paresis. This is the same child as in Video 7–13.

7–13.   Glottal stops in singing. This is the same child as in Video 7–12.

7–14.   Nasalization of oral sounds. This child has a submucous cleft with velopharyngeal insufficiency. She primarily uses nasal sounds and some glottal stops for all oral sounds.

7–15.   Compensatory articulation productions. On this segment, the patient demonstrates backing of anterior sounds. He has a large, midpalatal fistula. By producing sounds in the back of the mouth, he is able to make use of the air pressure before it is lost through the fistula. He also uses a pharyngeal fricative for sibilant sounds, most noticeable on /s/. (Note: He is talking about his dog going up to the mountains, and then about speech therapy.)

7–16.   Dysphonia. This child has multiple congenital anomalies, including a submucous cleft and unilateral vocal fold paralysis. He has nasal emission, which is partially masked by the dysphonia. Oral consonants are nasalized.

7–17.   Dysarthria. This child has cerebral palsy and mild dysarthria, primarily characterized by velopharyngeal incompetence.

7–18.   Dysarthria. This young man was in a motor vehicle accident and sustained a significant head injury. He has normal articulation placement, but there is severe hypernasality. There is also nasal emission, which causes the consonants to be very weak in intensity and pressure, and the utterance length to be short.

Notice the big breath before each utterance and the nasal grimace.

7–19. Apraxia. This child has motor difficulties that also affect velopharyngeal function. There is mild nasal emission and an occasional nasal rustle.

7–20. Apraxia. This child has hypernasality due to a submucous cleft, but also has apraxia of speech. Note the difficulty in even combining nasal sounds in the appropriate sequence.

7–21. Phoneme-specific hypernasality. This child demonstrates phoneme-specific hypernasality on the high vowel /i/ (eee), but not on other vowels. This is demonstrated by closing the nose while the child is producing the vowels. There should be no difference in the sound if the velopharyngeal valve is closed. On this video, a difference is noted when the child produces the /i/ vowel only, suggesting a velopharyngeal opening during production of that sound. This is a type of velopharyngeal mislearning.

7–22. Phoneme-specific nasal emission. This child has phoneme-specific nasal emission, in the form of a nasal rustle, on /s/ sounds. All other sounds (including other sibilants) are produced normally with no nasal emission. The nasal rustle is caused by the use of a posterior nasal fricative as a substitution for the correct placement. This is an articulation disorder due to velopharyngeal mislearning, rather than velopharyngeal insufficiency or incompetence. Therefore, it can be corrected easily with speech therapy.

7–23. Phoneme-specific nasal emission. This child has phoneme-specific nasal emission, in the form of a nasal rustle, on all sibilants (/s/, /z/, /sh/, /ch/, /j/). This is caused by the use of a posterior nasal fricative as a substitution for the correct placement. All other pressure-sensitive sounds are produced normally with no nasal emission.

CHAPTER 8

8–01. Ankylossed tongue. This patient has significant limitation of lingual movement for elevation, protrusion, and lateralization due to removal of a hemangioma. However, all lingual-alveolar sounds, including /l/, are produced without any distortion.

8–02.   Severe glossoptosis. Note that in this fMRI (functional magnetic resonance imaging) study, the tongue base is very close to the pharyngeal wall during breathing.

CHAPTER 9

9–01.   Obligatory production. This child has normal tongue position for the /s/ sound. However, due to an anterior crossbite with maxillary retrusion, the tongue tip is in front of the maxillary incisors during production. This is an obligatory production and in this case, it results in very little distortion.

9–02.   Middorsum palatal stops (palatal-dorsal productions). This child is producing lingual-alveolar sounds with the middle part of the tongue, rather than the tongue tip. This is a compensatory error due to an anterior crossbite and maxillary retrusion, which results in less space for movement of the tongue tip.

9–03.   Middorsum palatal stops (palatal-dorsal productions). Middorsum palatal stops are being used for lingual-alveolars due to anterior crowding that occurs with maxillary retrusion.

CHAPTER 12

12–01.   Speech evaluation procedures.

12–02.   Counseling parents about VP function.

CHAPTER 13

13–01.   Submucous cleft. Note the "V" shape during phonation. The uvula is square with a line in the middle. This is just as typical as a clearly bifid uvula is.

13–02.   Fistula and tongue flap from an oral view.

CHAPTER 14

14–01.   Nasometry preparation procedures.

14–02.   Demonstration of SNAP Test administration.

The following are nasometry tests on various patients. The passage (or speech sample) is indicated and the patient's mean nasalance score is noted. The mean (*M*) and standard deviation (*SD*) of the normative group for each passage are noted in the tables for comparison.

Case A: This child has normal speech and resonance. Nasalance (which measures resonance) comes from vowel sounds and voiced consonants. Voiceless consonants should be at baseline or 0. Note that the screen shots show how to determine the individual's mean nasalance for the passage.

Video #	Passage	Score	Norms
14–03	Bilabial Plosives	12	$M = 11$; $SD = 5$
14–04	Lingual-Alveolar Plosives	11	$M = 11$; $SD = 5$
14–05	Velar Plosives	12	$M = 13$; $SD = 6$
14–06	Sibilant Fricatives	14	$M = 12$; $SD = 15$
14–07	Nasals	54	$M = 54$; $SD = 9$

Case B: This child also has normal speech and resonance. The high vowel /i/ is usually about 10 percentage points higher than the low vowel /a/. (See Syllable Repetition/Prolonged Sounds Subtest of the SNAP Test.)

Video #	Passage	Score	Norms
14–08	Prolonged /a/	9	$M = 6$; $SD = 3$
14–09	Prolonged /i/	20	$M = 19$; $SD = 9$

Case C: This patient is status post tonsillectomy and adenoidectomy. He demonstrates a small velopharyngeal gap, causing a nasal rustle on pressure-sensitive phonemes.

Video #	Passage	Score	Norms
14–10	Bilabial Plosives	39	$M = 11$; $SD = 5$
14–11	Lingual-Alveolar Plosives	60	$M = 11$; $SD = 5$
14–12	Velar Plosives	61	$M = 13$; $SD = 6$
14–13	Sibilant Fricatives	60	$M = 12$; $SD = 15$

Case D: This child has a submucous cleft and small velopharyngeal opening, causing a nasal rustle. The nasalance score is higher on the sibilants sounds, which require higher pressure.

Video #	Passage	Score	Norms
14–14	Bobby–Bilabial Plosives (with nasals)	21	M = 16; SD = 5
14–15	Suzy–Sibilant Fricatives (without nasals)	40	M = 10; SD = 4

Case E: This child has a history of cleft palate. Speech is characterized by nasal emission, hypernasality, and glottal stops.

Video #	Passage	Score	Norms
14–16	Zoo	60	M = 16; SD = 5

Case F: This patient has severe nasal emission secondary to a submucous cleft palate. Note that the prolonged production of /s/, which is a voiceless consonant, should result in a 0 nasalance score. The score of 93 suggests a large velopharyngeal opening, causing significant nasal emission. Note that the nasalance values for the /si/ syllables are higher than for the /sa/ syllables, as would be expected.

Video #	Passage	Score	Norms
14–17	Prolonged /s/	93	M = 0; SD = 0
14–18	pa, pa, pa . . .	60	M = 7; SD = 5
14–19	si, si, si . . .	91	M = 17; SD = 8

Case G: This child has significant nasal emission secondary to a history of cleft palate.

Video #	Passage	Score	Norms
14–20	Sibilant Fricatives	68	$M = 12; SD = 5$

Case H: This patient has a history of cleft palate and velopharyngeal insufficiency. She had a pharyngeal flap. She now has hyponasality (in addition to upper airway obstruction and sleep apnea), suggesting that the lateral ports on either side of the pharyngeal flap are not open enough for breathing and nasal sound production. In addition, there is a nasal rustle, which suggests that there is not complete closure of one or both ports during production of pressure-sensitive consonants. The nasalance score would probably be lower if it weren't for the nasal rustle.

Video #	Passage	Score	Norms
14–21	Nasals	32	$M = 54; SD = 9$

Case I: This child has cul-de-sac resonance and hyponasality due to a scar band in the posterior pharynx wall. This band blocks sound energy from traveling superiorly into the oral and nasal cavities.

Video #	Passage	Score	Norms
14–22	Nasals	43	$M = 54; SD = 9$

CHAPTER 16

Note: On the AP and base views, "right" always refers to the patient's right, but is on the left side of the screen; and "left" always refers to the patient's left, but is on the right side of the screen.

16–01. Lateral and anterior-posterior (AP) view of normal velopharyngeal closure, as seen through videofluoroscopy. On the lateral view, the velum has good "knee action" and raises at the level of the hard palate. There is firm contact of the velum against the posterior pharyngeal wall. On the AP view, the lateral walls can be seen because they are coated with barium. On the oral level, the lateral walls appear to barely move. When the view is raised to the nasal level however, the lateral walls appear to come together against the septum (although in reality, they are well behind the septum).

16–02.   Lateral, anterior-posterior (AP), and base views of a patient with a nasal rustle. The coating of barium allows visualization of the lateral pharyngeal walls on the AP and base views. Although this study looks shows only normal closure, there is a small velopharyngeal opening that cannot be seen through videofluoroscopy. This is causing the nasal rustle that is heard periodically throughout the sample. The nasopharyngoscopy of this same patient can be seen in Video 17–07.

16–03.   Lateral view of a patient with nasal emission. A narrow velopharyngeal opening can barely be seen with this study.

16–04.   Lateral view of a patient with velopharyngeal incompetence. Note the occasional appearance of a Passavant's ridge as a projection on the posterior pharyngeal wall. Speech is characterized by hypernasality and nasalization of plosives, and barely audible nasal emission.

16–05.   Lateral, anterior-posterior (AP), and base views of a patient with a large velopharyngeal opening due to velopharyngeal incompetence, and the use of glottal stops for all pressure-sensitive phonemes. This type of opening can easily be seen through videofluoroscopy.

16–06.   Lateral, anterior-posterior (AP), and base views of a patient with severe velopharyngeal incompetence secondary to cerebral palsy. Speech is characterized by dysarthria, which includes hypernasality. This is the same patient as in Videos 7–17 and 18–11.

16–07.   Lateral view of a patient with severe apraxia. Notice the inconsistent velar movement and how the velum elevates but often drops down before the end of the word.

16–08.   Lateral, anterior-posterior (AP), and base views of a patient with a pharyngeal flap. A pharyngeal flap can be very difficult to see through videofluoroscopy unless there is a good coating of barium. This pharyngeal flap is too low for maximum benefit.

CHAPTER 17

Note: On all nasopharyngoscopy videos, "right" always refers to the patient's right, but is on the left side of the screen; and "left" always refers to the patient's left, but is on the right side of the screen.

17–01.   Normal velopharyngeal closure as seen through nasopharyngoscopy. Compare this view with what is seen through videofluoroscopy in Video 16–1 of the same speaker (this author). As can be seen from nasopharyngoscopy, there is firm and complete velopharyngeal closure during speech. From this view, the bulge of the musculus uvulae muscle can be seen during phonation. Also notice that there is no bubbling of secretions during speech, which would indicate a leak of air pressure.

17–02.   Touch closure just to the right of midline.

17–03.   Occult submucous cleft. This submucous cleft was not detected on the oral surface of the velum. However, on the nasal surface, there is a notch in the posterior border of the velum. During speech, there is a small, central velopharyngeal gap. The epiglottis can be seen at the beginning of the segment and the right tonsil (patient's right, left on the screen) can be seen protruding in the oropharynx.

17–04.   Submucous cleft. There is a notch in post border of velum. The epiglottis can be seen before she starts to speak. With speech, there is a small, midline opening. There is bubbling of secretions, causing the nasal rustle. This video illustrates the fact that frequently, children will cry at the start of the study. However, they usually calm down once the scope is in so that that a good study can be obtained.

17–05.   Submucous cleft. The musculus uvulae muscle is hypoplastic and the defect can be noted on the posterior border of the velum and all the way down the back of the uvula. A very low Passavant's ridge can be observed. Note that there was initially poor cooperation and therefore, true velopharyngeal function could not be determined. Once she stopped crying, better velopharyngeal function is noted. Despite that, she has a small velopharyngeal opening in the area of the submucous cleft defect. Note that there is a nasal rustle occasionally, which is associated with the bubbling of secretions.

17–06. Small gap. There is a small gap on the right of the adenoid pad. This results in nasal emission, particularly a nasal rustle due to the bubbling of secretions.

17–07. Small gap. There is a small, midline gap, resulting in nasal emission and a nasal rustle due to the bubbling. The video-fluoroscopic study of this same patient can be seen on Video 16–02.

17–08. Small opening at the midline. This results in nasal emission.

17–09. Small- to medium-sized gap. There is a coronal shape opening with nasal emission. Occasionally, there is midline closure with small lateral gaps. When this occurs, the gap size is smaller but the distortion is louder due to a nasal rustle.

17–10. Lateral gap. This patient has very low velopharyngeal closure. There is a gap on the right. A Passavant's ridge can be noted.

17–11. Lateral gaps. There is velar contact against the adenoid, but a lateral gap on both sides, resulting in a "bowtie" pattern.

17–12. Central gap. This patient achieves closure against adenoid tissue, but closure is not maintained. There is nasal emission as a result.

17–13. Small gap on the right side of midline. Note that the size is inconsistent. Closure can vary with speech sound, the length of an utterance, and with effort.

17–14. Small lateral gaps. There is a small gap on the left and occasionally on the right. There is touch closure in the midline.

17–15. Lateral gaps. There is touch closure against a small adenoid pad. There are gaps on each side of the midline, resulting in a "bowtie" pattern. There is nasal emission and hypernasality.

17–16. Irregular adenoids. A notch in middle of adenoid prevents a tight seal. In this case, the problem is the adenoid, not the velum. Therefore, a conservative adenoidectomy to smooth out the surface could be considered.

17–17. Large palatal fistula and coronal velopharyngeal opening. This is the same patient as in Video 13–02. There is a large palatal fistula that is viewed on the nasal surface of the hard palate through nasopharyngoscopy. During speech, the tongue can be seen rising in an attempt to partially occlude the fistula. In addition to the fistula, there is velopharyngeal insufficiency (short velum) resulting in a medium-sized coronal opening. Both the fistula and the velopharyngeal opening contribute to the nasal emission and hypernasality.

17–18.   Large opening. Note the projection of adenoid tissue and the Passavant's ridge.

17–19.   Large coronal opening. Closure is close to being complete with swallowing, due to the assistance of the tongue. Speech is hypernasal and oral consonants are nasalized.

17–20.   Large opening. There is a submucous cleft, characterized by a defect on the nasal surface of the velum. Note the epiglottis and adenoid pad. This child occasionally uses glottal stops.

17–21.   Large opening. This patient has a large opening, just to the left of center. Note the Passavant's ridge and large tonsils. Speech is characterized by hypernasality, nasal emission, and weak consonants.

17–22.   Large opening. This patient has a large velopharyngeal opening, but a narrow pharyngeal isthmus due to a history of Treacher Collins syndrome. This makes surgical correction difficult due to the risk of airway obstruction.

17–23.   Medialized carotid artery. This is a common finding in patients with velocardiofacial syndrome. Notice the epiglottis.

17–24.   Medialized carotid artery. This patient has velocardiofacial syndrome. There is a coronal gap with nasal emission that can be seen by the effect on the secretions. Note the adenoid pad, and the epiglottis at the end of the segment. Speech is characterized by hypernasality and nasal emission.

17–25.   Velopharyngeal incompetence. This patient has a history of head trauma. He has a consistent narrow opening on the left and in midline. On the right, there is a larger opening, resulting in nasal emission.

17–26.   Velopharyngeal incompetence. This patient has a history of myasthenia gravis. Velar elevation is poor, resulting in low closure that is not very firm. Lateral wall movement is also inadequate. There is mild nasal emission and consonants are weak.

17–27.   Velopharyngeal incompetence. This patient has a history of cerebral palsy. There is a very large velopharyngeal opening. As a result, she has severe nasal emission. This is the same patient as can be seen on Video 7–07. Note the adenoid pad.

17–28.   Normal closure. Note how the velum moves, but stays up during each speech segment. This video is to be compared with Video 17–29 (apraxia of speech).

17–29.   Apraxia of speech. This child has a normal velum. During speech, she is able to achieve closure, but cannot coordinate anterior or posterior (velopharyngeal) articulation. As a result, the velum often drops down inappropriately. This caused inconsistent hypernasality.

17–30.   Inconsistent closure. VPI ranges from a large opening on vowels to a very small opening on the right side of the adenoid. This patient is able to achieve complete closure. The velum is normal. Therefore, this suggests possibly mild apraxia as a cause. Speech therapy should be tried before considering surgical intervention.

17–31.   Phoneme-specific nasal emission. There child has normal closure for the production of almost all speech phonemes. Note the excellent lateral pharyngeal wall movement. During production of /s/, the velopharyngeal valve opens. This is due to velopharyngeal mislearning. See how this is corrected in Video 21–11.

17–32.   Phoneme-specific hypernasality. This child has fairly normal velopharyngeal closure. However, with the high /i/ (as in "eat"), the velum drops down, causing hypernasality.

17–33.   Stress incompetence with trumpet playing. Note that initially, there is firm closure. However, with continued playing, fatigue results in a small velopharyngeal opening, which is first seen as bubbling. The fatigue of playing the trumpet then affects speech because after playing the trumpet, there is a small velopharyngeal opening with speech that is not present before playing.

17–34.   Stress incompetence with clarinet playing. The leak is apparent through the bubbling of secretions.

17–35.   Normal vocal folds as seen through nasopharyngoscopy.

17–36.   Large bilateral vocal fold nodules at the anterior one-third point of the vocal cords.

17–37.   Large palatal fistula. This is a view of a large oronasal fistula as seen through nasopharyngoscopy. Note that during articulation, the tongue pushes against the fistula to compensate. This is the same patient that is seen in Video 13–02.

CHAPTER 18

Note: On all videofluoroscopy and nasopharyngoscopy videos, "right" always refers to the patient's right, but is on the left side of the screen; and "left" always refers to the patient's left, but is on the right side of the screen.

18–01. Pharyngeal flap as viewed on videofluoroscopy. On the lateral view, the pharyngeal flap can barely be seen. It is very low, near the base of the tongue, and can be seen as a slight shadow in the area where the velum appears to pull back and the posterior pharyngeal wall pulls forward. On the anterior-posterior (AP) view and the base view, the pharyngeal flap and pharyngeal walls are coated with barium. The position of the pharyngeal flap and the lateral ports is best appreciated after a swallow.

18–02. Pharyngeal flap as viewed on nasopharyngoscopy. The pharyngeal flap is in good position in the nasopharynx and is a good width. However, the lateral ports do not close completely during speech, leaving small openings on both sides. This is the same patient as in Video 18–01, but this study was done almost a year later.

18–03. Lateral port stenosis. The pharyngeal flap is in good position in nasopharynx. However, both ports are stenosed. Although the velopharyngeal insufficiency was corrected, speech is now characterized by hyponasality, and the obstruction is causing sleep apnea.

18–04. The pharyngeal flap is in good position in the nasopharynx and is a good width. Both ports open normally for nasal sounds and nasal breathing. However, the left port has a leak during the production of oral sounds.

18–05. Very narrow pharyngeal flap that is skewed to the right. The left port is very large.

18–06. Low, narrow pharyngeal flap. This pharyngeal flap is very low in the nasopharynx and also narrow. The pharyngeal flap has also torn, as noted on the patient's right side. A Passavant's ridge is actually noted above the level of the pharyngeal flap.

18–07. Low pharyngeal flap. This pharyngeal flap is of good width, but is low in the nasopharynx. There is a small opening on each side during speech.

18–08. Sphincter pharyngoplasty. This child has a bilateral sphincter pharyngoplasty. Evidence of the sphincter is noted on the right side and closure is good on that side. The sphincter is not noted on the left, and on that side, there is still a leak.

18–09. Secretions that obstruct the view. This pharyngeal flap is too low because it is below the point of maximum velar elevation. There is a leak in the left port. However, this is difficult to see due to the secretions. Sometimes, secretions can be cleared by asking the patient to sniff hard. At other times, it is necessary to suction the secretions in order to see the openings during speech.

18–10. Preoperative speech segment and postoperative speech results following a pharyngeal flap. Compare with Video 7–07, which was taken preoperatively. Note that fricatives are stronger with better pressure, and the nasal grimace less pronounced. There is very mild hyponasality, which is common for several months following placement of a pharyngeal flap.

18–11. Preoperative speech segment and postoperative speech results following a pharyngeal flap. This patient had a history of cerebral palsy. Although articulation placement was normal, speech was characterized by dysarthria with significant velopharyngeal incompetence. Note the increase in pressure for oral consonants in the postoperative video. In addition, the nasal grimace (indicating increased effort) is no longer noted.

18–12. Preoperative speech segment and postoperative speech results following a pharyngeal flap. This patient had a history of head trauma. Although articulation placement was normal, speech was characterized by dysarthria with significant velopharyngeal incompetence. In the preoperative video, note the need to take a deep breath before an utterance and the frequent breaths during counting. After the pharyngeal flap, there is an improvement in resonance, air pressure for consonants, and utterance length. The patient also reported a reduction in the fatigue that occurred with speech.

CHAPTER 21

21–01. Use of a listening tube for feedback of nasal emission.

21–02. Producing /p/ through a straw. This gives auditory feedback when there is oral air pressure.

21–03. Producing /s/ through a straw. This gives auditory feedback when there is oral air pressure.

21–04. Producing /s/ through a straw. This gives auditory feedback when there is oral air pressure.

21–05. Use of an "air paddle" to increase oral pressure.

21–06. Nose pinch (cul-de-sac) technique.

21–07. Use of the yawn technique to reduce nasal sound for /l/.

21–08. Use of /tssss/ technique to change nasal production of /s/ with nasal emission to an oral production with no nasal emission.

21–09. Use of /tssss/ technique to change nasal production of /s/ with nasal emission to an oral production with no nasal emission. This is the same patient as seen in Video 7–22.

21–10. Working on the transition from /s/ to the vowel. By inserting an /h/ between the consonant and vowel, this prevents nasal emission that often occurs during the transition in the initial stages of therapy.

21–11. This patient demonstrates phoneme-specific nasal emission (in the form of a nasal rustle) on all sibilant sounds (/s/, /z/, /sh/, /ch/, /j/) due to the use of a posterior nasal fricative. This is the result of velopharyngeal mislearning. He is very stimulable for correct production however, with the /tssss/ technique. This is the same patient as seen in Video 7–23.

21–12. Use of /tssss/ technique as seen through nasopharyngoscopy.

PREFACE

Anticipating the birth of a new baby is usually a very exciting time of life. The expectant couple does many things to prepare for the baby. This usually includes setting up a nursery, gathering baby clothes and diapers, and deciding on a name. The parents *expect* to have a normal baby, with ten fingers, ten toes, and an intact face. As a result, virtually nothing is done to prepare themselves for the possibility of a different outcome.

Unfortunately, not all babies are born with perfect structures. When a child is born with cleft lip/palate or craniofacial anomalies, this is a true shock, especially because it involves the face. This can be a devastating blow to the family. What was expected to be a very happy and exciting time becomes a very stressful and emotional time for the parents. It is impossible for the parents see their beautiful baby because the focus is on the abnormality.

Cleft lip or palate is the fourth most common birth defect and the first most common facial birth defect. In fact, about one in every 750 children born in the United States each year is born with a cleft of the lip or palate. About half of these children have other associated malformations that often occur with clefting. Cleft palate is a characteristic of over 200 recognized syndromes. In addition to clefts and their associated malformations, many children are born each year with other craniofacial anomalies.

Although current medical technology is not advanced enough to prevent the occurrence of these birth defects, most of the speech and physical impairments associated with craniofacial anomalies can be improved or even corrected with the help of a team of various professionals. To provide the type of care that these patients require, this group of professionals must be specialists within their field. In order to provide quality care, they must have a thorough understanding of the current methods of evaluation and treatment of this population.

Considering the prevalence of clefts and craniofacial anomalies in the population, however, general practitioners in all health care disciplines must also have knowledge about the management of this population. Considering the fact that these anomalies often have a significant effect on speech, speech-language pathologists in particular need to be trained in the basic evaluation, treatment, and referral of individuals with these anomalies. Certainly, school-based speech pathologists are very likely to have children in their caseloads with a history of cleft, craniofacial anomalies, or resonance disorders.

PURPOSE OF THIS BOOK

The purpose of this book is to inform, educate, and excite students in speech-language pathology and in the medical and dental professions regarding the management of individuals with a history of cleft or craniofacial anomalies. This book is designed to be a textbook for graduate students, and also a sourcebook for health care professionals who provide services in this area. My goal in writing this book was to provide readers with a great deal of information, but in a way that is both interesting and easy to read. As an active clinician myself, my intent was to make this book a very practical "how to do it" guide, as well as a source of didactic and theoretical information.

My ultimate goal with this book is to improve the knowledge of treating professionals who work with individuals who have a history of cleft or craniofacial anomalies—in order to positively impact the quality of care available to this population that I feel so passionate about!

ORGANIZATION

This book was written in a purposeful sequence so that the information from each chapter builds on the information from previous chapters. Part I of this text provides basic information on the normal anatomy of the orofacial structures and the normal physiology of the velopharyngeal valve. Once the normal structures and function are described, information on clefts and craniofacial anomalies is discussed in subsequent chapters. The various causes of these anomalies, including the genetic bases, are reviewed. Once the student has completed the first section, there should be a firm understanding of normal and abnormal facial and velopharyngeal features and the potential causes of abnormalities.

Part II of this text includes chapters on the various problems associated with clefts and craniofacial anomalies. In particular, this section covers the effects of these anomalies on feeding, dentition, language, cognition, phonology, articulation, resonance, hearing, and psychosocial development. After completing the second section, the reader will have an understanding of the number, types, and complexity of the problems that are secondary to clefts and craniofacial anomalies. It will then be apparent to the reader that there is a need for multidisciplinary management of these patients in an interdisciplinary setting. This leads naturally to the third section of this book where the importance of a team approach is covered.

Part III of this book is short, but important—because it emphasizes the fact that several disciplines are needed for these patients. The reader will complete this section with an understanding that quality patient care necessitates interdisciplinary interaction and collaboration in the assessment and treatment of patients with clefts and craniofacial anomalies.

Part IV of this text covers the various diagnostic methods for assessing speech, resonance, and velopharyngeal function. This section includes the perceptual examination of speech and resonance, the physical examination of the oral cavity, and instrumental measures for evaluating resonance and velopharyngeal function. The chapters on instrumentation ("Nasometry," "Speech Aerodynamics," "Videofluoroscopy," and "Nasopharyngoscopy") are very detailed and are written to provide specific information for the practicing clinicians who will be using these procedures. Professors of graduate students are advised to select sections from these chapters for their students. This will give the students an overview of the instrumentation that is available, without the detail of the procedures and interpretation.

Part V of this book discusses the treatment of speech and resonance disorders secondary to clefts, craniofacial anomalies, and velopharyngeal dysfunction. This section includes surgical management, prosthetic management, and speech therapy.

A glossary of terms is found at the back of the text. The first time that a technical or medical term is used in this book, it is printed in italics and a definition is given in the text. All of these words are also listed in the glossary. The student may find that studying the glossary of terms is helpful for learning much of the information in the book.

Finally, the reader will find appendices at the back of the book that contain resource information for parents. There is a list of publications for parents, and also a list of parent support groups.

FEATURES

- *Chapter outlines* help readers navigate through the content and find information quickly.

- Selected *technical and medical terms* are presented in italics and defined at first occurrence in the book and included in the *comprehensive glossary*.

- Over *250 photographs and illustrations* enhance comprehension of concepts discussed.

- *Case Studies* illustrate how chapter information applies to real-life situations.

- *Appendices* contain resource information for parents and guardians and include publications and lists of parent support groups.

NEW TO THIS EDITION

- Over 380 photographs and illustrations!

- A section for review, discussion, and critical thinking is included at the back of each chapter. These sections should help the reader to synthesize and apply information presented in the chapter.

- The *CD-ROM* packaged free at the back of the book contains over 100 video clips so readers can see and hear how speech and resonance can be affected by cleft palate, velopharyngeal dysfunction, or another type of craniofacial disorder. In addition, videofluoroscopy and nasopharyngoscopy videos are included to allow the user to see what is happening in the velopharyngeal valve when certain speech characteristics occur. These videos also help the reader to learn how these studies can be used to provide important diagnostic information that is necessary for treatment planning. There are several videos that illustrate specific therapy techniques. Each video in the CD-ROM illustrates more than one finding or speech characteristic. Therefore, a list of videos organized by topic has been provided. Users can access this list by going to the main menu of the CD-ROM and clicking on the link, "List of Videos Organized by Topic." A video icon located throughout several chapters cues the reader to the fact that one or more videos are available to illustrate that topic.

- At the end of each chapter, there is now a section entitled, "For Review, Discussion, and Critical Thinking." This section consists of questions and discussion items that cover the entire chapter. The purpose of this section is to help the student understand what is important to know, and to learn the information in a way that makes it practical and relevant to clinical work. This section should also be helpful to professors teaching a course, because the questions and discussion items can be used as a test for each chapter.

FORMAT NOTES

Service providers must be sensitive to the emotional and psychological needs of the patient. Sensitivity to the feelings of the patient is often overlooked by well-meaning service providers. It is easy to forget that we deal with real people, not just interesting cases. This lack of sensitivity is sometimes reflected in the terminology that is used in the literature and in daily use. I recall listening to a speech given by an adult who was born with a cleft palate. As he described his childhood, he pointed out that being called a "cleft palate child" evoked very negative feelings. Fortunately, this type of phrase is becoming "politically incorrect" at this point in time, just as the term "harelip" has in the past. Using the anomaly as an adjective to describe the individual is certainly insensitive to the feelings of the person who was born with this anomaly. Therefore, it is therefore preferable to use "patient-first" terminology as in "child with a cleft."

The reader will note that the word "child" is frequently used throughout the text for the individual with the anomaly. This is used since the speech and resonance disorders secondary to cleft lip/palate and craniofacial anomalies are usually addressed during childhood. However, it should be understood that this information also applies to adults with the same anomalies.

Finally, speech-language pathologists will observe that the International Phonetic Alphabet (IPA) and the complex symbols for compensatory articulation productions are not used in this book. This is by design. Common letters are used instead so that all readers, including those who are not speech-language pathologists, can read this information with understanding.

ACKNOWLEDGMENTS

There are so many people who need to be acknowledged for their help with this text. I have not been shy about asking others for opinions about specific chapters. Thanks to the following for reading chapters and giving me feedback: Alice Smith, Ph.D. ("Developmental Aspects"), Ronald Scherer, Ph.D. ("Resonance Disorders and Velopharyngeal Dysfunction"), Robert McClurkin from KayPENTAX ("Nasometry"), Janet H. Middendorf, M.A. ("Nasometry"), Janet Strife, M.D. ("Videofluoroscopy"), and J. Paul Willging, M.D. ("Nasopharyngoscopy"). A very special thank you goes to my friend and mentor, Linda Lee, Ph.D. Dr. Lee has been helpful in eliciting feedback from her students who used the first edition of this book. She has also given me excellent feedback and advice for this book and many other manuscripts over the years.

I would also like to acknowledge and thank April Johnson, M.A., who is a speech-language pathologist on my staff. She volunteered to read the entire book and make editing suggestions—all of which were excellent! Natalie Peters, B.A., is a graduate student who works in our department and she was very helpful in the preparation phase of the manuscript. Another special thank you goes to Janet H. Middendorf, M.A., who has helped me as a colleague and friend in many ways over the years. She covered many of my clinics so that I could work on this book! I'd also like to thank the members of the Craniofacial Anomaly Team at Cincinnati Children's Hospital for teaching me just about everything that I know regarding clefts and craniofacial conditions. Finally, I'd like to thank the reviewers of this text. Your comments were very valuable.

REVIEWERS

Dianne M. Altuna, M.S., CCC-SLP
Lecturer
University of Texas-Dallas
Speech Pathologist
Children's Medical Center
Dallas, TX

Monica C. Devers, Ph.D.,
CCC-SLP
Associate Professor and Chair
St. Cloud State University
St. Cloud, MN

Dennis Fuller, Ph.D., CCC-SLP
Associate Professor
Saint Louis University
St. Louis, MO

Linda Lee, Ph.D., CCC-SLP
Professor and Graduate Program
Director
University of Cincinnati
Cincinnati, OH

John Lowe III, Ph.D., CCC-SLP
Professor and Chair
University of Central Arkansas
Conway, AR

Tiana Pendleton, M.A., CCC-SLP
Speech-Language Pathologist
St. Peter's Hospital
Albany, NY

Nancye C. Roussel, Ph.D.,
CCC-SLP
Assistant Professor
University of Louisiana-Lafayette
Lafayette, LA

Christopher R. Watts, Ph.D.,
CCC-SLP
Associate Professor
James Madison University
Harrisonburg, VA

FEEDBACK

I would like to encourage the readers of this text to contact me by e-mail (ann.kummer@cchmc.org) or at Thomson Delmar Learning (info@delmar.com) with suggestions or comments about this text. My goal is to constantly improve this text over time.

FINAL WORDS

Speaking for myself and for all the contributors, we are grateful for the opportunity to present this information to you. We are hopeful that the readers will be educated, enlightened, and inspired to provide superior clinical services for individuals with a history of cleft or craniofacial conditions.

Ann W. Kummer

ABOUT THE AUTHOR

Ann W. Kummer, Ph.D., CCC-SLP, is Senior Director of Speech Pathology at Cincinnati Children's Hospital Medical Center (CCHMC) and Professor of Clinical Pediatrics at the University of Cincinnati Medical Center.

Under her direction, the speech pathology program at CCHMC has grown to be one of the largest and most respected in the country. Dr. Kummer gives frequent lectures on leadership and professional business practices. In addition to this text, she is one of the authors of the text entitled *Business Practices: A Guide for Speech-Language Pathologists,* published by the American Speech-Language-Hearing Association (ASHA) in 2004.

Dr. Kummer was one of the main developers of workflow software that won the 1995 International Beacon Award through IBM/Lotus. (Derivative software is marketed by Chart Links.)

As a clinician and researcher, Dr. Kummer specializes in speech and resonance disorders secondary to cleft palate, craniofacial anomalies, and velopharyngeal dysfunction. She is a member of the Craniofacial Team at CCHMC and at Shriners Hospital in Cincinnati, and also serves the Velopharyngeal Dysfunction Clinic at CCHMC. Dr. Kummer has served as Coordinator of American Speech-Language-Hearing Association's Division 5: Speech Science and Orofacial Anomalies, and is an active member of the American Cleft Palate-Craniofacial Association, serving on many committees.

Dr. Kummer gives many lectures and seminars on a national and international level. She is the author of many professional articles as well as 12 book chapters appearing in speech pathology and medical texts. In addition to this text, she the coauthor of the Simplified Nasometric Assessment Procedures (SNAP) test (1996) and author of the SNAP-R (2005) that is incorporated in the Nasometer equipment (KAYPentax, Lincoln Park, NJ). She has a patent on a device marketed as the Oral & Nasal Listener™ by Super Duper. This device amplifies the sound from the nasal cavity and oral cavity while the child is speaking, and allows both the child and the clinician (or parent) to hear this amplified sound in real time. She has also done two educational video seminars on resonance disorders for ASHA.

Dr. Kummer has received honors from the Southwestern Ohio Speech and Hearing Association (SWOSHA); honors from the Ohio Speech and Hearing Association (OSHA); a distinguished alumnus award from the Department of Communication Sciences and Disorders of the University of Cincinnati; the Director's Award for Excellence from her staff; and was elected Fellow of the American Speech-Language-Hearing Association (ASHA) in 2002. She was named one of the 25 most influential therapists in the United States by *Therapy Times* in 2006 and was named one of the 10 most inspiring women in Cincinnati by *Inspire Magazine* in 2007.

Dr. Kummer received her bachelor's degree and master's degree from Indiana University, and her Ph.D. from the University of Cincinnati.

CONTRIBUTORS

David A. Billmire, M.D.*
Associate Professor of Clinical
  Surgery
University of Cincinnati College
  of Medicine
Director, Plastic Surgery Division
Cincinnati Children's Hospital
  Medical Center
Address:
Cincinnati Children's Hospital
  Medical Center
3333 Burnet Avenue
Cincinnati, OH 45229-3039

**Richard Campbell, D.M.D.,
  M.S.***
Assistant Professor of Clinical
  Pediatrics
University of Cincinnati College
  of Medicine
Director, Orthodontics
Division of Pediatric Dentistry
Cincinnati Children's Hospital
  Medical Center
Address:
Cincinnati Children's Hospital
  Medical Center
3333 Burnet Avenue
Cincinnati, OH 45229-3039

Julia Corcoran, M.D.
Assistant Professor of Surgery
  (Plastic)
Feinberg School of Medicine,
  Northwestern University
Address:
Children's Memorial Hospital

Division of Pediatric Plastic Surgery
2300 Children's Plaza, Box 93
Chicago, IL 60614

Murray Dock, D.D.S., M.S.D.
Associate Professor of Clinical
  Pediatrics
University of Cincinnati, College
  of Medicine
Division of Pediatric Dentistry
Cincinnati Children's Hospital
  Medical Center
Address:
Cincinnati Children's Hospital
  Medical Center
3333 Burnet Avenue
Cincinnati, OH 45229-3039

Robert J. Hopkin, M.D.*
Assistant Professor of Clinical
  Pediatrics
University of Cincinnati College
  of Medicine
Division of Human Genetics
Cincinnati Children's Hospital
  Medical Center
Address:
Cincinnati Children's Hospital
  Medical Center
3333 Burnet Avenue
Cincinnati, OH 45229-3039

Claire K. Miller, Ph.D.
Speech Pathologist III
Speech Pathology Department
Cincinnati Children's Hospital
  Medical Center

Address:
Cincinnati Children's Hospital
  Medical Center
3333 Burnet Avenue
Cincinnati, OH 45229-3039

Howard M. Saal, M.D.*
Professor of Pediatrics
University of Cincinnati College
  of Medicine
Director, Clinical Genetics
Division of Human Genetics
Cincinnati Children's Hospital
  Medical Center
Address:
Cincinnati Children's Hospital
  Medical Center
3333 Burnet Avenue
Cincinnati, OH 45229-3039

Janet R. Schultz, Ph.D.*
Professor
Psychology Department
Xavier University
Address:
Xavier University
3800 Victory Parkway
Cincinnati, OH 45207-6511

J. Paul Willging, M.D.*
Professor
Department of Otolaryngology—
  Head and Neck Surgery
University of Cincinnati College
  of Medicine
Cincinnati Children's Hospital
  Medical Center
Address:
Cincinnati Children's Hospital
  Medical Center
3333 Burnet Avenue
Cincinnati, OH 45229-3039

David J. Zajac, Ph.D.
Associate Professor
Department of Dental Ecology
  and the Craniofacial Center
University of North Carolina
  at Chapel Hill
Address:
Craniofacial Center
CB# 7450
University of North Carolina
  at Chapel Hill
Chapel Hill, NC 27599

*Denotes current members of the team of The Craniofacial Center, Children's Hospital Medical Center, Cincinnati, Ohio.

PART 1

NORMAL AND ABNORMAL CRANIOFACIAL FEATURES

CHAPTER

1

ANATOMY AND PHYSIOLOGY: THE OROFACIAL STRUCTURES AND VELOPHARYNGEAL VALVE

CHAPTER OUTLINE

INTRODUCTION

The nasal, oral, and pharyngeal structures are all very important for normal speech and resonance. Unfortunately, these are the structures that are commonly affected by cleft lip and palate and other craniofacial anomalies. Before the speech-language pathologist can fully understand the effects of oral and craniofacial anomalies on speech and resonance, a thorough understanding of normal structure is important. In addition, knowledge about normal function of the oral structures and the velopharyngeal valve is essential before the speech-language pathologist will be able to effectively evaluate abnormal speech and velopharyngeal dysfunction.

This chapter reviews the basic anatomy of the structures of the orofacial and velopharyngeal complex as they relate to speech production. The physiology of the subsystems of speech, including the velopharyngeal mechanism, is also described. For more detailed information on anatomy and physiology of the speech articulators, the interested reader is referred to other sources (Cassell & Elkadi, 1995; Cassell, Moon, & Elkadi, 1990; Dickson, 1972, 1975; Dickson & Dickson, 1972; Dickson, Grant, Sicher, Dubrul, & Paltan, 1974, 1975; Huang, Lee, & Rajendran, 1998; Kuehn, 1979; Maue-Dickson, 1977, 1979; Maue-Dickson & Dickson, 1980; Maue-Dickson, Dickson, & Rood, 1976; Moon & Kuehn, 1996, 1997, 2004).

ANATOMY OF THE OROFACIAL STRUCTURES

Nose and Nasal Cavity

Although the facial structures are familiar to all, some aspects of the face are important to point out for a thorough understanding of congenital anomalies and clefting. The facial landmarks can be seen on Figure 1–1A and Figure 1–1B. Starting with the nose, the nasal root is where the nose begins at the level of the eyes. The nasal bridge, also known as the nasion, is the bony structure that is located between the eyes and corresponds with the nasofrontal suture. The nostrils are separated by the columella (little column), which is the tissue that is under the nasal tip and between the nostrils. The columella is at the lower end of the nasal septum and consists of cartilage and mucosa. Ideally, the columella is straight and backed by a straight nasal septum. It must also be long enough so that the nasal tip is not depressed or flattened.

The nostrils are frequently referred to as nares, although the individual nostril is a naris. The ala nasi (Latin for "wing") is the outside curved side of the nostril, which consists of cartilage. The alae are the two curved sides of the nostril. The alar rims surround the opening to the nostril on either side and the alar base is the area where the ala meets the upper lip. The nasal sill is the base of the nostril opening. The piriform aperture, which literally means pear-shaped opening, is the opening to the nostril or nasal cavity.

The nasal cavity is divided into two sections by the nasal septum. As can be seen in Figure 1–2, the nasal septum consists of the vomer bone, the perpendicular plate of the ethmoid, and the quadrangular cartilage. It is covered with

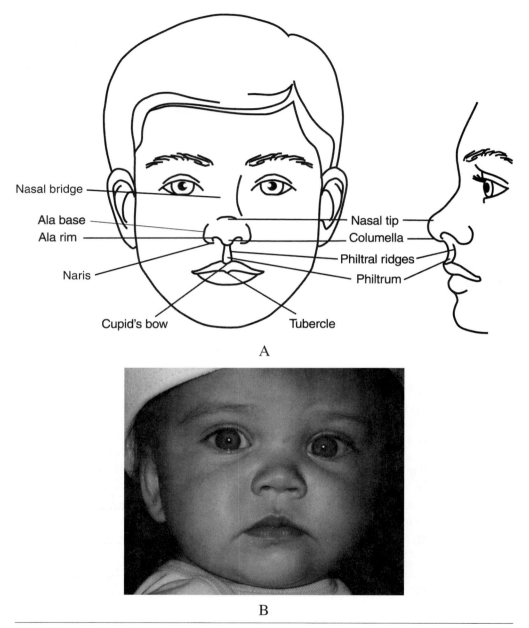

FIGURE 1–1 (A and B) Normal facial landmarks. A. Note the structures on the diagram. B. Normal face. Try to locate the same structures on this infant's face.

mucous membrane, which is the lining tissue of the nasal cavity, oral cavity, and the pharynx. The nasal septum consists of stratified squamous epithelium and lamina propria and is also known as mucosa. (This should not be confused with mucus, which is the clear, viscid secretion of the mucous membranes.) The vomer is positioned posteriorly and is perpendicular to the palate. As such, the lower portion of the vomer fits in a groove formed by the median

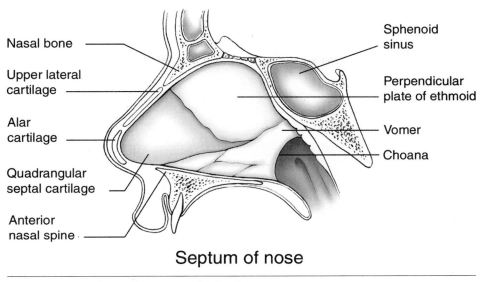

Septum of nose

FIGURE 1–2   The nasal septum and related structures.

palatine suture line on the nasal aspect of the maxilla. The perpendicular plate of the ethmoid is between the vomer and the quadrangular cartilage. It projects down to join the vomer. The quadrangular cartilage forms the anterior nasal septum and projects anteriorly to the columella. It is not uncommon for the nasal septum to be less than perfectly straight, particularly in adults. The anterior nasal spine is the anterior point of the maxilla that corresponds to the base of the columella.

Attached to the lateral walls of the nose are the superior, middle, and inferior turbinates (also called concha) (Figure 1–3). The turbinates are bony structures that are covered with mucosa. The superior and middle turbinates are parts of the ethmoid bone. The inferior turbinate, which is the largest, consists of part of the sphenoid bone. The superior, middle, and inferior nasal meatuses are the openings or passageways that lie directly under their respective turbinates. The purpose of the turbinates is to create turbulent airflow within the nose to increase humidification and to deflect air superiorly in

the nose for the sense of smell. The choana is a funnel-shaped opening at the back of the nasal cavity that leads to the nasopharynx. There is a choana on each side of the posterior part of the vomer.

Upper Lip

The features of the upper lip can be seen on Figure 1–1A. An examination of the upper lip reveals the philtrum, which is a long dimple or indentation that courses from the columella down to the upper lip. The philtrum is bordered by the philtral ridges on each side. These ridges are actually embryological suture lines that are formed as the segments of the upper lip fuse. The philtrum and philtral ridges course downward from the nose, and terminate at the edge of the upper lip.

The top of the upper lip is called the Cupid's bow due to its characteristic shape, which includes a rounded configuration with an indentation in the middle. The upper and lower lips are both highlighted by the white

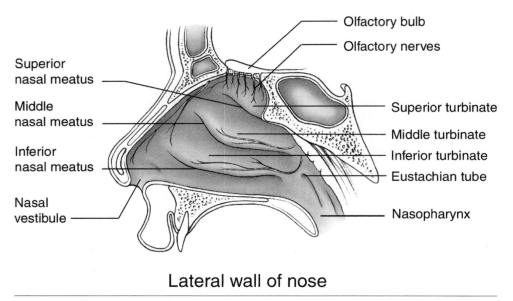

Lateral wall of nose

FIGURE 1–3   The lateral wall of the nose showing the turbinates.

roll. This white border tissue surrounds the red portion of the lip, which is called the vermilion. On the upper lip, the inferior border of the midsection of the vermilion comes to a point and is somewhat prominent. Therefore, it is referred to as the tubercle. In its naturally closed position, the upper lip rests over and slightly in front of the lower lip, although the inferior border of the upper lip is inverted. Figure 1–1A shows a diagram of the normal facial landmarks. The student is encouraged to identify the same structures on the photo of the normal infant face shown in Figure 1–1B.

Oral Cavity

Beginning with the gross anatomy first, the palate can be separated into two main parts: the hard palate and the soft palate (Figure 1–4). The hard palate is a bony structure that separates the oral cavity from the nasal cavity. The velum, frequently referred to as the soft palate, is the part of the palate that is muscular

and is located in the back of the mouth, just posterior to the hard palate. At the posterior edge of the velum is the pendulous uvula.

The tongue resides within the arch of the mandible and fills the oral cavity when the mouth is closed. With the mouth closed, the slight negative pressure within the oral cavity ensures that the tongue adheres to the palate and the tip rests against the alveolar ridge. The dorsum is the top of the tongue and the ventral surface is the lower surface of the tongue.

At the back of the oral cavity are bilateral paired curtain-like structures called faucial pillars (Figure 1–4). As the velum curves downward toward the tongue on both sides, it forms the anterior faucial pillar. Just behind the anterior pillar is the posterior faucial pillar. These structures contain muscles that assist with velopharyngeal and lingual movement. The palatine tonsils (or simply the tonsils) are found between the anterior and posterior faucial pillars on both sides. Although the tonsils are bilateral, differences in size are common, so that it is not unusual for one tonsil to be larger

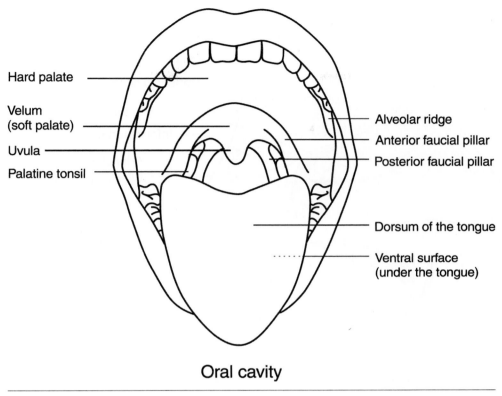

FIGURE 1–4   The structures of the oral cavity.

than the other. The lingual tonsils are masses of lymphoid tissue that are located at the base of the tongue and extend to the epiglottis (Figure 1–5). The oropharyngeal isthmus is the opening from the oral cavity to the pharynx and is bordered superiorly by the velum, laterally by the faucial pillars, and inferiorly by the base of the tongue. (See Chapter 8 for more information about tonsils and adenoids.)

Hard Palate

The hard palate forms a rounded dome on the upper part of the oral cavity called the palatal vault. In addition to serving as the roof of the mouth, it also serves as the floor of the nasal cavity. The outer portion of the hard palate is called the alveolar ridge, alveolus, or simply the gum ridge (see Figure 1–4). This ridge forms the base and the bony support for the teeth. The bony frame of the hard palate is covered by a mucoperiosteum. Mucoperiosteum consists of a mucous membrane and periosteum. As noted before, mucous membrane is a lining that consists of stratified squamous epithelium and lamina propria. Periosteum is a thick, fibrous tissue that covers the surface of bone. The mucosal covering of the hard palate has multiple ridges running transversely, which are called the rugae. There is a slight elevation of the mucosa in the middle of the anterior part of the hard palate, just in the area of the incisive foramen. This is called the incisive papilla. A narrow ridge, called the palatine

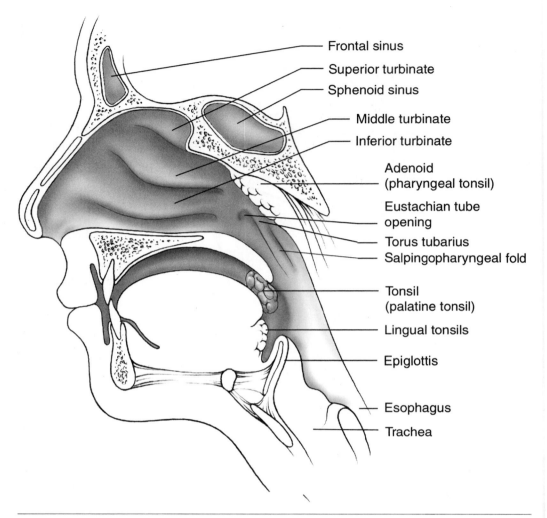

FIGURE 1–5   Lateral view of the nasal, oral and pharyngeal cavities and the structures in these areas.

raphe (pronounced "rayfay"), forms the midline of the hard palate and runs from the incisive papilla posteriorly over the entire length of the mucosa of the hard palate. At the junction of the hard and soft palate, bilateral midline depressions can often be seen. These are called the foveae palati and are the openings to minor salivary glands.

The hard palate is made up of fused bony segments that are separated by the incisive foramen and embryological fusion lines (Figure 1–6). By definition, a foramen is a hole or opening in a bony structure that allows blood vessels and nerves to pass through to the area on the other side. The incisive foramen is located in the alveolar ridge area of the maxillary arch, just behind the central incisors. This foramen is located at the tip of a triangular-shaped bone called the premaxilla. The premaxilla is bordered on either side by

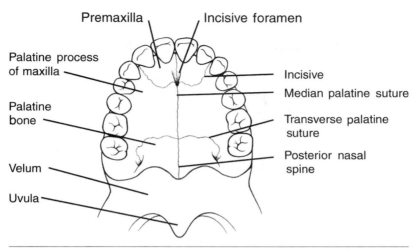

FIGURE 1–6 Bony structures of the hard palate.

the incisive suture lines. The dental arch of this bony segment contains the central and lateral maxillary incisors.

Behind the incisive suture lines are the paired palatine processes of the maxilla, which form the anterior three quarters of the maxilla. These paired bones terminate at the transverse palatine suture line (also known as the palatomaxillary suture line). Behind the transverse palatine suture line are the paired horizontal plates of the palatine bones. These bones form the posterior portion of the hard palate and end with the protrusive posterior nasal spine. The palatine processes of the maxilla and the horizontal plates of the palatine bones are both paired because they are separated in the midline by the median palatine suture (also known as the intermaxillary suture line). This suture line begins at the incisive foramen and ends at the posterior nasal spine. It should be noted that a prominent longitudinal ridge on the oral surface of the hard palate in the area of this suture line is sometimes found in some Caucasians, particularly those who are of northern European descent. It is also reportedly common in the

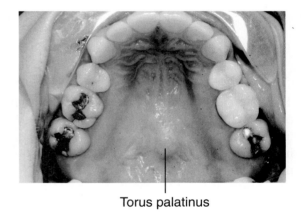

FIGURE 1–7 Small torus palatinus.

Native American and Eskimo populations. This is called a torus palatinus, or palatine torus (Figure 1–7). This finding is a normal variation rather than an abnormality.

The sphenoid and temporal bones provide bony attachment for the velopharyngeal musculature. The pterygoid process of the sphenoid bone contains the medial pterygoid plate, the lateral pterygoid plate, and the pterygoid hamulus, all of which provide attachments for muscles in the velopharyngeal complex (Figure 1–8).

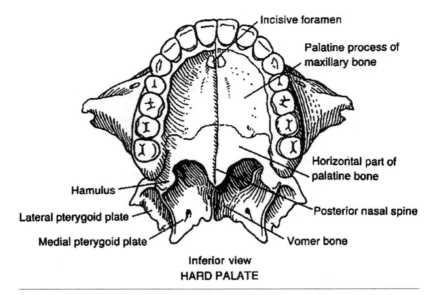

Inferior view
HARD PALATE

FIGURE 1–8 Inferior view of the hard palate. Note the hamulus, the lateral pterygoid plate and the medial pterygoid plate. (From *Human Vocal Anatomy,* by D.R. Dickson and W. Maue, 1970. Springfield IL: C.C. Thomas . Copyright 1970 C.C. Thomas. Reprinted with permission.)

Velum

The velum is attached to the posterior border of the hard palate and is held in place by its internal muscles. During normal nasal breathing, the velum drapes down from the hard palate and rests against the base of the tongue, thus opening the pharynx to the nasal cavity. (Figure 1–9A). The velum elevates during speech and other activities to close against the pharyngeal wall, thus closing off the nasal cavity (Figure 1–9B).

The velum has an oral surface and a nasal surface. The oral surface of the velum is covered by a mucous membrane and it has fine vessels under the mucosa. A thin white line, called the median palatine raphe, can be seen coursing down the midline of the velum on the oral surface. The nasal surface of the velum (Figure 1–10) consists anteriorly of pseudostratified, ciliated columnar epithelium, and posteriorly of stratified, squamous epithelium in the area where the velum contacts the posterior pharyngeal wall during closure

activities (Ettema & Kuehn, 1994; Kuehn & Kahane, 1990; Moon & Kuehn, 1996, 1997).

The anterior portion of the velum has very few muscle fibers. Instead, it consists of the tensor tendon, glandular tissue, adipose (fat) tissue, and the palatine (also called velar) aponeurosis (Figure 1–11). The palatine aponeurosis consists of a sheet of fibrous connective tissue and fibers from the tensor veli palatini tendon. It attaches to the posterior border of the hard palate and courses about one cm posteriorly through the velum. The velar aponeurosis provides an anchoring point for the velopharyngeal muscles and adds stiffness to that portion of the velum (Cassell & Elkadi, 1995; Ettema & Kuehn, 1994). The medial portion of the velum contains most of the muscle fibers; this will be described later in this chapter. The posterior portion consists of the same glandular and adipose tissue as can be found in the anterior portion. The muscle fibers taper off as they reach the posterior

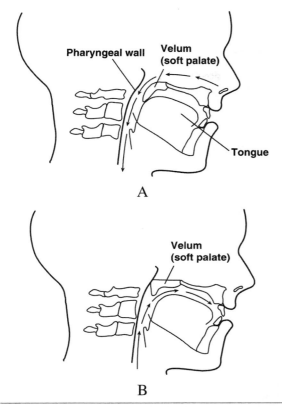

A

B

FIGURE 1–9 (A and B) Lateral view of the velum and posterior pharyngeal wall. A. The velum rests against the base of the tongue during normal nasal breathing, resulting in a patent airway. B. The velum elevates during speech and closes against the posterior pharyngeal wall. This allows the air pressure from the lungs and the sound from the larynx to be redirected from a superior direction to an anterior direction to enter the oral cavity for speech.

portion of the velum, so that few fibers are found in this section.

Uvula

The uvula is a teardrop-shaped structure that is typically long and slender (see Figure 1–4 and Figure 1–6). It hangs freely from the posterior border of the velum. The uvula consists of mucosa on the surface and connective, glandular, and adipose tissue underneath. The uvula is very vascular, with more vascular tissue than the connecting velum. It has been

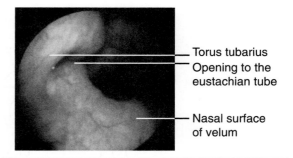

FIGURE 1–10 View of the nasal surface of the velum as seen through nasopharyngoscopy. Note the opening to the eustachian tube.

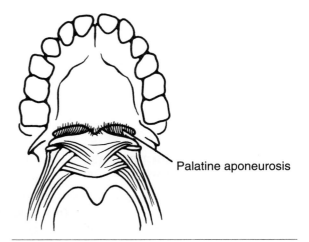

FIGURE 1–11 Position of the palatine (velar) aponeurosis. This is a sheet of fibrous tissue that is located just below the nasal surface of the velum and consists of periosteum, fibrous connective tissue, and fibers from the tensor veli palatini tendon. It provides an anchoring point for the velopharyngeal muscles and adds stiffness and velopharyngeal flexibility.

theorized that this vascularity provides a warming function for this pendulous structure. The uvula is not a contributor to velopharyngeal function and has no known function.

Pharynx

The throat area between the esophagus and the nasal cavity is called the pharynx. The

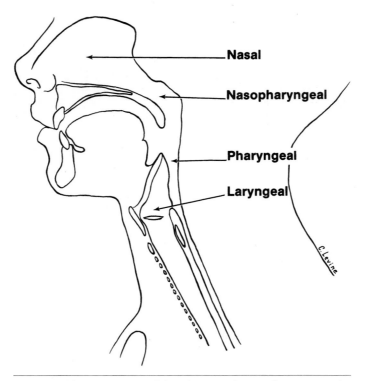

FIGURE 1–12 Sections of the pharynx. The *oropharynx* is at the level of the oral cavity or just posterior to the mouth. The *nasopharynx* is above the oral cavity and velum and is just posterior to the nasal cavity. The *hypopharynx* is below the oral cavity and extends from the epiglottis inferiorly to the esophagus.

pharynx is divided into several sections, as can be seen in Figure 1–12. These sections include the oropharynx, which is at the level of the oral cavity or just posterior to the mouth; the nasopharynx, which is above the oral cavity and velum and is just posterior to the nasal cavity; and the hypopharynx, which is below the oral cavity and extends from the epiglottis inferiorly to the esophagus. The back wall of the throat is called the posterior pharyngeal wall and the side walls of the throat are called the lateral pharyngeal walls. The adenoids (also called the pharyngeal tonsil) consist of lymphoid tissue and are found on the posterior pharyngeal wall

of the nasopharynx, just behind the velum. Adenoids are usually present in children, but they atrophy with age; therefore, adults have little, if any, adenoid tissue.

The eustachian tube connects the middle ear with the pharynx (see Figure 1–5 and Figure 1–10). On each side of the pharynx, the pharyngeal opening of the eustachian tube is lateral and slightly above the level of the velum during phonation. The torus tubarius (see Figure 1–5 and Figure 1–10) is a ridge that is located posterior to the eustachian tube opening and is caused by a projection of the cartilaginous portion of the tube. In the adult, the opening of the eustachian tube is about the size of the diameter of a pencil. The tube is closed at rest, but it opens whenever the individual swallows or yawns.

The salpingopharyngeal folds are found on both sides of the pharynx (see Figure 1–5). These folds originate from the torus tubarius at the opening to the eustachian tube and then course downward to the lateral pharyngeal wall. The folds consist primarily of glandular and connective tissue (Dickson, 1975).

Eustachian Tube

The *eustachian tube* is a membrane-lined tube that connects the middle ear space with the pharynx (see Figures 1–5 and 1–10). The pharyngeal opening of the eustachian tube is lateral (on both sides) and slightly above the level of the · velum during phonation. The eustachian tube is closed at rest, which helps prevent the inadvertent contamination of the middle ear by the normal secretions found in the pharynx and back of the nose. During swallowing and yawning, however, the velum raises and the tensor veli palatini muscle contracts to open the proximal end of the eustachian tube. This allows middle ear ventilation, which ensures that the pressure inside the ear remains nearly the same as ambient air pressure. In addition, the opening of the tube allows drainage of fluids and debris from the middle ear space.

In the infant or toddler, the eustachian tube is essentially horizontal and the opening is small, thus affecting the efficiency of middle ear ventilation and drainage. As the child grows, however, the tube changes in angle and the opening becomes larger. When the child becomes an adult, the eustachian tube is at about a 45-degree angle and the opening is about the size of the diameter of a pencil.

ANATOMY OF THE VELOPHARYNGEAL MECHANISM

Muscles of the Velopharyngeal Mechanism

The velopharyngeal sphincter requires the coordinated action of several different muscles, all of which are paired and are on each side of the midline (Moon & Kuehn, 1996) (Figure 1–13). Many of the muscles in the velopharyngeal complex have their attachments at the medial and lateral pterygoid plates and the pterygoid hamulus of the pterygoid process of the sphenoid bone. Each muscle has been studied extensively and its function defined. However, control of the velopharyngeal valve is very complex, requiring the interaction not only of these muscles, but also of the articulators, particularly the tongue. Therefore, much more remains to be learned about the dynamics of the muscles and their interactions during speech.

The levator veli palatini muscles provide the main muscle mass of the velum and are primarily responsible for velar elevation (Bell-Berti, 1973). The levator veli palatini muscles from each side of the head course medially to interdigitate in the middle of the velum and blend together to create the levator sling. Contraction of the levator muscles forces the free edge of the soft palate to move in a superior and posterior direction in order to close against the posterior pharyngeal wall. On each side of the nasopharynx, the levator veli palatini muscle originates from the apex of the petrous portion of the temporal bone at the base of the skull. The muscle then courses through an area that is anterior and medial to the carotid canal and inferior to the eustachian tube (Moon & Kuehn,

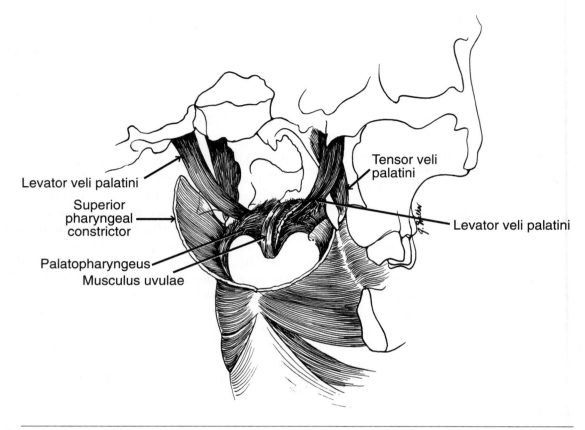

Levator veli palatini

Superior pharyngeal constrictor

Palatopharyngeus

Musculus uvulae

Tensor veli palatini

Levator veli palatini

FIGURE 1–13   The muscles of the velopharyngeal mechanism.

1996, 1997) so that it enters the velum at a 45° angle. The paired muscles then insert into the upper surface of the palatal aponeurosis and into the medial raphe of the velum. The levator veli palatini muscles take up the middle 40% of the entire velum (Boorman & Sommerlad, 1985).

The upper fibers of the superior constrictor muscles are thought to be responsible for the medial displacement of the lateral pharyngeal walls to effectively narrow the velopharyngeal port (Iglesias, Kuehn, & Morris, 1980; Shprintzen, McCall, Skolnick, & Lencione, 1975; Skolnick, McCall, & Barnes, 1973). The paired superior constrictor muscles are located in the upper pharynx and arise from the pterygoid hamulus, pterygomandibular raphe, posterior tongue,

posterior mandible, and palatine aponeurosis. They insert posteriorly in the pharyngeal raphe in the midline of the posterior pharyngeal wall.

The musculus uvulae muscles contract during phonation and create a bulge on the posterior part of the nasal surface of the velum. It has been postulated that the bulge serves two purposes (Kuehn, Folkins, & Linville, 1988; Moon & Kuehn, 1996, 1997). The first purpose is to provide additional stiffness to the nasal side of the velum during contraction, which prevents velar distortion. The second purpose is to fill in the area of contact between the velum and posterior pharyngeal wall in midline, which helps to assure a firm velopharyngeal seal (Huang, Lee, & Rajendran, 1997; Kuehn et al., 1988).

It has also been suggested that the musculus uvulae may have an extensor effect on the nasal aspect of the velum, displacing it toward the posterior pharyngeal wall (Huang et al., 1997). The paired musculus uvulae muscles overlie the levator sling in the midline of the posterior velum and originate from the area of the palatal aponeurosis. They are the only intrinsic muscles of the velum and, as such, they are contained solely within the velum and do not extend beyond its borders (Moon & Kuehn, 1996). They are positioned side by side and extend to the free edge of the soft palate, superficial to the levator veli palatini. It should be noted that the name of this muscle is somewhat misleading in that it does not exist within the uvula. In fact, the uvula contains very few muscle fibers and does not contribute to velopharyngeal closure (Ettema & Kuehn, 1994; Kuehn & Kahane, 1990; Moon & Kuehn, 1996, 1997).

The palatoglossus muscles act antagonistically to the levator veli palatini to depress the velum or elevate the tongue. As such, these muscles are felt to be responsible for the rapid downward movement of the velum during connected speech when a nasal consonant is produced. On each side, the palatoglossus muscle arises from the palatal aponeurosis of the anterior half of the soft palate and inserts into the posterior lateral aspect of the tongue. It is contained within the anterior faucial pillar, and may be subject to possible damage during tonsillectomy.

The function of the palatopharyngeus muscle is not well understood. The horizontal fibers of these muscles are thought to be associated with the sphincteric action of pulling the lateral pharyngeal walls medially to narrow the pharynx and assist with closure (Cassell & Elkadi, 1995). The vertical fibers may assist in the lowering of the velum, and could also assist with the elevation of the larynx and the lower portion of the pharynx (Moon & Kuehn, 1996,

1997). Some authors have suggested that this muscle functions as a muscular "hydrostat," which squeezes the posterior aspect of the velum so that it conforms to the shape of the posterior pharyngeal wall, thus resulting in a better velopharyngeal seal (Ettema & Kuehn, 1994; Moon & Kuehn, 1997; Smith & Kier, 1989). The palatopharyngeus muscle originates from the palatal aponeurosis and posterior border of the hard palate and then courses down through the posterior faucial pillars to the pharynx. A few of the vertical fibers of this muscle reach the thyroid cartilage of the larynx.

The paired salpingopharyngeus muscle cannot have a significant role in achieving velopharyngeal closure given its size and location. This muscle arises from the inferior border of the torus tubarius, which is at the upper level of the pharynx. It courses vertically along the lateral pharyngeal wall and under the salpingopharyngeal fold.

The tensor veli palatini muscles are responsible for opening the eustachian tubes in order to enhance middle ear aeration and drainage (Maue-Dickson, Dickson, & Rood, 1976). Although these muscles are the main contributors to the palatal aponeurosis, the tensor is not positioned in a way to either raise or lower the velum. Therefore, these muscles probably contribute little, if anything, to velopharyngeal closure. The tensor veli palatini muscle on each side originates from the membranous portion of the eustachian tube cartilage and the scaphoid fossa spine of the sphenoid bone (Barsoumian, Kuehn, Moon, & Canady, 1998). Additional slips arise from the lateral aspect of the medial pterygoid plate and the spine of the sphenoid. The tensor veli palatini muscle then courses vertically down from the skull base to pass around the pterygoid hamulus. This redirects the muscle tendon 90° medially where it contributes to the palatine aponeurosis in the superior and anterior region of the velum.

Although the velum is a main player in the velopharyngeal valve, muscle fibers (primarily those of the levator veli palatini) are found in only about 40% of this structure, and primarily in the midsection (Ettema & Kuehn, 1994). It is important to stress that the muscles of the velopharyngeal mechanism do not work in isolation. In fact, each motor movement is probably the result of the synergistic activities of several muscles. For example, the position and force of closure of the velopharyngeal valve varies with different activities, as will be discussed later. These variations are probably due to variations in the relative contribution of the levator veli palatini, palatoglossus, and palatopharyngeus muscles (Moon, Smith, Folkins, Lemke, & Gartlan, 1994). The complexity of the interaction of the muscles of the velopharyngeal mechanism has been studied, but further research is needed before this interaction is fully understood. The following list summarizes the velopharyngeal muscles.

Summary of Velopharyngeal Muscles

- **Levator Veli Palatini**—acts as a sling to pull the velum up and back toward the posterior pharyngeal wall.

- **Tensor Veli Palatini**—opens the eustachian tube during swallowing.

- **Musculus Uvulae**—forms the velar eminence on the nasal surface of the velum, adding bulk in the midline to assist with closure.

- **Superior Constrictor**—constricts the pharyngeal walls against the velum.

- **Palatopharyngeus**—narrows the pharynx by pulling the lateral pharyngeal walls upward and medially.

- **Palatoglossus**—brings the velum down for nasal consonants.

Velopharyngeal Motor and Sensory Innervation

The motor and sensory innervation of the velopharyngeal mechanism arises from the cranial nerves in the medulla. The following section describes the specific innervation for motor movement and sensation

Motor innervation for the muscles that contribute to velopharyngeal closure comes from the pharyngeal plexus (Figure 1–14). The pharyngeal plexus is a network of nerves that lies along the posterior wall of the pharynx and consists of the pharyngeal branches of the glossopharyngeal nerve (CN IX) and the vagus nerve (CN X). Innervation of the velar muscles with these nerves occurs through the brainstem nuclei ambiguus and retrofacialis (Cassell & Elkadi, 1995; Kennedy & Kuehn, 1989; Moon & Kuehn, 1996). The palatoglossus muscle has also been found to receive innervation from the hypoglossal nerve (CN XII) (Cassell & Elkadi, 1995). The tensor veli palatini, which does not contribute to velopharyngeal closure, receives motor innervation from the mandibular division of the trigeminal nerve (CN V).

Sensory innervation of both the hard and soft palate is believed to derive from the greater and lesser palatine nerves, which arise from the maxillary division of the trigeminal nerve (CN V). The faucial and pharyngeal regions of the oral cavity are innervated by the glossopharyngeal nerve (CN IX). The facial nerve (CN VII) and vagus nerve (CN X) might also contribute to sensory innervation. Although the peripheral distribution of sensory fibers may travel along different cranial nerve routes, they all appear to terminate in the spinal nucleus of the trigeminal nerve (Cassell & Elkadi, 1995). It has been reported that the cutaneous sensory nerve endings are more prolific in the anterior portion of the oral cavity, but diminish in quantity as they course toward the posterior regions of the

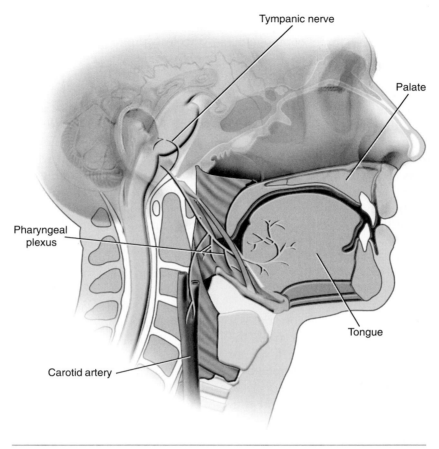

FIGURE 1–14   Position of the pharyngeal plexus.

mouth (Cassell & Elkadi, 1995). The following list summarizes velopharyngeal innervation.

Summary of Velopharyngeal Innervation

Motor Nerves of the Velum
- Glossopharyngeal (IX)
- Vagus (X)
- Accessory (XI)
- Trigeminal (V)
- Facial (VII)

Sensory Nerves of the Velum
- Vagus (X)
- Glossopharyngeal (IX)

PHYSIOLOGICAL SUBSYSTEMS FOR SPEECH

Speech is the result of the coordination of several physiological subsystems. These include respiration, phonation, resonance, and articulation. The velopharyngeal valve must function in coordination with the other subsystems of speech for speech to be produced normally and with good intelligibility. To understand the importance of these subsystems and the need for coordination, it may be helpful to review how sound is produced.

Every instrument that is capable of producing sound needs at least three components: (1) a vibrating mechanism that can be set in motion to produce sound, (2) a stimulating mechanism that can set the vibration in motion, and (3) a resonating mechanism to reinforce or amplify the sound. In human speech, the vocal folds are the vibrating bodies, the force of breath pressure is the stimulating force, and the cavities of the vocal tract provide the mechanism for resonating the sound energy (Baken, 1987). The acoustic product is then altered by the velopharyngeal valve and by changing the size and shape of the oral cavity through the movement and placement of the articulators.

Respiration

Respiration is essential for life support, but is it also important for speech. The air from the lungs is what provides the initiating force for phonation and the air pressure for articulation. During quiet breathing, the inspiratory and expiratory phases are relatively long and usually about equal in duration. During speech, however, inspiration occurs very quickly during times of purposeful pauses. Subglottic air pressure is then maintained under the vocal folds during the entire phrase or sentence. The expiratory phase is relatively long and varies; the variation depends on the length of the produced utterance. Both the inspiratory and expiratory phases must be controlled by the speaker during speech production.

Phonation

Phonation is the sound that is generated by the vocal folds as they begin to vibrate. This sound, called voice, is used for the production of all vowel sounds and about half of the consonant sounds. Some consonants are voiceless, however. Therefore, the vocal folds must vibrate

for voiced sounds, stop vibrating abruptly for voiceless sounds, and then vibrate again for the next vowel or voiced consonant (Kent & Moll, 1969). In the simple two-syllable phrase "a cup," the vocal folds vibrate on the vowel, stop on the /k/, vibrate on the vowel, and stop again on the /p/. This requires a great deal of neuromotor coordination and control.

Phonation is initiated when the vocal folds close and air from the lungs creates subglottic pressure. This air pressure forces the bottom of the vocal folds open and then continues to move upward to open the top of the vocal folds. The low pressure created behind the fast-moving air column causes the bottom of the folds to close, followed by the top folds. This is called the *Bernoulli effect*. The closure of the vocal folds cuts off the air column and releases a pulse of air. This completes one vibratory cycle. The cycles repeat for vocal fold vibration, resulting in a type of buzzing sound (which is later modified by resonance). During phonation, there is continuous adduction (or closing) of the vocal folds as they vibrate for voiced phonemes and periodic abduction (or opening) of the vocal folds as voiceless sounds are produced. Air pressure must be maintained throughout the utterance so that it can continue to provide the force for phonation.

Resonance

Once phonation has begun, the air pressure from the lungs and sound energy from the vocal folds travel in a superior direction in the vocal tract. The sound energy vibrates throughout the cavities of the supraglottic tract, beginning with the pharyngeal cavity and then including the oral cavity or nasal cavity. The resultant vibration of sound energy adds the resonance quality to the speech.

Several factors can affect the vibration and the overall acoustic product of the voice. These factors include the size and shape of the cavities of the vocal tract. This effect can be compared to what happens when you blow across the lip of a bottle. When the bottle is mostly full, the resonating space is small, and the resulting sound is high in pitch. When the bottle is almost empty and therefore leaves a larger resonating cavity, the sound is deeper in pitch. The variations among individuals in size and shape of the resonating cavities is often determined by age and gender. For example, infants have very small resonating cavities; thus, the vocal quality is very high in pitch. Women and children usually have a shorter vocal tract than men; therefore, they have higher formant frequencies in their vocal product. An additional consideration is the wall thickness of the cavities. A thick pharyngeal wall can absorb sound, whereas a thinner wall can reflect sound. The changes in vibration that result from all of these factors enhance the resonance and give the perception of timbre or vocal quality (Sataloff, 1992).

Once the sound energy and air pressure reach the pharyngeal cavity, the velopharyngeal valve regulates and directs the focus of resonance. During the production of oral speech sounds (all sounds with the exception of /m/, /n/, and /ng/), the velopharyngeal valve closes, thus blocking off the nasal cavity from the oral cavity. This allows the sound energy and air pressure to be directed anteriorly into the oral cavity. The velopharyngeal valve opens with the production of nasal sounds. This allows the nasal cavity to be *coupled* (sharing acoustic energy) with the oral and pharyngeal cavities, so that the sound energy can resonate primarily in the nasal cavity. The velopharyngeal valve is therefore very important for normal speech because it is responsible for regulating and directing the transmission of sound energy and air pressure in the cavities of the vocal tract.

Articulation

The sound that results from phonation and resonance is further altered for individual speech sounds by the articulators. The articulators are structures that include the lips, the jaws (including the teeth), the tongue, and even the velum. The articulators alter the acoustic product for different speech sounds in two ways. First, they can vary the size and shape of the oral cavity through movement and articulatory placement. In addition, the articulators can modify the manner in which the sound, and particularly the airstream, is released.

Both vowels and oral consonants require oral resonance for production, and many consonants also require oral air pressure. For the production of vowels, the tongue and jaws modify the size and shape of the oral cavity, but there is no constriction of the sound energy or air pressure. The differentiation of vowel sounds is determined by tongue height (high, mid, or low), tongue position (front, central, back), and lip rounding (present or absent). On the other hand, consonants are produced by partial or complete obstruction of the oral cavity, which results in a build-up of air pressure in the oral cavity. Intraoral air pressure provides the force for the production of all pressure-sensitive consonants (plosives, fricatives, and affricates). Plosive sounds (/p/, /b/, /t/, /d/, /k/, /g/) are produced with a build-up of intraoral pressure and then a sudden release. Fricative sounds (/f/, /v/, /s/, /z/, /sh/, /zh/, /th/) require a gradual release of air pressure through a small or restricted opening. Affricate sounds (/ch/, /j/) are a combination of plosive and fricative sounds (/ch/ = /t/ + /sh/ and /j/ = /d/ + /zh/). As such, affricate sounds require a build-up of intraoral air pressure and then a gradual release through a narrow opening. Consonants are differentiated not only by the manner of production (plosives, fricatives, affricates, liquids, and glides), but also by the place of production (bilabial, labiodental, linguoalveolar, palatal, velar, and glottal) and voicing (voiced or voiceless).

Stress and Intonation

In connected speech, articulation is influenced by the stress of individual phonemes and the intonation of the utterance. Stress is related to increased laryngeal and subglottic pressure during the production of a syllable. Stressed syllables are higher in pitch and intensity, longer in duration, and produced with greater articulatory precision as compared with unstressed syllables. Intonation refers to the frequent changes in pitch throughout an utterance, as controlled by subtle changes in vocal fold length and mass. These changes influence the rate of vibration of the vocal folds and the tension of the muscles of the larynx. Although there are changes in pitch throughout connected speech, the pitch of the voice tends to drop to a lower frequency at the end of each statement and rise to a higher frequency at the end of a question. Both stress and intonation are used for emphasis and also to help to convey meaning. For example, the words "desert" and "dessert" have different meanings that are conveyed through differences in the place of stress. When the sentence "Well that's just fine" is uttered as if it has an exclamation point, it has a different meaning than when it is spoken as if it has a period at the end. The differences in meaning are conveyed by differences in the intonation and stress.

Coordination of Processes

Speech is a very complicated process that requires the coordination of the subsystems of respiration, phonation, resonance, and articu-

lation. During speech, all movements must be done quickly and with good accuracy. In addition, the action of every muscle is influenced by the actions of other muscles in the system, the movements of each structure are influenced by movements of other structures, and every phoneme is influenced by other phonemes around it (Lubker, 1975). It is almost as if each subsystem is a player on a "team." Each player must be able to execute its own role, and also learn how to work with the other players. If it is a good player, the other team players will be more effective as well. If it is a poor player however, this will make the job of the other team players much more difficult and they will function less effectively. Overall, the complexity of speech production cannot be overstated.

PHYSIOLOGY OF THE VELOPHARYNGEAL VALVE

Normal velopharyngeal closure is accomplished by the coordinated action of the velum (soft palate), the lateral pharyngeal walls, and the posterior pharyngeal wall (Moon & Kuehn, 1996). These structures function as a valve that serves to close off the nasal cavity from the oral cavity during speech, as well as during singing, whistling, blowing, sucking, swallowing, gagging, and vomiting. Although the relative contributions of these structures to closure can vary among individuals, all are important for normal velopharyngeal function.

Velar Movement

When inactive, the velum is low in the pharynx and rests against the base of the tongue (see Figure 1–9A). This position contributes to a patent pharynx, which is important for the unobstructed movement of air between the nasal cavity and lungs during normal nasal breathing. During the production of oral speech, the velum raises in a superior and posterior direction to contact the posterior pharyngeal wall or, in some cases, the lateral pharyngeal walls (Figure 1–9B). As it elevates, it has a type of "knee action" where it bends to provide maximum contact with the posterior pharyngeal wall over a large surface. The point where the velum bends is called the *velar dimple.* This "dimple" is formed by the contraction of the levator muscles where they interdigitate. The velar dimple is usually located at a point that is about 80% of the distance from the hard palate to the end of the velum (Mason & Simon, 1977) and can be seen through an intraoral examination. An examination of the nasal surface of the velum through endoscopy would reveal a muscular bulge on that side of the velar dimple, called the velar eminence. This bulge results from the contraction of the musculus uvulae muscles. In fact, it could be said that the musculus uvulae muscles form the "patella" of the levator "knee." The contraction of the musculus uvulae muscles is felt to provide internal stiffness to the velum. In addition, the bulk that this bulge provides in this area helps to achieve velopharyngeal closure in the midline.

As the velum elevates, it also elongates through a process called velar stretch (Bzoch, 1968; Mourino & Weinberg, 1975; Pruzansky & Mason, 1962; Simpson & Austin, 1972; Simpson & Chin, 1981; Simpson & Colton, 1980). Due to this stretch factor, the velum is actually longer during function than it is at rest. Therefore, the effective length of the velum is the distance between the posterior border of the hard palate and the point on the posterior pharyngeal wall where it contacts during speech. This is measured in a line on the same plane as the hard palate (Mason & Simon, 1977). The amount of velar stretch and effective length of the velum varies among individuals and is dependent on the size and configuration of the pharynx. Simpson and Colton (1980) reported that the amount of velar stretch is highly correlated with the "need ratio," which they defined as the pharyngeal depth divided by the velar length at rest.

When nasal phonemes are produced, the velum is pulled down so that the sound energy can enter the nasal cavity. The lowering of the velum is the result of contraction of the palatoglossus muscles, and to a lesser extent, gravity and tissue elasticity (Fritzell, 1979; Kuehn & Azzam, 1978; Moon & Kuehn, 1996, 1997). Given the speed with which the velum must be lowered for nasal phonemes and then raised for oral phonemes, gravity alone would not be effective.

Lateral Pharyngeal Wall Movement

The lateral pharyngeal walls contribute to velopharyngeal closure by moving medially to close against the velum or, in some cases, to meet in midline behind the velum (Figure 1–15). Both lateral pharyngeal walls move during closure, but there is great variation among normal speakers as to the extent of movement (Shprintzen, Rakoff, Skolnick, & Lavorato, 1977). In addition, there is often asymmetry in movement so that one side may move significantly more than the other side. Although some lateral wall movement can be noted from an intraoral perspective, the point of greatest medial displacement occurs near the level of the hard palate (Iglesias et al., 1980) and velar eminence (Shprintzen et al., 1975). This area is well above the area that can be seen from an intraoral inspection. In fact, at the oral cavity level, the lateral walls may actually appear to bow outward during speech.

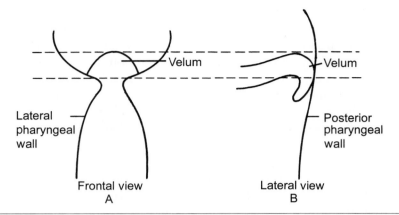

FIGURE 1–15 (A and B) A. Frontal view of the lateral pharyngeal walls. The lateral pharyngeal walls move medially to close against the velum on both sides. B. Lateral view of the velum as it contacts the posterior pharyngeal wall (PPW). (From "Lateral Defects in Velopharyngeal Insufficiency," by R. T. Cotton and F. Quattromani, 1977, *Archives of Otolaryngology, 103,* p. 469. Reprinted with permission.)

Posterior Pharyngeal Wall Movement

During velar movement, the posterior pharyngeal wall may move forward to assist in achieving contact, although this forward movement may be slight (Iglesias et al., 1980). Some posterior pharyngeal wall movement is noted in most normal speakers, but its contribution to closure seems to be much less than that of the velum and lateral pharyngeal walls. Some normal as well as abnormal speakers have a defined area on the posterior pharyngeal wall that bulges forward during speech. This is called Passavant's ridge, and is discussed in the next section.

Passavant's Ridge

A Passavant's ridge, first reported by Gustav Passavant in the 1800s, is a shelf-like ridge that projects from the posterior pharyngeal wall into the pharynx (Figure 1–16). Passavant's ridge

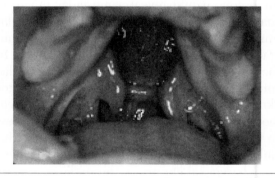

FIGURE 1–16 Passavant's ridge as noted during phonation. This patient has an open palate due to surgery for maxillary cancer. During phonation, the Passavant's ridge presents as a ridge of muscle on the posterior pharyngeal wall.

occurs in coordination with velopharyngeal closure. Its presence is associated with active lateral pharyngeal wall motion and is also synchronous with velar movement (Glaser, Skolnick, McWilliams, & Shprintzen, 1979). Passavant's ridge occurs in both normal and abnormal speakers. Reports of the prevalence of Passavant's ridge in normal speakers range from as little as 9.5% to as high as 80% (Calnan, 1957; Casey & Emrich, 1988; Finkelstein et al., 1991; Massengill, Walker, & Pickrell, 1969; Skolnick & Cohn, 1989; Skolnick, Shprintzen, McCall, & Rakoff, 1975). This variation in the reported prevalence may be due to the fact that Passavant's ridge is more prominent, and therefore is more easily identified, when the head is hyperextended (Glaser et al., 1979). In a look at the collective results of several studies, Casey and Emrich (1988) found that Passavant's ridge probably occurs in about 23% of individuals with a history of cleft and in 15% of normal speakers.

Passavant's ridge is discussed in the physiology section of this chapter rather than in the anatomy section because it is not a permanent structure. Instead, it is a dynamic structure that occurs inconsistently in some individuals during velopharyngeal activities such as speech, whistling, blowing, and swallowing (Glaser et al., 1979), but disappears during nasal breathing or when velopharyngeal activity ceases (Skolnick & Cohn, 1989). Because Passavant's ridge is a localized projection, it should not be confused with the generalized anterior movement of the posterior pharyngeal wall during speech.

Passavant's ridge is thought to be formed by the contraction of specific fibers of the superior constrictor muscles, and possibly of fibers of the palatopharyngeus muscles in the posterior pharynx (Dickson & Dickson, 1972; Finkelstein et al., 1993). This forms the muscular ridge, which projects from the posterior pharyngeal wall. Passavant's ridge extends from one lateral pharyngeal wall to the other lateral pharyngeal wall on the opposite side. The vertical location of the ridge is variable among individuals. Although it is across from the free margin of the velum, it is often well below the site of velopharyngeal

contact. A study by Glaser et al. (1979) of 43 individuals found that the ridge was located opposite the velar eminence in 5% of this group, opposite the vertical portion of the velum in 58%, opposite the uvula in 25%, and below the uvula in 12%. The orientation of the ridge is also variable among individuals. The ridge can be found to point in a superior, anterior, or inferior direction.

Although the location and orientation of the ridge is variable among different speakers, it appears to be in a consistent location for each individual speaker. However, the size of the ridge appears to vary according to the speech sound being produced and the overall degree of velar activity (Skolnick & Cohn, 1989). The size has also been found to be affected by fatigue (Calnan, 1957).

Passavant's ridge is not a prerequisite for normal velopharyngeal function, and it is probably not a compensatory mechanism either. When it is found in individuals with velopharyngeal dysfunction, it does not seem to be correlated with gap size or type of cleft palate (Massengill et al., 1969). In addition, the formation of Passavant's ridge does not appear to be associated with the degree of velopharyngeal closure necessary for the specific speech sound. Instead, it has been found to be closely related to the tongue position for vowel production (Honjo, Kojima, & Kumazawa, 1975). When an individual demonstrates a Passavant's ridge, it does not occur on all sounds all the time and when it does occur, it is often delayed, occurring after velopharyngeal closure has been achieved. It is often located well below the level of velar and lateral pharyngeal wall movement. Therefore, the appearance of Passavant's ridge is probably an insignificant finding because it does not indicate an abnormality and it is not relevant when considering appropriate treatment.

VARIATIONS IN VELOPHARYNGEAL CLOSURE

Variations in Closure among Normal Speakers

In looking at the entire velopharyngeal mechanism, it is important to recognize that this is a three-dimensional tube that includes the anterior-posterior dimension, the vertical dimension, and the horizontal dimension. During closure, there must be coordinated movement of all structures in all dimensions so that the velopharyngeal valve can achieve closure like a sphincter. This can be seen in Figure 1–17, which shows an inferior view of the entire sphincter.

The relative contribution of the velopharyngeal structures to closure varies among both normal and abnormal speakers. In fact, distinct patterns of velopharyngeal closure can be identified, based on the extent of movement of the soft palate and pharyngeal walls (Croft, Shprintzen, & Rakoff, 1981; Finkelstein, Talmi, Nachmani, Hauben, & Zohar, 1992; Igawa, Nishizawa, Sugihara, & Inuyama, 1998; Shprintzen et al., 1977; Siegel-Sadewitz & Shprintzen, 1982; Skolnick & Cohn, 1989; Skolnick et al., 1973; Witzel & Posnick, 1989). These basic patterns of closure can be seen in Figure 1–18.

The coronal pattern of closure is the most common and is accomplished by the posterior movement of the soft palate closing against a broad area of the posterior pharyngeal wall. There may also be anterior movement of the posterior pharyngeal wall. With this closure pattern, there is minimal contribution of the lateral pharyngeal walls to closure. Witzel and Posnick (1989) studied 246 individuals who underwent nasopharyngoscopy for evaluation of velopharyngeal function. (Nasopharyngoscopy is an endoscopic procedure in which a scope is

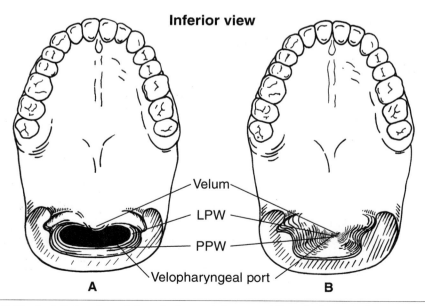

Inferior view

Velum

LPW

PPW

Velopharyngeal port

A

B

FIGURE 1–17 (A and B) An inferior view of the velopharyngeal port. A. The velopharyngeal port is open for nasal breathing. B. The velopharyngeal port is closed for speech.

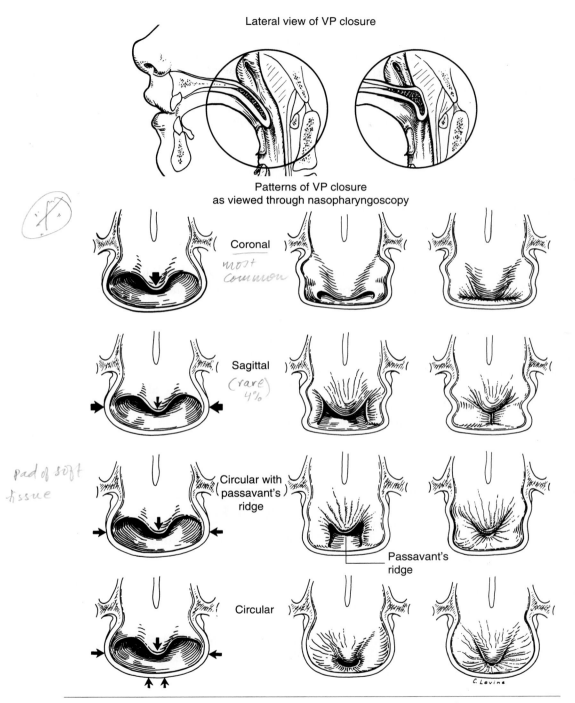

FIGURE 1–18 Patterns of velopharyngeal closure as viewed through nasopharyngoscopy.

inserted through the nose until it reaches the nasopharynx, allowing visual observation and analysis of the velopharyngeal mechanism. See Chapter 17 for more information.) In this study, they found that 68% of their patients demonstrated a coronal pattern of closure.

The next most common pattern of closure is the circular pattern. This pattern occurs when the soft palate moves posteriorly, the posterior pharyngeal wall moves anteriorly, and the lateral pharyngeal walls move medially. In this case, all the velopharyngeal structures contribute to closure, and the closure pattern resembles a true sphincter. Witzel and Posnick (1989) found this pattern in 23% of the individuals in their study. Another 5% had a circular pattern with Passavant's ridge. Although Passavant's ridge seems to be most common in individuals with a circular pattern of closure, it is also found with the other patterns of velopharyngeal closure (Skolnick & Cohn, 1989).

The least common pattern of closure is the sagittal pattern. This was found in only 4% of the patients in the Witzel and Posnick study (1989). With this pattern, the lateral pharyngeal walls move medially to meet in midline behind the velum. There is minimal posterior displacement of the soft palate to effect closure. Of note is the fact that the prevalence of the different patterns of closure is similar in frequency in both normal and abnormal speakers (Croft, Shprintzen, & Rakoff, 1981).

To try to explain the differences in movement patterns, Finkelstein and colleagues studied 42 consecutive individuals who were undergoing uvulopalatopharyngoplasty (UPPP), which is the partial excision of the velum and uvula to resolve sleep apnea. The velopharyngeal valve was studied through an oral examination and also through an endoscopic examination. They found that individuals with a deep oropharynx tended to show a sagittal or circular pattern of closure, while individuals

with a flat oropharynx showed a coronal pattern of closure. These researchers concluded that there must be minor differences in muscular orientation among individuals to account for the different pharyngeal configurations at rest and during speech (Finkelstein et al., 1992, 1993).

The variations in the basic patterns of closure among individuals are important to recognize and understand. This is particularly true in the evaluation process, because the basic pattern of closure may have an impact on the diagnosis of velopharyngeal dysfunction and on the type of intervention that is ultimately recommended (Siegel-Sadewitz & Shprintzen, 1982; Skolnick et al., 1973). For example, on a lateral videofluoroscopy (which is a radiographic procedure), it may appear as if there is inadequate velopharyngeal closure with the sagittal pattern of closure, even when closure is complete, since the velum does not close against the posterior pharyngeal wall. Therefore, evaluating all of the velopharyngeal structures and their contribution to closure is important so that the basic closure pattern can be identified and considered when making treatment recommendations.

Variations in Closure with Type of Activity

Velopharyngeal closure occurs in activities other than speech. If these activities are categorized into pneumatic and nonpneumatic functions, a characteristic and distinct closure pattern can be identified for each category (Flowers & Morris, 1973; Matsuya, Yamaoka, & Miyasaki, 1979; McWilliams & Bradley, 1965; Shprintzen, Lencione, McCall, & Skolnick, 1974). In fact, there seems to be a separate neurological mechanism for closure during nonspeech activities versus closure for speech.

Nonpneumatic activities include swallowing, gagging, and vomiting. With these activities, the velum raises very high in the pharynx and the lateral pharyngeal walls close tightly along their entire length. Closure appears to be almost exaggerated and is very firm, as viewed through videofluoroscopy. This type of closure is necessary because the purpose of closure in these cases is to allow substances to pass through the oral cavity—while preventing nasal regurgitation. In swallowing, velopharyngeal closure is further assisted by the back of the tongue, which raises against the velum, thus pushing the velum up and back (Flowers & Morris, 1973). It is important to note that velopharyngeal closure may be complete for nonpneumatic activities, but insufficient for speech or other pneumatic activities (Shprintzen et al., 1975).

Pneumatic activities are those that utilize air pressure (both positive and negative) as a result of velopharyngeal closure. Positive pressure is necessary for blowing, whistling, singing, and speech. Negative pressure is needed for sucking and kissing. With these activities, closure occurs lower in the nasopharynx and appears to be less exaggerated than with nonpneumatic activities.

It would be tempting to assume that closure for all pneumatic activities is about the same. If that were true, then the use of blowing and sucking exercises would be beneficial in improving velopharyngeal function for speech. Unfortunately, the closure patterns for all of these pneumatic activities are also physiologically different from each other (McWilliams & Bradley, 1965). Blowing, for example, requires generalized movements of the velopharyngeal structures—and levator activity for blowing is higher than for speech (Kuehn & Moon, 1994). On the other hand, speech requires precise, rapid movements of these structures; the point of contact even varies during speech, as will be discussed in the next section. When comparing velopharyngeal closure during singing and speech, the velopharyngeal port is closed longer and tighter in singing than in speech, particularly on the higher pitches (Austin, 1997).

Variations in Closure due to Timing

Voice onset and velopharyngeal closure must be closely coordinated during speech. Velar movement for oral sounds must begin prior to the onset of phonation so that the velopharyngeal valve is completely closed when phonation begins. If complete closure is not achieved before activation of the sound source, then hypernasal resonance may be noted (Ha, Sim, Zhi, & Kuehn, 2004).

The timing of closure for an oral sound has been found to be somewhat dependent on the type of phoneme. Kent and Moll (1969) found evidence to suggest that the velar elevating gesture for a stop begins earlier and is executed more rapidly when the stop is voiceless rather than voiced. The production of nasal consonants during an utterance has an additional effect on velopharyngeal function and timing. The velum remains elevated and closure is maintained throughout the utterance as long as oral consonants or vowels are being produced. As a nasal consonant (/m/, /n/, /ng/) is produced, the velum lowers quickly and the pharyngeal walls move away from midline, thus opening the velopharyngeal valve to allow for nasal resonance. Vowels that precede or follow the nasal consonant will be slightly affected by the anticipatory lowering of the velum just before the nasal consonant and by the slight delay in raising the velum just after the nasal consonant (Bunnell, 2005). Therefore, the timing of closure requires constant fine adjustments throughout an utterance, depending on the phonemic needs.

In addition, missed timing may have implications for the perception of resonance or nasality.

Variations in Closure with Phonemes

Even as velopharyngeal closure is maintained throughout oral speech, there are slight variations in both velar contact height and closure force. This variation is due primarily to the type of phoneme being produced and its phonetic environment (Flowers & Morris, 1973; McWilliams & Bradley, 1965; Moll, 1962; Moon & Kuehn, 1997; Shprintzen et al., 1975; Simpson & Chin, 1981).

The height of velar closure is affected by the movement and height of the tongue during articulation of the sound, and also by the phoneme's requirements for intraoral air pressure (Tom, Titze, Hoffman, & Story, 2001). In general, velar heights are slightly greater for consonants than for vowels. High-pressure consonants (plosives, fricatives, and affricates), especially those that are voiceless, have the greatest heights when compared to other consonants. High vowels have a higher velar height than low vowels (Moll, 1962; Moon & Kuehn, 1997), possibly due to the elevation of the tongue during the production of these sounds.

The same factors that increase the height of velar contact during speech also increase the firmness of closure. Therefore, velopharyngeal closure force is greater on consonants than on vowels and it is greatest on high pressure consonants, particularly fricatives (Kuehn & Moon, 1998). High vowels are associated with a greater degree of closure force than low vowels (Kuehn & Moon, 1998; Moll, 1962; Moon, Kuehn, & Huisman, 1994). Moll (1962) has shown that vowels adjacent to a nasal consonant, particularly when preceding the consonant, have less closure force than those adjacent to oral consonants. A decline in overall closure force occurs with fatigue (Kuehn & Moon, 2000).

Considering all of these factors, changes in velar position are the result of the interaction of a number of variables, including vowel height and the type of consonant (Lubker, 1975; Seaver & Kuehn, 1980). Therefore, velar position must be changed and coordinated with each syllable production (Karnell, Linville, & Edwards, 1988).

Variations in Closure due to Rate and Fatigue

Rapid speech can affect the efficiency of velar movement, thus compromising velopharyngeal closure. It has been shown that when speech rate increases, the height of closure decreases and is less firm (Moll & Shriner, 1967), presumably due to the difficulty in achieving appropriate height and contact with the rapid rate. Therefore, as speech rate increases, it can become more hypernasal. Even blowing can result in velar fatigue (Tachimura, Nohara, Satoh, & Wada, 2004).

Muscular fatigue can also affect the height and firmness of closure. Even normal speakers become "nasal" when they are tired. Young children are often described as "whiny" at the end of the day, especially when they are tired. The term "whiny" actually describes an increase in hypernasality due to velar fatigue.

CHANGES IN VELOPHARYNGEAL FUNCTION WITH GROWTH AND AGE

The maturational changes in the craniofacial skeleton result in changes in the relationships of the pharyngeal structures and the size of the cavities of the vocal tract (pharyngeal, oral, and nasal). The differences in the vocal tract anatomy between an infant, child, and adult are significant and account for the differences in the quality of the "voice" at different stages of development.

Although the cranium approaches adult size relatively early in childhood, the facial bones continue to grow into adolescence or early adulthood. The growth of the mandible and maxillary bones is somewhat affected by the development of dentition. As these structures grow and mature, they move down and forward relative to the cranium. Both the maxilla and mandible are similar in size in males and females until around 14 years of age. After that age, these facial bones continue to grow in males until around age 18, whereas there is very little additional growth in females (Ursi, Trotman, McNamara, & Behrents, 1993). Although there are changes in the size of these bony structures, these changes occur with relatively minor changes in shape, despite occlusal stages (Kent & Vorperian, 1995).

The size of the pharynx changes greatly during maturation. The newborn pharynx is estimated to be approximately 4 cm long. In fact, the velum and epiglottis are in close proximity, resulting in a very short pharynx (which accounts for the infant's high-pitched voice). In contrast, the adult pharynx is approximately 20 cm long. It has been shown that with age and height, there is a linear increase in the length of the pharynx for both boys and girls (Rommel et al., 2003; Stellzig-Eisenhauer, 2001).

In addition to the increase in length, there is increase of approximately 80% in the volume of the nasopharynx from infancy to adulthood (Bergland, 1963). Because there is more vertical than horizontal growth, there is very little change in the anterior-posterior dimension of the nasopharynx (Bergland, 1963; Kent & Vorperian, 1995; Tourne, 1991). However,

there is significant change in the angle of the posterior pharyngeal wall. In a newborn, the nasopharynx curves gradually to meet the oropharynx. At around age 5, the posterior pharyngeal wall of the nasopharynx and oropharynx meet at an oblique angle. By puberty and through adulthood, these sections of the posterior pharyngeal wall meet at almost a right angle (Kent, 1976; Kent & Vorperian, 1995). Although the velum moves down and slightly forward with the growth of the maxilla, the angle of the pharyngeal wall changes at the same time. In addition, the velum increases in both length and thickness and tends to stretch more to make up any difference in the structural relationships. As a result, the competency of velopharyngeal closure is maintained.

Another factor that changes the relative dimensions of the pharyngeal space and can introduce some instability in velopharyngeal function is the presence and size of the adenoid tissue. The adenoid pad is positioned on the posterior pharyngeal wall in the area of velopharyngeal closure. In many young children, the adenoid tissue assists with closure to a degree—so that closure is actually veloadenoidal (Croft, Shprintzen, & Ruben, 1981; Kent & Vorperian, 1995; Skolnick et al., 1975; Subtelney & Koepp-Baker, 1956). In young children, the adenoid pad can be prominent in size. A gradual process of involution and atrophy begins before puberty, but a more sudden involution may occur with puberty.

For the reasons noted above, the velopharyngeal mechanism is usually able to adapt to the anatomic changes that occur with adenoid atrophy in such a way that velopharyngeal function is maintained. In addition, there may be an increase in velopharyngeal movement following adenoid involution—so that a more mature pattern of velopharyngeal closure is adopted (Kent & Vorperian, 1995). However, if there was a history from the start of cleft palate or tenuous velopharyngeal closure, these compensations may not be possible. In these individuals, the changes that occur in the adenoid pad as the individual moves through puberty may result in the onset of velopharyngeal insufficiency that requires surgical intervention (Mason & Warren, 1980; Siegel-Sadewitz & Shprintzen, 1986; Van Demark & Morris, 1983).

Finally, the effect of aging on velopharyngeal function has been studied. One study has shown that changes can occur in velopharyngeal closure patterns with the onset of puberty and with adenoid involution (Siegel-Sadewitz & Shprintzen, 1986). Hoit and colleagues (1994) found no differences in nasal airflow in ages up to 80 years, suggesting that velopharyngeal function does not deteriorate with age alone.

SUMMARY

The anatomy of the face, oral cavity, and velopharyngeal valve is well documented, and is easy to describe and to understand. On the other hand, the physiology of the velopharyngeal mechanism, particularly as it relates to speech, is very complex and not well understood. There is still much to be learned regarding the roles of the various muscles, the interaction of velopharyngeal function with articulation, and the neuromotor controls required for coordination of velopharyngeal function with the other subsystems of speech. This information would help us understand not only normal speech production, but also the causes and possible treatment of disordered speech.

FOR REVIEW, DISCUSSION, AND CRITICAL THINKING

1. Why is it important to understand what is considered normal structure when working with individuals with a history of cleft lip and palate?

2. What are the facial landmarks and structures that may be relevant to the study of cleft lip?

3. Describe the internal nasal structures. Why do you think an understanding of the internal nasal structures might be relevant to a study of cleft lip and palate?

4. List the oral structures that can be seen when looking in the mouth.

5. List the suture lines of the hard palate. Why do you think they are called "suture" lines? Explain how they are formed.

6. Describe the movement of the velopharyngeal structures and the role of the velopharyngeal muscles in closing and opening the velopharyngeal valve.

7. What are the physiological subsystems of speech and how do they interact with each other for normal speech? Describe how a problem with one subsystem may affect other subsystems.

8. What are the types of velopharyngeal closure patterns among normal and abnormal speakers? Why do you think it is important to understand the basic patterns of speech when evaluating abnormal speakers?

9. Discuss the effects of type of activity, type of phoneme, rate of speech, and fatigue on velopharyngeal closure. Given the known effect of these factors on velopharyngeal closure, how would this affect the way you evaluate velopharyngeal function for speech?

10. How does velopharyngeal closure change with growth and adenoid involution? How could these changes potentially affect speech?

REFERENCES

Austin, S. F. (1997). Movement of the velum during speech and singing in classically trained singers. *Journal of Voice, 11*(2), 212–221.

Baken, R. J. (1987). *Clinical measurement of speech and voice.* Boston: College-Hill Press.

Barsoumian, R., Kuehn, D. P., Moon, J. B., & Canady, J. W. (1998). An anatomic study of the tensor veli palatini and dilatator tubae muscles in relation to the eustachian tube and velar function. *Cleft Palate-Craniofacial Journal, 35*(2), 101–110.

Bell-Berti, F. (1973). The velopharyngeal mechanism: An electromyographic study. Unpublished doctoral dissertation, City University of New York, NY.

Bergland, O. (1963). The bony nasopharynx. *Acta Odontologica Scandinavia, 21*(Suppl. 35), 1–137.

Boorman, J. G., & Sommerlad, B. C. (1985). Levator palati and palatal dimples: Their anatomy, relationship, and clinical significance. *British Journal of Plastic Surgery, 38*(3), 326–332.

Bunnell, H. T. (2005). The acoustic phonetics of nasality: A practical guide to acoustic analysis. *Perspectives on Speech Science and Orofacial Disorders, 15*(2), 3–10.

Bzoch, K. F. (1968). Variations in velopharyngeal valving: The factor of vowel changes. *Cleft Palate Journal, 5,* 211–218.

Calnan, I. (1957). Modern views on Passavant's ridge. *British Journal of Plastic Surgery, 10,* 89.

Casey, D. M., & Emrich, L. J. (1988). Passavant's ridge in patients with soft palatectomy. *Cleft Palate Journal, 25*(1), 72–77.

Cassell, M. D., & Elkadi, H. (1995). Anatomy and physiology of the palate and velopharyngeal structures. In R. J. Shprintzen & J. Bardach (Eds.), *Cleft palate speech management: A multidisciplinary approach* (pp. 45–62). St. Louis, MO: Mosby.

Cassell, M. D., Moon, J. B., & Elkadi, H. (1990). Anatomy and physiology of the velopharynx. In J. Bardach & H. L. Morris (Eds.), *Multidisciplinary management of cleft lip and palate.* Philadelphia: Saunders.

Croft, C. B., Shprintzen, R. J., & Rakoff, S. J. (1981). Patterns of velopharyngeal valving in normal and cleft palate subjects: A multi-view videofluoroscopic and nasendoscopic study. *Laryngoscope, 91*(2), 265–271.

Croft, C. B., Shprintzen, R. J., & Ruben, R. J. (1981). Hypernasal speech following adenotonsillectomy. *Otolaryngology—Head & Neck Surgery, 89*(2), 179–188.

Dickson, D. R. (1972). Normal and cleft palate anatomy. *Cleft Palate Journal, 9,* 280–293.

Dickson, D. R. (1975). Anatomy of the normal velopharyngeal mechanism. *Clinics in Plastic Surgery, 2*(2), 235–248.

Dickson, D. R., & Dickson, W. M. (1972). Velopharyngeal anatomy. *Journal of Speech and Hearing Research, 15*(2), 372–381.

Dickson, D. R., Grant, J. C., Sicher, H., Dubrul, E. L., & Paltan, J. (1974). Status of research in cleft palate anatomy and physiology, Part 1. *Cleft Palate Journal, 11,* 471–492.

Dickson, D. R., Grant, J. C., Sicher, H., Dubrul, E. L., & Paltan, J. (1975). Status of research in cleft lip and palate: Anatomy and physiology, Part 2. *Cleft Palate Journal, 12*(1), 131–156.

Ettema, S. L., & Kuehn, D. P. (1994). A quantitative histologic study of the normal human adult soft palate. *Journal of Speech and Hearing Research, 37,* 303–313.

Finkelstein, Y., Lerner, M. A., Ophir, D., Nachmani, A., Hauben, D. J., & Zohar, Y. (1993). Nasopharyngeal profile and velopharyngeal valve mechanism. *Plastic & Reconstructive Surgery*, 92(4), 603–614.

Finkelstein, Y., Talmi, Y. P., Kravitz, K., Bar-Ziv, J., Nachmani, A., Hauben, D. J., & Zohar, Y. (1991). Study of the normal and insufficient velopharyngeal valve by the "Forced Sucking Test." *Laryngoscope*, 101(11), 1203–1212.

Finkelstein, Y., Talmi, Y. P., Nachmani, A., Hauben, D. J., & Zohar, Y. (1992). On the variability of velopharyngeal valve anatomy and function: A combined peroral and nasendoscopic study. *Plastic & Reconstructive Surgery*, 89(4), 631–639.

Flowers, C. R., & Morris, H. L. (1973). Oral-pharyngeal movements during swallowing and speech. *Cleft Palate Journal*, 10, 181–191.

Fritzell, B. (1979). Electromyography in the study of the velopharyngeal function—A review. *Folia Phoniatrica*, 31(2), 93–102.

Glaser, E. R., Skolnick, M. L., McWilliams, B. J., & Shprintzen, R. J. (1979). The dynamics of Passavant's ridge in subjects with and without velopharyngeal insufficiency—A multi-view videofluoroscopic study. *Cleft Palate Journal*, 16(1), 24–33.

Ha, S., Sim, H., Zhi, M., & Kuehn, D. P. (2004). An acoustic study of the temporal characteristics of nasalization in children with and without cleft palate. *Cleft Palate-Craniofacial Journal*, 41(5), 535–543.

Hoit, J. D., Watson, P. J., Hixon, K. E., McMahon, P., & Johnson, C. L. (1994). Age and velopharyngeal function during speech production. *Journal of Speech and Hearing Research*, 37(2), 295–302.

Honjo, I., Kojima, M., & Kumazawa, T. (1975). Role of Passavant's ridge in cleft palate speech. *Archives of Otorhinolaryngology*, 211(3), 203–208.

Huang, M. H., Lee, S. T., & Rajendran, K. (1997). Structure of the musculus uvulae: Functional and surgical implications of an anatomic study. *Cleft Palate-Craniofacial Journal*, 34(6), 466–474.

Huang, M. H., Lee, S. T., & Rajendran, K. (1998). Anatomic basis of cleft palate and velopharyngeal surgery: Implications from a fresh cadaveric study. *Plastic & Reconstructive Surgery*, 101(3), 613–627; Discussion 628–629.

Igawa, H. H., Nishizawa, N., Sugihara, T., & Inuyama, Y. (1998). A fiberscopic analysis of velopharyngeal movement before and after primary palatoplasty in cleft palate infants. *Plastic & Reconstructive Surgery*, 102(3), 668–674.

Iglesias, A., Kuehn, D. P., & Morris, H. L. (1980). Simultaneous assessment of pharyngeal wall and velar displacement of selected speech sounds. *Journal of Speech and Hearing Research*, 23, 429–446.

Karnell, M. P., Linville, R. N., & Edwards, B. A. (1988). Variations in velar position over time: A nasal videoendoscopic study. *Journal of Speech and Hearing Research*, 31(3), 417–424.

Kennedy, J. G., & Kuehn, D. P. (1989). Neuroanatomy of speech. In D. P. Kuehn, M. L. Lemme, & J. M. Baumgartner (Eds.), *Neural bases of speech, hearing, and language* (pp. 111–145). Boston: College-Hill Press.

Kent, R. D. (1976). Anatomical and neuromuscular maturation of the speech mechanism: Evidence from acoustic studies. *Journal of Speech and Hearing Research*, 19(3), 421–447.

Kent, R. D., & Moll, K. L. (1969). Vocal-tract characteristics of the stop cognates. *Journal of the Acoustical Society of America*, 46(6), 1549–1555.

Kent, R. D., & Vorperian, H. K. (1995). Development of the craniofacial-oral-laryngeal anatomy: A review. *Journal of Medical Speech-Language Pathology*, 3(3), 145–190.

Kuehn, D. P. (1979). Velopharyngeal anatomy and physiology. *Ear, Nose, and Throat Journal*, 58(7), 316–321.

Kuehn, D. P., & Azzam, N. A. (1978). Anatomical characteristics of palatoglossus and the anterior faucial pillar. *Cleft Palate Journal*, 15, 349–359.

Kuehn, D. P., Folkins, J. W., & Linville, R. N. (1988). An electromyographic study of the musculus uvulae. *Cleft Palate Journal*, 25 (4), 348–355.

Kuehn, D. P., & Kahane, J. C. (1990). Histologic study of the normal human adult soft palate. *Cleft Palate Journal*, 27, 26–34.

Kuehn, D. P., & Moon, J. B (1994). Levator veli palatini muscle activity in relation to intraoral air pressure variation. *Journal of Speech & Hearing Research*, 37(6), 1260–1270.

Kuehn, D. P., & Moon, J. B (1998). Velopharyngeal closure force and levator veli palatini activation levels in varying phonetic contexts. *Journal of Speech, Language, & Hearing Research*, 41(1), 51–62.

Kuehn, D. P., & Moon, J. B (2000). Induced fatigue effects on velopharyngeal closure force. *Journal of Speech, Language, & Hearing Research*, 43(2), 486–500.

Lubker, J. F. (1975). Normal velopharyngeal function in speech. *Clinics in Plastic Surgery*, 2(2), 249–259.

Mason, R. L., & Simon, C. (1977). Orofacial examination checklist. *Language, Speech, and Hearing Services in the Schools*, 8, 161–163.

Mason, R. M., & Warren, D. W. (1980). Adenoid involution and developing hypernasality in cleft palate. *Journal of Speech & Hearing Disorders*, 45(4), 469–480.

Massengill, R., Jr., Walker, T., & Pickrell, K. L. (1969). Characteristics of patients with a Passavant's pad. *Plastic & Reconstructive Surgery*, 44(3), 268–270.

Matsuya, T., Yamaoka, M., & Miyasaki, T. (1979). A fiberoscopic study of velopharyngeal closure in patients with operated cleft palates. *Plastic & Reconstructive Surgery*, 63(4), 497–500.

Maue-Dickson, W. (1977). Cleft lip and palate research: An updated state of the art. Section II. Anatomy and physiology. *Cleft Palate Journal*, 14(4), 270–287.

Maue-Dickson, W. (1979). The craniofacial complex in cleft lip and palate: An update review of anatomy and function. *Cleft Palate Journal*, 16(3), 291–317.

Maue-Dickson, W., & Dickson, D. R. (1980). Anatomy and physiology related to cleft palate: Current research and clinical implications. *Plastic & Reconstructive Surgery*, 65(1), 83–90.

Maue-Dickson, W., Dickson, D. R., & Rood, S. R. (1976). Anatomy of the eustachian tube and related structures in age-matched human fetuses with and without cleft palate. *Transactions of the American Academy of Ophthalmology and Otolaryngology*, 82(2), 159–164.

McWilliams, B. J., & Bradley, D. P. (1965). Ratings of velopharyngeal closure during blowing and speech. *Cleft Palate Journal*, 2 (1), 46–55.

Moll, K. (1962). Velopharyngeal closure on vowels. *Journal of Speech and Hearing Research*, 5, 30–37.

Moll, K. L., & Shriner, T. H. (1967). Preliminary investigation of a new concept of velar activity during speech. *Cleft Palate Journal, 4,* 58.

Moon, J. B., & Kuehn, D. P. (1996). Anatomy and physiology of normal and disordered velopharyngeal function for speech. *National Center for Voice and Speech, 9* (April), 143–158.

Moon, J. B., & Kuehn, D. P. (1997). Anatomy and physiology of normal and disordered velopharyngeal function for speech. In K. R. Bzoch (Ed.), *Communicative disorders related to cleft lip and palate* (4th ed., pp. 45–47). Austin, TX: Pro-Ed.

Moon, J. B., & Kuehn, D. P. (2004). Anatomy and physiology of normal and disordered velopharyngeal function for speech. In K. R. Bzoch (Ed.), *Communicative disorders related to cleft lip and palate* (5th ed.), Austin, TX: Pro-Ed.

Moon, J., Kuehn, D. P., & Huisman, J. (1994). Measurement of velopharyngeal closure force during vowel production. *Cleft Palate-Craniofacial Journal, 31,* 356–363.

Moon, J., Smith, A., Folkins, J., Lemke, J., & Gartlan, M. (1994). Coordination of velopharyngeal muscle activity during positioning of the soft palate. *Cleft Palate-Craniofacial Journal, 31,* 45–55.

Mourino, A. P., & Weinberg, B. (1975). A cephalometric study of velar stretch in 8- and 10-year-old children. *Cleft Palate Journal, 12,* 417–435.

Pruzansky, S., & Mason, R. (1962). The "stretch factor" in soft palate function. *Journal of Dental Research, 48,* 972.

Rommel, N., Bellon, E., Hermans, R., Smet, M., De Meyer, A. M., Feenstra, L., Dejaeger, E., Veereman-Wauters, G. (2003). Development of the orohypopharyngeal cavity in normal infants and young children. *Cleft Palate-Craniofacial Journal, 40*(6), 606–11.

Sataloff, R. T. (1992, December). The human voice. *Scientific American,* 108–115.

Seaver, E. J., & Kuehn, D. P. (1980). A cineradiographic and electromyographic investigation of velar positioning in nonnasal speech. *Cleft Palate Journal, 17*(3), 216–226.

Shprintzen, R. J., Lencione, R. M., McCall, G. N., & Skolnick, M. L. (1974). A three-dimensional cinefluoroscopic analysis of velopharyngeal closure during speech and nonspeech activities in normals. *Cleft Palate Journal, 11,* 412–428.

Shprintzen, R. J., McCall, G. N., Skolnick, M. L., & Lencione, R. M. (1975). Selective movement of the lateral aspects of the pharyngeal walls during velopharyngeal closure for speech, blowing, and whistling in normals. *Cleft Palate Journal, 12*(1), 51–58.

Shprintzen, R. J., Rakoff, S. J., Skolnick, M. L., & Lavorato, A. S. (1977). Incongruous movements of the velum and lateral pharyngeal walls. *Cleft Palate Journal, 14*(2), 148–157.

Siegel-Sadewitz, V. L., & Shprintzen, R. J. (1982). Nasopharyngoscopy of the normal velopharyngeal sphincter: An experiment of biofeedback. *Cleft Palate Journal, 19*(3), 194–200.

Siegel-Sadewitz, V. L., & Shprintzen, R. J. (1986). Changes in velopharyngeal valving with age. *International Journal of Pediatric Otorhinolaryngology, 11*(2), 171–182.

Simpson, R. K., & Austin, A. A. (1972). A cephalometric investigation of velar stretch. *Cleft Palate Journal, 9,* 341–351.

Simpson, R. K., & Chin, L. (1981). Velar stretch as a function of task. *Cleft Palate Journal, 18*(1), 1–9.

Simpson, R. K., & Colton, J. (1980). A cephalometric study of velar stretch in adolescent subjects. *Cleft Palate Journal, 17*(1), 40–47.

Skolnick, M. L., & Cohn, E. R. (1989). *Videofluoroscopic studies of speech in patients with cleft palate*. New York: Springer-Verlag.

Skolnick, M. L., McCall, G., & Barnes, M. (1973). The sphincteric mechanism of velopharyngeal closure. *Cleft Palate Journal*, *10*, 286–305.

Skolnick, M. L., Shprintzen, R. J., McCall, G. N., & Rakoff, S. (1975). Patterns of velopharyngeal closure in subjects with repaired cleft palate and normal speech: A multi-view videofluoroscopic analysis. *Cleft Palate Journal*, *12*, 369–376.

Smith, K. K., & Kier, W. M. (1989). Trunks, tongues, and tentacles: Moving with the skeletons of muscle. *American Scientist*, *77*, 29–35.

Stellzig-Eisenhauer, A. (2001). The influence of cephalometric parameters on resonance of speech in cleft lip and palate patients. An interdisciplinary study. *Journal of Orofacial Orthopedics*, *62*(3), 202–223.

Subtelney, J. D., & Koepp-Baker, H. (1956). The significance of adenoid tissue in velopharyngeal function. *Plastic & Reconstructive Surgery*, *17*, 235–250.

Tachimura, T., Nohara, K., Satoh, K., & Wada, T. (2004). Evaluation of fatigability of the levator veli palatini muscle during continuous blowing using power spectra analysis. *Cleft Palate-Craniofacial Journal*, *41*(3), 320–326.

Tom, K., Titze, I. R., Hoffman, E. A., & Story, B. H. (2001). Three-dimensional vocal tract imaging and formant structure: Varying vocal register, pitch, and loudness. *Journal of the Acoustical Society of America*, *109*(2), 742–747.

Tourne, L. P. (1991). Growth of the pharynx and its physiologic implications. *American Journal of Orthodontics and Dentofacial Orthopediatrics*, *99*(2), 129–139.

Ursi, W. J., Trotman, C. A., McNamara, J. A., Jr., & Behrents, R. G. (1993). Sexual dimorphism in normal craniofacial growth. *Angle Orthodontist*, *63*(1), 47–56.

Van Demark, D. R., & Morris, H. L. (1983). Stability of velopharyngeal competency. *Cleft Palate Journal*, *20*(1), 18–22.

Witzel, M. A., & Posnick, J. C. (1989). Patterns and location of velopharyngeal valving problems: Atypical findings on video nasopharyngoscopy. *Cleft Palate Journal*, *26*(1), 63–67.

CHAPTER

2

CLEFTS OF THE LIP AND PALATE

INTRODUCTION

Cleft lip and palate is the fourth most common birth defect and the most common congenital defect of the face. The prevalence of clefts is usually quoted as one in every 750 live births (Cleft Palate Foundation, 1999), although this varies with racial background. This estimate does not include the prevalence of bifid uvula, submucous cleft palate, or congenital palatal incompetence. Note that in epidemiology, the term *incidence* refers to the number of new cases of a disease or disorder in a given population, such as the number of persons becoming ill with a certain disease. On the other hand, the term *prevalence* refers to a measure of existing cases of a disorder in a given population. Therefore, prevalence refers to the number of cases of clefts in the general population.

In addition to isolated clefts, there are about 300 recognized syndromes that include cleft palate as one of its features. When the cleft palate occurs as part of a syndrome, there are usually other associated craniofacial malformations (Jones, 1988; Rollnick & Pruzansky, 1981; Shprintzen, Schwartz, Daniller, & Hoch, 1985). In addition to cleft lip and palate, there are many other types of congenital craniofacial anomalies, which can affect communication abilities.

This chapter begins with a general description of a cleft and its associated malformations. It then goes on to describe the embryological development of the lip and palate, and the various types of clefts that can occur when there is a disruption in this development. The effect of the cleft on the anatomy of the lip, palate, and adjacent structures is described. Particular emphasis is placed on submucous cleft palate because this anomaly can cause significant problems with speech and resonance, but is not always easy to identify.

WHAT IS A CLEFT?

A *cleft* is an abnormal opening or a fissure in an anatomical structure that is normally closed. A cleft lip is the result of failure of parts of the lip to come together early in the life of a fetus. Cleft palate occurs when the parts of the roof of the mouth do not fuse normally during fetal development, leaving a large opening between the oral cavity and the nasal cavity. Clefts can vary in length and in width, depending on the degree of fusion of the individual parts. It is important to note that when there is a cleft lip and/or palate, the structures are all present but have not fused together normally. In addition, the structures may be *hypoplastic*, or under-developed, in their formation.

A cleft of the lip and/or palate is a congenital malformation that occurs in utero during the first trimester of pregnancy. Because a cleft is due to a disruption in embryological development, clefts typically follow the normal embryological fusion lines. The interference in embryological development of the midface and oral cavity is often associated with malformations of the nose, eyes, and other facial structures as well. When other congenital anomalies occur along with the cleft lip and palate, they usually have a genetic etiology and are part of a multiple malformation syndrome (Jones, 1988).

A cleft lip presents with more serious cosmetic concerns than cleft palate, but a cleft palate presents with more serious functional problems, particularly problems with speech. Individuals born with both cleft lip and cleft palate are at risk for problems with aesthetics, feeding, speech, resonance, and hearing. Although there are many commonalties in the appearance of the basic clefting conditions, clefts also give rise to unique anatomical and functional deviations. These deviations are due to variations in etiology, but are also due to the various forms of treatment to which the patient has been subjected. Therefore, the severity in aesthetics and function ranges from barely noticeable to severely affected and malformed.

CAUSES OF CLEFTS AND BASIC CLASSIFICATION

Before discussing the types and causes of clefts, it is important to have a basic knowledge of embryological development and the sequence of lip and palate formation. With this understanding, it is easy to see why clefts occur as they do. In addition, knowledge of the embryological sequence provides a foundation for clinicians to describe and classify various types of clefts.

Embryological Development of the Lip and Palate

Embryological development of the face and palate is dependent on the formation of neural crest cells in the embryo. These cells migrate at different rates to form the structures of the skull and face. If migration of the neural crest cells fails to take place or if the migration is delayed, this can affect the formation of facial structures and can cause clefts or other craniofacial anomalies.

Embryological development of the lip and alveolus begins at around 6 to 7 weeks of gestation and starts at the incisive foramen. Figure 2–1 shows the direction of embryological closure of the sutures lines. Fusion begins at the incisive foramen and then proceeds in an anterior direction to form the alveolus through the fusion of the bilateral incisive suture lines. Closure then proceeds to form the base of the anterior nose and finally the upper lip. The median and two lateral lip segments are then fused, forming the philtrum and philtral lines which completes the formation of the upper lip.

Embryological development of the palate starts at around 8 to 9 weeks of gestation. Prior to palate formation, the tongue is high and in the area of the nasal cavity. The palatal shelves are vertical and positioned on each side of the tongue. Around the seventh or eighth week of gestation, the tongue begins to gradually drop down. When this occurs, the palatal shelves move slowly from a vertical to a horizontal position and fuse, first with the premaxilla at the incisive foramen, and then with each other. As can be noted in Figure 2–1, the process of fusion begins and the incisive foramen and then proceeds between the palatal shelves, moving in a posterior direction along the median palatine suture line. This completes the formation of the hard palate. The vomer, forming a portion of the nasal septum, moves downward and fuses with the superior surface of the hard palate, thus completing the separation of the nasal cavity. Once the hard palate is formed, the velum and finally the uvula are formed. This process is usually complete by 12 weeks of gestation.

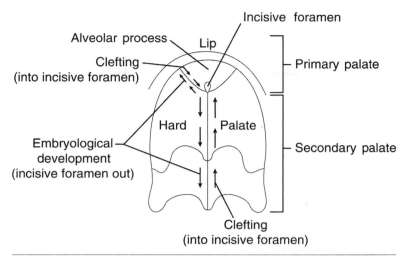

FIGURE 2–1 Embryological development and patterns of clefting. Embryological development proceeds from the incisive foramen out to the periphery. Clefting patterns begin at the periphery and follow the lines of normal embryological fusion toward the incisive foramen to the point of that disruption. The classification of clefts as affecting either the primary palate or secondary palate is based on embryological development, with the incisive foramen as the dividing point between the two.

Causes of Clefts

Since embryological development goes from the incisive foramen out, anything that disrupts that process of fusion will cause a cleft from that point all the way to the periphery (lip or uvula). Therefore, as can be seen in Figure 2–1, clefting patterns begin at the periphery and follow the lines of normal embryological fusion toward the incisive foramen to the point of that disruption. A "complete" cleft is one that follows the embryological fusion line all the way through to the incisive foramen.

Clefts can occur due to disruptions or delays in cell migration or palatal shelf movement. There are several basic causes of clefts and related craniofacial anomalies. These include chromosomal disorders and genetic disorders, which are both *endogenous* (internal) factors. Recently, older parental age has also been linked with an increased risk for both cleft lip

and cleft palate (Bille, Skytthe, Vach, Knudsen, Andersen, & Murray, 2005). In addition, clefts can be caused by environmental teratogens or by mechanical factors in utero. These are both considered *exogenous* (external) factors.

Environmental *teratogens* are substances that can cause congenital malformations. Teratogens that have been associated with cleft lip/palate include cigarette smoke (Honein, Paulozzi, & Watkins, 2001), phenytoin (Dilantin), thalidomide, valium, lead pollution (Vinceti et al., 2001), and systemic corticosteroid treatment (Edwards et al., 2003). Certain viruses, including rubella and even influenza (Metneki, Puho, & Czeizel, 2005), have been found to be risk factors for the pathogenesis of clefts. Even maternal nutritional deficiencies have been implicated in causing malformations. Lack of maternal vitamin B-6 has been associated with clefting (Munger et al., 2004). Folic acid deficiency has been suggested as a cause of orofacial clefts because it is thought to be important for normal embryonic and fetal development. However, recent studies have found that folic acid fortification during pregnancy has not reduced the prevalence of clefting in large populations (Bille, Knudsen, & Christensen, 2005; Castilla et al., 2003; Hashmi, Waller, Langlois, Canfield, & Hecht, 2005; Munger et al., 2004; Ray, Meier, Vermeulen, Wyatt, & Cole, 2003). Although the evidence linking low levels of folic acid to clefting is presently equivocal, there is stronger evidence for the role of folic acid in the prevention of neural tube defects (Simmons, Mosley, Fulton-Bond, & Hobbs, 2004). Finally, maternal obesity has even been found to cause an increased risk for orofacial clefts (Moore, Singer, Bradlee, Rothman, & Milunsky, 2000).

There is evidence to show that there are differences between males and females in the timing of embryological fusion and also in the types of clefts typically presented. Cleft lip, with or without cleft palate, occurs about twice as often in males than in females and is usually more severe in males. On the other hand, cleft palate occurs about twice as frequently in females as in males (Jensen, Kreiborg, Dahl, & Fogh-Andersen, 1988; Oka, 1979; Warkany, 1971). Although the reason for these differences between males and females is not clearly understood, it has been speculated that it could be related to differences in the timing of the development of the lip and palate in the embryo. Burdi and Silvey (1969) found that, in the male human embryo, the horizontal positioning and subsequent closure of the secondary palate occurs earlier than in the female embryo. Because the palatal shelves are open longer in the female, there is a greater period of time during which there is susceptibility to environmental teratogens.

Mechanical interference can also affect embryonic development and cause clefts. In the case of Pierre Robin sequence, crowding in utero can cause the head to be down and the mandible to be retracted, thus restricting oral cavity space. This prevents the tongue from dropping down into the oral cavity. Because of the interference of the tongue when the palate is formed, the result is a wide, bell-shaped cleft palate.

Although various causes of clefts have been identified, the etiology of clefting in a single individual is complex and may involve a combination of factors. Several genes can contribute to clefting. These genes may lead to a genetic predisposition for a cleft, but may not cause expression of the cleft unless combined with certain environmental factors. In fact, in most cases the cause of the cleft is not due to just one factor, but instead is due to the interaction of several factors. This is called *multifactorial inheritance*.

Classification of Clefts

Because there are different types of clefts with different combinations, the naming and classification of clefts can be a challenge. Although several classification systems have been proposed over the years, the system that has gained the most universal acceptance is the one proposed by Kernahan and Stark (1958). Kernahan and Stark recommended that clefts be classified based on embryological development with two basic categories: clefts of the primary palate and clefts of the secondary palate with the incisive foramen as the dividing point between the two. This division can be viewed schematically on the right side of Figure 2–1.

The *primary palate* includes the structures that are anterior to the incisive foramen. These are the structures that fuse around 7 weeks of gestation and include the alveolus and also the lip (even though the terminology is primary "palate"). The *secondary palate* includes the structures that are posterior to the incisive foramen. These are the structures that fuse around 9 weeks of gestation and include the hard palate (excluding the alveolus) and the velum. Clefts can be of either the primary or secondary palate, or of both.

Summary of Classification of Clefts

Primary Palate (also called the prepalate or intermaxillary segment)
- Anterior to the incisive foramen
- Includes lip and alveolus

Clefts include the following:
- Complete (through to the incisive foramen) or incomplete (such as lip only)
- Unilateral or bilateral

Secondary Palate
- Posterior to the incisive foramen
- Includes hard and soft palate

Clefts include the following:
- Complete (including the hard palate to the incisive foramen), incomplete (such as a portion of the velum only), or submucous
- Hard palate can be unilateral or bilateral

Although this basic classification system is used most commonly by professionals, a modification of the Kernahan and Stark classification system was later proposed by Kernahan (1971). Because clefts vary in severity, this system is more detailed. It uses a "striped–Y" figure as a means of identifying the extent of the cleft classification in Figure 2–2. The upper arms of the Y represent the primary palate and the base of the Y represents the secondary palate. The Y form is divided into sections that are numbered. The upper stems of the Y are divided into three segments with the right side numbered as 1, 2, and 3 and the left side numbered as 4, 5, and 6. The most anterior

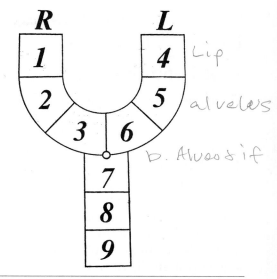

FIGURE 2–2 The Kernahan striped Y for cleft classification. The upper arms of the Y represent the primary palate and the base represents the secondary palate. The most anterior segment represents the lip, the middle segment represents the alveolus, and the posterior segment represents the area between the alveolus and the incisive foramen. The secondary palate (hard and soft palate) is also divided into sections to represent the areas of the velum and hard palate. The segments affected by the cleft are darkened on the diagram so that a visual representation can be made of the type and extent of the cleft. If there is a submucous cleft, the affected segments are marked with crosshatch marks. (From "The Striped Y—A Symbolic Classification for Cleft Lip and Palate," by Desmond A. Kernahan, 1971. *Plastic & Reconstructive Surgery, 47*(5), p. 469. Reprinted with permission.)

segment represents the lip, the middle segment represents the alveolus, and the posterior segment represents the area between the alveolus and the incisive foramen. The secondary palate (hard and soft palate) is also divided into three sections and these are numbered as 7, 8, and 9. When the segments affected by the cleft are darkened on the diagram, a visual representation can be made of the type and extent of the cleft. If there is a submucous cleft, the affected segments are marked with crosshatch marks. Using this figure, the extent of a cleft can be described or illustrated using the diagram.

CLEFTS OF THE PRIMARY PALATE (LIP AND ALVEOLUS)

Types and Severity

There are various types of clefts of the primary palate and various degrees of severity, as can be seen in Figure 2–3. A cleft of the primary palate can be "complete," which means that it extends through the entire lip, nostril sil, and alveolus to the incisive foramen. When the term "complete cleft lip" is used, it often refers to a complete cleft of the primary palate. If the cleft does not extend to the incisive foramen, it is considered "incomplete." An incomplete cleft lip can be as minor as a small, subcutaneous notch in the vermilion, or it may involve the entire lip, but not the alveolus.

In addition to incomplete or complete, a cleft of the primary palate can be unilateral (on the right or the left side) or bilateral (on both sides). If the cleft is unilateral, it most often occurs on the left side (Jensen et al., 1988; McWilliams, Morris, & Shelton, 1990). Figure 2–4 (A and B) illustrates examples of a unilateral incomplete cleft of the lip and alveolus. Figure 2–5(A through D) shows examples of a unilateral complete cleft of the primary palate (lip and alveolus). Figure 2–6(A through D) shows examples of bilateral

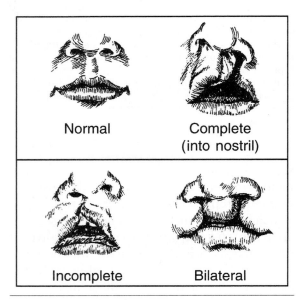

FIGURE 2–3 A normal lip and basic types of cleft lip. On the drawings of clefts, note the short columella and the distortion of the ala. (From *Your Cleft Lip and Palate Child: A Basic Guide for Parents*, by G. Snyder, S. Berkowitz, K. Bzoch, and S. Stool, 1980, Fig. 1. Evansville, IN: Meade Johnson & Co. Copyright Meade Johnson and Co. 1980. Reprinted with permission.)

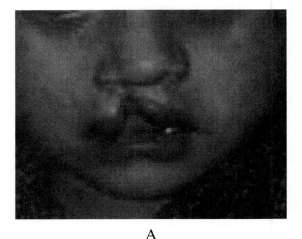

A

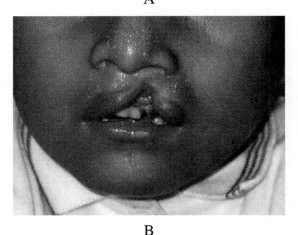

B

FIGURE 2–4 (A and B) Patients with a unilateral incomplete cleft of the primary palate (lip and alveolus).

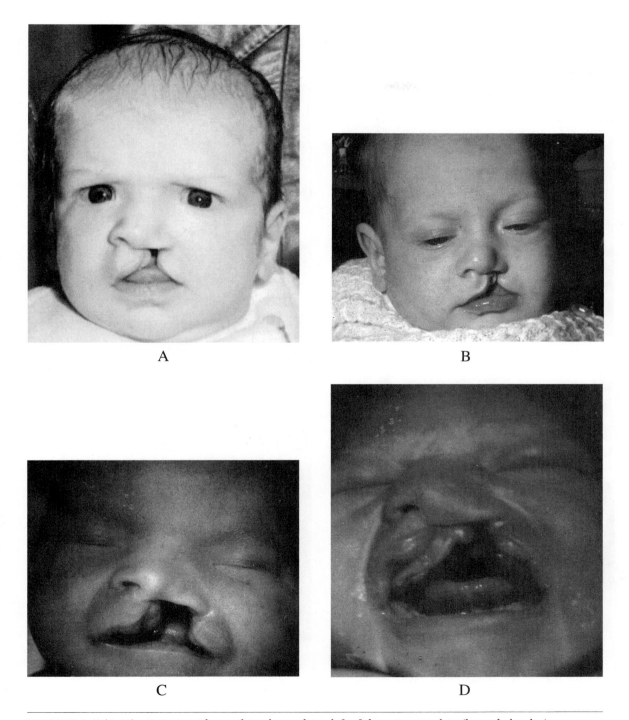

A

B

C

D

FIGURE 2–5 (A–D)   Patients with a unilateral complete cleft of the primary palate (lip and alveolus).

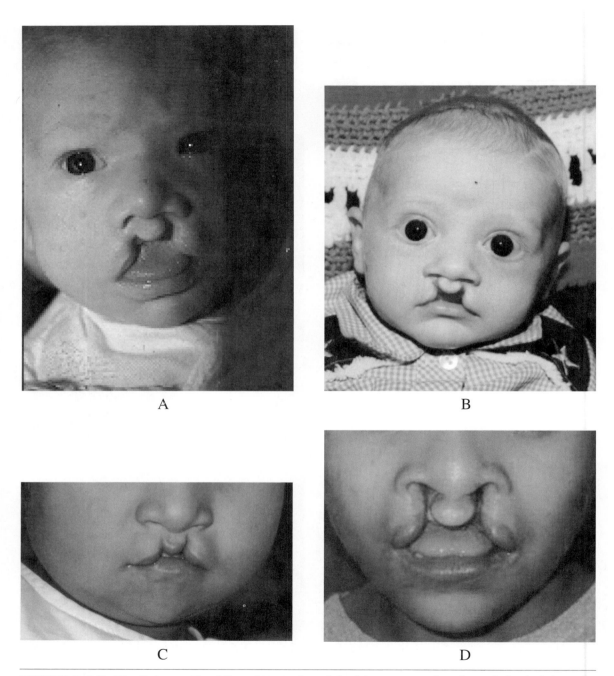

A

B

C

D

FIGURE 2–6 (A–D) Patients with a bilateral incomplete cleft of the primary palate (lip and alveolus). Note the distortion of the nose.

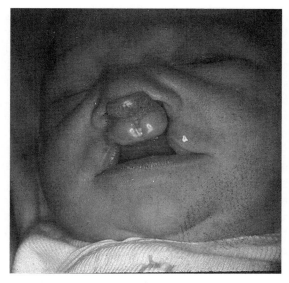

A

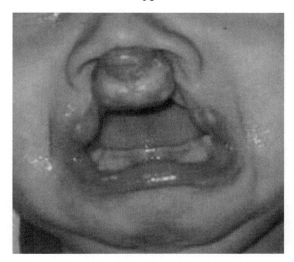

B

FIGURE 2–7 (A and B) Patients with a bilateral complete cleft lip.

segment that is isolated due to the bilateral cleft is called the *prolabium*. When a bilateral cleft courses through the lip and through both incisive suture lines in the alveolus to the incisive foramen, it separates the triangle-shaped premaxilla bone. Therefore, when there is a complete bilateral cleft of the lip and alveolus, both the prolabium and the premaxilla are separated. In many cases, these structures are positioned in an extremely anterior position at birth so that they appear to extend from the tip of the nose. In Figure 2–7 (A and B), the prolabium appears as tissue that is attached to the tip of the nose and the premaxilla is isolated and in an anterior position.

By examining an unrepaired cleft lip closely, one can see that all the structures are present, including the philtral dimple and both of the philtral ridges. The cleft passes just to the lateral side of the philtral ridge. On the cleft side, the lip is short and the Cupid's bow is twisted up into the cleft. Although cleft lip can occur in isolation, it is more often found to be associated with a cleft palate.

In rare cases, a *form fruste* (or *microform cleft*) may occur (Figure 2–8). A form fruste is a partial or arrested form of a cleft lip. In

incomplete cleft of the lip. Finally, Figure 2–7 (A and B) shows infants with bilateral complete cleft of the primary palate.

A bilateral cleft of the lip results in the complete separation of the tissue that would normally form the philtrum. The philtral tissue

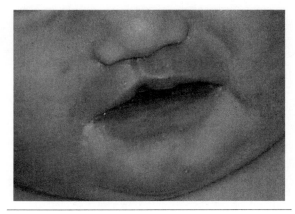

FIGURE 2–8 Patient with a forme fruste (or microform cleft). This is a partially arrested form of cleft lip.

Figure 2–8, the overlying skin is intact but the underlying muscle, nasal cartilage, and oral sphincter function usually are significantly affected. Whether the cleft is complete or incomplete, if it extends through the nostril sil, it will cause distortion of the nose. Another infrequent finding with regard to the cleft lip is a *Simonart's band* (Figure 2–9), which is a strand of soft tissue in the area of the cleft. A Simonart's band is due to partial, yet incomplete embryonic fusion of the upper lip; it has no particular clinical significance and the treatment is the same as in a complete cleft lip.

Effects on Structure and Function

Because a complete cleft of the lip and alveolus courses through the nostril sil, the nose can be adversely affected. The nose may appear to be very wide and flattened due to the separation of the *orbicularis oris muscle*, which is the

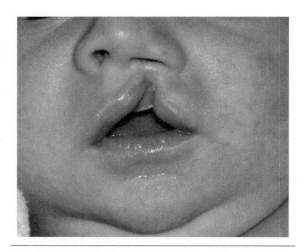

FIGURE 2–9   Patient with a Simonart's band, which is a strand of soft tissue in the area of the cleft due to partial, yet incomplete embryonic fusion of the upper lip.

muscle that encircles the mouth and functions by closing the lips. This muscle is not only divided, but it is misaligned and curves upward along the edges of the vermilion. The wide space within the cleft can further distort the nose by spreading the nasal ala. In fact, the wider the cleft, the more distorted the nasal features will be.

The formation of the columella may also be adversely affected by a cleft lip, causing it to be abnormally short. If the cleft is unilateral, the columella will be shortest on the cleft side and it will be positioned obliquely, with its base deviated toward the noncleft side. When the cleft is bilateral and complete, the columella may be so short that it is virtually nonexistent, giving the appearance that the prolabium and premaxilla are attached to the tip of the nose. In less common cases, as in the case of a forme fruste, the lip is essentially intact but there may be evidence of the nasal deformity and the muscle discontinuity that are typically found with cleft lip.

Clefts of the primary (and secondary) palate often result in nasal cavity deformities that tend to reduce the size of the nasal airway. The airway is smallest in individuals with unilateral cleft lip and palate and is largest in those with bilateral clefts. Although the nose continues to grow with age, it remains about 30% smaller than the noncleft nose (Drake, Davis, & Warren, 1993). The lip repair can also cause nasal obstruction if it results in stenosis of the nasal vestibule. In fact, surgical correction of labial, nasal, palatal, and pharyngeal structures have the potential to compromise breathing further (Hairfield & Warren, 1989). As a result of nasal cavity deformities and surgical correction, upper airway obstruction is noted more frequently in the cleft population than in the noncleft population (Drake, Davis, & Warren, 1993; Hairfield, Warren, & Seaton, 1988;

Liu, Warren, Drake, & Davis, 1992; Warren & Drake, 1993). This obstruction can also cause abnormal resonance.

A complete cleft of the primary palate may result in occlusal abnormalities as the dentition is developed. This can cause specific articulation errors, particularly on anterior speech sounds. The production of anterior sounds is often affected by dental interference of tongue tip movement or crowding in the anterior portion of the oral cavity.

CLEFTS OF THE SECONDARY PALATE (HARD PALATE AND VELUM)

Types and Severity

As with cleft lip, a cleft palate can be either incomplete or complete and can occur with various degrees of severity. This is shown in Figure 2–10. An incomplete cleft palate can be

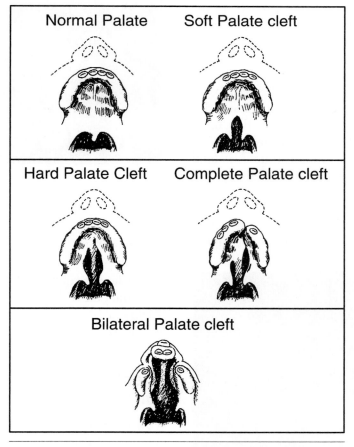

FIGURE 2–10 A normal palate and various types of cleft palate.
(From *Your Cleft Lip and Palate Child: A Basic Guide for Parents*, by G. Snyder, S. Berkowitz, K. Bzoch, and S. Stool, 1980, p. 2. Evansville, IN: Meade Johnson & Co. Copyright Meade Johnson and Co. 1980. Reprinted with permission.)

as slight as a bifid uvula or the cleft can extend farther into the velum. A complete cleft of the secondary palate goes through the uvula and the velum, and then follows the median palatine suture line through the hard palate, all the way to the incisive foramen. The vomer bone, which is the bottom part of the nasal septum, is usually attached to the larger of the two palatal segments in a unilateral cleft, and is not attached to either segment in a bilateral cleft. A cleft palate can occur with or without a cleft lip. Isolated cleft palate (with no involvement of the lip) is more frequently associated with a syndrome, and thus with other anomalies. Figure 2–11 shows an unrepaired complete cleft of the palate with no involvement of the primary palate. Figure 2–12(A and B) shows examples of infants with a bilateral complete cleft lip and palate. The prolabium and premaxilla are isolated and in an anterior position. The vomer portion of the nasal septum can be viewed through the palate.

Some patients will demonstrate a *palatal fistula* or hole in the palate after the palate is repaired. Although this may look like a partial cleft, it is actually due to a partial dehiscence (or breakdown) of the cleft repair. The fistula can be located anywhere in the

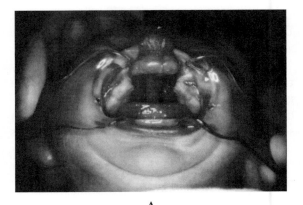

A

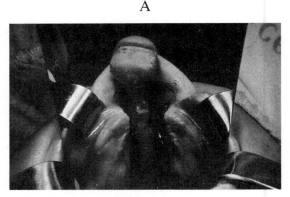

B

FIGURE 2–12 (A and B)   Patients with a bilateral complete cleft of the lip and palate (primary and secondary palate). Note the prolabium, premaxilla, and the nasal septum.

hard palate or velum, but will always be located along the embryological or surgical suture lines (Figure 2–13). For more information on palatal fistulas, see Chapters 7 and 8.

Effects on Structure and Function

With cleft palate there are additional abnormalities of the anatomy other than the obvious. If the cleft goes entirely through the velum, the velar aponeurosis is conspicuously absent (Dickson, 1972; Koch, Grzonka, & Koch,

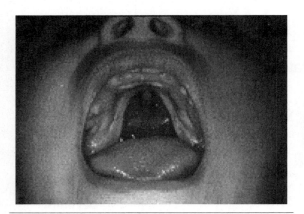

FIGURE 2–11   Wide unrepaired complete cleft of the secondary palate (hard palate and velum).

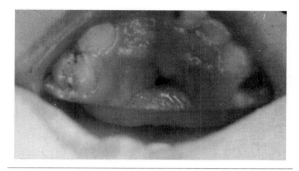

FIGURE 2–13 Palatal fistula. A palatal fistula is a hole in the palate that occurs due to a partial dehiscence (or breakdown) of the cleft repair. The fistula can be located anywhere in the hard palate or velum, but will always be located along the embryological or surgical suture lines.

1998) and the orientation of the muscles is necessarily altered. Although the muscle origins are normal, the muscle insertions are abnormal due to the open cleft. Because of the cleft, the levator veli palatini muscle cannot interdigitate (interlock like fingers) in the midline. Instead, this paired muscle and the palatopharyngeus muscles are inserted onto the posterior border of the cleft hard palate, rendering them essentially nonfunctional (Dickson, 1972; Dickson, Grant, Sicher, Dubrul, & Paltan, 1974, 1975; Kriens, 1975; Maue-Dickson, 1979; Maue-Dickson & Dickson, 1980). As a result, rather than being amuscular, the anterior one-third of the velum contains the muscle fibers of both the levator veli palatini and the palatopharyngeus muscles (Dickson, 1972). This configuration of muscles has been referred to as the *cleft muscle of Veau*. Figure 2–14A shows the orientation of the velar muscles in a normal palate and velum. Figure 2–14B shows the abnormal orientation of the muscles when there is a cleft.

One goal of cleft palate surgery is to correct the orientation of the muscles in order to achieve normal function. Despite surgical attempts to normalize the muscle orientation, individuals with a repaired cleft of the velum have great variability in the insertion point of the muscles and in the muscle mass (Moon & Kuehn, 1997). Therefore, the function of the muscles following surgery can be difficult to predict. In addition, the velum may be abnormally short due to the absent aponeurosis and hypoplasia of the levator veli palatini muscles (Dickson, 1972). It has been estimated that about 20% to 30% of individuals with a history of cleft palate are likely to have velopharyngeal dysfunction (Bardach, 1995) due to either poor velar movement or a short velum. Velopharyngeal dysfunction causes defective speech and resonance and can also cause nasal regurgitation of liquids in some cases.

Individuals with a history of cleft palate are also at high risk for otitis media and associated conductive hearing loss. This is due to malfunction of the *eustachian tube* (Bluestone, Beery, Cantekin, & Paradise, 1975; Doyle, Cantekin, & Bluestone, 1980; Paradise, Bluestone, & Felder, 1969), which connects the middle ear to the posterior pharynx. The eustachian tube is normally closed in its resting position. In response to changes in external air pressure, the individual usually swallows (or yawns) to relieve the pressure in the ears. The act of swallowing or yawning causes the tensor veli palatini muscle to contract to open the pharyngeal end of the tube. As the eustachian tube opens, it allows fluids to drain from the middle ear into the pharynx. It also results in the equalization of air pressure between the middle ear and the environment. If the tensor veli palatini muscle does not function normally, as is common when there is a history of cleft palate, this results in poor ventilation of the middle ear. This can lead to bacterial infection, inflammation, and the accumulation of fluids. The build-up of fluids impairs the conduction

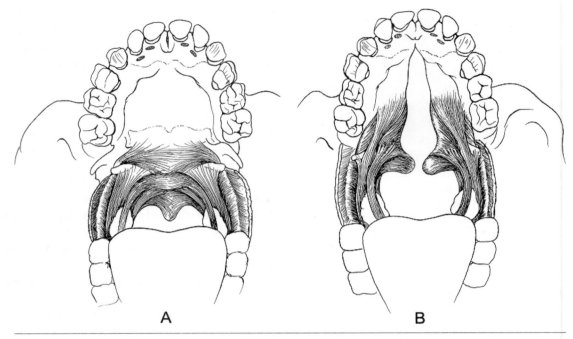

FIGURE 2–14 (A and B) A. Illustration of normal velar musculature. Note the orientation of the muscles in midline. B. Abnormal muscle orientation due to a cleft palate. As a result of the cleft, the anterior one-third of the velum contains the muscle fibers of the levator veli palatini and the palatopharyngeus muscles. Instead of inserting into the midline of the velum, these muscles are inserted into the posterior border of the hard palate. This abnormal orientation is called the *cleft muscle of Veau.*

of sound through the ossicles, resulting in a conductive hearing loss. If this fluid build-up and inflammation become chronic, permanent damage to the middle ear, to the surrounding structures, and to hearing can result.

As noted previously, the nasal cavity space can be compromised by developmental defects secondary to cleft lip and palate. Cleft palate alone can include abnormalities of both the cartilaginous and bony septum, causing a nasal septal deviation that can alter nasal cavity size (Wetmore, 1992). The nasopharyngeal anatomy also appears to be altered in individuals with a history of cleft palate. Smahel and colleagues (Smahel, Kasalova, & Skvarilova, 1991; Smahel & Mullerova, 1992) conducted a morphometric assessment of the pharynx of individuals with repaired cleft lip and/or palate using X-ray films. Their findings revealed significant nasopharyngeal differences in individuals with a history of cleft palate. These differences included a reduction of the nasopharyngeal airway due to a decrease in depth of the nasopharyngeal bony framework and the posterior displacement of the maxilla. The findings of reduced nasal cavity size and reduced nasopharyngeal depth can explain the high incidence of both upper airway obstruction and mouth breathing in the cleft palate population (Rose, Thissen, Otten, & Jonas, 2003; Warren, Hairfield, & Dalston, 1990, 1991).

SUBMUCOUS CLEFT PALATE

A *submucous cleft palate* is a congenital defect that affects the underlying structure of the palate, while the oral surface mucosa is intact. This defect often involves the muscles and nasal surface of the velum. Depending on the extent of the defect, it can also involve the bony structure of the hard palate. Therefore, a submucous cleft can range in severity from a bifid uvula to a complete cleft under the oral mucosa that extends to the area of the incisive foramen.

Like an overt cleft palate, a submucous cleft often occurs as part of a generalized syndrome of multiple malformations (Lewin, Croft, & Shprintzen, 1980). Although a submucous cleft represents partial fusion of the structures, the exact pathogenesis is not clearly understood.

Types and Severity

Overt Submucous Cleft

An *overt submucous cleft palate* is one that can be identified through an intraoral examination. The diagnosis is made by observation of one or more of the classic stigmata, which include bifid uvula, zona pellucida, and a notch in the posterior border of the hard palate. A bifid uvula may have two distinct pendulous structures (Figure 2–15A) instead of a single pedicle, or it may appear as one structure with a line down the middle (Figure 2–15B). In other cases, the uvula may merely have an indentation in the inferior border. At times, a bifurcation is not easily appreciated, but the uvula will appear to be hypoplastic (small and underdeveloped) (Figure 2–15C).

A bifid uvula can be an isolated anomaly with no submucous cleft of the velum and normal speech. This makes sense when one remembers that embryological development of the palate starts at the incisive foramen and finishes with the uvula. However, the observation of a bifid or hypoplastic uvula suggests that embryological development was disrupted at some point. Therefore, bifid uvula is frequently associated with a submucous cleft that extends into the velum (and even into the hard palate) and can result in velopharyngeal insufficiency with hypernasal speech (Shprintzen et al., 1985).

In addition to a bifid uvula, an inspection of the velum may reveal a *zona pellucida* (see Figure 2–15, A and B). This is a bluish area in the middle of the velum and is the result of thin mucosa with a lack of the normal underlying muscle mass. The velum may also appear to be in the shape of an inverted "V" at rest, but especially with phonation (see Figure 2–15D). This shape is due to the *diastasis* (separation) of the paired levator veli palatini muscle with abnormal insertion of these muscles into the posterior border of the hard palate, rather than into the midline of the velum. With phonation, this abnormal muscle insertion makes the velum appear to "tent up" toward the hard palate. The submucous cleft can extend into the hard palate, all the way to the incisive foramen. When this is the case, the "V" shaped abnormality can be viewed underneath the surface of the mucoperiosteum. Sometimes, the defect is not as obvious and may just look like a minor defect in the velum (Figure 2–15E).

At times, it is difficult to see evidence of a submucous cleft on the oral surface of the velum. In fact, a submucous cleft palate may be present, even when an intraoral examination shows an intact uvula and velum (Shprintzen et al., 1985). Palpation of the palate may reveal an abnormality that cannot be appreciated though visual inspection alone. (For information on palpation of the palate, see Chapter 13, "Orofacial Examination.") Figure 2–16 shows various degrees of severity

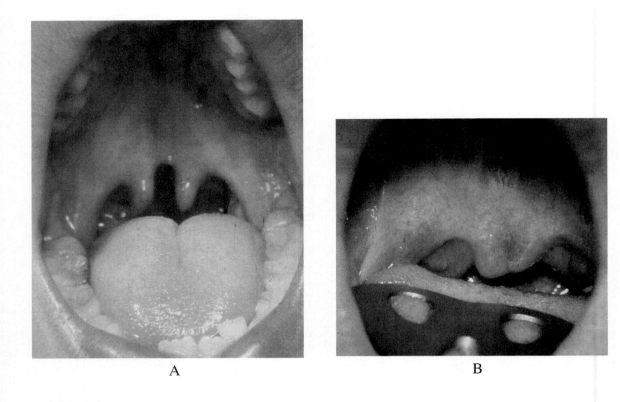

A

B

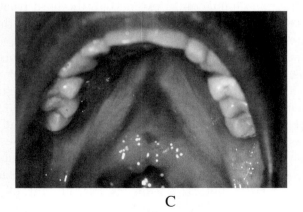

C

FIGURE 2–15 (A–E) A. Submucous cleft palate with bifid uvula and zona pellucida. B. Submucous cleft that is more subtle, but still very noticeable. Note the hypoplastic uvula with a faint line in the middle, and the zona pellucida. C. Submucous cleft with obvious diastasis of the velar musculature. Note how the muscles insert into the hard palate, resulting in an inverted "V" shape. (*continues*)

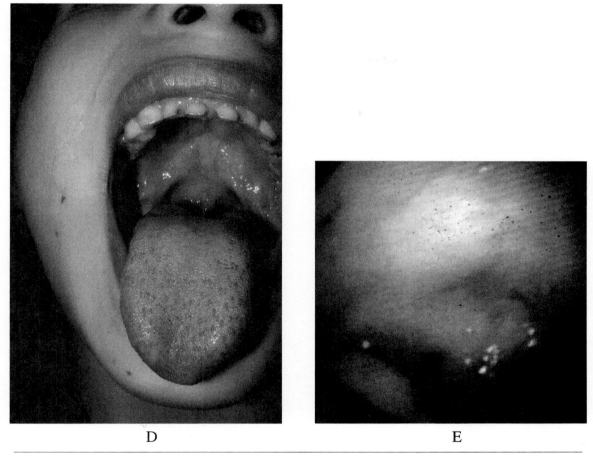

D   E

FIGURE 2–15 (A–E) (*continued*) D. Submucous cleft that is noted only during phonation. Note the subtle inverted "V" during velar elevation, indicating an abnormality in the insertion of the levator veli palatine muscle. E. Submucous cleft that is characterized by a hypoplastic uvula with a thin line in the middle.

of a submucous cleft and the effect of the defect on the musculature. Some individuals demonstrate a combination of an overt cleft and a submucous cleft. This may appear as a bifid uvula with an overt cleft that extends into the velum, and then as a submucous cleft that extends farther forward.

Occult Submucous Cleft

An *occult submucous cleft* is a defect in the velum that is not apparent on the oral surface (Kaplan, 1975; Minami et al., 1975). In fact, it can only be appreciated by viewing the nasal surface of the velum through nasopharyngoscopy. Because the word "occult" means "hidden" or "not revealed," this malformation is aptly named. The occult submucous cleft is not embryologically or genetically different from other variations of the submucous cleft. Instead, the occult submucous cleft represents a point on the continuum of submucous cleft defects and cleft palate.

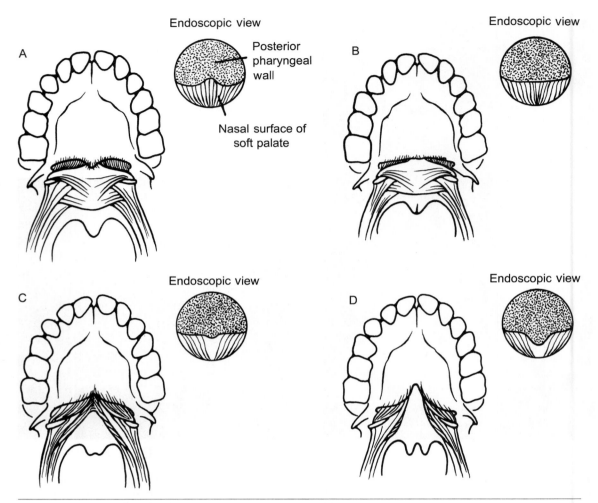

FIGURE 2–16 (A–D) Degrees of severity of a submucous cleft palate and the effect on the uvula and velar musculature. The endoscopic view of the nasal surface of the velum can be seen in the circles. A. A normal velum and uvula with normal velar musculature. B. A bifid uvula but normal velum with no involvement of the velar musculature. This type of submucous cleft is unlikely to affect velopharyngeal function. C. A bifid uvula and submucous cleft that extends through the velum to the hard palate. This type of submucous cleft affects the muscle orientation of the velum and could affect velopharyngeal function and thus speech. D. A bifid uvula and submucous cleft that extends through the velum and partially through the hard palate. This type of submucous cleft affects the velar musculature and has the potential to affect speech.

The diagnosis of occult submucous cleft is only pursued if the patient has velopharyngeal insufficiency of unknown etiology, as there is no obvious physical abnormality of the velum. McWilliams et al. (1990) used the term *congenital palatal insufficiency* (CPI) to describe characteristics of velopharyngeal insufficiency with no history of cleft palate, no apparent evidence of submucous cleft, or other known etiology. It is possible that individuals previously identified with CPI actually have an occult submucous cleft. With the help of

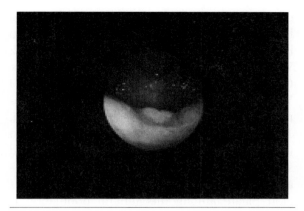

FIGURE 2–17 An endoscopic view of the velum showing the nasal surface. It can be seen that the edge of the velum has a depression rather than a rounded bulky muscle mass, thus indicating an occult submucous cleft.

nasopharyngoscopy, which is an endoscopic procedure, it is now possible to identify the velar abnormalities that commonly occur on the nasal surface only and could not be viewed through videofluoroscopy.

Figure 2–17 is an endoscopic view of the velum showing the nasal surface. It can be seen that on the posterior edge of the velum, there is a small indentation, and on the nasal surface, there is a depression rather than a rounded bulky mass of the musculus uvulae muscle. These characteristics, and the absence of an abnormality on the oral surface, are typical of an occult submucous cleft. Previously unidentified abnormalities on the nasal surface of the velum are frequently found by surgeons as the velum is dissected for a pharyngeal flap. In a study of 52 patients without overt cleft palate who were undergoing pharyngeal flap surgery, Trier (1983) found that 48 patients (92%) demonstrated abnormal anatomy of the velum, which explained the velopharyngeal incompetence.

Most individuals with an occult submucous cleft have the same abnormalities as those with an overt submucous cleft. The musculus uvulae muscles are either absent or deficient (Croft, Shprintzen, Daniller, & Lewin, 1978) and there is abnormal insertion of the muscles into the hard palate. This can often be seen through nasopharyngoscopy as a V-shaped midline defect, with a flattening or depression in the area of the velar eminence.

Effects on Structure and Function

The effect of a submucous cleft on structure and function is similar to that of an overt cleft. It also depends greatly on the type and extent of the defect. Abnormalities in the morphology of the velum can particularly affect velopharyngeal function and, therefore, speech. These abnormalities can also cause nasal regurgitation with swallowing, especially during the first year of life. With submucous cleft palate, there is an increased risk for middle ear disease with conductive hearing loss due to abnormalities of the tensor veli palatini muscle, which can cause eustachian tube malfunction (Garcia Velasco, Ysunza, Hernandez, & Marquez, 1988; Saad, 1980; Schwartz, Hayden, Rodriquez, Shprintzen, & Cassidy, 1985; Sheahan, Miller, Earley, Sheahan, & Blayney, 2004).

Although individuals with a submucous cleft are at risk for dysfunction of the velopharyngeal valve, many people with this abnormality have normal speech, normal middle ear function, and no history of nasal regurgitation with swallowing. McWilliams (1991) studied a group of 130 patients with submucous cleft, and found that 44% remained asymptomatic into adulthood. Therefore, the mere presence of a submucous cleft should not be a concern if there is normal speech. It is important, however, that the individual and the family be counseled regarding this abnormality for several reasons. The family should be informed that a full adenoidectomy with a submucous cleft is usually contraindicated due to the risk that this will cause velopharyngeal insufficiency (Shprintzen et al., 1985). In addition, the family should be counseled regarding the genetic risk for additional offspring with cleft palate or associated syndromes.

Prevalence of Submucous Cleft

Gorlin, Cervenka, and Pruzansky (1971) reported that 1 in 80 Caucasians, or about 1.2%, have a bifid uvula. Wharton and Mowrer (1992) evaluated 709 children and found some form of uvular cleft in 2.26% of the children, while a complete bifid uvula was found in only 0.3% of the children. Bagatin (1985) found the prevalence of bifid uvula to be 0.2% in Yugoslavian children. Saad (1980) found bifid uvula in 1% of a population of 1500 children. Meskin, Gorlin, and Isaacson (1964) reported bifid uvula in about 1 of 76 people in the general population, or 1.3%. Shapiro, Meskin, Cervenka, and Pruzansky (1971) compared the occurrence of bifid uvula in four races. They reported bifid uvula to be prevalent in 10.25% (sample size of 605) of Native American Chippewa; 9.96% (sample size of 4726) of Japanese; 1.44% (sample size of 9701) of whites; and 0.27% (sample size of 2968) of blacks. It is interesting that this relative frequency by race is similar to the relative frequency of cleft lip and palate. Although these studies reported the prevalence of bifid uvula, it is important to note that children with bifid uvula often have the additional characteristics of submucous cleft palate, including velopharyngeal insufficiency and hypernasal speech (Shprintzen et al., 1985).

Several studies have attempted to determine the prevalence of submucous cleft in the general population. In a large sample of over 10,000 Denver schoolchildren, the prevalence of a complete submucous cleft (including a bony defect of the hard palate) was found to be 0.08% (Stewart, Otet, & Lagace, 1972; Weatherly-White, Sakura, Brenner, Stewart, & Ott, 1972). In a study of almost 10,000 Yugoslavian children, the prevalence of submucous cleft was found to be 0.05% (Bagatin, 1985). Gosain, Conley, Marks, and Larson (1996) summarized the results of several surveys in the literature and stated that prevalence of the classic stigmata of submucous cleft palate among the general population is between 0.02% and 0.08%.

Although a submucous cleft may be noticed at birth or soon after, especially if there are early feeding problems, an occult submucous cleft is usually not discovered until the child begins to speak and has evidence of hypernasality. In some cases, the defect is not noted for years or is never discovered, especially if it is asymptomatic and not causing any problems with speech. Therefore, the prevalence of occult submucous cleft is not known.

The prevalence of submucous cleft palate in individuals with clefts of the primary palate has been found to be significantly greater than the prevalence of submucous cleft palate found in the general population (Gosain, Conley, Santoro, & Denny, 1999; Kono, Young, and Holtmann, 1981). Because of this increased risk, it is important for individuals with cleft lip to be thoroughly examined for submucous cleft. Early detection of submucous cleft associated with cleft lip is important for the prevention of middle ear problems and for the proper management of velopharyngeal insufficiency, if it occurs.

Individuals with submucous cleft palate are at high risk for velopharyngeal dysfunction resulting in hypernasality. The occurrence of velopharyngeal dysfunction in individuals with submucous cleft has been studied with various results. Garcia Velasco and associates (1988) reported a 53% occurrence; Stewart et al. (1972) reported a 28% occurrence; Kono and colleagues (1981) reported a 44% occurrence: and Bagatin (1985) found a 25% occurrence. Overall, it is safe to say that one-fourth to one-half of individuals with submucous cleft will have associated velopharyngeal dysfunction. On the other hand, it is important to recognize that most individuals with a submucous cleft will have normal speech (Shprintzen et al., 1985; Stewart et al., 1972).

Treatment of Submucous Cleft

The literature and most professionals do not support the prophylactic surgical correction of the physical stigmata of submucous cleft palate, because many individuals with a submucous cleft have normal speech, swallowing, and middle ear function. Instead, surgical correction is indicated only if there is evidence of velopharyngeal dysfunction that is affecting speech (Chen, Wu, & Noordhoff, 1994; Garcia Velasco et al., 1988; Gosain et al., 1996). It is therefore important to wait until speech has fully developed before considering surgical correction so that speech and velopharyngeal function can be adequately evaluated. For optimal speech results, however, it is best to surgically correct the defect as soon as a velopharyngeal dysfunction has been diagnosed (Abyholm, 1976).

When surgical correction is necessary and the child is still very young, a palatoplasty is often done to improve the orientation of the muscles for better function. If this is not effective, if the individual is older, or if there is significant velopharyngeal dysfunction, a common procedure for correction is the pharyngeal flap, either alone or in combination with a palatoplasty, for the best speech results (Porterfield, Mohler, & Sandel, 1976).

FACIAL CLEFTS

Most clefts follow the embryological suture lines of the lip and palate. However, other types of clefts can occur due to failure of neural crest cell migration, which results in the lack of fusion of the facial processes, including the branchial arches. In addition, *amniotic bands* (loose strands of tissue that have ruptured from the amnion) are thought to be responsible for certain types of facial clefts (Hukki et al., 2004; Rintala, Leisti, Liesmaa, & Ranta, 1980). Facial clefts are usually very severe and are accompanied by many other anomalies. The exact incidence of facial clefts is unknown, and estimates vary greatly because of the rarity of their occurrence and the lack of standard methods of data collection (Darzi & Chowdri, 1993).

Types and Severity

One type of facial cleft is the oblique cleft, which can be mostly unilateral (Figure 2–18A) or bilateral (Figure 2–18, B through D). This is an extremely disfiguring congenital anomaly of the face that affects the skeletal and soft tissue structures (Darzi & Chowdri, 1993). An oblique cleft begins at the mouth and then courses laterally, horizontally, and upward so that it may affect the facial bones, nasal structures, orbits, and even the ears.

Another type of facial cleft is the midline (median) cleft (Figure 2–19, A through E). This type of cleft can be very mild, so that there is only a notch in the midline of the vermillion or a slight cleft of the upper lip (Figure 2–19A). However, midline clefts are often associated with a spectrum of other midline anomalies, such as bifid nose (Miller, Grinberg, & Wang, 1999), frontonasal *dysplasia* (abnormal tissue development) (Hodgkins et al., 1998), and *hypertelorism*, which is wide

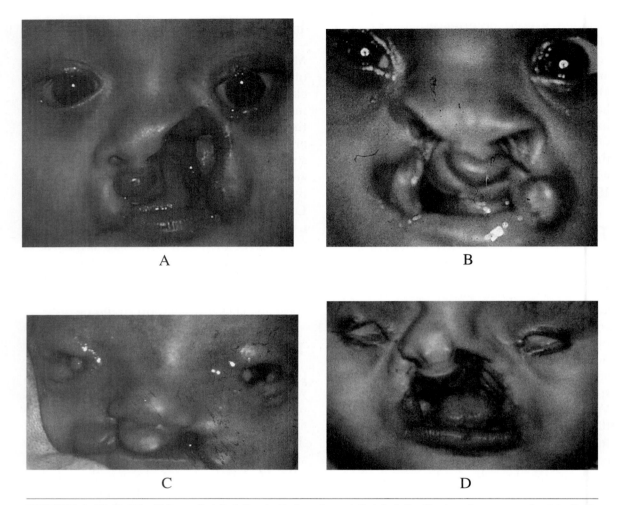

FIGURE 2–18 (A–D) Oblique facial clefts. A. Left unilateral facial cleft affecting the nose and orbit. B–D. Bilateral facial clefts. Note the wide nasal bridge and the effect on the eyes.

spacing between the eyes (Figure 2–19, B through E). Midline clefts can also affect brain development, causing cranial base anomalies, an *encephalocele* (which is a congenital gap in the skull with herniation of brain tissue into the nose or palate), or an absent *corpus callosum* (nerve fibers that allow communication between the cerebral hemispheres). In severe cases, a midline cleft may be associated with *holoprosencephaly*, which is failure of the forebrain to divide into two hemispheres (Figure 2–19F).

Facial clefts are often severe and may be accompanied by other significant craniofacial anomalies or other medical conditions. In addition to affecting the aesthetics, facial clefts can cause many functional problems. Fortunately, these types of clefts are very rare.

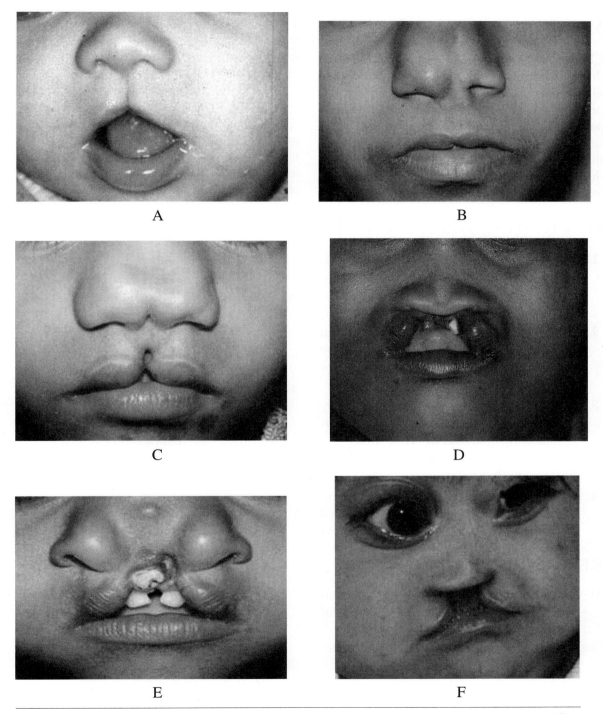

FIGURE 2–19 (A–F) Midline facial clefts of varying severity. A. Mild midline cleft of the lip only. B–E. Midline facial clefts that affect the nose. F. Midline facial cleft with holoprosencephaly, a condition in which there is failure of the forebrain to divide into the two hemispheres.

SUMMARY

Cleft lip and palate is a common birth defect that presents in a variety of ways. There are different types of clefts, such as clefts of the primary palate and clefts of the secondary palate. There are also different degrees of severity. A submucous cleft is a type of cleft that is not readily apparent because it affects the underlying structures of the velum while leaving the oral surface intact. When a cleft occurs, it is the result of a disruption in embryological development. Many craniofacial syndromes include cleft palate as part of the phenotype.

As will be noted in subsequent chapters, cleft lip and cleft palate can affect the development of communication skills in a variety of ways. Therefore, health care providers, particularly members of a cleft palate or craniofacial team, need to be aware of this so that appropriate intervention can be initiated.

FOR REVIEW, DISCUSSION, AND CRITICAL THINKING

1. Beginning with the incisive foramen, describe the process and direction of embryological development of the lip and palate.

2. What are possible causes of clefts? Given these causes, what do you think could be done to reduce the risk of clefting in a population?

3. What is meant by the terms "primary palate" and "secondary palate"? What structures are included? How does this classification system relate to embryological development?

4. List different types of clefts of the primary palate. What are the potential functional problems with regard to these clefts? What professional disciplines may be involved in treatment?

5. List different types of clefts of the secondary palate. What are the potential functional problems with regard to these clefts? What professional disciplines may be involved in treatment?

6. Describe the possible characteristics of a submucous cleft palate. Why is this type of cleft often undetected at birth? Discuss the occurrence of submucous cleft as it relates to embryological development.

7. What structures may be involved in a facial cleft? In addition to the obvious aesthetic concerns, what are some reasons that these types of clefts are of particular concern?

REFERENCES

Abyholm, F. E. (1976). Submucous cleft palate. *Scandinavian Journal of Plastic and Reconstructive Surgery, 10*(3), 209–212.

Bagatin, M. (1985). Submucous cleft palate. *Journal of Maxillofacial Surgery, 13*(1), 37–38.

Bardach, J. (1995). Secondary surgery for velopharyngeal insufficiency. In R. J. Shprintzen & J. Bardach (Eds.), *Cleft palate speech management: A multidisciplinary approach* (pp. 277–294). St. Louis, MO: Mosby.

Bille, C., Knudsen, L. B., & Christensen, K. (2005). Changing lifestyles and oral clefts occurrence in Denmark. *Cleft Palate-Craniofacial Journal, 42*(3), 255–259.

Bille, C., Skytthe, A., Vach, W., Knudsen, L. B., Andersen, A. M., Murray, J. C., et al. (2005). Parent's age and the risk of oral clefts. *Epidemiology, 16*(3), 311–316.

Bluestone, C. D., Beery, Q. C., Cantekin, E. I., & Paradise, J. L. (1975). Eustachian tube ventilatory function in relation to cleft palate. *Annals of Otolology, Rhinology, and Laryngology, 84*(3, Pt. 1), 333–338.

Burdi, A. R., & Silvey, R. G. (1969). Sexual differences in closure of the human palatal shelves. *Cleft Palate Journal, 6,* 1.

Castilla, E. E., Orioli, I. M., Lopez-Camelo, J. S., Dutra Mda, G., & Nazer-Herrera, J. (2003). Preliminary data on changes in neural tube defect prevalence rates after folic acid fortification in South America. *American Journal of Medical Genetics Part A. 123*(2), 123–128.

Chen, K. T., Wu, J., & Noordhoff, S. M. (1994). Submucous cleft palate. *Chang Keng I Hsueh: Chang Gung Medical Journal, 17*(2), 131–137.

Cleft Palate Foundation. (1999). Available on Web site: http://www.cleft.com.

Croft, C. B., Shprintzen, R. J., Daniller, A. I., & Lewin, M. L. (1978). The occult submucous cleft palate and the musculus uvulae. *Cleft Palate Journal, 15,* 150–154.

Darzi, M. A., & Chowdri, N. A. (1993). Oblique facial clefts: A report of Tessier numbers 3, 4, 5, and 9 clefts. *Cleft Palate-Craniofacial Journal, 30*(4), 414–415.

Dickson, D. R. (1972). Normal and cleft palate anatomy. *Cleft Palate Journal, 9,* 280–293.

Dickson, D. R., Grant, J. C., Sicher, H., Dubrul, E. L., & Paltan, J. (1974). Status of research in cleft palate anatomy and physiology, Part 1. *Cleft Palate Journal, 11,* 471–492.

Dickson, D. R., Grant, J. C., Sicher, H., Dubrul, E. L., & Paltan, J. (1975). Status of research in cleft lip and palate: Anatomy and physiology, Part 2. *Cleft Palate Journal, 12,* 131–156.

Doyle, W. J., Cantekin, E. I., & Bluestone, C. D. (1980). Eustachian tube function in cleft palate children. *Annals of Otology, Rhinology, and Laryngology Supplement, 89*(3, Pt. 2), 34–40.

Drake, A. F., Davis, J. U., & Warren, D. W. (1993). Nasal airway size in cleft and noncleft children. *Laryngoscope, 103*(8), 915–917.

Edwards, M. J., Agho, K., Attia, J., Diaz, P., Hayes, T., Illingworth, A., et al. (2003). Case-control study of cleft lip or palate after maternal use of topical corticosteroids during pregnancy. *American Journal of Medical Genetics Part A. 120*(4), 459–463.

Garcia Velasco, M., Ysunza, A., Hernandez, X., & Marquez, C. (1988). Diagnosis and treatment of submucous cleft palate: A review of 108 cases. *Cleft Palate Journal, 25*(2), 171–173.

Gorlin, R. J., Cervenka, J., & Pruzansky, S. (1971). Facial clefting and its syndromes. *Birth Defects Original Article Series, 7*(7), 3–49.

Gosain, A. K., Conley, S. F., Marks, S., & Larson, D. L. (1996). Submucous cleft palate: Diagnostic methods and outcomes of surgical treatment. *Plastic & Reconstructive Surgery, 97*(7), 1497–1509.

Gosain, A. K., Conley, S. F., Santoro, T. D., & Denny, A. D. (1999). A prospective evaluation of the prevalence of submucous cleft palate in patients with isolated cleft lip versus controls. *Plastic & Reconstructive Surgery, 103*(7), 1857–1863.

Hairfield, W. M., & Warren, D. W. (1989). Dimensions of the cleft nasal airway in adults: A comparison with subjects without cleft. *Cleft Palate Journal, 26*(1), 9–13.

Hairfield, W. M., Warren, D. W., & Seaton, D. L. (1988). Prevalence of mouthbreathing in cleft lip and palate. *Cleft Palate Journal, 25*(2), 135–138.

Hashmi, S. S., Waller, D. K., Langlois, P., Canfield, M., & Hecht, J. T. (2005). Prevalence of nonsyndromic oral clefts in Texas: 1995–1999. *American Journal of Medical Genetics* Part A. *134*(4), 368–372.

Hodgkins, P., Lees, M., Lawson, J., Reardon, W., Leitch, J., Thorogood, P., et al. (1998). Optic disc anomalies and frontonasal dysplasia. *British Journal of Ophthalmology, 82*(3), 290–293.

Honein, M. A., Paulozzi, L. J., & Watkins, M. L. (2001). Maternal smoking and birth defects: Validity of birth certificate data for effect estimation. *Public Health Reports, 116*(4), 327–335.

Hukki, J., Balan, P., Ceponiene, R., Kantola-Sorsa, E., Saarinen, P., & Wikstrom, H. (2004). A case study of amnion rupture sequence with acalvaria, blindness, and clefting: Clinical and psychological profiles. *Journal of Craniofacial Surgery, 15*(2), 185–191.

Jensen, B. L., Kreiborg, S., Dahl, E., & Fogh-Andersen, P. (1988). Cleft lip and palate in Denmark, 1976–1981: Epidemiology, variability, and early somatic development. *Cleft Palate Journal, 25*(3), 258–269.

Jones, M. C. (1988). Etiology of facial clefts: Prospective evaluation of 428 patients. *Cleft Palate Journal, 25*(1), 16–20.

Kaplan, E. N. (1975). The occult submucous cleft palate. *Cleft Palate Journal, 12*, 356–368.

Kernahan, D. A. (1971). The striped Y–A symbolic classification for cleft lip and palate. *Plastic & Reconstructive Surgery, 47*(5), 469–470.

Kernahan, D. A., & Stark, R. B. (1958). A new classification for cleft lip and cleft palate. *Plastic & Reconstructive Surgery, 22*, 435.

Koch, K. H., Grzonka, M. A., & Koch, J. (1998). Pathology of the palatal aponeurosis in cleft palate. *Cleft Palate-Craniofacial Journal, 35*(6), 530–534.

Kono, D., Young, L., & Holtmann, B. (1981). The association of submucous cleft palate and clefting of the primary palate. *Cleft Palate Journal, 18*(3), 207–209.

Kriens, O. (1975). Anatomy of the velopharyngeal area in cleft palate. *Clinical Plastic Surgery, 2*(2), 261–288.

Lewin, M. L., Croft, C. B., & Shprintzen, R. J. (1980). Velopharyngeal insufficiency due to hypoplasia of the musculus uvulae and occult submucous cleft palate. *Plastic & Reconstructive Surgery, 65*(5), 585–591.

Liu, H., Warren, D. W., Drake, A. F., & Davis, J. U. (1992). Is nasal airway size a marker for susceptibility toward clefting? *Cleft Palate-Craniofacial Journal, 29*(4), 336–339.

Maue-Dickson, W. (1979). The craniofacial complex in cleft lip and palate: An update review of anatomy and function. *Cleft Palate Journal, 16*(3), 291–317.

Maue-Dickson, W., & Dickson, D. R. (1980). Anatomy and physiology related to cleft palate: Current research and clinical implications. *Plastic & Reconstructive Surgery, 65*(1), 83–90.

McWilliams, B. J. (1991). Submucous clefts of the palate: How likely are they to be symptomatic? *Cleft Palate-Craniofacial Journal, 28*(3), 247–249; Discussion 250–251.

McWilliams, B. J., Morris, H. L., & Shelton, R. L. (1990). *Cleft palate speech*. Philadelphia: B. C. Decker.

Meskin, L., Gorlin, R., & Isaacson, R. (1964). Abnormal morphology of the soft palate: The prevalence of a cleft uvula. *Cleft Palate Journal, 3*, 342–346.

Metneki, J., Puho, E., & Czeizel, A. E. (2005). Maternal diseases and isolated orofacial clefts in Hungary. *Birth Defects Research*, *73*(9), 617–623.

Miller, P. J., Grinberg, D., & Wang, T. D. (1999). Midline cleft. Treatment of the bifid nose. *Archives of Facial Plastic Surgery*, *1*(3), 200–203.

Minami, T., Kaplan, E. N., Wu, G., & Jobe, R. P. (1975). Velopharyngeal incompetence without overt cleft palate. A collective review and experience with 98 patients. *Plastic & Reconstructive Surgery*, *55*(5), 573–587.

Moon, J. B., & Kuehn, D. P. (1997). Anatomy and physiology of normal and disordered velopharyngeal function for speech. In K. R. Bzoch (Ed.), *Communicative disorders related to cleft lip and palate.* Austin, TX: Pro-Ed.

Moore, L. L., Singer, M. R., Bradlee, M. L., Rothman, K. J., & Milunsky, A. (2000). A prospective study of the risk of congenital defects associated with maternal obesity and diabetes mellitus. *Epidemiology*, *11*(6), 689–694.

Munger, R. G., Sauberlich, H. E., Corcoran, C., Nepomuceno, B., Daack-Hirsch, S., & Solon, F. S. (2004). Maternal vitamin B-6 and folate status and risk of oral cleft birth defects in the Philippines. *Birth Defects Research*, *70*(7), 464–471.

Oka, S. W. (1979). Epidemiology and genetics of clefting: With implications for etiology. In H. K. Cooper, R. L. Harding, W. M. Krogman, M. Mazaheri, & Millard, R. T. (Eds.), *Cleft palate and cleft lip: A team approach to clinical management and rehabilitation of the patient.* Philadelphia: W. B. Saunders.

Paradise, J. L., Bluestone, C. D., & Felder, H. (1969). The universality of otitis media in 50 infants with cleft palate. *Pediatrics*, *44*(1), 35–42.

Porterfield, H. W., Mohler, L. R., & Sandel, A. (1976). Submucous cleft palate. *Plastic & Reconstructive Surgery*, *58*(1), 60–65.

Ray, J. G., Meier, C., Vermeulen, M. J., Wyatt, P. R., & Cole, D. E. (2003). Association between folic acid food fortification and congenital orofacial clefts. *Journal of Pediatrics*, *143*(6), 805–807.

Rintala, A., Leisti, J., Liesmaa, M., & Ranta, R. (1980). Oblique facial clefts: Case report. *Scandinavian Journal of Plastic & Reconstructive Surgery*, *14*(3), 291–297.

Rollnick, B. R., & Pruzansky, S. (1981). Genetic services at a center for craniofacial anomalies. *Cleft Palate Journal*, *18*(4), 304–313.

Rose, E., Thissen, U., Otten, J. E., & Jonas, I. (2003). Cephalometric assessment of the posterior airway space in patients with cleft palate after palatoplasty. *Cleft Palate-Craniofacial Journal*, *40*(5), 498–503.

Saad, E. F. (1980). The underdeveloped palate in ear, nose, and throat practice. *Laryngoscope*, *90*(8, Pt. 1), 1371–1377.

Schwartz, R. H., Hayden, G. F., Rodriquez, W. J., Shprintzen, R. J., & Cassidy, J. W. (1985). The bifid uvula: Is it a marker for an otitis prone child? *Laryngoscope*, *95*(9, Pt. 1), 1100–1102.

Shapiro, B. L., Meskin, L. H., Cervenka, J., & Pruzansky, S. (1971). Cleft uvula: A microform of facial clefts and its genetic basis. *Birth Defects Original Article Series*, *7*(7), 80–82.

Sheahan, P., Miller, I., Earley, M. J., Sheahan, J. N., & Blayney, A. W. (2004). Middle ear disease in children with congenital velopharyngeal insufficiency. *Cleft Palate-Craniofacial Journal*, *41*(4), 364–367.

Shprintzen, R. J., Schwartz, R. H., Daniller, A., & Hoch, L. (1985). Morphologic significance of bifid uvula. *Pediatrics*, *75*(3), 553–561.

Simmons, C. J., Mosley, B. S., Fulton-Bond, C. A., & Hobbs, C. A. (2004). Birth defects in Arkansas: Is folic acid fortification making a difference? *Birth Defects Research*, 70(9), 559–564.

Smahel, Z., Kasalova, P., & Skvarilova, B. (1991). Morphometric nasopharyngeal characteristics in facial clefts. *Journal of Craniofacial Genetics and Developmental Biology*, 11(1), 24–32.

Smahel, Z., & Mullerova, I. (1992). Nasopharyngeal characteristics in children with cleft lip and palate. *Cleft Palate-Craniofacial Journal*, 29(3), 282–286.

Stewart, J. M., Otet, J. E., & Lagace, R. (1972). Submucous cleft palate: Prevalence in a school population. *Cleft Palate Journal*, 9, 246–250.

Trier, W. C. (1983). Velopharyngeal incompetency in the absence of overt cleft palate: Anatomic and surgical considerations. *Cleft Palate Journal*, 20(3), 209–217.

Vinceti, M., Rovesti, S., Bergomi, M., Calzolari, E., Candela, S., Campagna, A., et al. (2001). Risk of birth defects in a population exposed to environmental lead pollution. *Science of the Total Environment*, 278(1–3), 23–30.

Warkany, J. (1971). *Congenital malformations: Notes and comments*. Chicago: Year Book.

Warren, D. W., & Drake, A. F. (1993). Cleft nose. Form and function. *Clinics in Plastic Surgery*, 20(4), 769–779.

Warren, D. W., Hairfield, W. M., & Dalston, E. T. (1990). The relationship between nasal airway size and nasal-oral breathing in cleft lip and palate. *Cleft Palate Journal*, 27(1), 46–51; Discussion 51–42.

Warren, D. W., Hairfield, W. M., & Dalston, E. T. (1991). Nasal airway impairment: The oral response in cleft palate patients. *American Journal of Orthodontics & Dentofacial Orthopedics*, 99(4), 346–353.

Weatherly-White, R. C. A., Sakura, C. Y., Brenner, L. D., Stewart, J. M., & Ott, J. E. (1972). Submucous cleft palate incidence, natural history, and implications for treatment. *Plastic & Reconstructive Surgery*, 49, 297–304.

Wetmore, R. F. (1992). Importance of maintaining normal nasal function in the cleft palate patient. *Cleft Palate-Craniofacial Journal*, 29(6), 498–506.

Wharton, P., & Mowrer, D. E. (1992). Prevalence of cleft uvula among school children in kindergarten through grade five. *Cleft Palate-Craniofacial Journal*, 29(1), 10–12; Discussion 13–14.

CHAPTER

3

GENETICS AND PATTERNS OF INHERITANCE

ROBERT J. HOPKIN, M.D.

CHAPTER OUTLINE

INTRODUCTION

Craniofacial anomalies, like many other conditions, tend to recur in families. The risk for recurrence, however, is variable, depending on interactions of multiple environmental and genetic factors. The purpose of this chapter is to briefly review the modes of inheritance that may influence the occurrence of craniofacial anomalies. The first part of the chapter reviews DNA, genes, chromosomes, and the cell cycle. (See Figure 3–1 for a diagram of a cell's genetic material.) The second part of the chapter discusses the principles of Mendelian inheritance, including autosomal recessive, autosomal dominant, and X-linked patterns. The last portion of the chapter focuses on complex, or non-Mendelian, inheritance. Particular attention is placed on multifactorial inheritance, the pattern associated with most cases of cleft palate—or cleft lip with or without cleft palate.

DEOXYRIBONUCLEIC ACID (DNA) AND GENES

Deoxyribonucleic Acid (DNA)

For centuries, scientists wondered how the information needed to organize and direct the development of an organism was transmitted from a single cell to a mature individual with complex organs and tissues. Then in 1869, Friedrich Miescher discovered a substance in cell nuclei that he called "nuclein." The name was eventually changed to deoxyribonucleic acid or DNA. In 1944, Avery, Macleod, and McCarthy demonstrated that DNA is the substance that carries hereditary information in bacteria. It is now known that the genetic information of all cells is carried on DNA (McKusick, 1997).

Deoxyribonucleic acid, or DNA, is a nucleic acid made up of building blocks called *nucleo-tides.* Nucleotides consist of a 5-carbon sugar (deoxyribose) chemically bonded to a phosphate group and a nitrogenous base. The nitrogenous bases can be divided into two groups: *purines* (adenine and guanine) and *pyrimidines* (thymine and cytosine). The nucleotides are linked

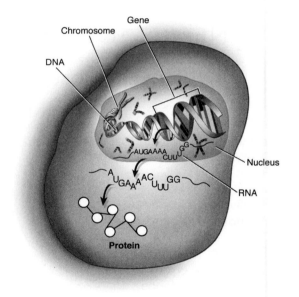

FIGURE 3–1 Diagram of a cell demonstrating that genetic material in the form of **DNA** is organized into **chromosomes**. Each chromosome contains thousands of **genes**. A gene is transcribed into **RNA**. The messenger RNA is transported outside the nucleus and translated into an amino acid sequence. The aminoacid "polypeptide" is then modified into a functional **protein**. This sequence of events occurs for the vast majority of genes. Changes in the DNA sequence of a gene are called mutations. Mutations can change the structure of the protein and interfere with its normal function. (From U.S. Department of Energy Human Genome Program, http://www.ornl.gov/hgmis.)

together through the phosphate groups at the 5th and 3rd carbons of the sugar to form long unbranching polymers. These are arranged in an antiparallel (going in opposite directions) *double helix* (coiled ladder) such that the nitrogenous bases are paired according to specific rules. A purine is always paired with a pyrmidine. In fact adenine (A) is always paired with thymine (T), and guanine (G) is always paired with cytosine (C). For example, if one strand contains the sequence 5′GGATTCG3′, the complementary sequence would be 3′CCTAAGC5′. The numbers 5′ and 3′ indicate the direction of the strand. The strands are held together by hydrogen bonds between A-T pairs and C-G pairs (Strachan & Read, 1996).

Replication

The complementary nature of the double helix allows DNA to serve as a template for its own *replication*. Replication, which is the process of making two identical DNA molecules from one, is a process resulting in two double strands, each containing one original and one complimentary newly synthesized strand of DNA. This process is complex and carefully controlled, but it must take place quickly to allow for rapid cell division and growth. In humans, over 3.5×10^4 nucleotides must be precisely matched for each cell division. The process starts at several sites along a DNA molecule simultaneously. When DNA is replicated, a replication bubble forms as the double helix is unwound and the complementary strands are separated. Nucleotides are then added sequentially, forming new complementary strands. The final result is two identical double helix molecules of DNA (Strachan & Read, 1996).

The process of replicating DNA is very carefully controlled to prevent errors. In addition, there are proofreading and repair mechanisms

to preserve the exact sequence of nucleotides (Strachan & Read, 1996). Fortunately errors are rare; however, they do occur. When a change in the sequence of a molecule of DNA occurs, it is referred to as a *mutation*. The mutation can be as small as a substitution of a single base pair or as large as the deletion of an entire chromosome. Mutations may have important consequences for the cell and for the individual.

Genes

Long strands of DNA are organized into shorter functional units known as genes. A *gene* is a submicroscopic functional unit of heredity. It consists of a discrete segment of a DNA molecule that resides within the *chromosome*. A chromosome is a single, linear double strand of DNA with associated proteins that function to organize and compact the DNA and/or function in regulating gene activity. Thousands of genes are found in each chromosome. The order of the nucleotides in the DNA of an individual gene determines the information coded by that gene. Each gene consists of a promoter region that functions as the starting point for the gene's activity and serves as an on/off switch, a coding region that contains the information needed to make a functional protein, and regulatory elements that determine how much of that protein will be made.

Even small changes in the coding region of a gene may lead to changes in function through several mechanisms. Disease-causing mutations may disrupt gene function, leading to early termination of translation and often to an unstable or nonfunctional product. A change in the DNA can lead to disease if the change results in a change of function for the protein. For example, the mutations in the MSX2 gene that cause craniosynostosis do not lead to decreased protein production but to a gain of function in the protein that is produced. This results in craniosynostosis. Loss of function for the same gene leads to a very different disorder characterized by delayed closure of cranial sutures and persistence of fontanels into adulthood (Wilkie et al., 2000).

Deletions and insertions of one or more nucleotides can disrupt gene function by changing, adding, or deleting important amino acids. Changes in DNA can also lead to disease by changing the regulation of gene expression. Both over- and underexpression of genes can lead to abnormal function. Nevertheless, with the exception of identical twins, no two individuals share exactly the same DNA sequence. In fact, much of the DNA in humans is variable. This variability is called polymorphism. Polymorphisms are very common (seen in virtually all genes) and contribute to the uniqueness of each individual. Mutations lead to new variations in the DNA. New variants that do not contribute to disease or that improve function may become more common over time, while changes that lead to disease will tend to remain rare or be eliminated (Cummings, 1997).

Ribonucleic Acid (RNA)

The processes controlled by the genes take place outside the nucleus in the cytoplasm of the cell. However, the DNA is found primarily in the nucleus of the cells. The genetic information is transported from the nucleus to the cytoplasm as strands of *ribonucleic acid* (RNA). The DNA in a gene serves as a template for *transcription*, which is the process of creating a strand of RNA that is complementary to a given strand of DNA. RNA is similar to DNA in that it is a linear polymer composed of a 5-carbon

sugar (although ribose is the sugar in RNA) bound to a phosphate group and a nitrogenous base. The nitrogenous bases differ slightly from those in DNA because RNA contains the pyrimidine uracil in place of thymine. The other nitrogenous bases are the same as in DNA. However, RNA is a single-stranded molecule in living cells. The RNA sequence of a gene is read in the cytoplasm and determines which amino acids will be incorporated into the protein. Each amino acid is specified by a group of three nucleotides called a codon. Most amino acids can be coded by more than one codon. Thus some changes in the nucleotide sequence may not result in changes in the amino acid sequence of the protein. These changes are called conservative mutations (Cummings, 1997).

The portions of a gene that determine the amino acid sequence for a polypeptide are referred to as the *coding region*. The coding region is divided into segments called *exons*. *Introns* are the segments between exons. They are removed or "spliced out" from the RNA following transcription. The exons are then spliced together to form a continuous RNA coding sequence. It is critical that the process of removing introns and splicing the remaining RNA segments together starts and stops at the correct point. An error of one nucleotide can result in an RNA transcript that codes for a nonfunctional protein.

RNA that has had the introns removed is called *messenger RNA* or *mRNA*. mRNA is transported from the nucleus to the cytoplasm to function as a template for protein synthesis. In the cytoplasm of the cell, *ribosomes* (organelles within the cell that function in protein synthesis) attach to the mRNA and translate the nucleotides into the specified amino acid sequence, forming a polypeptide. The polypeptides are then processed to form the functional proteins (Mange & Mange, 1999).

The flow of genetic information, therefore, proceeds from DNA through transcription to RNA. RNA is then translated into an amino acid sequence, forming a protein. In addition, it has recently been discovered that transporting genetic information to the cytosol of the cell for translation is only one of the functions of RNA. Several genes have been discovered that produce RNA transcripts but no protein. Some of these have been shown to specifically regulate other genes. In fact, functional RNA is now thought to play an important role in regulating gene expression (Kim & Nam, 2006).

CHROMOSOMES

As noted previously, chromosomes are single, linear double strands of DNA with associated proteins that function to organize and compact the DNA in a cell for cell division. The genetic material, DNA, is organized in human cells into 46 chromosomes in most cells. This can be seen in a *karotype*, which is a chromosome analysis that is done by drawing blood, growing the cells in a culture, analyzing the white blood cells, photographing the chromosomes, and then arranging the chromosomes in pairs for display and assessment. A karotype of normal human chromosomes can be seen in Figure 3–2.

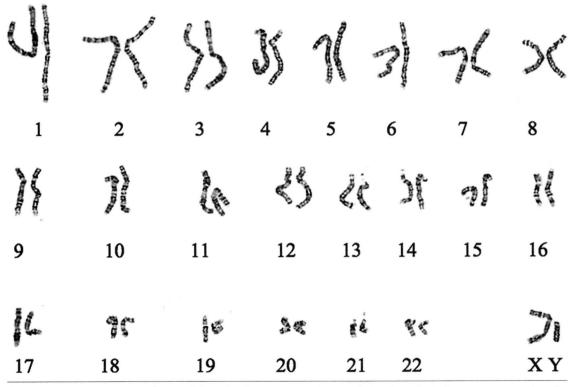

FIGURE 3–2   Karyotype of normal human chromosomes. It is traditional to align chromosomes so that the parm is on top. (Karyotype provided by R. Blough, Ph.D., Division of Human Genetics, Children's Hospital Medical Center, Cincinnati, Ohio.)

Together the chromosomes contain the complete set of instructions for cell replication and differentiation. This complete set of instructions is called the *genome* (Cummings, 1997).

Each chromosome has a narrowed region called a *centromere*. The centromere is critical for normal cell division; however, the location of the centromere is quite variable. In some cases it is in the middle of the chromosome, dividing it into approximately equal halves. Chromosomes with a centrally located centromere are referred to as *metacentric*. The centromere may also be off-center, leading to a short (p) arm. The "p" refers to *petit*, the French word for "small." The long arm is referred to as the q arm. The "q" is simply the letter after "p." Chromosomes with this structure are referred to as *submetacentric*. Finally, the centromere may be very close to one end of the chromosome. These chromosomes are *acrocentric*. The location of the centromere and the length of the chromosome give each chromosome a characteristic shape, which allows them to be distinguished from one another. Traditionally chromosomes are labeled according to length, with the longest being number 1.

Each of 22 chromosomes has two copies, one from each parent. These chromosomes are called *autosomes* (and include all chromosomes with the exception of the two *sex chromosomes*). The 23rd pair of chromosomes are referred to as the sex chromosomes (X and Y) because of their role in gender determination. If a person inherits two X chromosomes (one from each parent), that person will be female. If an X (from the mother) and a Y (from the father) are inherited, the person will be male. The normal chromosomal make-up is written as 46,XX for a female or 46,XY for a male (Keagle & Brown, 1999).

Chromosomes can be specially stained to reveal a pattern of light- and dark-colored bands. This allows specific segments of the chromosome to be identified. The bands are labeled by the chromosome number followed

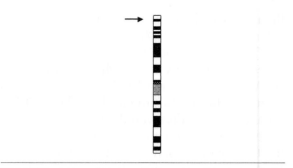

FIGURE 3–3 Ideogram (schematic drawing of the banding pattern) of chromosome 1: Note the light and dark bands. Each chromosome has a unique but consistent banding pattern that allows it to be distinguished from other chromosomes. The arrow indicates band 1p36.

by "p" or "q" to indicate which arm the band is on. Each band is also given a number that indicates its location relative to the centromere and the other bands on that arm of the chromosome. This system is used to describe the rough location of genes in gene mapping studies. For example, a gene may be mapped to 1p36. This means that the gene is found on the short arm of chromosome 1 in the band labeled 36. Figure 3–3 shows an *ideogram* (a schematic drawing of the banding pattern of a chromosome) for chromosome 1. The bands can be further subdivided in some cases, allowing for more specific localization to be described. Even with the best current staining techniques, it is not possible to identify individual genes on a chromosome. The smallest bands that can be distinguished still contain multiple genes (Mange & Mange, 1999).

Cell Cycle

Cells in the body alternate between states of active division and states of nondivision. When a cell is dividing, it goes through a sequence of events called the *cell cycle*, which is the process of preparing for and undergoing cell division. The frequency of the cell cycle depends on the type of cell and the rate of growth of the organism at the time. The steps in each cycle are very similar for all types of somatic cells.

Cell division can be divided into two major processes: *mitosis*, which is the process of separating duplicated chromosomes and reconstitution of two cell nuclei, and *cytokinesis*, which is the separation of the cell cytoplasm to form two distinct cells with separate cell membranes. During mitosis, a complete identical set of chromosomes is distributed to each daughter cell. It is critical for the process to be accurate and precise in order for the cells to function normally. The chromosomes contain the genes and therefore the instructions that govern cell function. If errors (mutations) occur in either the process of DNA replication or in the separation of the chromosomes, they often have serious consequences for the cell. The process of division takes about one hour. The time between cell divisions is called *interphase*. Cells spend much more time in interphase than in active division.

Mitosis takes place in the somatic cells and results in daughter cells that have the same number of chromosomes (46) as the parent cell. In contrast, *meiosis* results in 23 chromosomes rather than 46. Meiosis occurs only in the production of *gametes*, which are sperm from the testes and eggs from the ovaries. If sperm and eggs each contained 46 chromosomes at conception, the new cell would contain double that number or 92 chromosomes. This number would double with each generation. During meiosis cells undergo one round of DNA replication but two rounds of cell division. This produces four cells, each with a single copy of each chromosome (Griffiths, Miller, Suzuki, Lewontin, & Gelbart, 1996).

In men, meiosis occurs continuously following puberty and produces four sperm cells per original cell. This results in the availability of large numbers of mature sperm on a continual basis. In women, meiosis starts in fetal life but then arrests until puberty. Following puberty, one oocyte per menstrual cycle completes meiosis. Errors in meiosis may have serious consequences because they result in abnormalities in every cell in a developing organism (Keagle & Brown, 1999).

Chromosomal Abnormalities

Chromosomal mutations may include changes in the number of copies of an individual chromosome. Loss of one copy of a chromosome results in *monosomy*, which is the presence of a single copy of a chromosome. The gain of one extra copy of a chromosome (for a total of three chromosomes) results in *trisomy*. Figure 3–4 shows a karotype of trisomy 13. Most monosomies and trisomies end in early miscarriage.

The only monosomy that commonly results in the birth of living infants is monosomy X. This results in Turner syndrome. Turner syndrome is characterized by short stature, webbed neck, and lack of sexual maturation. The presence of the Y chromosome with no X results in early miscarriage.

Survival is possible for several trisomies, including trisomy for X, 13, 18, or 21. Individuals born with trisomy X or with 47,XXY may be relatively healthy and undistinguishable from the general population. The presence of extra copies of the Y chromosome is also compatible with healthy survival. Those with trisomy 21 have Down syndrome, which is associated with mental retardation, congenital heart disease, low muscle tone, and distinct facial features. Trisomy 13 and 18 may result in live born infants; however, these infants are born with multiple severe birth defects and rarely survive more than a few weeks. Trisomy 13 is frequently associated with cleft lip and palate and other craniofacial malformations. Trisomy 18 can lead to Pierre Robin sequence and cleft palate in addition to many other malformations. Trisomies for other chromosomes result in early miscarriage.

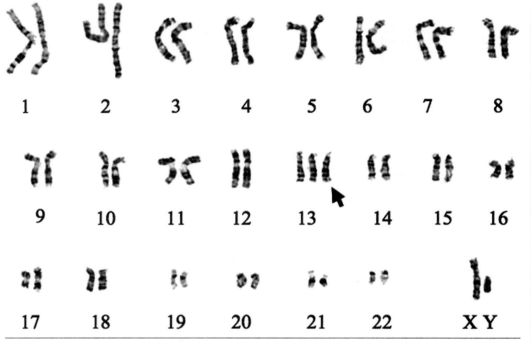

FIGURE 3–4 Karyotype of human chromosomes demonstrating trisomy 13. (Karyotype provided by R. Blough, Ph.D., Division of Human Genetics, Children's Hospital Medical Center, Cincinnati, Ohio.)

Trisomies and monosomies result from a failure in meiosis. The abnormal number of chromosomes results from *nondisjunction*, which is the failure of one or more chromosomes to separate in cell division. Nondisjunction can be seen in both sperm and egg development. The cause of nondisjunction is not known, but the risk for nondisjunction and related chromosomal abnormalities increases with advancing maternal age. For example, the risk for trisomy 21 (which causes Down syndrome) in a pregnancy to a 20-year-old woman is approximately 1:2000. The risk for a pregnancy to a 45-year-old woman is approximately 1:20. The risk for nondisjunction rises slowly with age at first but increases more rapidly after age 35. For this reason, pregnant women over age 35 are offered chromosomal analysis through amniocentesis. The risk for nondisjunction in men remains relatively stable with advancing age (Randolph, 1999).

Mosaicism is the presence of cells with two or more different genetic contents in a single individual. This may be caused by nondisjunction in mitosis. Because errors in mitosis affect only the daughter cells descended from the cell in which the error occurred, in many cases the abnormal cells may simply be eliminated or the functions of the cell may not be seriously impaired. However, if nondisjunction occurs in mitosis early in embryonic development, it may result in serious malformations. The effect of the abnormal cells will depend on the ratio of normal versus abnormal cells and the distribution of the each cell type (Mange & Mange, 1999).

Chromosomal abnormalities, other than the gain or loss of an entire chromosome, can also occur. These include deletions, duplications, inversions, and translocations.

When part of a chromosome becomes separated and lost, this is called a *deletion*.

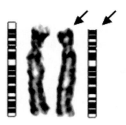

FIGURE 3–5 Normal and deleted human chromosome 4 with ideograms. The arrows indicate the deleted segment at 4p16. This deletion is associated with Wolf-Hirschhorn syndrome. (Photographs of chromosomes provided by R. Blough, Ph.D., Division of Human Genetics, Children's Hospital Medical Center, Cincinnati, Ohio.)

Deletions have been reported for all chromosomes. The location of the deletion is designated by the chromosome number, a "p" (for the short arm) or "q" (for the long arm), and the number of the band where the break occurred. For example, a deletion of the short arm of chromosome 4 with a break point in band 16 in a female could be written 46,XXdel(4)(p16). Figure 3–5 shows ideograms of a normal and a deleted chromosome 4. This deletion would result in Wolf-Hirschhorn syndrome (see Chapter 4). Deletions are often accompanied by multiple malformations, including facial clefts or other craniofacial malformations. However, unlike the example above, many deletions do not result in recognizable genetic syndromes.

Pure *duplications* of part of a chromosome are rare. Like deletions, chromosomal duplications are usually associated with multiple malformations and developmental handicaps. The pattern of malformations and severity of developmental disability depend on the size and location of the duplication. Even when the size and location are known, it can be difficult to predict what malformations will result and the long-term outcome for an individual patient. Combinations of deletion and duplication frequently result from unbalanced translocations (Kaiser-Rogers & Rao, 1999) and will be discussed later in this chapter.

Inversions occur when a portion of a chromosome is turned 180° from its usual orientation. *Translocations* are the result of a transfer of genetic material between two or more chromosomes. Inversions and translocations may not be associated with any abnormalities in the individual because the total amount of genetic material may be unchanged. In that case, a problem will result only if the break points are located in areas that disrupt a gene or genes. Inversions and translocations that do not result in the gain or loss of DNA have approximately a 10% risk for associated malformations or developmental disabilities. This is not surprising, as only approximately 10% of our DNA is in genes. Translocations and inversions may, however, increase the risk for infertility or birth defects in the children of an asymptomatic individual who carries the chromosomal rearrangement.

All of the types of chromosomal abnormalities discussed above can be associated with cleft palate, cleft lip, or other craniofacial malformations. Chromosomal abnormalities involve both large changes in the genome and multiple genes. Because they involve large amounts of DNA, the changes are relatively easy to detect. It is important to identify people with chromosomal abnormalities because their needs and associated risks may be different from those of patients with isolated craniofacial malformations or single gene disorders. However, chromosomal abnormalities account for only a small portion of birth defects and genetic diseases. Smaller mutations involving only single genes are collectively common even though the individual disorders are often rare.

Chromosome Analysis

In order to discover abnormalities in the chromosomes, they must be visualized. The chromosomes are condensed enough to be easily viewed under a microscope only during certain stages of the cell cycle. Fortunately, by stimulating white blood cells to divide simultaneously, large numbers of cells can be expected to reach the same stage of the cell cycle at about the same time. This greatly improves the efficiency of chromosomal analysis. There are also chemicals that lead to arrest of cell division at certain stages of the cell cycle. Thus, the cell cycle can be controlled to maximize the number of cells appropriate for analysis (Keagle & Gersen, 1999).

Some chromosomal rearrangements involve only very short segments that are too small to be seen using routine chromosomal analysis. With special techniques, such as *fluorescence in situ hybridization,* or FISH, some submicroscopic segments of DNA can be identified by a cytogenetic laboratory. (*Cytogenetics* is the branch of genetics that is concerned with the structure and function of the cell, particularly the chromosomes within the cell.) This procedure involves the use of a nucleic acid probe labeled with a fluorescent dye that localizes a specified DNA segment. For example, the deletion of chromosome 22q11.2, associated with velocardiofacial syndrome (see Chapter 4), is usually not visible on chromosomal analysis, but is seen using FISH in the majority of cases. Syndromes caused by deletions large enough to contain several genes, but too small to be seen on routine cytogenetic analysis, are referred to as *contiguous gene syndromes.* In most, if not all cases, the problems associated with the syndrome are caused by the loss of function of several important genes (Kaiser-Rogers & Rao, 1999). See Table 3–1 for a list of some microdeletion contiguous gene syndromes. Until recently, it has only been possible to look for submicroscopic deletions by ordering site-specific testing for specific changes that were suspected based on the pattern of malformations. In other words, some one had to recognize the condition to find the change. New technology using SNPs (single nucleotide polymorphisms) and CGH (comparative genomic hybridization) microarray

TABLE 3–1	Examples of microdeletion contiguous gene syndromes.
Velocardiofacial syndrome	del 22q11.2
Wolf-Hirschhorn syndrome	del 4p16.3
Cri du chat syndrome	del 5p15
Prader-Willi syndrome	del 15q11q13
Miller-Dieker syndrome	del 17p13.3
Langer-Giedion syndrome	del 8q24
Smith-Magenis syndrome	del 17p11.2
Kallmann syndrome	del Xp22.3
X-linked ichthyosis	del Xp22.3
Jacobsen syndrome	del 11q24.1
Williams syndrome	del 7q11.23

analysis allows analysis of thousands of loci simultaneously (Le Caignec, 2005; Schoumans et al., 2005; Ting et al., 2006). This is expected to greatly increase the ability to detect small cytogenetic rearrangements that lead to malformation syndromes.

MENDELIAN INHERITANCE

The common patterns of inheritance and the rules that govern them were first outlined by Mendel in 1866 in his studies on peas (McKusick, 1997). The patterns he described are known as Mendelian inheritance and include autosomal recessive, autosomal dominant, and X-linked patterns. Mendel described four rules of inheritance. He discovered that:

1. Genes come in pairs, one from each parent.

2. Genes can have different *alleles*, which are variations of a gene. Some of these are dominant, and will exert their effects over the effects of the other allele. Other alleles will be manifest only when the genes are *homozygous* (having two similar alleles). They are called recessive.

3. At meiosis, alleles segregate from each other; each gamete carries only one allele.

4. The segregation of alleles for one trait is independent of the segregation of alleles from other genes for other traits.

These principles have remained valid (with only a few modifications) since they were first described.

Pedigrees

In determining a pattern of inheritance for a condition in a family, it is helpful to have a systematic way of collecting and recording the family history. A system has been developed, called a *pedigree*, which is a pictorial representation of family members and their line of descent. This system is used to record the inheritance of traits or anomalies affecting several members of a family. It allows the important findings to be recorded in a short period of time. Most families can be easily described for three to four generations on a single page. In addition, with minimal training and a little practice, pedigrees can be simply and quickly drawn by hand during the course of a brief interview (Mange & Mange, 1999). Three sample pedigrees are illustrated in Figure 3–6.

Autosomal Recessive Inheritance

All people carry genes with mutations that are capable of causing disease. Fortunately, we inherit two copies of each gene, one from each parent, and in many cases, one copy that functions normally is sufficient. There are approximately 30,000 different genes in each cell, but each person carries on average six to seven potentially disease-causing mutations. Therefore, the chance that both members of a couple will carry mutations in the same gene is small. Individuals who have one abnormal copy of a gene and are without detectable abnormalities are referred to as carriers. They are *heterozygous* (having two different alleles of a gene). Traits that are manifest only when mutations are present in both copies of a gene are recessive traits. If a gene causing a recessive trait is on one of the autosomes, the trait is *autosomal recessive*.

Autosomal recessive traits tend to occur more frequently in isolated populations or in cases of *consanguinity*, which is mating between related individuals. The parents of affected individuals are usually unaffected. Recurrences between siblings are common, but recurrences in multiple generations of a family are rare in the absence of consanguinity. Autosomal recessive conditions are seen in both males and females in equal numbers.

The probability of two people carrying abnormalities in the same genes is increased if they are related. This is because relatives share genetic material. The closer the relationship, the more shared genetic material two individuals will have in common. Thus, consanguinity leads to increased risk for both members of a couple to carry disease-causing mutations in the same genes. This is one explanation for the high incidence of genetic disorders in isolated or inbred populations. In some populations, a relatively small number of original ancestors has led to a high frequency of carriers for certain disorders. This is known as a founder effect. In some cases, it is possible to trace family lines to a single common ancestor who brought a trait into a population. More frequently, a founder effect is implied by a high frequency of a few mutations in a large population. For example, three mutations account for 98% of Tay-Sachs disease in the Ashkenazi Jewish population (Rutledge & Percy, 1997).

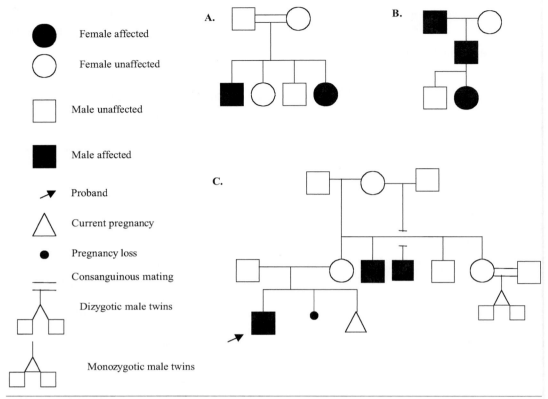

FIGURE 3–6 (A–C) Symbols used in pedigree construction with three sample pedigrees. A. demonstrates probable autosomal recessive inheritance. Note recurrence in siblings with unaffected parents and consanguinity. Multifactorial inheritance cannot be ruled out based on the information given. B. demonstrates autosomal dominant inheritance. Note father-to-son transmission and recurrence in several generations. C. demonstrates X-linked recessive inheritance. Note occurrence of multiple males born to unaffected female relatives over multiple generations. In drawing a pedigree, horizontal lines connecting two individuals indicate mating between them. Children are indicated by vertical lines with squares or circles to indicate the sex of the child. If more than one child is born to a couple, a horizontal line intersects the vertical line to allow each child to be appropriately recorded. If a parent has children with more than one partner additional lines can be drawn as seen in the first generation of family C. Divorce or separation can be indicated by as hash mark and space in the line connecting two individuals (not shown). If more than one trait is being recorded in a family, the affected individuals can be indicated by shading only one quadrant, for example the upper left for trait 1, the lower left for trait 2, etc. If still more traits are recorded, different colors or patterns of shading can be added.

The chance of having an affected child is 25% for each pregnancy resulting from mating between two heterozygous carriers of an autosomal recessive condition. The other possibilities are 50% that a child will be a carrier of a single copy of the mutation and 25% that the child will be a noncarrier. This is because each parent has an approximately equal probability of passing on either the normal or abnormal allele. If two individuals with the same autosomal recessive condition have children together, all of their children will be affected because the parents only have abnormal alleles to pass on (Mueller & Cook, 1997).

Recurrence in more than one generation is uncommon because carrier frequency is low for most autosomal recessive conditions. For example, cystic fibrosis is one of the most common autosomal recessive disorders, affecting 1:2000 live births among populations of Northern European descent. The carrier frequency in that population is 1:25. That means a carrier would have a 24/25 probability of reproducing with a noncarrier in a population with random choice of partners. Testing is available for carrier status of some of the more common autosomal recessive diseases, such as cystic fibrosis, sickle cell anemia, and Tay-Sachs disease. This can help couples in making reproductive decisions if they are from a high-risk population or if there is a family history of the disorder that indicates a high probability that one or both partners may be carriers for that condition. Prenatal testing that can distinguish affected individuals from carriers is also available for some autosomal recessive conditions.

Occasionally two people with the same autosomal recessive trait will have children but the children will be unaffected. An example of this would be autosomal recessive hearing loss. This can be explained by *heterogeneity*, which occurs when mutations in different genes lead to the same abnormality or *phenotype* (Mueller & Cook, 1997). See Table 3–2 for a list of some autosomal recessive conditions that can be associated with cleft lip or cleft palate.

Autosomal Dominant Inheritance

In autosomal dominant disorders, heterozygous individuals have a recognizable phenotype, which is the group of characteristics associated with the genetic condition. Homozygous individuals also show the phenotype, but may be more severely affected. Pedigrees from families with autosomal dominant conditions demonstrate

TABLE 3–2 Examples of autosomal recessive craniofacial syndromes.

Smith-Lemli-Opitz syndrome

Meckel-Gruber syndrome

Baller-Gerold syndrome

Oral-facial-digital syndrome type II

Insley-Astley syndrome

Dubowitz syndrome

Roberts syndrome

Toriello-Carey syndrome

Varadi-Papp syndromes

different findings than are seen with autosomal recessive inheritance.

Autosomal dominant pedigrees will frequently show that a parent is affected. If neither parent is affected, the affected individual is presumed to carry a new mutation that is causing the condition. For some autosomal dominant conditions, the new mutation rate is high and may account for a large percentage of affected individuals, as in Pfieffer syndrome (Winter & Baraitser, 1996). The chance that the offspring of an individual with a dominant condition and an unaffected partner will have an affected child is 50% for each pregnancy. The number of affected males and females is approximately equal.

Because there are relatively few genes on the Y chromosome and the only Y-linked traits are male gender and sperm production, the transmission of other traits from a father to his son is considered diagnostic of autosomal dominant inheritance. Two individuals with the same autosomal dominant disorder may have affected and unaffected children because each parent would have one normal and one abnormal allele. *Homozygotes* (persons with two abnormal alleles) for autosomal dominant disorders often have a more severe phenotype than heterozygotes. For example, achondroplasia is the most common form of short-limbed dwarfism. Homozygous offspring of parents with achondroplasia have a severe phenotype, with a small chest and pulmonary hypoplasia that is incompatible with survival beyond the first few days of life (Winter & Baraitser, 1996).

Many autosomal dominant conditions have *variable expressivity* (variation in the phenotype associated with a single condition). This may cause affected individuals to be missed if the phenotype is not appropriately defined. For example, in Van der Woude syndrome, affected members of the same family may have cleft lip, cleft palate, lip pits, or a combination of these. Obviously, an individual with isolated lip pits could be missed if only individuals with cleft lip are identified when a family history is obtained. Most, if not all, autosomal dominant conditions demonstrate some degree of variable expressivity (Mueller & Cook, 1997).

Incomplete penetrance is the lack of a recognizable phenotype in an individual who carries a gene for an autosomal dominant trait. This is also common in autosomal dominant conditions. At times it may be difficult to distinguish between minimal expression due to variable expressivity and true incomplete penetrance. Some families have members who have no abnormal findings (nonpenetrance), but have transmitted the trait to their children. Other individuals may have only one feature of a condition (variable expressivity), but may transmit the complete condition to their children. The factors that determine the penetrance and expressivity for a given trait are not well understood, but include different mutations in the same gene, modifying genes that interact with the gene that causes the disorder, environmental influences, and random variation (Mueller & Cook, 1997; Murray, 1995).

Many genes have more than one function and may therefore be associated with multiple seemingly unrelated abnormalities. For example,

TABLE 3–3 Examples of autosomal dominant craniofacial syndromes.

Apert syndrome

Branchio-oto-renal syndrome

Crouzon syndrome

Distichiasis-lymphedema syndrome

Ectrodactyly ectodermal dysplasia clefting syndrome

Opitz Frias syndrome

Stickler syndrome

Treacher-Collins syndrome

Van der Woude syndrome

Waardenburg syndrome

neurofibromatosis type 1 is associated with growth of large nerve sheath tumors, called neurofibromas, pigmentary abnormalities of the skin, bony dysplasias, and learning disabilities. This *pleiotropy* (the phenomenon where a single mutant gene can affect multiple, unrelated systems) can contribute to the variability in genetic syndromes because each function of a gene can have either variable expression or nonpenetrance (Mueller & Cook, 1997).

For examples of autosomal dominant disorders that are associated with craniofacial malformations, see Table 3–3.

X-Linked Inheritance

X-linked inheritance refers to conditions caused by genes on the X chromosome. There are many X-linked recessive conditions and a few X-linked dominant conditions. X-linked inheritance is unique because males inherit only one copy of the X chromosome while females inherit two copies. Therefore, if a mutation occurs in an X-linked recessive gene, a female is likely to have mild or no effects. A male who inherits that gene is likely to be more severely affected because he has only one allel (copy) of each gene. X-linked

TABLE 3-4 Examples of X-linked recessive craniofacial syndromes.
Chitayat syndrome
X-linked cleft palate
Oro-facial-digital syndrome type VIII
VATER with hydrocephaly
Lenz microphthalmia
Lowe syndrome
Oto-palato-digital syndrome type II
Simpson-Golabi-Behmel syndrome
SCARF syndrome
Say-Meyer syndrome

TABLE 3-5 Examples of X-linked dominant syndromes.
Aarskog syndrome
Goltz syndrome
Conradi chondrodysplasia punctata
Oral-facial-digital syndrome type I
Melnick-Needles ostoedysplasty
Aicardi syndrome
Alport syndrome
Incontinentia pigmenti
X-linked hypophosphataemic rickets
Rett syndrome

recessive disorders affect males almost exclusively. Transmission occurs from carrier females to 50% of their sons—and 50% of their daughters will be carriers. Affected males pass the gene to 100% of their daughters. There is no father-to-son transmission because fathers do not give an X chromosome to their sons (Mueller & Cook, 1997). See Table 3–4 for examples of X-linked recessive disorders.

X-linked dominant inheritance is rare, with only a few disorders demonstrated. X-linked dominant disorders are characterized by having all of the daughters of affected males inherit the disorder. Sons of affected males never inherit the disorder, again because they receive the Y chromosome from the father. Affected females can transmit the disorder to offspring of both sexes. There is an excess of affected females in pedigrees for X-linked dominant disorders. Many X-linked dominant disorders are lethal to affected males. See Table 3–5 for a list of X-linked dominant disorders.

There are a number of X-linked conditions that cannot be clearly categorized as either X-linked recessive or X-linked dominant. They often have effects on females who are heterozygous, but they may affect males more severely. This group of disorders is often lumped with X-linked recessive disorders in the medical literature, but should more appropriately be referred to simply as X-linked. Some examples of this pattern include Coffin-Lowry syndrome, fragile X syndrome, and Fabry disease. This group of disorders is characterized by variable expressivity and high levels of nonpenetrance in females, but with complete penetrance and more uniform expression in males.

NON-MENDELIAN INHERITANCE

Many disorders that tend to recur in families do not follow the basic rules of Mendelian inheritance. The remainder of this chapter reviews some of the mechanisms involved in the inheritance of these disorders.

Multifactorial Inheritance

Some human disorders result from an interaction of multiple genes with environmental influences. This is called *multifactorial inheritance*. Environmental factors known to increase risks for birth defects are called *teratogens* (Murray,

1995). Common examples of teratogens include ethanol, cigarette smoke, anti-epileptic medications, maternal diabetes, and congenital infections. Most, if not all, teratogens exert their effects by interfering with the regulation of gene expression.

Multifactorial disorders can be divided into two categories: traits that demonstrate continuous variation and threshold disorders.

Some traits that exhibit continuous variation include height, weight, intelligence, and blood pressure. Abnormalities involving continuous traits are not easily distinguished from normal variation since, by definition, there will be large numbers of people on the border between normal and abnormal. The boundary therefore becomes subjective and a matter of definition. In many cases, "abnormal" is defined as greater than two standard deviations from the mean. Although this can be used to define abnormality, it may or may not be significant to the affected individual.

The second group of multifactorial disorders is threshold traits, such as cleft lip, pyloric stenosis, and neural tube defects. For these disorders, the trait is either present or absent; therefore, the abnormality is usually not difficult to distinguish. For example, one either has a cleft lip or does not have a cleft lip. With a threshold disorder, as the number of risk factors for the trait increases, the additive risk may cross a boundary or threshold, resulting in expression of the trait.

In the case of cleft lip only, a few of the possible risk factors that contribute to the total risk have been identified. Recent evidence has led to the estimate that variations in 4 to 12 genes contribute most of the genetic risk for cleft lip with or without cleft palate. Candidate genes include TGFA, RARA, BCL3, and END1 (Lidral & Moreno 2005). Some environmental influences that affect risk for cleft lip have also been identified. Maternal smoking, for example

raises the risk for cleft lip (Shaw et al., 1996); whereas maternal supplementation of folic acid appears to decrease recurrence risk in at least some studies (Tolarova & Harris, 1995). The interaction between genes and environmental factors may be additive in multifactorial disorders. For example, the risk attributed to a rare polymorphism of the TGFA gene is small (one- to twofold). The risk associated with maternal smoking is also small (1.5- to twofold). In a recent study, when both heavy maternal smoking and the high-risk allele of TGFA were present, the risk jumped to three- to elevenfold compared to the control group risk (Shaw et al., 1996).

The risk for recurrence of a multifactorial trait in family members can be estimated by doing population studies and gathering empirical data by looking at variables that may correlate with risk for the condition in question. In the case of cleft lip only, a few of the possible risk factors that contribute to the total risk have been identified. For example, cleft lip is more common in boys than girls. It is therefore predicted by the multifactorial model that, if a woman has cleft lip, the recurrence risk in the family will be higher than the risk if a man has cleft lip, and that the brothers of an affected individual will be at higher risk than sisters. Both of these predictions have been studied, but the results have been inconsistent. If both parents have cleft lip, the recurrence risk should be still higher because risk factors could be inherited from each parent. In fact, the more affected relatives, the higher the predicted risk. This prediction has been verified in cleft lip and cleft palate families. The estimated recurrence risk for future children in a family with one individual with cleft palate is 3% to 5%. If there are two affected first-degree relatives, the risk goes up to approximately 9% to 15%, depending on which family members have cleft lip (Curtis, Fraser, & Warburton, 1961; Wyszynski, Zeiger, Tilli, Bailey-Wilson, & Beaty, 1998).

The severity of the defect is also predicted to impact the recurrence risk. For example, one would predict that the recurrence risk in a family with a child who has a bilateral cleft lip would be higher than if the child had a unilateral cleft because the bilateral cleft is a more severe defect. Most studies have supported this prediction. The presence of cleft palate with cleft lip, on the other hand, has not been found to correlate well with recurrence risk in spite of being clinically more difficult to manage (Crawford & Sofaer, 1987).

The risk for multifactorial disorders is increased in close relatives because they tend to share similar genetic backgrounds and similar environmental risk factors. However, recurrences do not occur in a predictable pattern and are usually lower than the 25% or 50% that is predicted for Mendelian disorders. The risk is often in the range of 3% to 5% for first-degree relatives in families with one family member who has cleft lip, and much lower for more distant relatives. In consanguinous matings and inbred populations, recurrence risk is increased for multifactorial disorders because the amount of shared genetic material, and therefore the genetic risk, will be higher. Isolated populations will also share many environmental exposures as well.

There are several variations of the multifactorial model. These include the *oligogenic model*. According to this model, a trait may be determined by the interaction of multiple genes and little environmental influence. Usually a small number of genes contribute most of the risk. For example, one model of risk for cleft palate estimates that six major genes contribute most of the risk for nonsyndromic cleft palate (Fitzpatrick & Farrall, 1993). The major gene model assumes that abnormalities in one of several genes known to influence risk for a trait contribute most of the risk, but that the remaining risk is defined by environmental factors. This model has been suggested for

TABLE 3–6 Examples of multifactorial traits.

Cleft lip with or without cleft palate

Cleft palate

Velo-pharyngeal insufficiency (VPI)

Diabetes mellitus

Alzheimer disease

Alcoholism

Athrosclerotic heart disease

Mental retardation

Colon cancer

Bipolar disease

isolated cleft lip recurrence risk estimation (Farrall & Holder, 1992).

Multifactorial inheritance is very difficult to study because it is complicated by heterogeniety, small effects of each risk factor, incomplete penetrance, and complex interactions. On the other hand, some of the most common human diseases demonstrate multifactorial inheritance. See Table 3–6 for examples of human diseases demonstrating multifactorial inheritance.

Recent advances in informatics and genetics have greatly increased the ability to study the additive effects of multiple genetic factors or of interacting factors relating to specific birth defects. This is referred to as genomics. It involves searching for interactive effects throughout the genetic material. This differs from traditional genetics, which focuses on specific effects due largely or entirely to the effects of a single gene. This area of study is now possible only with the advent of the Human Genome Project. There are few current applications that are available, but there is intriguing evidence that this will be a powerful tool in elucidating the etiology of multifactorial disorders. In some microdeletions there are specific genes associated with various aspects of the disorder. For example, the heart disease in Williams syndrome is due to the loss of the elastin gene. However, there has been no gene identified that explains the developmental abnormalities in velocardiofacial syndrome. Some recent studies have provided evidence that the interactions between several of the deleted genes contribute additively to these abnormalities such that loss of any one gene may not cause any recognized problems, but loss of several causes a recognizable pattern of abnormality (Vitelli & Baldini, 2003). This is a small example of genomics (interactions between multiple genes) leading to a specific phenotype.

Anticipation

Some inherited disorders show a tendency to have more severe manifestations or an earlier age of onset with succeeding generations. This phenomenon is known as *anticipation*. For many years, anticipation was assumed to be due to sampling errors or ascertainment bias. Recent discoveries have proven that there is a genetic basis for anticipation in some diseases. All disorders with proven anticipation have a common mechanism. They are all caused by large expansions of nucleotide repeats. Most of these have repeats consisting of three nucleotides. The triplet repeat most commonly involved is CAG, which codes for glutamine. As the number of repeats expands, it becomes unstable so that in the next generation there is a tendency for the number of repeats to be greater. This, in turn, leads to an earlier age of onset and a more severe phenotype. Disorders caused by CAG repeats include Huntington's disease, spinocerebellar ataxias, and other adult-onset neurodegenerative disorders. A second group of diseases is caused by unstable expansion of untranslated triplet repeats. Fragile X syndrome, the most common inherited form of mental retardation, is caused by a large

expansion of an untranslated CGG repeat (Lindblad & Schalling, 1996).

Imprinting

Historically, it was assumed that having two working copies of each gene was always normal and that the two copies had equivalent function. However, some genes function differently, depending on whether they were inherited maternally or paternally. This phenomenon is called *imprinting* (Butler, 2002; Tilghman, 1999). It has only been demonstrated in a small number of disorders. These include Beckwith-Weidemann syndrome, Prader-Willi syndrome, Angelman syndrome, and Russell-Silver syndrome. If a gene is maternally imprinted, the allele inherited from the mother is not expressed. The opposite is true for genes that are paternally imprinted. It appears that imprinting is important in growth control and brain development (Butler, 2002). It may also play an important role in carcinogenesis (Tilghman, 1999).

SUMMARY

The principles of inheritance and genetics that are covered in this chapter are fundamental to the understanding of most human malformations. Accurate counseling for parents and other family members concerning long-term prognosis and recurrence risks depends on correct diagnosis and identification of the appropriate patterns of inheritance. In addition, an understanding of the basis of malformation syndromes often changes management. For example, the needs of a child with cleft lip caused by an unbalanced chromosomal translocation are likely to differ from those of a child with cleft lip due to multifactorial inheritance. As new insights are discovered into the causes of genetic disease, it will become increasingly important to understand these principles in order to optimize the treatment of each patient according to their individual risks and needs.

FOR REVIEW, DISCUSSION, AND CRITICAL THINKING

1. Describe the "anatomy" of a chromosome and all of its contents.

2. Define DNA and RNA and list their contents. What are their similarities and differences?

3. How many chromosomes are in human cells? Describe how the 23rd pair of chromosomes determines gender.

4. What is meant by "monosomy" and "trisomy"? What common syndrome is due to trisomy 21?

5. Which is likely to cause more abnormalities— a chromosomal defect or genetic defect? Why do you think that is?

6. Cleft palate is often described as the result of multifactorial inheritance. Explain what that means and what the factors might be that can cause cleft palate.

7. What is X-linked inheritance? Will it be more serious in boys or girls? Why?

8. What can a pedigree tell you and why should it be done for individuals with a craniofacial anomaly?

9. What is a phenotype? How does it relate to variable expressivity? Why is it important to know about variable expressivity when evaluating a genetic syndrome in a family?

REFERENCES

Butler, M. G. (2002). Imprinting disorders: Non-Mendelian mechanisms affecting growth. *Journal of Pediatric Endocrinology*, 15(Suppl 5), 1279–1288.

Crawford, M., & Sofaer, J. (1987). Cleft lip with or without cleft palate: Identification of sporadic cases with a high level of genetic predisposition. *Journal of Medical Genetics*, 24, 163–169.

Cummings, M. (1997). *Human heredity* (4th ed.). Eagan, MN: West/Wadsworth.

Curtis, E., Fraser, F., & Warburton, D. (1961). Congenital cleft lip and palate. *American Journal of Diseases in Childhood*, 102, 853–857.

Farrall, M., & Holder, S. (1992). Familial recurrence-pattern analysis of cleft lip with or without cleft palate. *American Journal of Human Genetics*, 50, 270–277.

Fitzpatrick, D., & Farrall, M. (1993). An estimation of the number of susceptibility loci for isolated cleft palate. *Journal of Craniofacial Genetics and Developmental Biology*, 13, 230–235.

Griffiths, A., Miller, J., Suzuki, D., Lewontin, R., & Gelbart, W. (1996). *An introduction to genetic analysis* (6th ed.). New York: W. H. Freeman and Company.

Kaiser-Rogers, K., & Rao, K. (1999). Structural chromosomal rearrangements. In S. Gersen & M. Keagle (Eds.), *The principles of clinical cytogenetics* (pp. 191–228). Totowa, NJ: Humana Press.

Keagle, M., & Brown, J. (1999). DNA, chromosomes, and cell division. In S. Gersen & M. Keagle (Eds.), *The principles of clinical cytogenetics* (pp. 11–30). Totowa, NJ: Humana Press.

Keagle, M., & Gersen, S. (1999). Basic laboratory procedures. In M. Keagle & S. Gersen (Eds.), *The principles of clinical cytogenetics* (pp. 71–90). Totowa, NJ: Humana Press.

Kim, N. V., & Nam, J. W., (2006). Genomics of microRNA. Trends in Genetics [Epub ahead of print].

Le Caignec, C., Boceno, M., Saugier-Veber, P., Jacquemont, S., Joubert, M., David, A., Frebourg, T., & Rival, J. M. (2005). Detection of genomic imbalances by array-based comparative genomic hybridization in fetuses with multiple malformations. *Journal of Medical Genetics*, *42*, 121–128.

Lidral, A. C., & Moreno L. M. (2005). Progress toward discerning the genetics of cleft lip. *Current Opinion in Pediatrics*, *17*, 731–739.

Mange, E., & Mange, A. (1999). *Basic human genetics* (2nd ed.). Sunderland, MA: Sinauer Associates, Inc.

McKusick, V. (1997). History of medical genetics. In D. Rimoin, J. Connor, & R. Pyeritz (Eds.), *Emery and Rimoin's principles and practice of medical genetics* (3rd ed., Vol. 1, pp. 1–30). New York: Churchill Livingstone, Inc.

Mueller, R., & Cook, J. (1997). Mendelian inheritance. In D. Rimoin, J. Connor, & R. Pyeritz (Eds.), *Emery and Rimoin's principles and practice of medical genetics* (3rd ed., Vol. 1, pp. 87–102). New York: Churchill Livingstone.

Murray, J. C. (1995). Face facts: Genes, environment, and clefts [Comment]. *American Journal of Human Genetics*, *57*(2), 227–232.

Randolph, L. (1999). Prenatal cytogenetics. In S. Gersen & M. Keagle (Eds.), *The principles of clinical cytogenetics* (pp. 259–316). Totowa, NJ: Humana Press.

Rutledge, S., & Percy, A. (1997). Gangliosidoses and related lipid storage diseases. In D. Rimoin, J. Connor, & R. Pyeritz (Eds.), *Emery and Rimoin's principles and practice of medical genetics* (3rd ed., Vol. 2, pp. 2105–2130). New York: Churchill Livingstone.

Schoumans, J., Ruivenkamp, C., Holmberg, E., Kyllerman, M., Anderlid, B. M., & Nordenskjold, M. (2005). Detection of chromosomal imbalances in children with idiopathic mental retardation by array-based comparative genomic hybridization (array-CGH). *Journal of Medical Genetics*, *42*, 699–705.

Shaw, G., Wasserman, C., Lammer, E., O'Malley, C., Murray, J., Basart, A., & Tolarova, M. M. (1996). Orofacial clefts, parental cigarette smoking, and transforming growth factor-alpha gene variants. *American Journal of Human Genetics*, *58*, 551–561.

Strachan, T., & Read, A. (1996). *Human molecular genetics*. New York: Wiley-Liss.

Tilghman, S. M. (1999). The sins of the fathers and mothers: Genomic imprinting in mammalian development. *Cell*, *96*(2), 185–193.

Ting, J. C., Ye, Y., Thomas, G. H., Ruczinski, I., & Pevsner, J. (2006). Analysis and visualization of chromosomal abnormalities in SNP data with SNPscan. *Bioinformatics*, *7*(1), 25.

Tolarova, M., & Harris, J. (1995). Reduced recurrence of orofacial clefts after periconceptional supplementation with high-dose folic acid and multivitamins. *Teratology*, *51*, 71–78.

Vitelli, F., & Baldini, A. (2003). Generating and modifying DiGeorge syndrome–like phenotypes in model organisms: Is there a common genetic pathway? *Trends in Genetics*, *19*, 588–93.

Wilkie, A. O., Tang, Z., Elanko, N., Walsh, S., Twigg, S. R., Hurst, J. A., Wall, S. A., Chrzanowska, K. H., & Maxson, R. E., Jr. (2000). Functional haploinsufficiency of the human homeobox gene MSX2 causes defects in skull ossification. *Nature Genetics*, 24(4), 387–390.

Winter, R., & Baraitser, M. (1996). *London dysmorphology database* (1) [Compact Disc]. London: Oxford Medical Databases.

Wyszynski, D. F., Zeiger, J., Tilli, M. T., Bailey-Wilson, J. E., & Beaty, T. H. (1998). Survey of genetic counselors and clinical geneticists regarding recurrence risks for families with nonsyndromic cleft lip with or without cleft palate. *American Journal of Medical Genetics*, 79(3), 184–190.

CHAPTER

4

THE GENETICS EVALUATION AND COMMON CRANIOFACIAL SYNDROMES

HOWARD M. SAAL, M.D.

CHAPTER OUTLINE

Miscellaneous Syndromes
Hemifacial Microsomia (Oculoauriculovertebral
   Dysplasia)
CHARGE Syndrome
Treacher Collins Syndrome
Beckwith-Wiedemann Syndrome

Summary
For Review, Discussion, and Critical Thinking
References

INTRODUCTION

Congenital anomalies occur in 3% to 5% of all live births. They are among the most common causes of hospitalization in childhood. There are numerous causes of congenital anomalies, with contributions from both genetic and environmental factors. Craniofacial disorders make up a significant number of congenital anomalies, with 1 in 700 children born with cleft lip with or without cleft palate and 1 in 2000 children born with cleft palate (Gorlin, Cohen, & Hennekam, 2001; Wyszynski, Beaty, & Maestri, 1996). Other craniofacial anomalies frequently encountered are craniosynostosis, hemifacial microsomia, submucous cleft palate, and velopharyngeal insufficiency. Because there is usually a significant genetic component to the pathogenesis of most craniofacial disorders, it is important for each child born with these conditions to have a complete genetic evaluation and follow-up evaluations as the child grows and develops.

The purpose of this chapter is to first describe the components of the genetics evaluation and the information that is important to obtain in order to arrive at a genetics diagnosis. The reader will then learn about the types and causes of dysmorphology. This chapter includes a description of the genetics of clefting and the incidence of clefts. Finally, common craniofacial syndromes will be described.

THE GENETICS EVALUATION

The purpose of the genetics evaluation is as follows: (1) to make a diagnosis; (2) to determine the natural history of a condition, which will assist with anticipatory management for medical and developmental issues; (3) to determine recurrence risks for the parents and other close family members, which may include information regarding availability of prenatal diagnosis for future pregnancies; and (4) to provide genetic psychosocial counseling and family support, which is often the most important function of the genetic evaluation.

It is clear that the genetics evaluation is an important component of the early management of the child born with a craniofacial disorder and the findings can significantly influence long-term medical and educational management.

The genetics evaluation is somewhat different from the standard medical evaluation. Greater emphasis is placed on pregnancy history and family history. Additionally, most cases of craniofacial disorders are treated as chronic conditions with a need for long-term integrated management, although occasional acute interventions are required (see Table 4–1).

TABLE 4–1 Elements of the Clinical Genetics Evaluation

Major Elements	Contributing Elements
History of present illness	Pregnancy history, complications, exposures
	Birth weight and length
	Perinatal history and complications
	Feeding history
	Identification of other anomalies
Past medical history	Major illnesses
Review of systems	Hospitalizations
	Surgeries
	Growth
	Feeding difficulties
	Other medical problems and illnesses
	Medications
Developmental history	Major milestones
	Developmental interventions
	School performance
	Therapeutic interventions
Family history	Four-generation pedigree
	Consanguinity
	Birth defects
	Infertility
	Pregnancy loss
	Mental retardation
	Major illness
Physical examination	Growth parameters: height, weight, head circumference
	Dysmorphology examination
	Complete physical examination
Medical counseling	Diagnosis
	Prognosis
	Additional testing
	Additional referrals
Laboratory testing and referrals as indicted	Chromosomes
	Other genetic studies as indicated
	Brain imaging studies
	Ophthalmology examination
	EEG
	Developmental evaluation
	Other medical consultations

(continues)

TABLE 4–1 *(continued)*

Major Elements	Contributing Elements
Genetic counseling	Diagnosis
	Prognosis
	Medical interventions
	Developmental interventions
	Recurrence risks
	Prenatal diagnosis
Psychosocial genetic counseling	Family support and education
	Identification of related local support groups
	Identification of national support groups
Follow-up genetics evaluations	Diagnosis
	Medical management
	Genetic counseling
	Family support

Prenatal History

The prenatal history is an essential component of the genetics evaluation. In particular, it is important to determine if the fetus had any exposure to teratogens. A *teratogen* is a chemical or physical agent that can interfere with the normal embryological processes. Teratogens can include viruses, drugs, radiation, or any other outside agent that can result in abnormal fetal development. Therefore, information regarding maternal illnesses during pregnancy, such as infections or diabetes, or medications taken can be helpful in determining a diagnosis.

Several common medications can act as teratogens and cause orofacial and other disorders if taken during pregnancy (Spranger et al., 1982). Some of these medications are still prescribed to pregnant women, even though they are known teratogens with potential risks for the fetus. For example, anticonvulsants such as hydantoin and valproic acid, are still prescribed during pregnancy because it is assumed that their benefit in controlling seizures outweighs

the risks for fetal anomalies. Alcohol is another significant teratogen. In addition to causing developmental disabilities and growth delays, its use has been associated with cleft lip, cleft palate, and Pierre Robin sequence. For certain at-risk individuals, smoking cigarettes can increase the risk for having a child with a cleft lip.

Medical and Feeding History

The medical history of the newborn with a craniofacial disorder is usually straightforward and uncomplicated. Any and all perinatal complications should be noted, especially if there are any respiratory problems, seizures, heart defects, or congenital anomalies. Knowledge of birth weight, length, and head circumference can give valuable clues to diagnosis, since many syndromes are associated with low birth weight or small head size. Other disorders, such as Beckwith-Wiedemann syndrome, are associated with large body size for gestational age. The infant who is small or large for gestational age often has other underlying medical issues that require greater attention. Although any congenital anomaly can give a clue to diagnosis, specific birth defects, which are often associated with genetic conditions, include structural heart anomalies, seizures, eye anomalies, and genital anomalies.

Early feeding problems are common in infants with cleft palate, but they are usually resolved quickly with simple feeding modifications. They become significant if they persist beyond the first week of life. Children who have normal neurological status rarely have prolonged feeding problems, however.

Developmental History

The developmental history is important and should include comprehensive information about early developmental milestones, especially those regarding gross motor and language development. A history of early developmental interventions, especially those related to speech and physical therapy, should be determined. School performance information should obtained, including the history of special therapies, the need for special education, and the results of any developmental or intelligence testing. It should also be noted which grades were repeated if any, and for what reasons.

Family History

What really distinguishes the genetics evaluation from a standard medical evaluation is the comprehensiveness of the family history. A *pedigree* is developed, which is a pictorial representation of family members and their line of descent. This can be used by the geneticist to analyze inheritance, particularly for certain traits or anomalies. It is important to extend the pedigree to four generations, if information is available (Figure 4–1). Any and all medical problems in relatives are noted, with special attention to birth defects, includ-

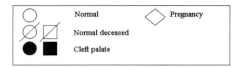

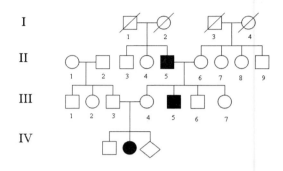

FIGURE 4–1 A pedigree, which is a pictorial representation of family members and their line of descent.

ing cleft lip, cleft palate, and congenital heart defects. Developmental disabilities and mental retardation are recorded, as are miscarriages and early deaths. It can be valuable to identify if the parents are related in any way (this is called *consanguinity*), since this can give insight into rare autosomal recessive disorders.

Physical Examination

The physical examination of the child with a craniofacial disorder is straightforward. As with any examination, attention is given to the growth parameters (weight, height or length, and head circumference). *Microcephaly*, which is a small head size, can indicate poor brain growth or development. Children with microcephaly often have underlying genetic conditions and are at greater risk for developmental disabilities. Poor weight gain may indicate poor feeding or possibly a genetic condition associated with small stature, such as a chromosome disorder.

In addition to the standard physical examination, the clinical geneticist is trained to perform a dysmorphology examination. Here, the physician examines the child for features that may not be familial, but rather, specific to that child and often indicative of specific disorders or syndromes. This may include measurements of the eyes, ears, mouth, nose, and numerous other structures. It may be helpful to identify specific *dermatoglyphics,* which are creases on the hands or changes in the fingerprints, which can give clues to early developmental problems. The neurologic examination is especially helpful, since this may give insight regarding the child's muscle tone, level of function, and degree of social interaction. Photographs are taken of the patient at each visit. It is often helpful to look at earlier photographs that the parents bring to the visit, as well at photographs of other family members. It is also helpful to examine the parents and often siblings for features similar to those of the patient.

Laboratory Studies

After the history is reviewed and the examination is completed, it becomes necessary to determine if any laboratory studies are needed to help make a diagnosis or to confirm clinical suspicions about a diagnosis. Chromosome studies can be helpful in identifying known common and rare syndromes. Usually, children with chromosome anomalies have multiple anomalies; however, there are some conditions in which there may be few specific clinical features. For example, velocardiofacial syndrome, which will be discussed later in greater detail, is associated with cleft palate and/or velopharyngeal insufficiency and may present with very few features. This condition is diagnosed by finding a deletion of the long arm of chromosome 22. Many children with chromosome disorders have rare deletions or duplications, adding to the challenge of genetic counseling.

In addition to the laboratory studies, it may be helpful to obtain X-rays to determine bone maturation or to identify specific skeletal syndromes. An MRI scan of the brain can be helpful in identifying structural anomalies in children with serious developmental disorders, microcephaly, or neurological problems.

Referral to other physicians may be necessary as part of a complete genetics assessment. An ophthalmology examination should be done for all children with cleft palate, since the discovery of nearsightedness is a clue to the diagnosis of Stickler syndrome. All children with suspected heart defects, such as those with velocardiofacial syndrome, should be evaluated by a cardiologist.

Genetic Counseling

After all the above are completed, it is time to sit with the family for genetic counseling. This is usually the longest part of the genetics evaluation, since it is necessary to educate the family regarding issues of heredity and development. Part of the process involves discussion of natural history of the suspected condition and planning for medical interventions. Since many genetic disorders have associated developmental disabilities, it is important to plan for developmental testing; this should include a speech and language evaluation. It is also important to plan for developmental or school interventions, with referrals to community agencies or the school system for special services as deemed necessary.

As part of the genetic counseling process, families often have questions regarding cause of the condition and the recurrence risks for themselves, their child, and for other family members. For many genetic disorders, recurrence risks are known and can be shared with the family.

In addition to discussing recurrence risks, it is also important to identify the prenatal testing for the condition and reproductive options. Amniocentesis can be performed for prenatal identification of chromosome anomalies and specific known genetic disorders using molecular analysis. For some birth defects, such as cleft lip with or without cleft palate, fetal ultrasound studies are the only test available for prenatal diagnosis. Unfortunately, prenatal therapy for most birth defects is not available.

Psychosocial Counseling

Last, the genetics evaluation should include both recognition of the difficulty of having a child with a birth defect and offers of psychosocial support for the family. It is essential to identify community and national resources for the family, such as local, state, and national support groups and meetings. Specific Web sites can be shared with the families to help them to identify educational and support resources.

DYSMORPHOLOGY

Dysmorphology is the study of abnormal shape or form. Any clinical abnormalities that are of significant medical or cosmetic consequence, especially those requiring medical intervention, are considered major anomalies. On the other hand, those abnormal features that have clinical diagnostic implications but are of minimal medical or cosmetic significance and require no intervention are considered minor anomalies. Minor anomalies occur in less than 5% of the population. The diagnosis of many genetic and craniofacial disorders depends upon the identification of specific dysmorphic features—both major and minor anomalies. It is important to understand the underlying pathogenesis of congenital anomalies.

Morphogenesis is the process of embryonic tissue formation. *Dysmorphogenesis* describes errors in this process. These errors result in *dysmorphic* (abnormally formed) features (Spranger et al., 1982). Factors that can cause these abnormalities can be related to external non-genetic forces, usually attributable to abnormal fetal environment, disruption of normal development, or intrinsic genetic or developmental abnormalities.

Malformations and Deformations

Most craniofacial anomalies are malformations. A *malformation* is a morphologic anomaly that results from an intrinsically abnormal developmental process (Spranger et al., 1982) and is due to a genetic etiology. Cleft lip and many cases of cleft palate are examples of malformations. Mental retardation may also be a malformation if it results from a genetic etiology or from a brain malformation. Genetic factors can cause a *dysplasia*, which refers to an abnormal organization of cells into tissues and to the outcome of the process (Spranger et al., 1982), and this leads to the malformation. The *craniosynostoses* are the commonly encountered dysplasias. These usually represent the abnormal development of the cranial skeleton, with other skeletal structures or tissues often being affected as well.

Some birth defects may arise as a result of abnormal mechanical forces on an otherwise normal structure. An anomaly that is caused by physical forces in the fetal environment is called a *deformation* or *deformity*. Deformations usually result in the abnormal shape or form of a completely formed organ or structure (Spranger et al., 1982). Classic examples of fetal deformations include clubfoot and *plagiocephaly* (abnormal skull shape).

Deformations occur when external forces disrupt the development of an intrinsically normal structure. A *disruption* causes a morphologic defect due to an extrinsic breakdown or interference with a normal developmental process (Spranger et al., 1982). Since teratogens interfere with the normal embryological processes, they are often implicated in disruptions. Examples of teratogens that cause birth defects include alcohol, anticonvulsants (such as hydantoin, valproic acid, and carbamazipine), and vitamin A analogs (such as retinoic acid), which can cause ear anomalies, hearing loss, brain anomalies, and congenital heart defects. Physical disruption of normal development can also occur. For example, *amniotic bands* occur when the *amnion*, the membrane surrounding the embryo and fetus, ruptures, leaving strands of tissue floating in the amniotic cavity. These strands can attach to limbs, the head, or other body parts and act as tourniquets, cutting off blood supply to developing structures. This results in amputations of limbs and digits, cleft lip, and encephalocele if the cranium is involved. Even some maternal illnesses can result in disruptions, such as maternal diabetes, which can result in vertebral, heart, and even brain anomalies.

Syndromes, Sequences, and Associations

A *syndrome* is a pattern of multiple anomalies that are pathogenically related, and therefore have a common known or suspected cause (Spranger et al., 1982). Since craniofacial syndromes affect the facial features, they can cause affected individuals to look alike, even when there is no family relationship. An example of this is Down syndrome. Many children with craniofacial conditions have underlying syndromes as the cause of the specific craniofacial anomaly. Recognizing a specific syndrome is important for medical management and is a focus of genetic counseling.

In contrast to a syndrome, a *sequence* is an anomaly or a pattern of multiple anomalies that arise from a single known or presumed prior anomaly or mechanical factor (Spranger et al., 1982). As a result, one anomaly occurs due to the presence of a preexisting anomaly. The best known and perhaps one of the best understood examples is the Pierre Robin sequence. This sequence usually includes a wide, U-shaped cleft palate; *micrognathia*, which is a small jaw or mandible; and *glossoptosis*, which is the posterior displacement of the tongue. The initiating event for this sequence is the interference with normal development of the mandible at 9 weeks gestation. The small mandible then forces the tongue to remain high in the oral cavity, thereby interfering with closure of the velum. After birth, the upper airway may be obstructed, causing life-threatening respiratory distress. A cleft palate is not always seen in Pierre Robin sequence, but is present in the majority of cases.

An *association* is a nonrandom occurrence of a pattern of multiple anomalies in two or more individuals that are not a syndrome or sequence (Spranger et al., 1982). In an association, the pathogenesis is not known, and therefore a genetic etiology cannot be discerned. An association is a diagnosis of exclusion; in other words, a genetic, developmental, or teratogenic etiology must first be excluded before making the diagnosis of an association. Since no genetic etiology can be discerned, the recurrence risks for associations are no greater than the risks for the general population. One example of an association is VATER association. In VATER association, one can see vertebral anomalies; anorectal anomalies (imperforate anus); tracheoesophageal fistula; and renal, radial, and other limb anomalies. In VATER association, the etiology is not known and there appears to be no increased recurrence risk.

GENETICS OF CLEFT LIP (WITH OR WITHOUT CLEFT PALATE)

As has been noted, cleft lip with or without cleft palate (CL/P) is a very common birth defect with a prevalence of 10.48 in 10,000 live births (MMWR, 2006). Boys are affected more frequently than girls by a ratio of 3:2 (Wyszynski et al., 1996). A left-sided cleft lip is more common than a right-sided cleft, and both occur more frequently than bilateral CL/P.

Although most cases of CL/P are isolated— that is, there are no associated syndromes or other birth defects—there still is a substantial underlying genetic pathogenesis. This is supported by the fact that the recurrence risk for CL/P is elevated for individuals with CL/P, for parents of a child with CL/P, and even for siblings of an individual born with CL/P. For parents of a child with CL/P and for the individual who is born with CL/P, the recurrence risk with each future pregnancy is in the range of 3% to 5%—in other words a 30- to 45-fold increase over baseline risk. After a second child is born with CL/P, the recurrence risk rises to 10% to 15%, consistent with an increased genetic contribution. With the birth of a third first-degree relative that is affected, the recurrence risk increases to 25% to 50%, consistent with dominant or recessive inheritance. The recurrence risk is also influenced by the severity of the CL/P. For a child born with bilateral cleft lip and cleft palate, the recurrence risk is 5.6% for a bilateral cleft lip and palate, 4.1% for a unilateral cleft lip and cleft palate, and 2.6% for a unilateral cleft lip without cleft palate (Fraser, 1970).

In some families, there are multiple individuals affected with CL/P. This can represent a more significant underlying genetic influence or predisposition. In these families, the inheritance may appear to be autosomal dominant. One syndrome has been identified with autosomal-dominant inheritance of clefts, and this is the Van der Woude syndrome. In addition to having cleft lip and/or cleft palate, most individuals with this disorder also have bilateral pits in the lower lip. Because this is an autosomal dominate syndrome, the recurrence risk with Van der Woude syndrome is 50%

rather than the typical 3% to 5% when there is a nonsyndromic cleft.

There are significant racial differences in the incidence of CL/P. For African-Americans it is only 1 in 2000, for Caucasian populations the incidence is 1 in 800, and for Asians it is 1 in 500. The incidence of CL/P appears to be highest in Native Americans, with 1 in 300 being affected. Even with these data, recurrence risks are similar among all racial and ethnic groups (Gorlin et al., 2001; Wyszynski et al., 1996).

Although most cases of CL/P are isolated birth defects, a substantial number are caused by underlying genetic syndromes or are part of a multiple congenital anomaly disorder. There are over 219 different syndromes that have CL/P as a component (Winter & Baraitser, 1996). At the Craniofacial Center at Cincinnati Children's Hospital Medical Center, approximately 27% of cases are isolated and 73% are syndromic or associated with other birth defects. A great variety of disorders are associated with CL/P (Table 4–2).

TABLE 4–2 Syndromes Associated with Cleft Lip (with or without Cleft Palate)

Syndrome	Inheritance
Opitz syndrome	Autosomal dominant; X-linked recessive
Trisomy 13	Chromosomal (usually sporadic)
Wolf-Hirshhorn syndrome	Chromosomal (usually sporadic)
Hemifacial microsomia	Sporadic
Amniotic bands	Sporadic
Diabetic embryopathy	Teratogenic (maternal illness)
Fetal alcohol syndrome	Teratogenic
CHARGE association	Sporadic
Van der Woude syndrome	Autosomal dominant
Popliteal pterygium syndrome	Autosomal dominant
Orofaciodigital syndrome Type I (OFD I)	X-linked dominant

The most common birth defects encountered in the Cincinnati Craniofacial Center are congenital heart defects, sensorineural hearing loss, microcephaly, and *colobomas* (a congenital defect of the eye, which often involves a notch of the eyelid margin and usually affects the lower lid or causes defects in the iris and/or retina). Brain anomalies, including brain cysts and seizures, are also common (Table 4–2). Some patients have CL/P with multiple anomalies in what appears to be an underlying syndrome, although a diagnosis cannot be made because the pattern of anomalies is not one that has been previously described. Approximately 40% to 50% of patients seen by a geneticist have syndromes which are either rare or possibly unique. These patients are diagnosed as having *provisionally unique syndromes* until other patients with the same syndromic pattern are identified and reported.

A great deal of research is underway that searches for the genes that cause or predispose to isolated CL/P (Murray, 1995; Stein et al., 1995). Specific genes that are active during early craniofacial development have been implicated in the etiology of CL/P, including transforming growth factor-alpha retinoic acid receptor, transforming growth factor beta, MSX1 (Lidral et al., 1998), and IRF6, the gene responsible for Van der Woude syndrome and isolated CL/P (Zucchero et al., 2004).

SYNDROMES ASSOCIATED WITH CLEFT LIP (WITH OR WITHOUT CLEFT PALATE)

Trisomy 13

Trisomy 13 (Figure 4–2) is a disorder where the baby is born with 47 chromosomes instead of the normal number of 46 due to an extra copy of chromosome 13. The incidence of this

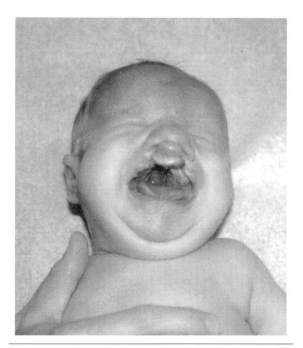

FIGURE 4–2 A newborn male infant with trisomy 13 and bilateral cleft lip and palate. Other typical findings include a broad nose and microphthalmia.

disorder is about 1 in 5000 live births (Jones, 2006). Trisomy 13 is associated with multiple serious life-endangering birth defects, including severe brain anomalies, congenital heart defects, polydactyly (extra fingers and/or toes), spina bifida, and severe eye defects. CL/P is seen in 60% to 80% of cases (Jones, 2006). Many infants with trisomy 13 will have a midline cleft lip and midline facial deformities (Figure 4–3). This usually denotes the presence of *holoprosencephaly*, which is the failure of the brain to divide into the two hemispheres. Other infants have unilateral or bilateral CL/P. This is a lethal disorder, with over 90% of individuals dying before their first birthday, usually from a central nervous system or cardiac event. For this reason most patients with trisomy 13 are rarely seen in a craniofacial center. On rare occasions, a child may survive

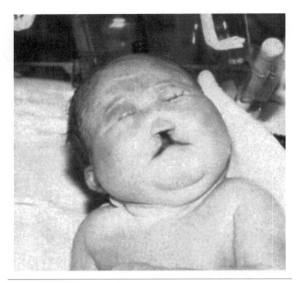

FIGURE 4–3 A newborn female with trisomy 13 and holoprosencephaly. Note the midline cleft lip and cleft palate.

for several years. These long-term survivors are usually severely to profoundly mentally retarded and require a great deal of intervention and supervision. Feeding difficulties are usually seen in these patients, most of whom require *nasogastric feeding* through a tube that is placed through the nose to the stomach.

Wolf-Hirschhorn Syndrome

Wolf-Hirschhorn syndrome is a rare chromosome disorder that is caused by a deletion or missing portion of the short arm of chromosome 4. These patients have a very distinctive facial appearance, likened to a Greek helmet because of the presence of *hypertelorism* (widespaced eyes) and a prominent nasal bridge. CL/P is a common feature. Most patients are very small, grow poorly, and have microcephaly. They may have heart defects, and seizures are very common. Developmental disabilities are universal in this disorder, with most patients having severe to profound mental retardation

(Jones, 2006). Most patients are expected to have significant communication disorders.

Opitz G Syndrome

Opitz G syndrome is a condition that has many names, including hypertelorism-hypospadias syndrome, Opitz BBB syndrome, and Opitz-Frias syndrome. The typical manifestations are hypertelorism, and *hypospadias* in affected males (where the orifice of the penis is proximal to its normal location). Other features which may be seen include imperforate anus, *cryptorchidism* (undescended testes), congenital heart defects, inguinal hernias, and developmental disabilities. One characteristic that may be very serious is that of the presence of a laryngeal cleft. This abnormality in the development of the larynx can lead to swallowing and speech disorders, aspiration pneumonia, and often will require long-term tracheostomy management. CL/P is frequently seen, and the Opitz G syndrome is the second-most common identifiable cause of syndromic CL/P at the Craniofacial Center at Cincinnati Children's Hospital Medical Center. Opitz G syndrome is genetically *heterogeneous*, meaning that there is more than one gene that can cause the same clinical features. A gene for Opitz G syndrome has been found on chromosome 22, which is associated with autosomal dominant inheritance (Robin et al., 1996). A second gene for Opitz G syndrome is on the X chromosome and is associated with X-linked recessive inheritance (Robin et al., 1996). Patients with Opitz syndrome are at risk for mental retardation as well as for learning disabilities.

Those patients with Opitz G syndrome and normal development are not at increased risk for speech and language problems, other than those related to the cleft palate. Those with laryngeal clefts may need additional services related to any problems with voice or feeding.

Individuals with developmental disabilities are not at risk for any specific speech or language disorders, but remain at risk for similar speech and language difficulties encountered in others with developmental problems.

Van der Woude Syndrome

Van der Woude syndrome is among the most common syndromic causes of CL/P. Some reports suggest that this disorder may be responsible for up to 3% of all cases of cleft lip (Murray et al., 1990). This is an autosomal dominant disorder. The gene for this condition is interferon regulatory growth factor 6 (IRF6) which has been mapped to the long arm of chromosome 1 (Kondo et al., 2002). The major manifestations are the presence of pits of the lower lip and cleft lip, cleft palate, or both (Figure 4–4). Approximately 80% of

gene carriers will have lip pits (Jones, 2006). Other features described in Van der Woude syndrome include neonatal teeth and missing teeth. Development is usually normal and speech problems are usually related to issues related to the cleft palate.

Orofaciodigital Syndrome Type I (OFD I)

Orofaciodigital syndrome type I (OFD I) is one of many genetic disorders where a single mutant gene can affect multiple unrelated systems. This phenomenon is called *pleiotropy*. The gene for this condition is on the X chromosome, and the inheritance for this condition is X-linked dominant. Therefore, affected females can have affected daughters. This is presumed to be lethal in males, and this is supported by the paucity of males reported with this condition, the severe phenotype of affected males, and the diminished number of sons born to affected women (Goodship, Platt, Smith, & Burn, 1991). Infants born with this condition often have a midline cleft lip with multiple oral frenulae (oral tissue webs), cleft palate, and tongue abnormalities that include lobulations and notching of the tongue (Figure 4–5). There is hypertelorism with a broad

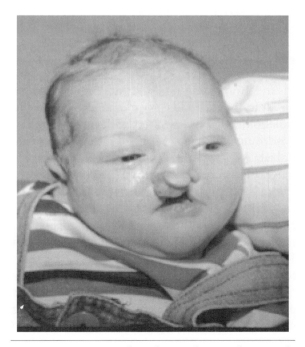

FIGURE 4–4 A male infant with Van der Woude syndrome and bilateral cleft lip and cleft palate. The lip pits of the lower lip are a diagnostic feature of this syndrome.

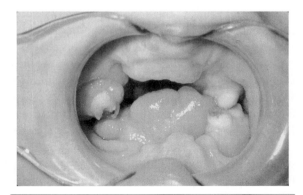

FIGURE 4–5 Lobulations and fissures of the tongue. This is a common characteristic of patients with orofaciodigital syndrome type I.

nose and the hair is coarse and often sparse. The teeth may be abnormal with decreased enamel and often there are missing teeth. Digital anomalies include asymmetric short fingers, variable degrees of *syndactyly* (fusion or webbing of the digits), or *clinodactyly* (curved or bent digits). Renal anomalies may be seen, including the presence of renal cysts. Brain anomalies have been reported, including hydrocephalus and absence of the corpus callosum (Jones, 2006).

Developmental disabilities are commonly seen in this population, especially in the presence of brain anomalies (Jones, 2006). Speech and language difficulties are generally related to the cleft palate and developmental disabilities.

GENETICS OF CLEFT PALATE

Cleft palate (CP) has a prevalence of 6.39 per 10,000 live births (MMWR, 2006). In contrast to CL/P, CP is much more likely to be associated with an underlying syndrome or other congenital anomalies. A prospective analysis of all cases of CP seen in the Craniofacial Center at Cincinnati Children's Hospital shows that approximately 55% of cases are syndromic or associated with additional anomalies. Since it can be difficult to distinguish between the malformation of cleft palate and cleft palate as a disruption of normal development, all cases of cleft palate, including those caused by Pierre Robin sequence, will be discussed as a single group of disorders.

CP is a component of numerous syndromes (Table 4–3). The London Dysmorphology Database, a computerized database of over 3,000 different non-chromosomal disorders, lists 485 syndromes, excluding chromosome disorders, in which CP may be seen, many of which are quite rare (Winter & Baraitser, 2003). Cleft palate may occur as a malformation, but it may also be seen as part of a sequence, particularly Pierre Robin sequence.

TABLE 4–3 Syndromes Associated with Cleft Palate

Syndrome	Inheritance
Stickler syndrome	Autosomal dominant
Velocardiofacial syndrome	Autosomal dominant
Fetal alcohol syndrome	Teratogenic
Fetal hydantoin syndrome	Teratogenic
Kabuki syndrome	Possible autosomal dominant
Van der Woude syndrome	Autosomal dominant
Hemifacial microsomia	Sporadic
CHARGE association	Sporadic
Treacher Collins syndrome	Autosomal dominant
Diabetic embryopathy	Teratogenic

SEQUENCE AND SYNDROMES ASSOCIATED WITH CLEFT PALATE

Pierre Robin Sequence

Pierre Robin sequence is a common cause of cleft palate. This sequence can occur in isolation, but is associated with an underlying syndrome in over 50% of cases (Tomaski, Zalzal, & Saal, 1995). This condition is not a diagnosis unto itself, but rather encompasses the pathogenesis of the cleft palate and, when recognized, gives some critical clues to how a newly diagnosed infant should be managed. As noted earlier in this chapter, infants born with Pierre Robin sequence are born with their tongues positioned posteriorly, often causing blockage of the pharynx and airway, a process called glossoptosis. This affects both breathing and feeding. There are many approaches to airway management in infants with Pierre Robin sequence, and often the treatment must be individualized for each child. The first approach is to place the infant in a prone position. Gravity will then allow the tongue to fall forward, and this can relieve the glossoptosis for some infants. Sometimes it becomes necessary to place a tube in the nose of the infant in such a way that one end of the tube is placed below the region of tongue obstruction and the other end sticks out of the nose. This tube is called a *nasopharyngeal airway*, and some infants with Pierre Robin sequence will require such management until 3 or 4 months of age (Tomaski et al., 1995). Some infants will not respond adequately to such conservative treatments and will require a *tracheostomy*, which is surgical placement of a tube directly in the trachea in order to bypass the area of upper airway obstruction (Tomaski et al., 1995). Usually the tracheostomy will remain in place until after the palate is repaired, usually until 14 months. Unfortunately, the presence of the tracheostomy prevents or interferes with most vocalizations, often leading to further speech issues in addition to those related to the cleft palate.

A newer procedure which has been shown to be successful in selected patients with Pierre Robin sequence with obstructive apnea is mandibular osteogenic distraction (Fritz et al., 2004; Sidman et al., 2001). With this procedure, an *osteotomy* (fracture) is created on both sides of the manible and the two segments of the mandible are separated and pulled apart gradually (over several days or weeks) until there is adequate lengthening of the mandible to prevent *glossoptosis* (blockage of the airway with the tongue). This procedure can be done in early infancy and usually results in normal respiration and feeding. (See Chapter 19 for more information.)

Most infants with Pierre Robin sequence also have early feeding problems, often due to difficulty coordinating breathing, sucking, and swallowing. Some of these infants respond to short periods of feeding with *nasogastric tube*, a tube placed through the nose into the stomach. Some infants will need a tracheostomy in order to feed adequately by mouth. Some infants will require a *gastrostomy* tube (G-tube), which is a tube that is placed directly into the stomach for feeding.

Stickler Syndrome

Stickler syndrome is by far the most common identifiable cause of cleft palate. This is an autosomal dominant disorder with *variable expressivity*; in other words, there is a great deal of variability in the clinical presentation of patients with this disorder. Individuals with this condition may have just a few or all of the clinical features associated with this disorder.

The classic presentation of Stickler syndrome (Figure 4–6) is Pierre Robin sequence, including cleft palate; early onset osteoarthritis, often in early adulthood but sometimes in later childhood; and *myopia* (nearsightedness) (Snead & Yates, 1999; Spranger, 1998). The eye problems associated with Stickler syndrome can be very severe, with most patients having moderate to high myopia. The myopia is usually progressive; patients with Stickler syndrome and myopia are at high risk for retinal detachments, and therefore must be followed closely for any vision changes (Naiglin et al., 1999). In addition, sensorineural hearing loss is very common in Stickler syndrome. Most individuals have hearing loss in the high frequencies, but the loss may occasionally fall within the voice range (Nowak, 1998). Sensorineural hearing loss is also complicated by the conductive hearing loss that can be seen secondary to middle ear effusion that more commonly occurs with a history of cleft palate. For these reasons, individuals with Stickler syndrome should be followed with serial audiograms. Many individuals with Stickler syndrome

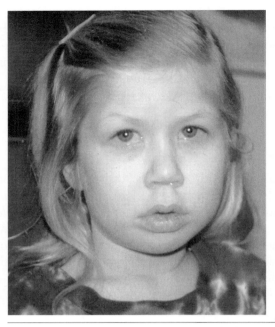 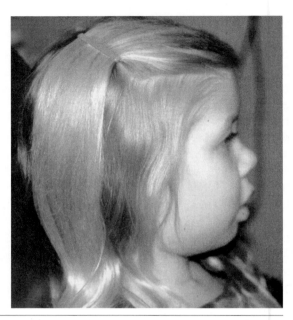

FIGURE 4–6 This girl has the typical findings of Stickler syndrome. Characteristic features are the flat facial profile, small nose, and flat nasal bridge. She was born with Pierre Robin sequence.

also have characteristic facial features including micrognathia in infancy, a flat facial profile, *epicanthal folds* (folds of skin over the medial portion of the openings of the eyes or palpebral fissures), and midface hypoplasia. The nasal bridge is often flat, even in adulthood.

Development is usually normal in Stickler syndrome. These individuals do not appear to be at increased risk for any particular learning disabilities. Speech and language problems are usually related to the cleft palate, hearing loss, and in some instances, problems related to tracheostomy.

Stickler syndrome is a genetically heterogeneous disorder, meaning that mutations of different genes can cause the same clinical features. At least three different genes may cause a form of Stickler syndrome. Stickler syndrome type I is the most common type and is characterized by Pierre Robin sequence, high myopia, and osteoarthritis.

It is associated with mutations in the gene for a particular collagen, collagen 2A1. This is a ubiquitous protein present in the craniofacial skeleton, the eye, and cartilage (Snead & Yates, 1999; Spranger, 1998). Stickler syndrome type II is also characterized by Pierre Robin sequence, high myopia, and osteoarthritis. However, it is associated with mutations in the gene for collagen 11A1 (Richards et al., 1999). Sticker syndrome type III is characterized by the typical facial features, Pierre Robin sequence, and hearing loss. However, ocular manifestations are not present. Stickler syndrome type III is caused by mutations of collagen 11A2, which maps to chromosome 6p21 (Brunner et al., 1994). Clinical testing is available for gene collagen 2A1 and collagen 11A1 mutations, but if negative, these tests do not exclude the other genetic causes of Stickler syndrome. Therefore, diagnosis is generally made by clinical evaluation.

Deletion 22q11.2 Syndrome (Velocardiofacial Syndrome)

Deletion 22q11.2 syndrome is a relatively common condition with an incidence of approximately 1 in 4000 live births (Demczuk & Aurias, 1995; Motzkin, Marion, Goldberg, Shprintzen, & Saenger, 1993). This disorder is caused by an interstitial deletion of chromosome 22q11.2 as demonstrated by fluorescence in situ hybridization (FISH) studies. This is a highly variable condition with many names, including DiGeorge syndrome, conotruncal face syndrome, and velocardiofacial syndrome. More than 180 different associated features have been reported. The most common anomalies are palate anomalies (cleft palate and/or velopharyngeal insufficiency), congenital heart defects, hypocalcemia, immunodeficiency, and dysmorphic facial features (Goldmuntz, 2005; Shprintzen et al., 1978; Vantrappen et al., 1999).

This is a highly variable condition, with over 160 different associated features having been reported. The most common anomalies are palate anomalies (cleft palate and/or velopharyngeal insufficiency), congenital heart defects, and dysmorphic facial features (Shprintzen, 1994, 2000).

The most common characteristic of deletion 22q11.2 is velopharyngeal insufficiency. At the Velopharyngeal Insufficiency Clinic at Cincinnati Children's Hospital, velocardiofacial syndrome is diagnosed in about 20% of individuals with velopharyngeal insufficiency in the absence of overt cleft palate, although some patients will have submucous cleft palate (Dyce et al., 2002). Deletion 22q11.2 syndrome is also the third most common cause of cleft palate. The cleft palate is often associated with Pierre Robin sequence, and therefore, these infants must be monitored for the respiratory and feeding complications.

Approximately 75% of all children with deletion 22q11.2 syndrome followed in the Division of Human Genetics at Children's Hospital Medical Center of Cincinnati are born with congenital heart defects. These are specific defects affect the formation of the aorta, the ventricular septum (the tissue which separates the two lower chambers of the heart), the pulmonary artery, and the pulmonary valve. The group of heart defects seen in velocardiofacial syndrome, characterized by abnormalities of the heart's chambers or blood vessels, are called *cronotruncal defects*, because of their location and development. In the population of children born with conotruncal heart defects, 10% to 15% have a deletion of chromosome 22 and deletion 22q11.2 syndrome (Goldmuntz, 2005; Motzkin et al., 1993).

In addition to the cardiac anomalies, vascular anomalies have also been reported with deletion 22q11.2 syndrome. In particular, tortuosity and medial displacement of the carotid arteries is commonly seen in this population (D'Antonio & Marsh, 1987; Finkelstein et al., 1993; MacKenzie-Stepner et al., 1987; Ross, Witzel, Armstrong, & Thomson, 1996; Witt, Miller, Marsh, Muntz, & Grames, 1998). The pulsation of the carotid arteries can often be viewed on the pharyngeal wall through nasopharyngoscopy. Knowledge of this syndrome and the potential for displacement of the carotid arteries in the posterior pharyngeal wall is important for the surgeon prior to placement of a pharyngeal flap.

The facial characteristics associated with velocardiofacial syndrome include microcephaly, narrow *palpebral fissures* (eye slits), a wide nasal root, a bulbous nose, vertical maxillary excess, a thin upper lip, a long face, micrognathia, and minor auricular anomalies (Dyce et al., 2002) (Figure 4–7 and Figure 4–8). Additional physical features include short stature, usually below the 10th percentile, and long, tapered fingers.

Individuals with deletion 22q11.2 syndrome can have myriad medical problems, and these can include kidney or urinary tract anomalies

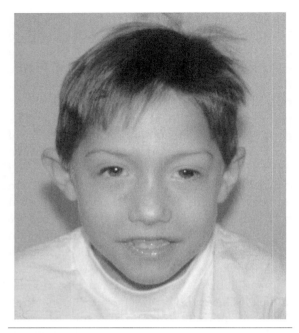

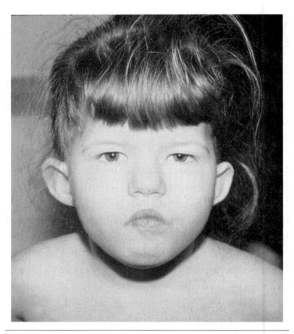

FIGURE 4–7 A boy with velocardiofacial syndrome. Note the narrow face and broad nasal tip.

FIGURE 4–8 A girl with velocardiofacial syndrome. She has a long oval face, broad nasal tip, and small mouth.

(Ryan et al., 1997), obesity, and failure to thrive in infancy. A subgroup of patients will have what is termed the DiGeorge sequence (Stevens, Carey, & Shigeoka, 1990). This condition is characterized by not only the conotruncal heart defects, but also hypoplasia or absence of the thymus (the organ in the chest which is the source of T-lymphocytes), and absence or hypoplasia of the parathyroid glands (glands responsible for making parathyroid hormone, which helps regulate calcium levels in the blood). These individuals can have seizures from hypocalcemia and serious infections from abnormal T-lymphocyte function and abnormal immune response (Motzkin et al., 1993; Ryan et al., 1997).

Chronic recurrent otitis media is also a common problem. One study demonstrated that chronic middle ear problems were seen in approximately 50% of patients with deletion 22q11.2 syndrome (Dyce et al., 2002). Airway problems may also be seen in infancy, occa-

sionally caused by presence of narrow airway and in some cases laryngotracheal anomalies, including laryngeal web (Dyce, 2002).

Infants with velocardiofacial syndrome often demonstrate hypotonia, and oral apraxia is often evident, even in early infancy. Most of these children will have problems with sucking because of poor oral-motor skills and abnormal palate function. Later feeding problems include difficulty with chewing and swallowing. Drooling is often noted due to difficulty in handling oral secretions (Rommel et al., 1999). When speech develops, articulation disorders are common and are caused by a combination of velopharyngeal insufficiency or incompetence, and oral-motor dysfunction. If a pharyngoplasty is needed for velopharyngeal dysfunction, the prognosis for total correction is somewhat guarded due to the pharyngeal hypotonia and oral-motor problems.

Developmental disabilities are characteristic for velocardiofacial syndrome. Most individuals with this disorder will have some degree of learning problems or mental retardation (Kok & Solman, 1995; Swillen et al., 1997). Intelligence tends to be in the low-to-normal range (Golding-Kushner, Weller, & Shprintzen, 1985), although mild to moderate mental retardation is relatively common (Ryan et al., 1997). Language and learning disabilities are also common, with most patients having difficulty with reading comprehension and extemporaneous speech (Golding-Kushner et al., 1985). Educational goals must therefore focus on the development of language and communication skills.

Specific abnormalities of behavior and socialization are common with velocardiofacial syndrome (Swillen et al., 1997). In addition, psychiatric problems are seen in many of these individuals. There is an increased incidence of schizophrenia and schizo-affective disorders, often beginning in the second decade (Heineman-de Boer, Van Haelst, Cordia-de Haan, & Beemer, 1999; Karayiorgou et al., 1995). In addition, there is an increased incidence of depression, usually related to bipolar illness. Exactly how these conditions are related to velocardiofacial syndrome has yet to be determined.

Velocardiofacial syndrome has been shown to be associated with a 22q11 deletion, which is a deletion of part of band 11 on the long arm of chromosome 22. This is determined through *fluorescent in situ hybridization* (FISH) *techniques*. Although most individuals with velocardiofacial syndrome demonstrate this deletion, approximately 10% of patients with velocardiofacial syndrome will not have a demonstrable deletion on chromosome 22. It is assumed that these individuals have a mutation or genetic rearrangement of the critical gene or genes in the velocardiofacial syndrome region on chromosome 22 that cannot be detected by routine established diagnostic tests. Most identified cases represent new deletions with no prior family history, but in between 10% and 20% of cases, one of the parents will have a deletion of chromosome 22 and will have phenotypic features of velocardiofacial syndrome.

The diagnosis of velocardiofacial syndrome is usually straightforward. However, any child with a cleft palate or velopharyngeal insufficiency and a congenital heart defect should be evaluated for this disorder. Not all patients will have the classic presentation, and some patients may present with just velopharyngeal insufficiency and learning disabilities. Also, any child with a conotruncal heart defect should be tested for a deletion on chromosome 22 as well (Goldmuntz, 2005; Ryan et al., 1997).

Fetal Alcohol Syndrome (FAS)

The efforts of Jones and colleagues demonstrated the teratogenic potential of alcohol, and they described the specific syndromic characteristics associated with in utero alcohol exposure (Jones & Smith, 1973). These investigators recognized that alcohol exposure in utero was a common occurrence and that the effects could be very severe and debilitating for the fetus. This condition, called fetal alcohol syndrome, is caused by in utero exposure to significant amounts of alcohol during gestation, with the most sensitive period of exposure being the first trimester of pregnancy, although significant exposure at any time during pregnancy can have adverse effects. It is generally accepted that women who take two alcoholic drinks daily are at risk for having babies with smaller birth size; however, with the intake of between four and six drinks per day, many additional clinical features become apparent (Jones, 2006).

Fetal alcohol syndrome is one of the more common causes of Pierre Robin sequence and cleft palate. It can also be associated with cleft lip, with or without cleft palate. The most striking features of children with fetal alcohol syndrome are the small size at birth, microcephaly, short *palpebral fissures* (eye slits), short nose, flat philtrum, and thin upper lip. Congenital heart defects are relatively common, with the most common anomalies being *ventricular septal defect* (VSD), which is discontinuity of tissue that separates the lower chambers of the heart, and *atrial septal defect* (ASD), which is discontinuity in the tissue that separates the upper chambers of the heart.

Fetal alcohol syndrome is a common cause of mental retardation (Jones, 1986). The average intelligence quotient in this population has been estimated to be 63 (Jones, 2006). In addition to developmental disabilities, older children with fetal alcohol syndrome often have severe behavior problems including hyperactivity, distractibility, poor judgment, and difficulty interpreting social cues (Jones, 2006; Streissguth et al., 1991).

Genetics of Craniosynostosis

Craniosynostosis is the premature fusion of one or more cranial sutures. Although not as common as cleft lip or cleft palate, it is nonetheless a relatively common condition, with an incidence of 1 in 2000 to 1 in 2500 live births (Hunter & Rudd, 1976, 1977). Most cases are isolated, limited to the fusion of a single suture with no other associated anomalies, and these cases are usually sporadic without a genetic etiology. When craniosynostosis involves more than one suture or if there are associated congenital anomalies, the likelihood that there is an underlying syndrome or genetic etiology is greatly increased.

Craniosynostosis is a feature in over 150 syndromes (Cohen, 1979, 1991; Gorlin et al., 2001). Craniosynostosis syndromes include involvement of multiple cranial sutures and additional clinical features (Table 4–4). Most are inherited in an autosomal dominant manner. Recently, the genes that cause the common craniosynostosis syndromes have been identified. Most fall within the category of what are called the fibroblast growth factor receptors. These receptors, which are located on the cell surface, bind the fibroblast growth factors, which help to regulate cell proliferation, differentiation, and migration (Robin, 1999; Wilkie, 1997).

The premature fusion of the cranial suture lines in craniosynostosis causes the skull to grow abnormally, resulting in a misshapened head. The resultant distortion of the skull depends on the sutures that are involved. If the sagittal suture is involved, the lateral growth of the skull will be prevented. Therefore, the growth occurs in an anterior-posterior (AP) direction, resulting in frontal bossing and *scaphacephaly,* where the skull is oblong from front to back. On the other hand, if the coronal suture is involved, the skull cannot expand in the AP direction, causing *brachycephaly,* which is a short skull. When multiple sutures are involved, there may be asymmetry of the skull, called *plagiocephaly. Dolichocephaly* is the long, narrow skull that is often seen with prematurity, and typically resolves on its own.

Children with isolated craniosynostosis have no associated malformations, and have an excellent prognosis with regard to health, growth, and neurodevelopment. The prognosis for children who have a craniosynostosis syndrome is more guarded and depends upon the specific syndrome diagnosed. If brain development is impaired by the cranium or there is an increase in intracranial pressure (ICP), mental retardation can result. Craniotomy and skull reshaping procedures are often required, both for normal brain development and function, and also to improve the aesthetics.

TABLE 4–4 Common Craniosynostosis Syndromes[1]

Syndrome	Craniofacial Features	Gene (Chromosome)	Additional Anomalies
Crouzon syndrome	Coronal synostosis	FGFR2 (10q26)	Occasional hydrocephalus
	Shallow orbits		Occasional hearing loss
	Hypertelorism		
	Exophthalmos		
Apert syndrome	Coronal synostosis	FGFR2 (10q26)	Syndactyly
	Hypertelorism		Mental retardation
	Beaked nose		
	Occasional cleft palate		
	Occasional upper airway obstruction		
Pfeiffer syndrome	Coronal synostosis	FGFR1 (8p11.2- p11.1)	Broad toes and thumbs
	Cloverleaf skull (type 2)	FGFR2 (10q26)	Mild syndactyly
	Shallow orbits		Hearing loss
	Hypertelorism		Mental retardation (type 2 and type 3)
	Exophthalmos		Tracheal anomalies (type 2 and type 3)
Saethre-Chotzen syndrome	Coronal synostosis	TWIST gene (7p21)	Broad thumbs and great toes
	Hypertelorism		Mild syndactyly
	Ptosis		Occasional congenital heart defect
	Down-slanting palpebral fissures		
	Dysplastic ears		
	Occasional cleft palate		

[1] All of the listed disorders are autosomal dominant.

CRANIOSYNOSTOSIS SYNDROMES

Saethre-Chotzen Syndrome

Saethre-Chotzen syndrome (Figure 4–9) is probably the most common craniosynostosis syndrome, although many individuals with this disorder may not have craniosynostosis. The clinical features can be quite variable, but the most common presenting features are coronal synostosis; *ptosis* or drooping of the eyelids; midface hypoplasia; mild external ear anomalies; and mild digit anomalies, including mild syndactyly, mild brachydactyly or short fingers—and in some individuals, broad thumbs and/or great toes with medial deviation of the great toes. A small number of individuals will have cleft palate or submucous cleft palate. Recently, it has been postulated that more

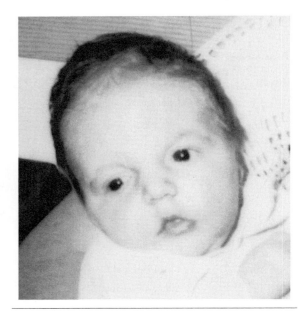

FIGURE 4–9 This male infant has Saethre-Chotzen syndrome. He has a depressed nasal bridge and down-slanting palpebral fissures.

severely affected individuals, especially those with developmental disabilities and/or cleft palate, have a complete or partial deletion of the TWIST gene, whereas more mildly affected individuals have point mutations of the gene (mutations involving one or a limited number of nucleotides) (Johnson et al., 1998; Robin, 1999).

Intelligence in Saethre-Chotzen syndrome is usually normal, although there is an increased risk for developmental disabilities, including mental retardation. Most patients do not have significant speech or language difficulties, unless there are extenuating factors including cleft palate or mental retardation.

Crouzon Syndrome

Crouzon syndrome (Figure 4–10) is another common craniosynostosis syndrome. The major clinical characteristics are limited to

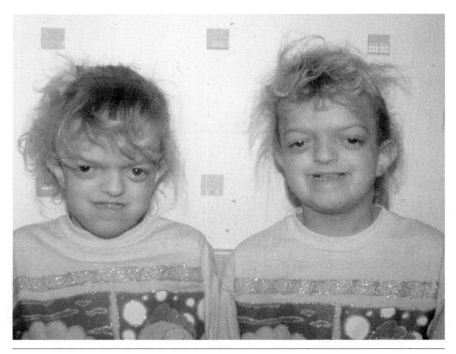

FIGURE 4–10 Monozygotic (identical) twin girls with Crouzon syndrome. They have shallow orbits with prominent eyes.

cranial and facial involvement. The craniosynostosis in Crouzon syndrome usually involves the coronal sutures. The orbits are shallow, causing *exophthalmos*, or protrusion of the eyeballs. There is also hypertelorism, strabismus, and midface hypoplasia. Development is usually normal, but there is a higher incidence of mental retardation. Developmental disabilities can be related to brain anomalies identified in some patients, including hydrocephalus and agenesis of the corpus callosum. Cleft palate and submucous cleft palate may be seen in some patients, but these are uncommon findings (Jones, 2006; Robin, 1999).

Apert Syndrome

Individuals with Apert syndrome (Figure 4–11) often look remarkably like patients with Crouzon syndrome, although the exophthalmos tends to be less pronounced, despite similar midface hypoplasia (Cohen & Kreiborg, 1992; Jones, 2006).

The nose is beaked, and strabismus is frequently seen. The palate is often narrow and cleft palate is seen more frequently in Apert syndrome than in Crouzon syndrome. The upper nasal and pharyngeal airway may be narrowed, causing respiratory obstruction and hyponasality in some patients. Choanal stenosis may also be present, causing significant upper airway obstruction. The main distinguishing feature between these syndromes, however, is that individuals with Apert syndrome have syndactyly, which is often mitten-like webbing of the fingers of the fingers and toes. The webbing may be of soft tissue, but it often includes the bone as well.

Most patients with Apert syndrome have some degree of developmental disability. Although normal intelligence is found in some patients, many others have mild to moderate mental retardation. Speech disorders are common, including articulation disorders due to the small oral cavity and narrow palate, and hyponasality secondary to upper airway obstruction.

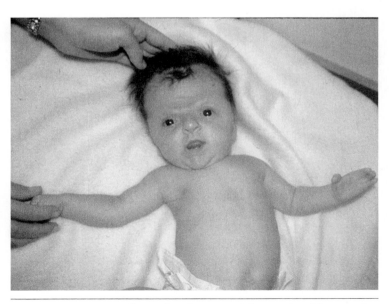

FIGURE 4–11 An infant girl with Apert syndrome. In addition to her craniosynostosis, she has syndactyly (webbing) of the fingers and toes of all four extremities.

Pfeiffer Syndrome

Pfeiffer syndrome (Figure 4–12) is a genetically heterogeneous autosomal dominant craniosynostosis syndrome, with mutations being identified in two different fibroblast growth factor receptor genes. Most are new mutations, especially those with Pfieffer syndrome type 2 or type 3. The severity and degree of craniofacial involvement and associated anomalies depends upon the specific gene mutation (Plomp et al., 1998).

In most patients with classic Pfeiffer syndrome, or Pfieffer syndrome type 1, the common craniofacial features are coronal craniosynostosis, midface hypoplasia, shallow orbits with exophthalmos, and hypertelorism (Figure 4–12A). Limb anomalies consist of broad thumbs and great toes with variable degrees of mild syndactyly (Figure 4–12B). Hearing loss has also been reported (Robin, 1999). Cleft palate is seen on rare occasions and there is no association with cleft lip. Intelligence is usually normal.

In Pfeiffer syndrome type 2 and type 3, the clinical features are much more pronounced and severe. The craniosynostosis may involve multiple sutures, giving the skull a cloverleaf appearance, hence the term cloverleaf skull. The exophthalmos is more pronounced and the midface hypoplasia more severe. Hearing loss is common. There can be severe airway compromise from tracheal anomalies and upper airway stenosis (Stone, Trevenen, Mitchell, & Rudd, 1990). Mental retardation is seen in almost all children with Pfeiffer syndrome type 2 and type 3, and is often severe. Death in early

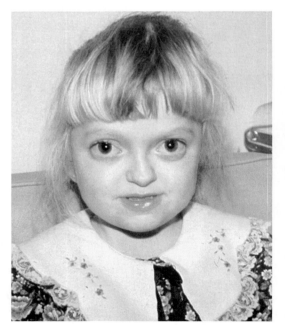

A

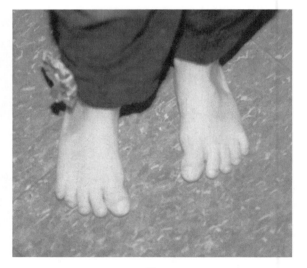

B

FIGURE 4–12 (A and B)   A girl with Pfeiffer syndrome. A. She has shallow orbits similar to those seen in Crouzon syndrome. B. She also has broad and deviated great toes.

childhood is common, especially in Pfeiffer syndrome type 2, which is more likely to be associated with cloverleaf skull and more serious upper airway obstruction.

MISCELLANEOUS SYNDROMES

Hemifacial Microsomia (Oculoauriculovertebral Dysplasia)

Hemifacial microsomia (Figure 4–13) is a condition with numerous names, most of which are descriptive. It is also known as oculoauriculovertebral dysplasia, facioauriculovertebral spectrum, and there is a variant called the Goldenhar syndrome. This is a relatively common multiple anomaly disorder with a birth incidence of 1 in 3000 to 5000 live births (Jones, 2006). Most cases appear to be sporadic, but there are rare reports of more than one affected first-degree family member. Most cases have unilateral involvement, but in 30% of the cases, bilateral hemifacial microsomia can be demonstrated (Gorlin et al., 2006). The right side tends to be affected more often than the left side and boys are affected more frequently than girls (Jones, 2006).

The primary features of hemifacial microsomia include facial asymmetry due to unilateral hypoplasia. This causes malar, maxillary, and especially mandibular hypoplasia on the affected side. With the mandibular involvement, there is hypoplasia of the mandibular ramus and often dysplasia or aplasia of the temporomandibular joint, limiting the excursion of the mandible and the opening of the mouth. There can also be weakness of cranial nerve VII on the affected side. The craniofacial involvement in hemifacial microsomia is often bilateral; however, the involvement of the

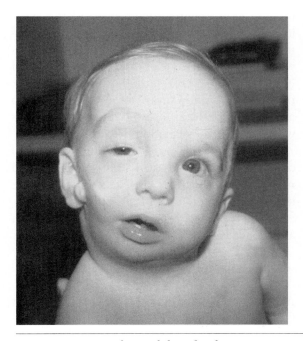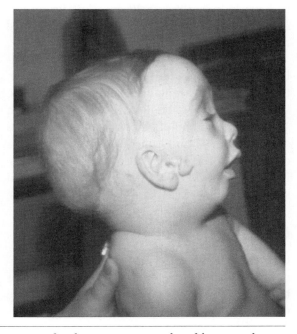

FIGURE 4–13 A boy with hemifacial microsomia. He has severe facial asymmetry exacerbated by cervical spine abnormalities and fusion. The lateral view shows severe dysplasia of the right ear and an ear tag.

facial skeleton, soft tissues and ears is usually more severe on one side. Evaluating both sides is essential.

There is usually ear involvement on the affected side, ranging from mild aplasia to *anotia* with absence of the external auditory canal. Anomalies of the eyes are often noted, including *colobomas* (notches) of the upper eyelid, *epibulbar lipodermoids* (fatty cysts on the eyeball, distinguishing the Goldenhar syndrome), colobomas of the retina, and *microphthalmia* (small eyes) (Figure 4–13).

Brain anomalies can be seen in this population and include hydrocephalus, *encephaloceles*, absence of the corpus callosum, and cell migration abnormalities. Vertebral anomalies are found in about 15% of cases, and usually involve the cervical vertebrae, although any segment of the spine may be affected. Heart defects also can be found with this syndrome and can be very serious, leading to significant morbidity. Some patients have also been found to have kidney abnormalities. Cleft lip and/or cleft palate is seen in about 15% of hemifacial microsomia patients.

Although most patients have normal intelligence, learning disabilities are common in this population. Mental retardation may also be seen, and is more likely in those patients with structural brain anomalies. Speech disorders are common, and contributing factors are orofacial clefts, cranial nerve VII weakness, inability to completely open the mouth, and in some cases, cleft palate or unilateral velar paresis.

CHARGE Syndrome

CHARGE syndrome is a genetically heterogeneous multiple congenital anomaly disorder that that is caused by a mutation of the gene chromodomain helicase DNA-binding protein-7 (CHD7) on chromosome 8 and mutations of the semaphorin-3E gene (SEMA3E) on chromosome 7 (Lalani et al., 2006; Vissers et al., 2004). CHARGE is an acronym for **c**oloboma, **h**eart defect, choanal **a**tresia, **r**etarded growth and/or development, **g**enitourinary anomalies, and **e**ar anomalies and/or deafness. In order for an individual to have CHARGE association, at least four of the six clinical features should be present, and at least one of these features must be the presence of coloboma and/or choanal atresia (Pagon, Graham, Zonana, & Yong, 1981).

The colobomas usually affect the retina of the eye, and many children have significant visual impairment as a result. The heart defects are often very serious and life threatening. Genitourinary anomalies are usually related to *micropenis* (small penis) or *cryptorchidism* (undescended testicles) in males. These may be related to pituitary abnormalities which may also be manifested in adolescence as delayed or absent puberty and amenorreha. External ear anomalies and deafness are very common as well. Brain anomalies are very common, and include abnormalities or absence of the pituitary gland, which will affect growth and genitourinary development. Although some individuals with CHARGE association will have normal intelligence, mental retardation is seen in most patients and is often severe to profound. Cleft lip and/or cleft palate is also seen in many patients with CHARGE association (Blake et al., 1998).

Speech and language management will depend upon the identification of associated medical complications. Speech and language disorders related to clefts are often complicated by the coexistence of mental retardation and deafness.

Treacher Collins Syndrome

Although not a common disorder, Treacher Collins syndrome (Figure 4–14) is an autosomal dominant condition with variable expressivity. This variability can be seen within a

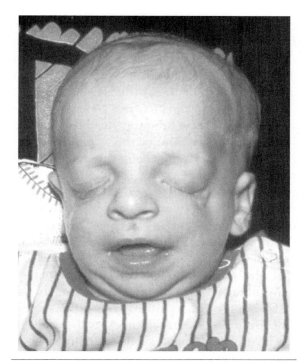

FIGURE 4–14 A male with Treacher Collins syndrome. He has micrognathia, severe hypoplasia of the zygomatic arches, and secondary low-set ears and down-slanting palpebral fissures.

family, making it difficult to predict outcome for offspring of affected individuals. The gene which causes Treacher Collins syndrome has been mapped to the long arm of chromosome 5 (5q32-q33.3) (Dixon et al., 1992).

The classic features of Treacher Collins syndrome include downward slanting palpebral fissures, colobomas of the lower eyelids, microtia or small dysplastic ears, hypoplastic zygomatic arches, and macrostomia or large mouth. Conductive hearing loss is extremely common because of frequent middle ear anomalies. There is also significant malar hypoplasia (Dixon, 1995). Treacher Collins syndrome usually includes Pierre Robin sequence, although most individuals with this condition do not have clefts, despite having pronounced micrognathia.

Intelligence is usually normal in this population. Speech disorders are common because of the hearing loss and micrognathia. The speech disorders are exacerbated when a cleft palate is present and there is also airway obstruction.

Beckwith-Wiedemann Syndrome

Beckwith-Wiedemann syndrome (Figure 4–15) is a genetic disorder that has as its primary features prenatal and postnatal overgrowth, neonatal *hypoglycemia* (or low blood sugar), macroglossia (or large tongue), and coarse facial features (Cohen, 1998). Often patients with Beckwith-Wiedemann syndrome have hemihypertrophy (Hoyme et al., 1998), where one side of the body grows faster than

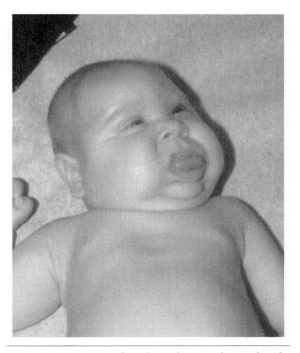

FIGURE 4–15 A female infant with Beckwith-Wiedemann syndrome. Note the macroglossia (large tongue), which can cause respiratory problems, feeding difficulties, and speech problems.

the other side, leading to asymmetry. Some individuals with this condition are also born with umbilical hernia or even an *omphalocele*, where part of the intestine is outside of the abdomen in the region of the umbilical cord. As noted, children with Beckwith-Wiedemann syndrome are usually born large for gestational age, some may even be more than 10 pounds at birth. They also are at risk for severe hypoglycemia, which can be life threatening. If blood sugar is low enough, it can result in seizures. Growth tends to be somewhat accelerated during early childhood. One very helpful diagnostic feature is the presence of macroglossia (Cohen, 1998). The tongue is sometimes large enough to interfere with normal breathing, leading to a Pierre Robin sequence (Figure 4–15). Rarely, a child with Beckwith-Wiedemann syndrome will have a cleft palate.

Children with Beckwith-Wiedemann syndrome have a significant risk of developing *Wilms tumor*, a malignant tumor of the kidney, and malignant tumors in the abdomen, including a liver tumor called *hepatoblastoma* (DeBaun, Siegel, & Choyke, 1998; DeBaun & Tucker, 1998; Hoyme et al., 1998; Schneid et al., 1997). The risk for developing such tumors is between 5% and 8%, with most cases occurring before 8 years. For this reason, each child with Beckwith-Wiedemann syndrome is closely followed for the development of these tumors with renal and abdominal ultrasound examinations at least every four months.

The genetic etiology of Beckwith-Wiedemann syndrome appears to be complex. This is a genetically heterogeneous disorder, although the genes that are involved in this disorder are responsible for imprinting and are located on the short arm of chromosome 11. Some children have been found to have a duplication of a portion of chromosome 11 (11p15.5) as the cause of their Beckwith-Wiedemann syndrome. For some individuals, the disorder is caused by inheriting both copies of chromosome 11 from the father (paternal disomy) with no maternal chromosome 11 contribution. In approximately 10% to 15% of cases, this is an autosomal dominant disorder (Cohen, 1998). There are growth regulatory genes on chromosome 11p15 that are influenced by genomic *imprinting*, where the expression of a particular gene depends on whether it was inherited maternally or paternally. There are two clusters of imprinted genes on the short arm of chromosome 11, each with its own imprinting center, called IC1 and IC2 (Cytrynbaum et al., 2005). In the first imprinting center, two genes are found; IGF2 is expressed on the paternally inherited chromosome and H19 on the maternally inherited chromosome. Expression of the IGF2 gene on the paternally and the maternally inherited chromosomes will result in Beckwith-Wiedemann syndrome. Similarly, in imprinting center 2, there are several genes, of which two have been implicated in Beckwith-Wiedemann syndrome: KCNQ10T1 and CKDN1C. Loss of maternal methylation of IC2 with expression of KCNQ10T1 in both parentally inherited alleles is seen in 50% to 60% of sporadic Beckwith-Wiedemann syndrome patients (Cooper et al., 2005).

Development in Beckwith-Wiedemann syndrome is usually normal, although children with duplication of chromosome 11p15.5 usually have developmental delays or mental retardation. There is also a risk for developmental disabilities if neonatal hypoglycemia is prolonged. The large tongue may also contribute to obstructive respiratory problems, eating disorders, and abnormal cranial and dental growth and development, including *prognathism* (having a large mandible). For these reasons, some children with Beckwith-Wiedemann syndrome require surgical reduction of the tongue.

Language disorders may be associated with cognitive impairment and speech is usually affected by the macroglossia. Resonance can be affected not only by the history of cleft palate, but also by the size of the tongue, which can block the transmission of acoustic energy in the oral cavity.

SUMMARY

Patients who present with craniofacial anomalies should be seen for a complete genetics evaluation. This is important so that an appropriate diagnosis can be made and recurrence risks can be determined. Identification of a genetic syndrome is also important because it allows the physician to counsel the family regarding the natural course of the disorder and the potential medical, developmental, and communication problems that are associated with the syndrome. Armed with this knowledge, the family, in collaboration with the medical professionals from the craniofacial team, can plan appropriate medical, surgical, therapeutic, and educational interventions in order to achieve the best possible outcome.

FOR REVIEW, DISCUSSION, AND CRITICAL THINKING

1. Why is a genetics evaluation recommended for children born with cleft lip and palate? Why is it particularly important for children born with cleft palate only (without cleft lip)?

2. What is the purpose of the genetics evaluation and how can the results affect the management of the child?

3. Describe the components of a genetics evaluation and why each component is important.

4. What is the difference between a deformation and malformation? What is the difference between a syndrome, sequence, and association? Describe the series of events that result in Pierre Robin sequence.

5. What is the approximate prevalence of cleft lip and palate? How does it vary with racial groups?

6. What syndromes are particularly associated with cleft lip?

7. What does the presence of bilateral lip pits indicate and why is it important to identify the lip pits?

8. Describe some syndromes that are associated with cleft palate.

9. What is the difference between Pierre Robin sequence and Stickler syndrome? Which is more serious and why?

10. What are the characteristics of velocardiofacial syndrome? Why do you think identification of this syndrome often occurs in the school years, rather than in infancy?

11. What is craniosynostosis and what are some syndromes that include this as a characteristic? What are potential functional problems with craniosynostosis syndromes?

REFERENCES

Blake, K. D., Davenport, S. L., Hall, B. D., Hefner, M. A., Pagon, R. A., Williams, M. S., Lin, A. E., & Graham, J. M., Jr. (1998). CHARGE association: An update and review for the primary pediatrician. *Clinical Pediatrics, 37*(3), 159–173.

Brunner, H. G., van Beersum, S. E. C., Warman, M. L., Olsen, B. R., Ropers, H. H., & Mariman, E. C. M. (1994). A Stickler syndrome gene is linked to chromosome 6 near the COL11A2 gene. *Human Molecular Genetics, 3*(9), 1561–1564.

Cohen, M. M., Jr. (1979). Craniosynostosis and syndromes with craniosynostosis: Incidence, genetics, penetrance, variability, and new syndrome updating. *Birth Defects: Original Article Series, 15*(5B), 13–63.

Cohen, M. M., Jr. (1991). Etiopathogenesis of craniosynostosis. *Neurosurgery Clinics of North America, 2*(3), 507–513.

Cohen, M. M., Jr., & Kreiborg, S. (1992). Upper and lower airway compromise in the Apert syndrome. *American Journal of Medical Genetics, 44*(1), 90–93.

Cooper, W. N., Luharia, A., Evans, G. A., Raza, H., Haire, A. C., Grundy, R., Bowdin, S. C., Riccio, A., Sebastio, G., Bliek, J., Schofield, P. N., Reik, W., Macdonald, F., & Maher, E. R. (2005). Molecular subtypes and phenotypic expression of Beckwith-Wiedemann syndrome. *European Journal of Human Genetics, 13*(9), 1025–1032.

Cytrynbaum, C. S., Smith, A. C., Rubin, T., & Weksberg, R. (2005). Advances in overgrowth syndromes: Clinical classification to molecular delineation in Sotos syndrome and Beckwith-Wiedemann syndrome. *Current Opinion in Pediatrics, 17*(6), 740–746.

D'Antonio, L. D., & Marsh, J. L. (1987). Abnormal carotid arteries in the velocardiofacial syndrome. *Plastic and Reconstructive Surgery, 80*(3), 471–472.

°Demczuk, S., & Aurias, A. (1995). DiGeorge syndrome and related syndromes associated with 22q11.2 deletions: A review. *Annals of Genetics, 38*(2), 59–76.

Dixon, M. J. (1995). Treacher Collins syndrome. *Journal of Medical Genetics, 32*(10), 806–808.

Dixon, M. J., Dixon, J., Raskova, D., Le Beau, M. M., Williamson, R., Klinger, K., & Landes, G. M. (1992). Genetic and physical mapping of the Treacher Collins syndrome locus: Refinement of the localization to chromosome 5q32-33.2. *Human Molecular Genetics, 1*(4), 249–253.

Dyce, O., McDonald-McGinn, D., Kirschner, R. E., Zackai, E., Young, K., & Jacobs, I. N. (2002). Otolaryngologic manifestations of the 22q11.1 deletion syndrome. *Archives of Otolaryngology–Head & Neck Surgery, 128*(12), 1408–1412.

Finkelstein, Y., Zohar, Y., Nachmani, A., Talmi, Y. P., Lerner, M. A., Hauben, D. J., et al. (1993). The otolaryngologist and the patient with velocardiofacial syndrome. *Archives of Otolaryngology—Head & Neck Surgery, 119*(5), 563–569.

Fraser, F. C. (1970). The genetics of cleft lip and cleft palate. *American Journal of Human Genetics, 22*(3), 336–352.

Fritz, M. A., & Sidman, J. D. (2004). Distraction osteogenesis of the mandible. *Current Opinion in Otolaryngology & Head & Neck Surgery, 12*(6), 513–518.

Golding-Kushner, K. J., Weller, G., & Shprintzen, R. J. (1985). Velocardiofacial syndrome: Language and psychological profiles. *Journal of Craniofacial Genetics & Developmental Biology, 5*(3), 259–266.

Goldmuntz, E. (2005). DiGeorge syndrome: New insights. *Clinics in Perinatology, 32*(4), 963–978.

Goodship, J., Platt, J., Smith, R., & Burn, J. (1991). A male with type I orofaciodigital syndrome. *Journal of Medical Genetics, 28*(10), 691–694.

Gorlin, R., Cohen, M. J., & Hennekam, R. C. M. (2001). *Syndromes of the head and neck* (4th ed.). New York: Oxford University Press.

Heineman-de Boer, J. A., Van Haelst, M. J., Cordia-de Haan, M., & Beemer, F. A. (1999). Behavior problems and personality aspects of 40 children with velocardiofacial syndrome. *Genetic Counseling, 10*(1), 89–93.

Hunter, A. G., & Rudd, N. L. (1976). Craniosynostosis. I. Sagittal synostosis: Its genetics and associated clinical findings in 214 patients who lacked involvement of the coronal suture(s). *Teratology, 14*(2), 185–193.

Hunter, A. G., & Rudd, N. L. (1977). Craniosynostosis. II. Coronal synostosis: Its familial characteristics and associated clinical findings in 109 patients lacking bilateral polysyndactyly or syndactyly. *Teratology, 15*(3), 301–309.

Johnson, D., Horsley, S. W., Moloney, D. M., Oldridge, M., Twigg, S. R., Walsh, S., Barrow, M., Njolstad, P. R., Kunz, J., Ashworth, G. J., Wall, S. A., Kearney, L., & Wilkie, A. O. (1998). A comprehensive screen for TWIST mutations in patients with craniosynostosis identifies a new micro-deletion syndrome of chromosome band 7p21.1 [see Comments]. *American Journal of Human Genetics, 63*(5), 1282–1293.

Jones, K. L. (1997). *Smith's Recognizable Patterns of Human Malformation* (5th ed.). Philadelphia: W. B. Saunders Company.

Jones, K. L. (2006). *Smith's recognizable patterns of human malformation* (5th ed.). Philadelphia: Elsevier, Inc.

Jones, K. L., & Smith, D. W. (1973). Recognition of the fetal alcohol syndrome in early infancy. *Lancet, 2*(7836), 999–1001.

Karayiorgou, M., Morris, M. A., Morrow, B., Shprintzen, R. J., Goldberg, R., Borrow, J., Gos, A., Nestadt, G., Wolyniec, P. S., Lasseter, V. K., et al. (1995). Schizophrenia susceptibility associated with interstitial deletions of chromosome 22q11. *Proceedings of the National Academy of Sciences of the United States of America, 92*(17), 7612–7616.

Kok, L. L., & Solman, R. T. (1995). Velocardiofacial syndrome: Learning difficulties and intervention. *Journal of Medical Genetics, 32*(8), 612–618.

Kondo, S., Schutte, B. C., Richardson, R. J., Bjork, B. C., Knight, A. S., Watanabe, Y., Howard, E., de Lima, R. L., Daack-Hirsch, S., Sander, A., McDonald-McGinn, D. M., Zachai, E. H., Lammer, E. J., Ayllsworth, A. S., Ardinger, H. H., Lidral, A. C., Pober, B. R., Moreno, L., Arcos-Burgos, M., Valencia, C., Houdayer, C., Bahuau, M., Moretti-Ferreira, D., Richieri-Costa, A., Dixon, M. J., & Murray, J. C. (2002). Mutations in IRF6 cause Van der Woude and popliteal pterygium syndromes. *Nature Genetics, 32*(2), 219–220.

Lalani, S. R., Safullah, A. M., Fernback, S. D., Harntyunyan, K. G., Thaller, C., Peterson, L. E., McPherson, J., Gibbs, R. A., White, L. D., Hefner, M., Davenprot, S. L., Graham, J. M., Bacino, C. A., Glass, N. L., Towbin, J. A., Craiagen, W. J., Neish, S. R., Lin, A. E., & Belmont, J. W. (2006). Spectrum of CHD7 mutations in 110 individuals with CHARGE syndrome and genotype-phenotype correlation. *American Journal of Human Genetics, 78*(2), 303–314.

Lidral, A. C., Romitti, P. A., Basart, A. M., Doetschman, T., Leysens, N. J., Daack-Hirsch, S., Semina, E. V., Johnson, L. R., Machida, J., Burds, A., Parnell, T. J., Rubenstein, J. L., & Murray, J. C. (1998). Association of MSX1 and TGFB3 with nonsyndromic clefting in humans. *American Journal of Human Genetics, 63*(2), 557–568.

MacKenzie-Stepner, K., Witzel, M. A., Stringer, D. A., Lindsay, W. K., Munro, I. R., & Hughes, H. (1987). Abnormal carotid arteries in the velocardiofacial syndrome: A report of three cases. *Plastic and Reconstructive Surgery, 80*(3), 347–351.

Marino, B., Digilio, M. C., Toscano, A., Giannotti, A., & Dallapiccola, B. (1999). Congenital heart defects in patients with DiGeorge/velocardiofacial syndrome and del22q11. *Genetic Counseling, 10*(1), 25–33.

Motzkin, B., Marion, R., Goldberg, R., Shprintzen, R., & Saenger, P. (1993). Variable phenotypes in velocardiofacial syndrome with chromosomal deletion. *Journal of Pediatrics, 123*(3), 406–410.

Murray, J. C. (1995). Face facts: Genes, environment, and clefts [Editorial; Comment]. *American Journal of Human Genetics, 57*(2), 227–232.

Murray, J. C., Nishimura, D. Y., Buetow, K. H., Ardinger, H. H., Spence, M. A., Sparkes, R. S., Falk, R. E., Falk, P. M., Gardner, R. J., Harkness, E. M., et al. (1990). Linkage of an autosomal dominant clefting syndrome (Van der Woude) to loci on chromosome Iq. *American Journal of Human Genetics, 46*(3), 486–491.

Naiglin, L., Clayton, J., Gazagne, C., Dallongeville, F., Malecaze, F., & Calvas, P. (1999). Familial high myopia: Evidence of an autosomal dominant mode of inheritance and genetic heterogeneity [In Process Citation]. *Annals of Genetics, 42*(3), 140–146.

Nowak, C. B. (1998). Genetics and hearing loss: A review of Stickler syndrome. *Journal of Communication Disorders, 31*(5), 437–453, 453–454.

Pagon, R. A., Graham, J. M., Jr., Zonana, J., & Yong, S. L. (1981). Coloboma, congenital heart disease, and choanal atresia with multiple anomalies: CHARGE association. *Journal of Pediatrics, 99*(2), 223–227.

Plomp, A. S., Hamel, B. C., Cobben, J. M., Verloes, A., Offermans, J. P., Lajeunie, E., Fryns, J. P., & de Die-Smulders, C. E. (1998). Pfeiffer syndrome type 2: Further delineation and review of the literature. *American Journal of Medical Genetics, 75*(3), 245–251.

Richards, M. S., Yates, J. R., Pope, M., & Snead, M. P. (1999). Stickler syndrome: Further mutations in COL11A1 and evidence for additional locus heterogeneity. *European Journal of Human Genetics, 7*(7), 807–814.

Robin, N. H. (1999). Molecular genetic advances in understanding craniosynostosis. *Plastic and Reconstructive Surgery, 103*(3), 1060–1070.

Robin, N. H., Opitz, J. M., & Muenke, M. (1996). Opitz G/BBB syndrome: Clinical comparisons of families linked to Xp22 and 22q, and a review of the literature. *American Journal of Medical Genetics, 62*(3), 305–317.

Rommel, N., Vantrappen, G., Swillen, A., Devriendt, K., Feenstra, L., & Fryns, J. P. (1999). Retrospective analysis of feeding and speech disorders in 50 patients with velocardiofacial syndrome. *Genetic Counseling, 10*(1), 71–78.

Ross, D. A., Witzel, M. A., Armstrong, D. C., & Thomson, H. G. (1996). Is pharyngoplasty a risk in velocardiofacial syndrome? An assessment of medially displaced carotid arteries. *Plastic and Reconstructive Surgery, 98*(7), 1182–1190.

Ryan, A. K., Goodship, J. A., Wilson, D. I., Philip, N., Levy, A., Seidel, H., Schuffenhauer, S., Oechsler, H., Belohradsky, B., Prieur, M., Aurias, A., Raymond, F. L., Clayton-Smith, J., Hatchwell, E., McKeown, C., Beemer, F. A., Dallapiccola, B., Novelli, G., Hurst, J. A., Ignatius,

J., Green, A. J., Winter, R. M., Brueton, L., Brondum-Nielsen, K., Scambler, P. J., et al. (1997). Spectrum of clinical features associated with interstitial chromosome 22q11 deletions: A European collaborative study. *Journal of Medical Genetics, 34*(10), 798–804.

Sidman, J. D., Sampson, D., & Templeton, B. (2001). Distraction osteogenesis of the mandible for airway obstruction in children. *Laryngoscope, 111*(7), 1137–1146.

Snead, M. P., & Yates, J. R. (1999). Clinical and molecular genetics of Stickler syndrome. *Journal of Medical Genetics, 36*(5), 353–359.

Spranger, J. (1998). The type XI collagenopathies. *Pediatric Radiology, 28*(10), 745–750.

Spranger, J., Benirschke, K., Hall, J. G., Lenz, W., Lowry, R. B., Opitz, J. M., Pinsky, L., Schwarzacher, H. G., & Smith, D. W. (1982). Errors of morphogenesis: Concepts and terms. Recommendations of an international working group. *Journal of Pediatrics, 100*(1), 160–165.

Shprintzen, R. J. (1994). Velocardiofacial syndrome and DiGeorge sequence. *Journal of Medical Genetics, 31*(5), 423–424.

Shprintzen, R. J. (2000). Velocardiofacial syndrome. *Otolaryngologic Clinics of North America, 33*(6), 1217–1240.

Stein, J., Mulliken, J. B., Stal, S., Gasser, D. L., Malcolm, S., Winter, R., Blanton, S. H., Amos, C., Seemanova, E., & Hecht, J. T. (1995). Nonsyndromic cleft lip with or without cleft palate: Evidence of linkage to BCL3 in 17 multigenerational families [see Comments; published Erratum appears in *American Journal of Human Genetics, 1996, 59*(3), 744]. *American Journal of Human Genetics, 57*(2), 257–272.

Stevens, C. A., Carey, J. C., & Shigeoka, A. O. (1990). DiGeorge anomaly and velocardiofacial syndrome. *Pediatrics, 85*(4), 526–530.

Stone, P., Trevenen, C. L., Mitchell, I., & Rudd, N. (1990). Congenital tracheal stenosis in Pfeiffer syndrome. *Clinical Genetics, 38*(2), 145–148.

Streissguth, A. P., Aase, J. M., Clarren, S. K., Randels, S. P., LaDue, R. A., & Smith, D. F. (1991). Fetal alcohol syndrome in adolescents and adults [see Comments]. *Journal of the American Medical Association, 265*(15), 1961–1967.

Swillen, A., Devriendt, K., Legius, E., Eyskens, B., Dumoulin, M., Gewillig, M., et al. (1997). Intelligence and psychosocial adjustment in velocardiofacial syndrome: A study of 37 children and adolescents with VCFS. *Journal of Medical Genetics, 34*(6), 453–458.

Tomaski, S. M., Zalzal, G. H., & Saal, H. M. (1995). Airway obstruction in Pierre Robin sequence. *Laryngoscope, 105*, 111–115.

Vantrappen, G., Devriendt, K., Swillen, A., Rommel, N., Vogels, A., Eyskens, B., Gewillig, M., Feenstra, L., & Fryns, J. P. (1999). Presenting symptoms and clinical features in 130 patients with the velocardiofacial syndrome. *Genetic Counseling, 10*(1), 3–9.

Vissers, L. E., van Ravenswaaij, C. M., Admiraal, R., Hurst, J. A., de Vries, B. B., Janssen, I. M., van der Vliet, W. A., Huys, E. H., de Jong, P. J., Hame, B. C., Schoenmakers, E. F., Brunner, H. G., Veltman, J. A. & van Kessel, A. G. (2004). Mutations in a new member of the chromodamoain gene family cause CHARGE syndrome. *Nature Genetics, 36*(9), 955–957.

Wilkie, A. O. (1997). Craniosynostosis: Genes and mechanisms. *Human Molecular Genetics, 6*(10), 1647–1656.

Winter, R. M., & Baraitser, M. (1987). The London Dysmorphology Database. *Journal of Medical Genetics, 24*(8), 509–510.

Winter, R. M., & Baraitser, M. (1996). *London Dysmorphology Database*. London: Oxford University Press.

Witt, P. D., Miller, D. C., Marsh, J. L., Muntz, H. R., & Grames, L. M. (1998). Limited value of preoperative cervical vascular imaging in patients with velocardiofacial syndrome. *Plastic and Reconstructive Surgery, 101*(5), 1184–1195; Discussion 1196–1189.

Wyszynski, D. F., Beaty, T. H., & Maestri, N. E. (1996). Genetics of nonsyndromic oral clefts revisited. *Cleft Palate-Craniofacial Journal, 33*(5), 406–417.

Zucchero, T. M., Cooper, M. E., Maher, B. S., Daack-Hirsch, S., Nepomuceno, B., Ribeiro, L., Caprau, D., Christensen, K., Suzuki, Y., Machida, J., Natsume, N., Yoshiura, K., Biera, A. R., Orioli, I. M., Castilla, E. E., Moreno, L., Arcos-Burgos, M., Lidral, A. C., Field, L. L., Liu, Y. E., Ray, A., Goldstein, T. H., Schultz, R. E., Shi, M., Johnson, M. K., Kondo, S., Schutte, B. C., Maraziata, M. L., & Murray, J. C. (2004). Interferon regulatory factor 6 (IRF6) gene variants and the risk of isolated cleft lip or palate. *New England Journal of Medicine, 351*(8), 769–780.

PROBLEMS ASSOCIATED WITH CLEFTS AND CRANIOFACIAL ANOMALIES

CHAPTER

5

FEEDING PROBLEMS OF INFANTS WITH CLEFT LIP/PALATE OR CRANIOFACIAL ANOMALIES

CLAIRE K. MILLER, PH.D.

ANN W. KUMMER, PH.D.

CHAPTER OUTLINE

INTRODUCTION

F eeding is the one the most immediate challenges parents face following the birth of their baby born with a cleft lip/palate or craniofacial anomaly. Obtaining input and good advice about feeding adaptations has been described by parents of cleft palate infants as being of high priority (Young, O'Riordan, Goldstein, & Robin, 2001). Fortunately, most feeding problems can be resolved using therapeutic interventions, including certain feeding adaptations and strategies.

An opening in the palate can have a profound effect on oral-motor mechanics, specifically in regard to the ability to generate the intraoral pressure necessary for effective sucking during infant feeding. In addition, difficulty with airway protection during swallowing may occur, and this can have serious implications for the infant's respiratory health. Sequelae of chronic aspiration during feeding include recurrent respiratory illness, pneumonia, and lung damage (Arvedson & Brodsky, 2002). Last, parental frustration as a result of difficulty with infant feeding can have a negative effect on the parent-infant bonding process (Johansson & Ringsberg, 2004). Generally, the more extensive the cleft, the greater the chance for significant oral feeding problems and, consequently, poor volume of oral intake. The volume of intake must be sufficient for adequate weight gain prior to the surgical repair of lip or palatal clefts. Therefore, early identification of feeding problems and subsequent modifications in the feeding method must be made so that the infant can receive adequate nutrition for growth.

This chapter focuses upon the disruptions in the normal feeding process that occur secondary to clefts and craniofacial anomalies. Assessment of feeding difficulties and the options for individualizing modifications to the feeding method are discussed.

Feeding and Swallowing Function

Feeding, which is accomplished in early infancy by sucking, provides nourishment for normal growth and development. The feeding process provides satisfaction from hunger and helps the infant to maintain homeostasis. The reflexive activity of both nutritive and nonnutritive sucking facilitates state regulation. Feeding serves other important functions as well, including opportunities for sensory and motor stimulation, mother or caregiver and infant bonding, and oral-motor skill development.

Feeding provides the infant with important sensory stimulation. The tactile input to the mouth initiates both the rooting and suck-swallow response in neurologically intact infants. The sensory input eliciting the sucking reflex represents the primary step in initiation of the suck-swallow-breathe synchrony central to the infant feeding process. The activity of feeding also serves as an important part of the bonding process between the caregiver and infant. The caregiver spends time holding and cuddling the infant during the feeding. In addition to the physical contact, there is mutual eye contact during feeding. The feeder learns to identify the infant's cues during feeding and respond appropriately. Mutual eye contact and the vocalizations of the parent help the infant to gain some of the prerequisite skills for communication development. The behaviors of both the caretaker and infant during feeding have been shown to contribute significantly to the overall success of the feeding interaction as well as to the feeding performance (Meyer et al., 1994).

The physical act of sucking requires the active use of the jaw, cheeks, lips, and tongue. The active movement of these oral structures during feeding helps to provide a basis for the movements that are later required for more mature feeding skills (Morris & Klein, 1987). The infant uses sucking to satiate hunger and quickly learns to use sucking for calming and self-regulation as well.

In summary, the early experience of feeding is the foundation for important developmental functions. The presence of a cleft has the potential to interrupt the normal feeding process, which can have significant implications for a successful feeding outcome. Adequacy of nutrition, caregiver interaction patterns, and oral-motor development all have the potential to be affected.

Normal Anatomy and Physiology of Infant Feeding

Oral/Pharyngeal/Laryngeal Anatomy of the Infant

There are distinct differences in location and size of the oral, pharyngeal, and laryngeal structures of the infant as compared with the adult. The anatomic relationships of these areas change significantly during the first several months of infancy as well as during the first two to three years of life (Figure 5–1). The infant's structures are smaller and are in close proximity. As the infant grows, the structures become larger and move apart. They become supported by increased amounts of connective tissue and by complex muscle control secondary to normal maturational development of the central nervous system (Bosma, 1985).

The small size and shape of the infant's oral cavity are ideal for sucking. The infant's tongue, which is relatively large, but only half the size of the adult tongue, fills the oral cavity. The infant's buccal pads are also relatively large and stabilize the lateral walls of the oral

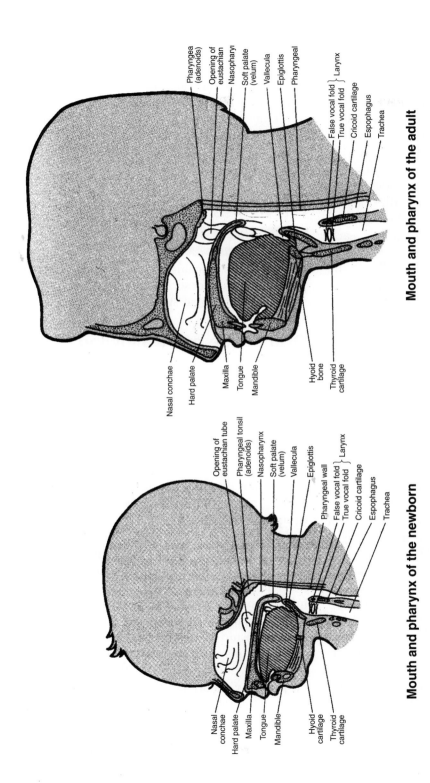

Mouth and pharynx of the newborn

Nasal conchae
Hard palate
Maxilla
Tongue
Mandible
Hyoid cartilage
Thyroid cartilage

Opening of eustachian tube
Pharyngeal tonsil (adenoids)
Nasopharynx
Soft palate (velum)
Vallecula
Epiglottis
Pharyngeal wall
False vocal fold
True vocal fold
Larynx
Cricoid cartilage
Esophagus
Trachea

Mouth and pharynx of the adult

Nasal conchae
Hard palate
Maxilla
Tongue
Mandible
Hyoid bone
Thyroid cartilage

Pharyngea (adenoids)
Opening of eustachian
Nasopharyn
Soft palate (velum)
Vallecula
Epiglottis
Pharyngeal
False vocal fold
True vocal fold
Larynx
Cricoid cartilage
Esophagus
Trachea

FIGURE 5–1 Anatomy of the head and neck as it relates to feeding in the infant as compared with the adult. (From *Prefeeding Skills*, by S. E. Morris and M. D. Klein, 1987. Tucson, AZ: Therapy Skill Builders, a division of Communication Skill Builders, Inc. Copyright Therapy Skill Builders 1987. Reprinted with permission.)

cavity. Because the infant has not yet developed teeth, the effective vertical dimension of the oral cavity is further reduced in size, causing the tongue to rest in a more anterior position than is typically seen in the adult. The tongue tip protrudes past the alveolar ridge and maintains contact with the lower lip. The temporomandibular joint does not allow much movement of jaw due to undeveloped connective tissue, causing the mouth opening to be smaller in the infant than in the adult. All of these oral characteristics facilitate early suckling, characterized by extension-retraction movements of the tongue, as well as the development of more mature up-down tongue movements that are characteristic of true sucking (Arvedson & Brodsky, 2002; Morris & Klein, 1987; Wolf & Glass, 1992).

The pharyngeal area in the newborn is also characterized by very little space between the structures. The soft palate is relatively large and has a large area of contact with the tongue. The tongue base, soft palate, and pharyngeal walls are all in close approximation. The inferior border of the uvula and velum rests in front of the epiglottis.

The position of the infant's larynx, which is one-third the adult size, is high in the hypopharynx, residing adjacent to cervical vertebrae C-1–C-3. In comparison, the larynx in the adult is located at the C-6–C-7 vertebral level. The high position of the infant larynx causes the epiglottis to pass superiorly to the free margin of the soft palate and project into the nasopharynx. The epiglottis is tubular, proportionally narrow, and more vertical in the infant as compared with the adult (Myer, Cotton, & Shott, 1995).

As the infant matures, the oral cavity gradually becomes larger, with concurrent mandibular growth and dental eruption. The tongue begins to descend and move back into the mouth, with the tip becoming positioned behind the alveolar ridge. The increased space facilitates the development of a range of oral-motor movements for feeding as well as for speech production. The pharynx begins to elongate and the larynx begins its gradual descent from C-3 to C-6, which is complete by age 3 (Sasaki, Levine, Laitman, Phil, & Crelin, 1977).

Physiology of Infant Feeding

The feeding process itself is dependent on smooth synchronization of sucking, swallowing, and breathing. Sucking and swallowing occur in phases generally described as the oral, pharyngeal, and esophageal stages of swallowing.

Oral Phase of Swallowing

The oral phase of swallowing in infants is composed of rhythmic sucking, during which the oral structures work together to stabilize the nipple, create pressure gradients for fluid flow, and control the bolus prior to swallowing initiation. The presence of the rooting reflex aids in the search for the nipple and the subsequent lip seal around the nipple. The sucking reflex is initiated as the tongue elevates to squeeze the nipple against the alveolar ridge and hard palate. The compression of the nipple against this bony surface creates positive pressure within the nipple and causes the release of a small amount of fluid. The infant then initiates sucking: a rhythmic forward-backward tongue motion. The tongue is cupped around the nipple and a depression in the center of the tongue forms a groove. As the tongue moves backward during sucking, the infant's jaw drops, thus enlarging the space in the oral cavity. This action generates negative pressure, resulting in suction and expression of fluid from the nipple into the infant's oral cavity. Therefore, both nipple compression and the

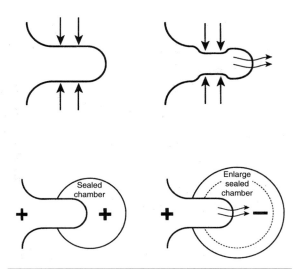

FIGURE 5–2 Comparison of positive pressure (compression) and negative pressure (suction) components during sucking. (From *Feeding and Swallowing Disorders in Infancy*, by L. Wolf and R. Glass, 1992, p. 17. Therapy Skill Builders, San Antonio, Texas, a division of Communication Skill Builders, Inc. Copyright Therapy Skill Builders 1992. Reprinted with permission.)

generation of negative pressure suction are essential for normal feeding (Figure 5–2).

To achieve compression of the nipple against the bony roof of the mouth, the palate must be intact in the area of the nipple. To achieve suction in the oral cavity, there must be adequate lip closure around the nipple, and the oral cavity must be closed off posteriorly with the back of the tongue against the soft palate. The hard palate, and to some extent the soft palate, serve to close off the nose from the mouth during feeding. Any opening in this cavity can reduce or eliminate the ability to create negative suction pressure.

Pharyngeal Phase of Swallowing

The pharyngeal phase of swallowing is initiated once the fluid bolus is channeled by the tongue into the pharynx. Because the pharynx serves as a conduit for food as well as respiratory air,

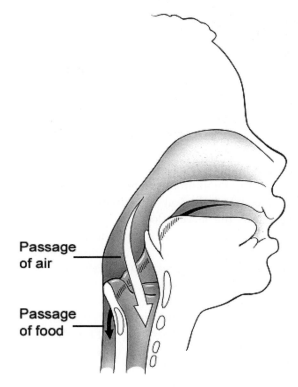

FIGURE 5–3 The pharynx as a conduit of food and air. (From *The Pediatric Airway: An Interdisciplinary Approach*, by C. M. Myer, R. T. Cotton, and S. R. Shott, 1995, p. 9. Philadelphia: J. B. Lippincott Company. Copyright J. B. Lippincott 1995. Reprinted with permission.)

precise coordination of breathing, sucking, and swallowing is necessary during the pharyngeal swallowing phase (Figure 5–3). There are significant differences in the pharyngeal phase of swallowing in infancy versus adulthood due to the size and location of the pharyngeal and laryngeal structures in the first several months.

When the liquid reaches the posterior oral cavity, the posterior pharyngeal wall, velum, and tongue base work together to provide the driving force for bolus transfer through the pharynx. The velum elevates and the velopharyngeal valve closes completely to close off the nasal cavity from the oral cavity. The tongue base moves back as negative pressure builds in the pharynx. The bolus diverts around the epiglottis as the pharynx fills and contracts sequentially for swallowing (Newman, Cleveland, Blickman, Hillman, & Jaramillo, 1991). Throughout the sucking action, the infant continues to maintain nasal breathing. To facilitate this, the epiglottis is positioned around the back of the velum, which keeps the pharynx open and allows the nasal cavity to be in direct contact with the glottis for a continuous patent airway. However, at the time of swallow initiation, respiration ceases as the larynx closes by adduction of the true and false vocal folds, the forward and medial movement of the arytenoids, and the subsequent retroversion of the epiglottis (Koenig, Davies, & Thach, 1990; Mathew, 1991). Additional respiratory effort is necessary to support the work of feeding. The normal infant is able to tolerate the decreased ventilation during feeding; however, this may not be the case in infants presenting with borderline respiratory reserve (Glass & Wolf, 1999; Mathew, 1988b; Mathew, Clark, Pronske, Luna-Solarzano, & Peterson, 1985).

Esophageal Phase of Swallowing

The bolus moves through the pharynx and into the esophagus, where the esophageal phase of swallowing is initiated. The upper part of the esophagus, commonly referred to as the *upper esophageal sphincter* (UES), is normally closed, but stretches open as the bolus travels through the hypopharynx and into the esophagus. The *lower esophageal sphincter* (LES) relaxes to allow the bolus to enter the stomach. After each swallow occurs, the velum drops down to the base of the tongue and in front of the epiglottis, the tongue returns to an anterior position, sucking and breathing resume, and both the upper and lower esophageal sphincters maintain a closed position.

Coordination of sucking and swallowing with breathing is precisely synchronized to prevent aspiration (entry of material into the airway). The suck-swallow-breathe ratio during bottle feeding is generally considered to be 1:1:1 or 2:1:1. Some variations to this pattern occur during the initial rapid sucking phase, generally described as the initial two to three minutes of feeding, as compared with the slower sucking rates occurring during the subsequent intermittent sucking phase (Bu'Lock, Woolridge, & Baum, 1990; Mathew, 1991; Wolf & Glass, 1992).

Changes in the Swallowing Process with Growth

The process of feeding and swallowing changes as the infant grows and matures. The oral cavity enlarges, the pharynx elongates, and the hyoid, epiglottis, and larynx descend. The increased size of the oral cavity supports the development of more refined oral-motor skills, such as chewing and cup drinking. Neuromuscular maturation as well as increased cartilage and connective tissue are reflected in the mobility of the hyoid and larynx, which must become more active during the swallowing process in order to maintain airway protection that was previously facilitated by the proximity of structures. The hyoid and larynx must be mobile enough to elevate and provide sphincteric closure during swallowing (Bosma & Donner, 1980).

CRANIOFACIAL ANOMALIES AND PEDIATRIC DYSPHAGIA

Any anatomical malformation in the oral cavity, pharynx, or larynx can cause or contribute to a feeding or swallowing problem. Anomalies that are associated with feeding problems include cleft lip and palate, *micrognathia* (small mandible), *macroglossia* (large tongue), pharyngeal *stenosis* (narrowing), laryngeal cleft, tracheoesophageal fistula, and vascular anomalies causing compression in the esophagus or airway. Cortical or cranial nerve involvement, as seen in some syndromes, may affect the neuromuscular coordination required for sucking and swallowing. Finally, conditions that can cause airway compromise, such as Pierre Robin sequence, midface retrusion, congenital heart or lung disease, or *choanal atresia* (congenital closure of the opening to the pharynx from the back of the nose) can interfere with the suck-swallow-breathe sequence. Of all of these anomalies, cleft palate is the most common.

Characteristics of Feeding Problems Due to Clefts

The feeding problems of infants who have a cleft will reflect the type and the severity of the cleft. The issues with feeding problems vary greatly depending on whether the cleft is of the lip or palate and if it is unilateral, bilateral, complete, or incomplete. The feeding problems typically encountered include poor oral suction, inadequate volume of intake, lengthy feeding times, *nasal regurgitation*, excessive air intake, and coughing or choking (Glass & Wolf, 1999). These difficulties are due to the structural problems in the oral cavity. In most cases, pharyngeal swallowing function is normal. Therefore, once the milk reaches the oropharynx, swallowing is initiated and coordinated with airway protection. However, problems with maintaining airway protection during the pharyngeal phase of the swallow can occur when pharyngeal, esophageal, or central nervous system abnormalities occur in conjunction with the cleft defect. Problems with airway protection can also occur when the timing of the oral phase

of swallowing is so disorganized that the integrity of airway protection is compromised.

Infants with a cleft of the lip usually do not have significant problems with feeding, especially if the cleft is unilateral. There may be some initial difficulty in learning how to latch onto the nipple. However, once the nipple is placed intraorally, the infant's tongue and jaw movements should be sufficient to produce compression of the nipple against the intact part of the alveolus and palate. There may be some difficulty in achieving negative pressure suction, depending on how much the lip seal on the nipple is compromised.

Infants with a minimal cleft of the soft palate are often able to feed without special modifications. With a small posterior cleft, the infant may actually occlude the cleft with the tongue during part of the sucking movement, so that negative pressure can be obtained normally.

Infants with a cleft of the hard and soft palate have more difficulty feeding for several reasons. Depending on the extent of the cleft, the infant may be unable to find a hard palatal surface to work against, making compression of the nipple impossible. This situation may result in the nipple being pushed into the area of the cleft if placement cannot be achieved against an area of hard palate. Another concern is that with an open cavity, the subsequent generation of suction is difficult and may be impossible to achieve. The extent of difficulty again depends on the size and location of the cleft. Posterior clefts may be occluded with the base of the tongue during the sucking movement. The more anterior the cleft is, the harder it is for the infant to achieve compression of the nipple and subsequent generation of negative pressure for efficient sucking.

The hard palate and the velum separate the oral cavity from the nasal cavity during feeding. With an open palate, nasal regurgitation, which is reflux of milk into the nasopharynx and nasal cavity, will often occur. This can cause discomfort and disorganization with regard to the coordination of breathing and feeding.

Due to difficulty with oral feeding, several secondary problems can occur. These include poor weight gain, excessive energy expenditure during feeding, lengthy feeding times, discomfort with feeding, and stressful feeding interactions between the infant and caretaker (Carlisle, 1998).

To support weight gain during the early months of infancy, it is important for infants with cleft palate to obtain adequate nutrition; this can be problematic if feeding problems are present (Glass & Wolf, 1999; Jones, 1988; Redford-Badwal, Mabry, & Frassinelli, 2003). A full-term newborn infant will generally need 2 to 3 ounces of breast milk or formula per pound of body weight per day in order to gain weight appropriately (The Cleft Palate Foundation, 1998). Therefore, an infant who weighs 10 pounds will require between 20 and 30 ounces per day; a significant amount for an infant having feeding difficulty. As the infant gains weight, his or her daily intake should increase accordingly. If the infant has a cleft palate, however, it is harder to achieve compression of the nipple to generate the suction needed for efficient ingestion of the amount of formula required for continued growth. In addition, nasal regurgitation must be subtracted from total intake of formula.

The infant with a cleft may take much longer to feed than an infant without a cleft yet still not get enough during each feeding to be satisfied or gain weight. To complicate this problem, the infant must work much harder to feed and therefore expends more calories during the feeding process than the average infant. Most infants can complete a feeding within 20 to 30 minutes. If the infant takes 45 minutes or longer to feed, with clearly increased effort and relatively little intake, consultation with a pediatrician, nutritionist, and feeding specialist (a speech-language pathologist or occupational therapist with special training in feeding) is indicated. Weight gain should be monitored closely by the pediatrician, especially during the first few months.

Because air continues to flow in through the nose and then the mouth during feeding due to the open cleft, this may result in excessive intake of air. This can cause the infant to become bloated or have episodes of frequent "spit up." Excess air intake needs to be monitored closely by the caretaker as it is a potential source of discomfort for the infant, both during and after feeding.

A final concern is for the parents. Normally, the feeding process serves as a loving and bonding experience between the caregiver and the infant. However, feeding an infant with cleft palate can be very time-consuming for the caregivers and often results in a great deal of frustration. Fortunately, with individualized feeding modifications most feeding problems can be avoided or minimized.

Feeding Problems Due to Other Anomalies

Pierre Robin Sequence

Patients with a diagnosis of Pierre Robin sequence (micrognathia, glossoptosis, and cleft palate) may have feeding problems due to the cleft palate as well as potential problems with the coordination of the suck-swallow-breathe triad (Lehman, Fishman, & Neiman, 1995; Shprintzen, 1992; van den Elzen et al., 2001). *Micrognathia* (small mandible) is often associated with a wide U-shaped cleft of the palate. The tongue is posteriorly positioned in relation to the oral cavity, a condition generally referred to as *glossoptosis*. The presence of glossoptosis creates the potential for upper airway obstruction, which may be exacerbated by the respiratory effort of feeding. Episodic or chronic airway obstruction can occur during the infant's effort to maintain sequential chain swallowing sequences (Shprintzen & Singer, 1992).

Moebius Syndrome

Moebius syndrome is a rare, genetic disorder that involves absence or underdevelopment of the abducent nerve (VI) and the facial nerve (VII). Eye movements and the muscles of facial expression are affected. Motor delays, breathing problems, hearing problems, and abnormalities in movements of the cheeks, lips, tongue, jaw, and limbs may be present. A high palatal vault or cleft palate may be present. Problems with feeding and swallowing are frequent due to the inability to suck. The weakness in the lips limits the infant's ability to achieve and maintain an adequate seal on the nipple and can cause excessive drooling. The high palatal vault may cause difficulty in establishing an adequate tongue-palate seal for efficient sucking. Anterior loss of formula is a common finding during the clinical feeding evaluation. A chronic open-mouth posture with limited range of movement in the jaw and tongue has a profound effect on the oral-motor mechanics necessary for efficient sucking (Arvedson & Brodsky, 2002).

Hemifacial Microsomia

Hemifacial microsomia results in various degrees of both unilateral mandibular hypoplasia and facial weakness. This generally results in limitations to the range of motion in the jaw, lips, and tongue on one side. Utilization of the stronger side of the mouth during feeding presentations while providing stabilization to the weaker side may work when attempting to establish a compensatory feeding pattern (Arvedson & Brodsky, 2002).

Treacher Collins Syndrome

The characteristics of Treacher Collins syndrome include underdevelopment of the zygomatic bones, malformation of the ears and the lower eyelids, and downward-slanting palpebral fissures. Oral-motor mechanics for sucking may be inefficient and require special feeding adaptations.

Other Congenital Anomalies

If the infant has other oral, tracheal, or laryngeal anomalies in addition to the cleft palate, feeding can become even more of a challenge. Micrognathia or a posterior tongue position associated with a variety of syndromes can result in problems with oral-motor mechanics and airway compromise which affects the ability to coordinate breathing and feeding. A tracheoesophageal fistula can cause aspiration during feeding secondary to communication between the esophagus and trachea. Hypotonia, hypertonia, or generalized oral-motor dysfunction secondary to weakness or myopathy all can affect the infant's ability to suck efficiently and coordinate the suck-swallow-breathe triad.

GENERAL FEEDING MODIFICATIONS

Unfortunately, there is no single feeding method that will be successful for infants with different types of clefts or craniofacial abnormalities. General feeding tips are summarized in Appendix 5–1. The infant's performance during the initial feedings will dictate which feeding method and technique is feasible (Wolf & Glass, 1992). Individualized modifications should allow the infant to feed with relative ease as well as to obtain an adequate amount of nutrition in a reasonable amount of time.

Infants who present with feeding problems that are not easily resolved postnatally by a simple adjustment in feeding method will benefit from a clinical oral-motor/feeding evaluation performed by a qualified speech-language pathologist or occupational therapist, or other feeding specialist. Such an evaluation can assess an infant's specific oral-motor strengths and weaknesses with the ultimate goals of:

- Maximizing the infant's ability to orally feed for adequate nutrition and weight gain by matching feeding modifications to oral-motor skills.

- Facilitating the suck-swallow-breathe synchrony for safe and efficient feeding.

The Issue of Breast Feeding

Most pediatricians and health care providers agree that breast milk is best for the newborn infant for several reasons. It contains the mother's antibodies against illnesses and therefore can provide the infant with some immunity. Early food allergies can also be avoided through the use of breast milk. It has been suggested that feeding with breast milk offers protection from otitis media (Aniansson, Svensson, Becker, & Ingvarsson, 2002; Paradise, Elster, & Tan, 1994). However, opinions regarding the feasibility of breast feeding a child with a cleft vary across centers (Alexander-Doelle, 1997; Biancuzzo, 1998; Crossman, 1998; Darzi, Chowdri, & Blat, 1996; Kogo, Okada, Ishii,

Shikata, Iida, & Matsuya, 1997). As with other feeding methods, the success of breast feeding will depend on the location and severity of the cleft.

Breast feeding is usually not a problem for the infant who has a cleft lip only, since the infant should still be able to achieve adequate suction. Even with a cleft in the lip and alveolus, the breast tends to fill the opening by molding to the shape of the oral cavity. Upright positioning while attempting breast feeding is generally recommended. Supplemental bottle feeding or a complete switch to the bottle may be necessary if difficulties with breast feeding are immediately apparent.

Breast feeding the infant with a cleft palate is very difficult, however, and this can be a particular disappointment for many new mothers. Breast feeding a child with a cleft palate can be done, but to be successful it requires specialized modifications (Wolf & Glass, 1992). Monitoring weight gain closely during a trial period of breast feeding will provide both objective evidence regarding its feasibility and definitive information as to whether a supplementary feeding method is needed.

If the mother wishes to try breast feeding, she should consult with a feeding specialist or lactation consultant who has experience with patients having special needs, particularly those with cleft lip or palate. If a trial of breast feeding proves unsuccessful and the mother still wishes to continue breast feeding, a supplemental nursing system may be an option. The supplemental nursing system utilizes a reservoir and tubing. The reservoir can be filled with formula or with milk that the mother has expressed. A thin tube, connected to the reservoir, is taped above the mother's breast and nipple. As the infant latches onto the breast for feeding, the mother supplements the breast milk with milk that is squeezed manually through the tube. The flow of milk needs to be simultaneous with the baby's efforts at sucking. With this method, the baby is supplemented at the breast, while maintaining the important physical contact for the infant and mother. In addition, this method stimulates the breast to continue to produce and maintain the milk supply. Drawbacks to the use of supplemental nursing systems include the potential for difficulty in maintaining the proper flow rate, though adjustable flow rate systems are available on some supplemental nursing systems. There is also the possibility that the baby will reject intraoral placement of the tube during breast feeding.

After attempting breast feeding with modifications, some mothers may find that bottle feeding using a modified bottle and/or a modified nipple is easier and more efficient. She can still use breast milk however, but in this case, the breast milk is given via the modified bottle or nipple.

Breast milk can be expressed through the use of a variety of breast pumps. Breast pumps are available for purchase or for rental through local home health suppliers. There are several kinds of breast pumps, including manual pumps, battery-operated pumps, and electric pumps. The electric pumps tend to be more efficient and faster than the manual pumps. An electric pump that allows both breasts to be pumped at the same time is particularly useful because it can greatly reduce the amount of time required to express the milk. This is a definite advantage, especially if breast milk is used exclusively. Breast pumps may be covered by the family's insurance plan, but this usually requires a signed prescription in the baby's name and a letter from the physician describing the special circumstances that make this equipment necessary.

Modified Nipples

If problems with feeding are immediately apparent, a variety of special bottles and nipples are available. Commonly used nipples and bottles are described in Table 5–1. Instructions for feeding using adapted nipples and bottles are described in Appendix 5–2. When considering what nipple to use for enhancement of sucking, there are four basic parameters to consider: pliability, nipple shape, nipple size, and hole type and size (Mathew, 1988a). Table 5–2 compares the characteristics of the commonly used nipples. The type of nipple chosen must be based on the type of cleft and the baby's oral-motor/feeding skills as determined by the initial feeding evaluation. Modified nipples, such as the Pigeon nipple or Ross nipple, can be fitted with either standard or flexible bottles.

Pliability

The nipple must be pliable enough to release breast milk or formula with limited compression and without creation of suction. At the same time, the nipple needs to be firm enough to provide an appropriate degree of proprioceptive input to stimulate sucking. A soft nipple tends to have a higher flow rate than a firmer nipple and thus requires less compression effort and suction. The degree of pliability must match the infant's strength of sucking and provide an appropriate flow rate to allow the baby to coordinate the suck-swallow-breathe sequence. This is important because an increased rate of fluid flow will require a faster rate of swallowing and greater respiratory effort (Glass & Wolf, 1999). A "preemie" nipple is often used for infants with cleft palate because it is designed to be very soft and pliable. A standard nipple can also be softened through boiling. A variety of

---

TABLE 5–1 Commercially Available Bottles and Nipples

- **Mead Johnson Cleft Lip/Palate Nurser:** This is a soft bottle that is easily squeezed and which also has a long soft cross-cut nipple. A standard nipple will also fit onto the Mead Johnson bottle and works well for some infants. The caregiver can help to regulate the liquid by assistive squeezing. The use of either the cross-cut nipple or a standard nipple with a modified hole will depend on the oral-motor skills of each particular infant.

- **Ross Cleft Palate Nurser:** This bottle has a long, thin nipple that delivers milk to the back of the throat. The small diameter of this nipple does not facilitate tongue movements for sucking. The long length may cause gagging in some infants. Fluid flow is steady and rapid and can be difficult for infants who cannot tolerate a rapid flow rate. This could result in disorganization of airway protection and possible aspiration.

- **Pigeon Nipple:** The pigeon nipple has one side with thinner walls, enabling the infant to express milk through a suckling motion. The thicker side of the nipple is placed against the roof of the mouth. The bottle can be squeezed by the feeder to assist with fluid flow. The nipple has a tendency to collapse because it does not vent rapidly due to its thin walls. The pigeon nipple can be used with bottles designed to prevent excessive air intake, such as the Playtex Ventair® or Dr. Brown® bottle.

- **Lamb's Nipple:** This nipple is long, wide, and soft, with compression occurring between the lateral alveolar ridges. The shape of this nipple does not facilitate normal sucking movements. The hole may be too large for infants who cannot tolerate a rapid fluid flow. The length of the nipple may induce gagging in some infants. This nipple, while used widely in the past, has been found to have a high nitrate level.

- **Haberman Feeder™:** The Haberman Feeder is designed to allow release of milk through the infant's compressions alone; no suction is required. There is a soft nipple that is filled with breast milk or formula prior to feeding. The nipple has a one-way valving component that prevents rapid fluid flow by only opening when the infant sucks. The valve is also designed to prevent excessive intake of air. Squeezing can be done to assist with fluid flow as needed. The nipple has a slit which allows flow control during feeding depending upon the orientation of the slit in the infant's mouth. The flow can therefore be easily regulated by the feeder. The Mini-Haberman™ is a smaller version of the feeder and is designed for smaller or premature babies with cleft palate or other special feeding problems.

- **Preemie Nipple:** This nipple is smaller, thinner, and softer than a standard nipple, making suction easier. This is a fast-flow nipple which should be used only by those infants who have demonstrated tolerance for the increased respiratory effort associated with increased swallowing associated with fast fluid flow.

- **Obturator Nipple:** The Obturator nipple, also referred to as the Brophy nipple, has a flap above the nipple, which is intended to occlude the cleft and facilitate normal sucking. This is rarely recommended as it has the potential to obstruct the oral cavity, irritate the nasopharyngeal space, and cause sucking-swallowing disorganization.

- **Standard Amber Nipple:** This nipple has a narrow base and has been shown to be effective when used in conjunction with a squeeze bottle while feeding infants who have demonstrated the ability to develop some suction independently. A slight enlargement of the nipple hole may be necessary.

- **NUK Nipple:** The NUK-style nipple has a wide-based nipple with a fast flow rate. It can be used with a squeeze bottle for infants who show good ability to rapidly coordinate suck-swallow and breathing.

- **Medela® SoftCup Feeder:** The SoftCup feeder is designed to be used with the Medela® 80-ml polypropylene bottle. Other bottles can be used, but some leakage may occur in the collar area. The SoftCup feeder does not require the infant to actively suck because fluid is delivered via a small flexible cup-like reservoir. The flow rate is controlled by the feeder.

---

specialized nipples and bottle systems, such as the Mead Johnson (Figure 5–4), Haberman Feeder™ (Figure 5–5), and Pigeon nipple (Figure 5–6), are designed specifically for infants with cleft palate.

Nipple Shape

Regardless of what nipple is used, the shape of the nipple needs to provide adequate contact between the nipple and the tongue for adequate compression. The shape also

TABLE 5–2 Characteristics of Commonly Used Nipples

Nipple Type	Pliability	Flow Rate	Shape	Hole Type
Preemie	Soft	Fast	Traditional	Hole and cross-cut
NUK-style	Soft	Fast	Broad, flat	Hole on top surface of tip
Ross Cleft	Soft	Fast	Long, thin	Large hole
Standard	Medium	Low	Traditional	Hole and cross-cut, several holes
Mead Johnson	Soft	Feeder regulated	Customized	Cross-cut
Haberman system	Soft	Feeder regulated	Customized	Slit

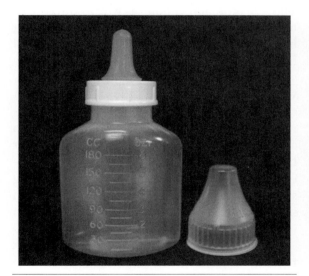

FIGURE 5–4   Mead Johnson Cleft Palate Nurser.

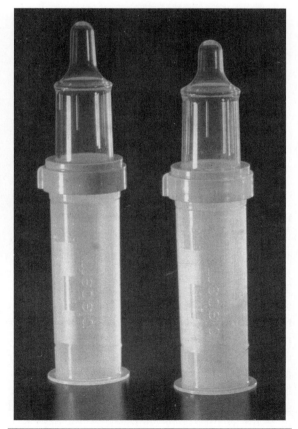

FIGURE 5–5   Haberman Feeder by Medela.

must support the oral-motor patterns desired during sucking. Numerous nipple designs are available; however, nipple shapes basically fall into two categories: traditional, straight-shaped nipples, and broad, flat nipples (Figure 5–7). The traditional nipple has a straight configuration, which gradually tapers to a flared base.

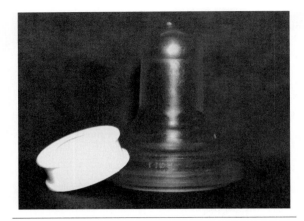

FIGURE 5–6 Pigeon nipple.

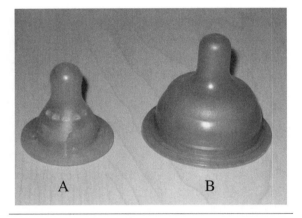

FIGURE 5–7 (A and B) Basic categories of nipples. A. Round cross-section. B. Broad, flat cross-section.

The broad, flat nipples, sometimes referred to as "orthodontic nipples," have bulb-type ends that flare to a large, wide base. This style is perhaps best known as the NUK nipple; however, many manufacturers, including Gerber and Playtex, now make nipples shaped similarly to the original NUK style. Such nipples are generally advantageous for infants with isolated cleft lip as they may conform to the cleft and prevent air leakage while sucking.

Nipple Size

Determining the appropriate-sized nipple to use should be based on the length needed to provide adequate contact between the nipple and tongue for effective tongue movements. Nipple length can vary substantially with regard to the type of base and the distance from the tip to the base, especially for those nipples that have tapered bases. The strength of the infant's suck, the degree of lip closure around the nipple, and the control the feeder provides to maintain the nipple position are all factors that should be considered.

Hole Type and Size

The size ofhe nipple hole, as well as the type of hole, determines flow rate. Two basic types of holes are found in standard nipples: standard holes and cross-cuts. The holes are usually very small openings in nipples and the size can vary widely across different styles of nipples. A cross-cut opening is basically an "X" configuration. A standard nipple hole can be modified to a cross-cut with a single-edged sterile razor blade. The size of the hole is generally considered to be indicative of flow rate during sucking (Mathew, 1990). The type of hole an infant should use is determined during an initial feeding assessment.

The cross-cut configuration allows the milk to flow only when the infant compresses the nipple to make the cross-cut open. This allows the infant to control the milk flow with the normal rhythm of sucking and swallowing and prevents the infant from getting too much liquid, which can cause choking. A nipple with a traditional hole should have an opening that is large enough so that, when the bottle is held upside down, the liquid drips out but does not run out rapidly. A standard nipple can be enlarged or slit to increase the fluid flow rate; however, the increased flow may cause the infant to have difficulty with coordination of swallowing and breathing.

Flexible Bottles with Modified Nipples

In considering the appropriate bottle, a flexible plastic squeeze bottle or plastic bottle liner can be used and can be paired with a specialized nipple as needed. Feeder-assisted squeezing for milk expression allows the infant to conserve energy and thus have less calorie expenditure during feeding. If a plastic liner is used, the caregiver can reduce the excess intake of air by pushing all the air out of the liner before beginning the feeding and by applying intermittent pressure to the liner to push milk out as the infant compresses the nipple (Barone & Tallman, 1998). The flow of milk can be difficult to modulate with a flexible bottle, which may make it more difficult for the infant to maintain organization of sucking, swallowing, and breathing.

A soft bottle, such as the Mead Johnson™ Cleft Palate Nurser or the Haberman Feeder™, may allow for more precision in the amount of milk squeezed. The Mead Johnson bottle is soft and easily held in the feeder's hand and requires the use of an assistive squeeze for release of the milk. The nipple of the Haberman Feeder allows milk release from the infant's compression alone and also allows for control of flow during feeding by changing the orientation of the nipple slit in the infant's mouth. The softness of the Haberman nipple also allows for assistive squeezing (Haberman, 1988).

Regardless of which device is used, the pressure applied to a squeeze bottle or plastic liner must be in rhythm with the infant's suck and swallow to ensure that the infant does not become discoordinated with the suck-swallow-breathe synchrony. The feeder must become skilled at providing the assistive squeeze in synchrony with the infant's sucking rhythm, allowing time for each swallow to take place. An inappropriately rapid rate or continuous squeezing will result in an increased rate of swallowing, which will decrease available breathing time. This may result in problems with maintaining an appropriate respiratory rate and may also result in discoordination of the suck-swallow-breathe synchrony with subsequent aspiration into the airway.

Overall, the device chosen must allow the infant to receive an adequate amount of intake for nutrition and weight gain. It should be easy enough so that the infant can conserve energy and fast enough so that it does not cause lengthy feeding times and eventual frustration for the caregiver. Consistency of nipple and bottle use is as important as the consistency of the feeder's method. The feeding system should allow the infant to experience some sucking for normal oral-motor development. Finally, the option chosen should be relatively inexpensive and readily available.

SPECIFIC FEEDING CONSIDERATIONS AND TECHNIQUES

Cleft Lip Only

Clefts of the lip may be unilateral or bilateral and may extend into the nares and alveolus. This may result in problems in achieving an adequate anterior lip seal on the nipple of the bottle or breast, which is needed to generate effective negative pressure during feeding.

Breast Feeding

Breast feeding often will work in cases of cleft lip only, as the breast tends to conform to and fill in the cleft area. If necessary, the mother can assist with lip closure by gently holding the upper lip together while the baby sucks. Positioning should be as upright as possible to allow gravity to pull the liquid into the pharynx. Consultation with a certified lactation consultant regarding strategies for assisting with breast feeding may also be advisable.

Bottle Feeding

Infants who present with a cleft lip only generally feed adequately; however, occasionally air leak from the cleft will interrupt the generation of negative pressure. The use of a soft, wide-based nipple, as depicted in Figure 5–6, will close the area of the cleft and allow suction generation.

Cleft Palate Only

A cleft of the palate may involve only the soft palate or it may also extend into the hard palate. Whatever the case, there will be compromise in the infant's ability to seal the oral cavity and create negative pressure for suction.

Breast Feeding

Generally, infants with a narrow or posterior cleft (soft palate only) will be able to breastfeed without undue difficulty. The infant will likely be able to develop adequate suction to form and position the nipple for adequate compression (Glass & Wolf, 1999). Infants with a complete cleft of the soft and hard palate are much more likely to have a difficult time with breast feeding due to the fact that they will simply be unable to create negative pressure for suction due to the large opening and lack of surface for the tongue to compress against.

Bottle Feeding

Generally, the options for bottle feeding include a system where the feeder assists with formula or breast milk delivery by squeezing a flexible bottle fitted with a modified nipple. Nipple modifications may include the use of a specialized cleft palate nipple, or the use of a soft wide-based, cross-cut nipple or soft nipple with a slightly enlarged single hole. The use of assisted feeding techniques (flexible bottles as opposed to rigid) has been shown to be more effective for infants with clefts (Shaw, Bannister, & Roberts, 1999).

Cleft Lip and Palate

The infant presenting with a cleft of the lip and palate will generally have significant difficulty with all aspects of feeding due to the inability to achieve an anterior seal with the lips, inability to compress the nipple due to the open palate, and failure to generate negative pressure suction. Significant nasopharyngeal reflux of liquid secondary to the open nasopharynx will also be present.

Breast Feeding

Infants with a cleft lip and palate will have a large area of cleft, which has a direct impact on the baby's sucking mechanics overall. Breast feeding is highly unlikely in this group of infants. Unlike the infant with just a cleft of the soft palate, there is no effective means for positioning or compressing the nipple. The use of a supplemental nursing system, such as the Medela Supplemental Nursing System™, may be of some benefit in supporting breast feeding; however, the infant's growth and hydration status should be closely monitored. Supplemental or exclusive transition to bottle feeding is highly likely.

Bottle Feeding

A variety of modified feeding devices, both nipples and bottles that assist in delivery of milk, will be necessary for the infant with cleft lip and palate. Assistive squeezing of the bottle by the feeder and the use of a soft nipple are often necessary. The feeder must control the flow of milk to give the infant time to swallow. Overall, as tongue movements during sucking are generally normal (anterior-posterior), efficient oral feeding can be successfully achieved by making the modifications to the feeding system in order to compensate for difficulty with complete compression and inability to generate negative pressure.

Pierre Robin Sequence and Orofacial Syndromes

The infant with Pierre Robin sequence often has breathing and feeding difficulties (Nassar, Marques, Trindade, & Bettiol, 2006). The infant's ability to compress the nipple adequately is often decreased secondary to the presence of micrognathia and a retracted tongue position. The habitual position of the tongue does not allow for positioning beneath the nipple to allow for compressive action. If the infant has Pierre Robin sequence including the typical U-shaped cleft palate, problems with generation of negative pressure also contribute to feeding difficulty. The presence of glossoptosis creates an airway obstruction, which may be exacerbated by the increased respiratory effort required during feeding. A patent airway must be confirmed prior to attempts at oral feeding (Bath & Bull, 1997). Some patients may require placement of a nasopharyngeal (NP) airway. Oral feedings can be done with the NP tube in place.

Despite the problems, feeding modifications can be made to help the infant with Pierre Robin sequence feed successfully (Nassar et al., 2006). If medical clearance is given for oral feedings, prone positioning may help to position the tongue anteriorly and facilitate tongue movements during feeding. However, if the infant has a cleft palate, prone positioning is generally not helpful, as the infant will not be able to move the milk to the back of the mouth for the initiation of swallowing. Using a semireclined or standard feeding position will help to minimize gravitational pull on the tongue. Sidelying positioning may be an option with use of either the Haberman Feeder or a Mead Johnson bottle. Success with feeding will need to be closely monitored with the possible need for supplemental feedings (Glass & Wolf, 1999). As with other infants with cleft palate, tongue movements during sucking are generally normal. However, these modifications to the feeding system help the infant to overcome the difficulty with both compression and the ability to generate negative pressure.

Modified feeding strategies may also be necessary when feeding infants with Treacher Collins syndrome, Moebius syndrome, or hemifacial microsomia. The feeding strategies used for patients with Pierre Robin sequence may also be helpful in patients with Treacher Collins if significant retrognathia or micrognathia is present. In patients with hemifacial microsomia, utilizing the stronger side of the mouth during feeding presentations while stabilizing the weaker side may work when attempting establish a compensatory feeding pattern (Arvedson & Brodsky, 2002). Modified presentation of fluid is necessary for infants with Moebius syndrome due to the significantly restricted range of movement in the jaw, lips, and tongue. The use of feeder-assisted squeezing or presentation by a specialized feeding nipple/bottle is likely necessary.

Breast Feeding

The success of breast feeding in the infant with Pierre Robin sequence will depend on the degree of micrognathia, the status of the airway, and whether the infant has a cleft. In infants without clefts and with mild retrognathia, breast feeding may be an option. It should be noted, however, that breast feeding will probably be difficult. The retracted tongue position may cause inadequate compression of the milk ducts in the breast, which will lead to limited milk flow, and ultimately less milk production. If micrognathia, upper airway obstruction, and a velar cleft are present, breast feeding is unlikely to be successful due to the inability to position the nipple, increased respiratory effort during feeding, and reduced sucking mechanics (Wolf & Glass, 1992).

Bottle Feeding

Generally, the nipple that will work most effectively in feeding the infant with micrognathia and a retracted tongue will need to be long enough to provide adequate contact between the nipple and tongue without causing gagging. A narrow base or standard nipple will allow full insertion of the nipple into the infant's mouth. The nipple should compress easily and be used in conjunction with a bottle that allows squeezing to assist with the flow of milk.

Feeding and Mandibular Distraction

Micrognathia and upper airway obstruction are treated in a variety of ways including positioning alone, mandibular distraction, tracheostomy, or tongue-lip adhesion (Schaefer, Stadler, & Gosain, 2004). Infants who undergo mandibular distraction to improve posterior airway space are unable to orally feed during the distraction procedure as their jaws are immobilized and they are unable to suck. During that time, they are usually fed through an NG tube. However, once the distraction procedure is completed, oral feeding can be resumed, and recent reports indicate immediate improvement of oral feeding following

the distraction procedure (Izadi, Yellon, Mandell, Smith, Song, Bidic, & Bradley, 2003; Mandell, Yellon, Bradley, Izadi, & Gordon, 2004; Schaefer et al., 2004).

Feeding after the Cleft Lip and Palate Repair

Postoperative feeding recommendations following cleft lip and palate repair vary among centers and remain a controversial topic (Cohen, Marschall, & Schafer, 1992). Immediate unrestricted feeding is allowed by some groups, while others recommend a restricted approach to facilitate good healing. For example, some centers discourage sucking following cleft lip and palate repair, and recommend the use of a cup or a spoon instead. Other centers may recommend supplemental tube feeding for a period of 7–10 days. In contrast, for a number of years some centers have implemented immediate, unrestricted feeding after the cleft repair without problems.

KEY ORAL-MOTOR FACILITATION TECHNIQUES

Positioning the Infant

Optimal positioning is central to successful feeding because it facilitates control of jaw, cheek, lip, and tongue movements for sucking/swallowing coordination (Morris & Klein, 1987). Feeding the infant with a cleft in an upright position of at least 60 degrees so that gravity can work to assist in swallowing is often helpful (Wolf & Glass, 1992). The baby's head should be supported in a chin-tuck position, with arms forward, trunk in midline, and the hips flexed. The use of this upright positioning can help to prevent nasal regurgitation. Placing the infant in a horizontal position increases the potential for nasal regurgitation, coughing, and sneezing. In addition, there may be flooding of the eustachian tube and reflux into the middle ear, causing middle ear effusion. The use of a bottle with an angled neck provides a downward flow of milk and simplifies feeding the infant in upright positioning.

Positioning the Nipple

Working with the baby during an initial feeding session to find the optimal intraoral position for the nipple is critical for feeding success. Studies have shown that the difference between success and failure of nipple placement for feeding effectiveness consists of only a few millimeters (Clarren, Anderson, & Wolf, 1987). It is important to position the nipple under a shelf of bone of the hard palate to provide the stable base needed to achieve compression. The use of the proper size and shape of the nipple, based on the patient's cleft, will facilitate proper positioning intraorally.

Pacing Intake

The caregiver should carefully pace the flow rate by providing fluid in rhythm with the infant's movements and reactions. Identifying the infant's cues during feeding is a learning process for both the caregiver and the infant. Eye widening, changes in facial expression, or a decrease in alertness are all signs the infant may give during feeding that may signal stress responses or subtle avoidance in response to feeding. If the infant begins feeding rapidly and then shows signs of swallowing disorganization, such as coughing or choking, the feeder will need to make adjustments in the feeding process, such as slowing the pace of fluid presentation. If the infant begins to slow down or stop sucking during the feeding, this may be an indication that the infant has tired and needs an imposed pause before continuing feeding. The infant may show signs of excessive air intake and need a pause in feeding to allow burping. The feeder must be able to deliver enough nutrition before the infant becomes tired; however, allowing enough time to facilitate safe feeding is vital to overall feeding success. Consulting a dietitian about the use of a higher calorie formula preparation with a lower volume intake requirement will allow the infant to spend less time feeding and to use a slower pace of intake while still ingesting an adequate amount of calories for growth (Kovar, 1997).

Oral Facilitation

It may be necessary for the feeder to provide oral facilitation techniques such as jaw and cheek support to increase the infant's oral control during feeding. The need for such strategies can be determined during an oral-motor/feeding assessment. The type of bottle used can support the use of certain strategies to increase oral control. For example, the use of a small diameter bottle, such as the infant Volu-Feed Disposable™ Nurser (60 ml capacity), will allow the feeder to use hand and finger positioning to facilitate support to the jaw and cheeks during feeding (Morris & Klein, 1987).

Preventing Excessive Air Intake

The caregiver may need to increase the frequency of burping, as the infant with a cleft will take in an increased amount of air with the liquid. If the infant is sucking vigorously, the feeder may need to impose a pause in feeding for burping to prevent excessive air intake and subsequent discomfort. As a general rule of thumb, the infant should be burped once every ounce to prevent the discomfort associated with the intake of air that inevitably will occur with each feeding.

CASE REPORT

Appropriate Positioning and Placement

Lydia was born with Pierre Robin sequence with the characteristic micrognathia, glossoptosis (posteriorly displaced tongue), and wide bell-shaped cleft palate. The potential for upper airway obstruction secondary to the posterior placement of the tongue was analyzed by continuous oxygen saturation monitoring and by a formal sleep study. The results of the sleep study were within normal limits and oxygen saturation levels were maintained, except during the mother's initial attempts at oral feedings. Lydia was described as being a poor feeder with little sucking, frequent gasping, and oxygen desaturations. Despite the mother's efforts, Lydia's intake was only minimal (5–10cc) before she would completely "shut down" and fall asleep, usually 10 minutes into the feeding.

A speech pathology oral motor/feeding consultation was requested. The results of the evaluation indicated normal oral reflexes with good rooting as well as the ability to initiate and sustain a rhythmical nonnutritive sucking pattern. Observation was then made of the mother as she demonstrated the methods she had been using while attempting oral feeding. The mother explained that she had already tried numerous nipples, including the cleft palate feeders, without success. She was observed positioning Lydia in a semireclined, cradle position as she offered her a standard nipple, which had been slit to assist with a faster milk delivery. She explained that she had been advised that the cleft would make sucking difficult and that she would need a nipple which would not require sucking.

Upon presentation of the nipple, Lydia made a few tentative sucking attempts as the milk rapidly flowed from the nipple. She coughed, sputtered, and pulled away from the nipple. An oxygen desaturation event was documented. The mother attempted to place the nipple intraorally again and had difficulty placing the nipple onto the tongue body. She continued with these attempts but the baby continued to resist, causing intermittent oxygen desaturations. Lydia then fell asleep after struggling to accept an intake of only 10 cc. The remainder of the feeding was then presented via oral gavage. The mother agreed to allow the speech pathologist to try interventional feeding techniques during the next feeding time.

Interventional techniques which were recommended included the use of upright positioning as opposed to the semireclined cradle position. Being upright helped Lydia avoid further posterior displacement of her tongue during her efforts at feeding. Non-nutritive oral stimulation was then provided with Lydia in upright positioning to help increase alertness and to help facilitate and organize oral movements for feeding. The Haberman Feeder was then presented intraorally. The longer size of this nipple made placement onto the tongue easier. In addition, there was no flow of liquid from the nipple prior to either active sucking or assistive squeezing, which allowed Lydia to become accustomed to the presence of the nipple without being flooded by formula. Once Lydia began to attempt sucking, a gentle assistive squeeze to deliver a small amount of formula was given in synchrony with her sucking attempts. Lydia was able to successfully transfer this small amount of formula without any clinical signs of swallowing dysfunction. A cycle of approximately eight assistive squeezes was completed before Lydia showed some disorganization by again pulling away from the nipple. After a brief pause, additional feeding trials revealed that Lydia could handle approximately five sequences of assistive squeeze for completion of suck-swallow before requiring a pause with repetition of the cycles for intake of approximately 30 cc. Gradually over a three-week time period, oral intake improved with toleration of longer cycles of assistive squeezing. Eventually the transition to complete oral feedings with maintenance of good oxygen saturation levels was accomplished.

Managing Nasal Regurgitation

Infants with a cleft palate often experience nasal regurgitation through the nose, and they may cough frequently during the feeding and seem to "choke." When nasal regurgitation occurs, the caregiver should stop feeding and allow the infant some time to cough or sneeze to clear the nasal passage. If nasal regurgitation occurs frequently during feeding, the caregiver should check positioning to assure that the infant is in an upright position that allows gravity to assist with downward flow of liquid. If coughing occurs frequently in conjunction with the nasal regurgitation, the feeder should consider using a slower flow nipple. Using pacing to additionally slow the presentation of fluid may help the infant to become more organized in maintaining synchrony of the sucking, swallowing, and breathing.

Consistency of Method

Consistency in how the baby is fed will contribute to overall feeding success. The baby should be fed in the same position, with the same nipple and bottle, and with the same technique during each feeding. The feeder must learn how to easily position the baby, how much of an assistive squeeze is required, how long to keep feeding, how often to burp the baby, and how to read the baby's cues related to feeding. If several different nipples and bottles are intermittently tried, and varying positions and different rates of assistive squeezing by a range of feeders are used, it is almost certain that feeding confusion and a poor feeding outcome will result. Fortunately, for the majority of infants, normal maturation and increased experience of the infant and caregiver with feeding helps to gradually ease the feeding process, in spite of variations in method which may occur.

Use of Feeding Obturators

A feeding obturator consists of an acrylic plate, which is inserted in the mouth and fits over the hard palate (refer to Figures 5–8A and 5–8B). It is retained in the crevices of the cleft and provides a seal between the mouth and the nasal cavity. This effectively closes the palatal defect and maintains a separation between the nasal cavity and oral cavity. (See Chapter 20 for more information.) The obturator can promote a more normal tongue position and it improves the infant's ability to achieve compression of the nipple against the plate. A pediatric dentist or prosthodontist is the professional who can construct the feeding appliance and check it frequently so that it can be modified periodically as the child grows. If the obturator is to be successful, it should be used within the first few days of life.

There are differing views regarding the use of palatal appliances for assisting with feeding in infants with palatal clefts (Choi, Kleinheinz, Joos, & Komposch, 1991; Crossman, 1998; Delgado, Schaaf, & Emrich, 1992; Kogo et al., 1997; Osuji, 1995; Savion & Huband, 2005; Selley & Boxall, 1986). Some craniofacial centers advocate the use of a palatal obturator or feeding appliance and recommend its use on a regular basis. There have been reports of increased weight gain in selected groups of infants who have been fitted with feeding appliances (Balluff & Udin, 1986). In other settings, infants are given a trial of oral feedings and are fitted with appliances only if significant feeding problems are demonstrated. In some settings, appliances are rarely recommended, as those professionals feel that, with modifications of the nipple or bottle, correct positioning, and appropriate feeding technique, the obturator simply is not necessary.

Disadvantages of the obturator include the expense and the difficulty of use. Because the infant has no teeth to stabilize the appliance, it may be hard to insert the appliance as well as

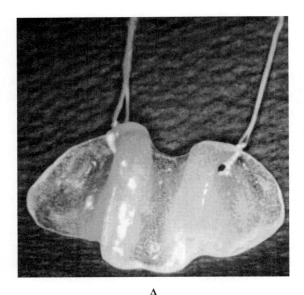

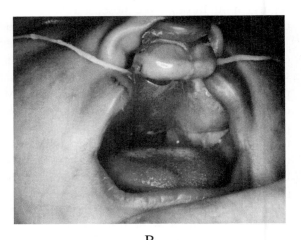

A   B

FIGURE 5–8 (A and B)   A. An infant feeding obturator. B. An infant feeding obturator in place. This type of obturator provides a separation of the nasal cavity from the oral cavity, which helps to eliminate the regurgitation of liquids into the nose. The feeding appliance also keeps the tongue from resting inside the cleft, and it provides a solid surface so that the tongue can achieve compression of the nipple in order to express the milk.

keep it in place. Other disadvantages include the possibility of irritation to the oral tissues and the need for ongoing replacement to accommodate growth. Hygiene may also be a concern if the appliance is not properly cleaned prior to insertion into the infant's oral cavity. Some maintain that, although the obturator can assist during feeding by helping the infant achieve compression of the nipple, the generation of negative pressure does not always occur (Choi et al., 1991). However, even without allowing suction, the opportunity to compress the nipple by providing a hard palatal surface is considered a distinct advantage by others (Crossman, 1998).

Oral Hygiene

With all infants, it is important to maintain good oral hygiene. Although the mouths of infants tend to be self-cleaning, it is particularly important to attend to the infant's oral hygiene if there is a cleft

lip or palate. With an open cleft, fluid will often enter the cleft area and nose. In addition, even with an upright feeding position, some nasal regurgitation is to be expected. The fluid can mix with mucous secretions from the mouth and nose and form a hard crust, which can become infected, causing irritation and soreness. Therefore, after each feeding, the caregiver should provide some water to the infant, and also cleanse the areas surrounding the cleft. The pediatrician may recommend using a washcloth, a small piece of gauze moistened with water, or water with hydrogen peroxide to gently wipe the mucous membrane in the oral cavity, with particular attention to that area that surrounds the cleft.

The caregiver should be careful not to cause discomfort or injury during this process; therefore, the use of a syringe or cotton swab is usually not recommended. However, it should be remembered that the cleft is not a wound, and therefore, it is not sore to touch. Gentle cleansing of this area will not cause discomfort or irritation.

FEEDING THE OLDER INFANT

Transitioning to a Cup

Most infants are ready for transition to the cup by 8 or 9 months of age. Some normally developing infants show readiness even earlier, between 6 to 8 months of age (Lang, Lawrence, & Orme, 1994). The initial response to the cup is generally sucking, with tongue protrusion and loss of liquid from the mouth. Gradually the infant will demonstrate increased oral skills for cup drinking and is able to take one or two sip-swallows as the cup is held by the caregiver. Using a slightly thickened liquid to slow the liquid flow during initial training with cup drinking is often beneficial.

There are a wide variety of cup options available for weaning from a bottle to a cup. Selecting a cup that does not promote continued sucking is important. A small open cup without a spout, straw, or valve is generally the best option for transitioning away from sucking and toward cup-drinking skills. Using the Medela SoftCup™ feeder is an alternative during the transitional period (Figure 5–9). Milk or breast milk is delivered through a narrow, flexible cup reservoir, facilitating development of oral skills for handling small amounts of liquid from a cup.

Most surgeons recommend weaning from the bottle to the cup prior to the palate repair. Immediately after the palate repair, sucking is discouraged because it can result in a breakdown of the repair. The palate repair is usually done around 9 to 10 months of age, so weaning to the cup should be done sometime before this age to avoid feeding problems postoperatively.

Introduction of Solid Foods

Solid foods can be introduced to the baby with an unrepaired cleft palate at about the

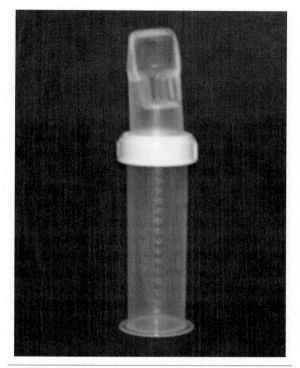

FIGURE 5–9 The Medela SoftCup feeder. This can be used as an alternative during the transitional period between a bottle and cup.

same time as with any infant. The timing of solid introduction is dependent upon the preferences of the pediatrician, parent, and the individual baby. Usually, spoon-feedings begin with rice cereals and strained foods at or around 4 to 6 months of age. The baby will respond to the spoon-feedings at first by suckling. This may result in food being pushed into the nasal cavity. As the baby becomes more skilled in eating and begins to use more mature tongue patterns, this will occur less often. Mixing the pureed fruit with the cereal provides a degree of thickness that may reduce the tendency for nasal reflux. The feeder should use a slow rate of presentation while spoon-feeding to allow the baby to gradually learn how to direct the food around the area of the cleft. The feeder should watch the baby for cues to know when to present the next bite. The baby's cues include leaning forward or opening the mouth in anticipation of the spoon. Leaving the spoon in the baby's mouth long enough to allow the baby to use his or her lips to clean the spoon will help to facilitate lip mobility. This is especially important following the surgery for cleft lip repair. Rapid spoon-feeding or presentation of large spoonfuls may cause more frequent nasal regurgitation as well as disorganized swallowing.

The transition to more textured foods, such as lumpy or bite-sized table foods, also can be introduced in the same sequence as for other children. Foods should initially be offered by spoon with the baby seated in an upright position to reduce nasal regurgitation. The baby should be provided with opportunities to practice finger feeding with small pieces of easily dissolvable solid foods such as easily dissolvable crackers or cookies. This will help to develop independence with self-feeding and give the baby practice with the tongue movements for diversion around the cleft and increase efficiency of skills needed for mastication. If food is observed passing from the nose or becomes lodged in the area of the cleft, it should be removed gently with either a finger or a swab. As the baby's oral-motor skills become more proficient, the baby will learn how to efficiently manage transfer of solids for swallowing.

Until the palate is repaired, cleansing the oral cavity by feeding the baby water after each meal is important for the maintenance of oral hygiene. In addition, foods that are acidic or spicy should be avoided prior to the palate repair as the lining of the nose is particularly sensitive to this kind of food.

Objective Studies for Assessment of Airway Protection during Feeding

When the feeding difficulties are significant, as characterized by clinical signs of airway compromise, further evaluation is needed. Clinical signs of feeding dysfunction and airway protection problems can include the inability to establish and maintain a coordinated suck-swallow-breathe sequence, coughing, choking, color change, increased respiratory rate, as well as oxygen desaturations during feedings. The infant may respond to feeding attempts with arching or refusal to accept the nipple. When these signs are noted, objective studies of swallowing function should be performed to assess the infant's ability to safely feed. These studies may also give information regarding the effect of compensatory strategies to improve the infant's feeding performance.

Videofluoroscopic Swallowing Study (VSS)

A *videofluoroscopic swallowing study,* also referred to as a *modified barium swallow,* is generally performed by a radiologist and a speech-language pathologist. The videofluoroscopic study allows an overall view of the oral, pharyngeal, and esophageal phases of swallowing as well as the interactions between the phases. Swallowing function, as well as the infant's ability to maintain airway protection during swallowing, is carefully assessed. The degree of nasopharyngeal reflux and the occurrence of penetration or aspiration can be documented. The infant's protective reaction to aspirated material can also be assessed. Compensatory strategies, such as positional adaptations, different nipples, and pacing of presentations, can be utilized to determine their effect on improving the feeding process (Kramer, 1985; Newman et al., 1991). Disadvantages to the videofluoroscopic study include radiation to the infant as well as the feeder during the study, the necessity of adding barium contrast to the formula (increases viscosity, unfamiliar taste), and the fact that the swallows viewed represent a relatively small sample of feeding overall.

Fiberoptic Endoscopic Evaluation of Swallowing (FEES)

Pediatric *fiberoptic endoscopic evaluation of swallowing* (FEES) involves the transnasal passage of an endoscope for viewing of the pharyngeal and laryngeal structures (Willging, 1995). The focus of this study is on assessing the integrity of airway protection during swallowing. FEES also provides information regarding sensory threshold in the pharynx and larynx (Aviv et al., 1998). Advantages of the FEES procedure include the ability to clearly visualize pharyngeal and laryngeal structures as well as the spontaneous swallowing of secretions. Feeding can be assessed using the infant's customary bottle and nipple and the usual formula. Green food coloring or liquid betacarotene is added to enhance visualization of the bolus during the study. Compensatory swallowing strategies can be tried during the FEES study without the time limitations of fluoroscopy. Disadvantages include the temporary loss of view that occurs as the velopharyngeal valve closes around the scope during swallowing. This is generally not a problem with single swallows as the structures quickly return to their resting position following the swallow, thus restoring the view. There is, however, a particular disadvantage while viewing the rapid chain swallowing sequences characteristic of early infancy because the view is obscured with more frequency.

MANAGEMENT OF SEVERE CASES

Alternative Feeding Methods for Severe Cases

When the feeding problem is not easily resolved with modifications of the nipple or bottle, supplemental feeding through an *orogastric* or *nasogastric (NG) tube* may be required for a period of time. During this time period, oral-motor treatment strategies for improving oral-motor function for feeding should be provided, as appropriate. If the feeding problems persist for a period of time and cannot be adequately resolved with other measures, *gastrostomy (G) tube* feeding may be considered. This is particularly indicated if the infant presents with abnormal oral reflexes or shows poor ability to coordinate airway protection with swallowing during a videofluoroscopic or endoscopic swallowing study. A gastrostomy tube is inserted in the stomach through a surgical procedure, and may remain in place for an extended period of time. Should the infant show considerable signs of progress with regard to feeding skill development and oral intake volume, the tube can be removed (Rudolph, 1994).

Interdisciplinary Feeding Team Evaluation

In more severe cases, an evaluation by a team of specialists may be indicated. Typically, an interdisciplinary feeding team consists of a core group of medical professionals that may include a gastroenterologist, nutritionist, nurse, speech-language pathologist, occupational therapist, behavioral psychologist, otolaryngologist, pulmonologist, and consulting radiologist. The composition of interdisciplinary feeding teams varies among centers (Lefton-Greif & Arvedson, 1997; Miller, Burklow, Santoro, Kirby, Mason,

& Rudolph, 2001; Rudolph, 1994). With the coordinated assessment of these specialists, management and long-term planning for treatment of complicated feeding problems can be accomplished.

SUMMARY

Whatever feeding method is chosen, it is important that the feeding process becomes relatively easy and efficient. The infant must receive adequate nutrition in a relatively short period of time and without undue effort. Weight gain should be monitored closely by the pediatrician. If there is any evidence of inadequate weight gain, the pediatrician may consider the need for assessment of feeding modifications as well as supplemental feedings if necessary. The two appendices at the end of this chapter provide feeding tips for parents as well as information on feeding infants with clefts using adapted nipples and bottles.

It is important that the feeding process is made to be a pleasurable experience for both the infant and the caregiver. It should not be forgotten that the time spent in feeding serves as an important part of the bonding process as well as the foundation for early sensorimotor and developmental experiences.

FOR REVIEW, DISCUSSION, AND CRITICAL THINKING

1. Describe the normal swallowing process and how it changes with growth.

2. What are reasons that cleft palate causes feeding difficulty? Why is there less of a problem with cleft lip?

3. What are some reasons that breast feeding is particularly difficult for a baby with cleft palate? How would you counsel the mother about alternative feeding methods?

4. What modifications can be made to a nipple in order to assist the baby with a cleft palate in feeding?

5. Describe different types of bottles that are commercially available for infants with cleft palate.

6. Discuss some oral-motor facilitation techniques that may be helpful for a child with feeding difficulties.

7. What are the reasons that an upright feeding position is preferable to a supine position?

8. How would you counsel the caregiver to deal with oral hygiene for the infant with a cleft?

REFERENCES

Alexander-Doelle, A. (1997). Breastfeeding and cleft palates. *AWHONN Lifelines, 1*(4), 27.

Aniansson, G., Svensson, H., Becker, M., & Ingvarsson, L. (2002). Otitis media and feeding with breast milk of children with cleft palate. *Scandinavian Journal of Plastic and Reconstructive Surgery, 36*, 9–15.

Arvedson, J., & Brodsky, L. (Eds.). (2002). *Pediatric swallowing and feeding: Assessment and management* (2nd ed.). San Diego, CA: Singular Publishing Group.

Aviv, J. E., Kim, T., Thomson, J. E., Sunshine, S., Kaplan, S., & Close, L. G. (1998). Fiberoptic endoscopic evaluation of swallowing with sensory testing (FEESST) in healthy controls. *Dysphagia, 13*(2), 87–92.

Balluff, M. A., & Udin, R. D. (1986). Using a feeding appliance to aid the infant with a cleft palate. *Ear, Nose, and Throat Journal, 65*(7), 316–320.

Barone, C. M., & Tallman, L. L. (1998). Modification of Playtex nurser for cleft palate patients. *Journal of Craniofacial Surgery, 9*(3), 271–274.

Bath, A. P., & Bull, P. D. (1997). Management of upper airway obstruction in Pierre Robin sequence. *Journal of Laryngology and Otology, 111*(12), 1155–1157.

Biancuzzo, M. (1998). Clinical focus on clefts. Yes! Infants with clefts can breastfeed. *AWHONN Lifelines, 2*(4), 45–49.

Bosma, J. D. (1985). Postnatal ontogeny of performances of the pharynx, larynx, and mouth. *American Review of Respiratory Disorders, 131*, S10–S15.

Bosma, J. D., & Donner, M. W. (1980). *Physiology of the pharynx.* Philadelphia: W. B. Saunders.

Bu'Lock, F., Woolridge, M. W., & Baum, J. D. (1990). Development of coordination of sucking, swallowing and breathing: Ultrasound study of term and preterm infants. *Developmental Medical Child Neurology, 32*(8), 669–678.

Carlisle, D. (1998). Feeding babies with cleft lip and palate. *Nursing Times, 94*(4), 59–60.

Choi, B. H., Kleinheinz, J., Joos, U., & Komposch, G. (1991). Sucking efficiency of early orthopaedic plate and teats in infants with cleft lip and palate. *International Journal of Oral Maxillofacial Surgery, 20*(3), 167–169.

Clarren, S. K., Anderson, B., & Wolf, L. S. (1987). Feeding infants with cleft lip, cleft palate, or cleft lip and palate. *Cleft Palate Journal, 24*(3), 244–249.

The Cleft Palate Foundation. (1998). *Feeding an infant with a cleft.* Chapel Hill, NC: Author.

Cohen, M., Marschall, M., & Schafer, M. (1992). Immediate unrestricted feeding of infants following cleft lip and palate repair. *Journal of Craniofacial Surgery, 3*(1). 30–32.

Crossman, K. (1998). Breastfeeding a baby with a cleft palate: A case report. *Journal of Human Lactation, 14*(1), 47–50.

Darzi, M. A., Chowdri, N. A., & Bhat, A. N. (1996). Breast feeding or spoon feeding after cleft lip repair: A prospective, randomised study. *British Journal of Plastic Surgery, 49*(1), 24–26.

Delgado, A. A., Schaaf, N. G., & Emrich, L. (1992). Trends in prosthodontic treatment of cleft palate patients at one institution: A twenty-one year review. *Cleft Palate-Craniofacial Journal, 29*(5), 425–428.

Glass, R. P., & Wolf, L. S. (1999). Feeding management of infants with cleft lip and palate and micrognathia. *Infants and Young Children, 12*(1), 70–81.

Haberman, M. (1988). A mother of invention. *Nursing Times, 84*, 52–53.

Izadi, K., Yellon, R., Mandell, D., Smith, M., Song, S., Bidic, S., & Bradley, J. (2003). Correction of upper airway obstruction in the newborn with internal mandibular distraction osteogenesis. *Journal of Craniofacial Surgery, 14*(4), 493–499.

Johansson, B., & Ringsberg, K. C. (2004). Parents' experiences of having a child with cleft lip and palate. *Journal of Advanced Nursing, 47*(2), 165–173.

Jones, J. E., Henderson, L., & Avery, D. R. (1982). Use of a feeding obturator for infants with severe cleft lip and palate. *Special Care in Dentistry, 2*(3), 116–120.

Jones, W. B. (1988). Weight gain and feeding in the neonate with cleft: A three-center study. *Cleft Palate Journal, 25*(4), 379–384.

Koenig, J. S., Davies, A. M., & Thach, B. T. (1990). Coordination of breathing, sucking, and swallowing during bottle feedings in human infants. *Journal of Applied Physiology, 69,* 1623–1629.

Kogo, M., Okada, G., Ishii, S., Shikata, M., Iida, S., & Matsuya, T. (1997). Breast feeding for cleft lip and palate patients, using the Hotz-type plate. *Cleft Palate–Craniofacial Journal, 34*(4), 351–353.

Kovar, A. J. (1997). Nutrition assessment and management in pediatric dysphagia. *Seminars in Speech and Language, 18*(1), 39–49.

Kramer, S. S. (1985). Special swallowing problems in children. *Gastrointestinal Radiology, 10,* 241–250.

Lang, S., Lawrence, C. J., & Orme, R. L. (1994). Cup feeding: An alternative method of infant feeding. *Archives of Diseases in Childhood, 71*(4), 365–369.

Lefton-Greif, M. A., & Arvedson, J. C. (1997). Pediatric feeding/swallowing teams. *Seminars in Speech and Language, 18*(1), 5–11; Quiz 12.

Lehman, J. A., Fishman, J. R., & Neiman, G. S. (1995). Treatment of cleft palate associated with Robin sequence: Appraisal of risk factors. *Cleft Palate-Craniofacial Journal, 32*(1), 25–29.

Mandell, D., Yellon, R., Bradley, J., Izadi, K., & Gordon, C. (2004). Mandibular distraction for micrognathia and severe upper airway obstruction. *Archives of Otolaryngology–Head & Neck Surgery, 130*(3), 344–348.

Mathew, O. P. (1988a). Nipple units for newborn infants: A functional comparison. *Pediatrics, 81*(5), 688–691.

Mathew, O. P. (1988b). Respiratory control during nipple feeding in preterm infants. *Pediatric Pulmonology, 5*(4), 220–224.

Mathew, O. P. (1990). Determinants of milk flow through nipple units: Role of hole size and nipple thickness. *American Journal of Diseases of Children, 144*(2), 222–224.

Mathew, O. P. (1991). Science of bottle feeding. *Journal of Pediatrics, 119*(4), 511–519.

Mathew, O. P., Clark, M. L., Pronske, M. L., Luna-Solarzano, H. G., & Peterson, M. D. (1985). Breathing pattern and ventilation during oral feeding in term newborn infants. *Journal of Pediatrics, 106*(5), 810–813.

Meyer, E. C., Coll, C. T., Lester, B. M., Boukydis, C. F., McDonough, S. M., & Oh, W. (1994). Family-based intervention improves maternal psychological well-being and feeding interaction of preterm infants. *Pediatrics, 93*(2), 241–246.

Miller, C., Burklow, K., Santoro, K., Kirby, E., Mason, D., & Rudolph, C. (2001). An interdisciplinary team approach to the management of pediatric feeding and swallowing disorders. *Children's Health Care, 30*(3), 201–218.

Morris, S. E., & Klein, M. D. (1987). *Prefeeding skills: A comprehensive resource for feeding development.* Tucson, AZ: Therapy Skill Builders.

Myer, C. M., Cotton, R. T., & Shott, S. R. (1995). *The pediatric airway: An interdisciplinary approach.* Philadelphia: J. B. Lippincott.

Nassar, E, Marques, I. L., Trindade, A. S., & Bettiol, H. (2006). Feeding-facilitating techniques for the nursing infant with Robin sequence. *Cleft Palate-Craniofacial Journal, 43*(1), 55–60.

Newman, L. A., Cleveland, R. H., Blickman, J. G., Hillman, R. E., & Jaramillo, D. (1991). Videofluoroscopic analysis of the infant swallow. *Investigative Radiology, 26*(10), 870–873.

Osuji, O. O. (1995). Preparation of feeding obturators for infants with cleft lip and palate. *Journal of Clinical Pediatric Dentistry, 19*(3), 211–214.

Paradise, J., Elster, B., & Tan, L. (1994). Evidence in infants with cleft palate that breast milk protects against otitis media. *Pediatrics, 94*(6), 853–860.

Redford-Badwal, D. A., Mabry, K., & Frassinelli, J. D. (2003). Impact of cleft lip and/or palate on nutritional health and oral-motor development. *Dental Clinics of North America, 47*(2), 305–317.

Rudolph, C. D. (1994). Feeding disorders in infants and children. *Journal of Pediatrics, 125*(6, Pt. 2), S116–S124.

Sasaki, C. T., Levine, P. A., Laitman, J. T., Phil, M., & Crelin, E. S. (1977). Postnatal descent of the epiglottis in man. *Archives of Otolaryngology, 103*, 169–171.

Savion, I., & Huband, M. (2005). A feeding obturator for a preterm baby with Pierre Robin sequence. *Journal of Prosthetic Dentistry, 93*(2), 197–200.

Schaefer, R., Stadler, J., & Gosain, A. (2004). To distract or not distract: An algorithm for airway management in isolated Pierre Robin sequence. *Plastic and Reconstructive Surgery, 113*(4), 1113–1125.

Selley, W. G., & Boxall, J. (1986). A new way to treat sucking and swallowing difficulties in babies. *Lancet, 1*(8491), 1182–1184.

Shaw, W., Bannister, R., & Roberts, C. (1999). Assisted feeding is more reliable for infants with clefts: A randomized trial. *Cleft Palate-Craniofacial Journal, 36*(3), 262–268.

Shprintzen, R. J. (1992). The implications of the diagnosis of Robin sequence. *Cleft Palate-Craniofacial Journal, 29*(3), 205–209.

Shprintzen, R. J., & Singer, L. (1992). Upper airway obstruction and the Robin sequence. *International Anesthesiology Clinics of North America, 30*(4), 109–114.

Willging, J. P. (1995). Endoscopic evaluation of swallowing in children. *International Journal of Pediatric Otorhinolaryngology, 32* (Suppl.), S107–S108.

Van den Elzen, A., Semmekrot, B., Bongers, E., Huygen, P., & Marres, H. (2001). Diagnosis and treatment of Pierre Robin sequence: Results of a retrospective clinical study and review of literature. *European Journal of Pediatrics, 160*, 47–53.

Wolf, L. S., & Glass, R. P. (1992). *Feeding and swallowing disorders in infancy: Assessment and management*. Tucson, AZ: Therapy Skill Builders.

Young, J., O'Riordan, M., Goldstein, J., & Robin, N. (2001). What information do parents of newborns with cleft lip, palate, or both want to know? *Cleft Palate-Craniofacial Journal, 38*(1), 55–58.

Appendix 5–1

General Feeding Tips for Parents

By Claire K. Miller, Ph.D.

Relax

Most parents report feeling anxious about learning how to feed their baby with a cleft, but find the problems to be fewer than expected and easy to overcome when using the right type of nipple, bottle, and technique.

Feeding Equipment and Methods

A particular method of feeding is usually recommended shortly after birth by a nurse, speech pathologist, or occupational therapist. Try to use the adapted nipples, bottles, and feeding methods that are recommended, and be sure not to hesitate to call the nurse or speech pathologist if any questions arise about how to use the equipment.

Using Appropriate Positioning

Feeding a baby with cleft palate in an upright position as opposed to the traditional cradle or reclined position will reduce the amount of liquid that can escape up into the nose during feeding. Try using a pillow or small foam wedge to support the baby against you in an upright position.

Dealing with Nasal Regurgitation

If milk does have a tendency to come from the baby's nose even while using an upright position, the flow of the liquid may be too fast. Try using a nipple with a slower flow rate such as a smaller cross-cut or slit.

Feeding Refusal

- The baby may seem to be refusing to breast- or bottle-feed. Try to problem-solve what might be happening by considering the length of time between feedings. If the feedings are too close together, the baby may not be hungry enough to be motivated to feed.

- Consider the size of the nipple hole (is the baby working too hard to extract the fluid?). This is a common problem. Explore using a nipple that either has a faster flow rate or that is flexible enough for assistive squeezing.

- If breast feeding, the baby may be overwhelmed with the initial milk let-down during feeding and demonstrate avoidance. Experiment with hand-expressing some milk before beginning to breast-feed.

- Experiment with the temperature of the formula if bottle feeding. Although not proven by research, many infants seem to prefer warm formula as opposed to room temperature.

- Try to be consistent with the method being used for feeding. Train others who may be feeding the baby to use the same positioning, the same feeding equipment, and the same type of strategies you use when feeding your baby. For example, demonstrate how to use assistive squeezing or how often you give the baby breaks for resting or burping during a feeding.

MANAGING AIR INTAKE DURING FEEDING

Babies with clefts will tend to swallow some extra air while feeding. After intake of every ounce (or so), giving the baby a pause from feeding and chance to burp may help to alleviate discomfort associated with excessive air intake.

PERSISTENT ORAL FEEDING PROBLEMS

Most feeding problems can be easily resolved. If your baby continues to have trouble feeding and you are concerned, consult your pediatrician for a referral to a speech pathologist or occupational therapist experienced with the special feeding issues associated with cleft lip/palate or other craniofacial anomalies.

Appendix 5–2

Feeding Infants with Clefts Using Adapted Nipples and Bottles

By Claire K. Miller, Ph.D.

Bottle Feeding Using the Mead Johnson™ Cleft Palate Nurser

- Position baby in a semi-upright position in your lap. Hold the Mead Johnson bottle in your right hand, using your left arm/hand to support the baby's head and shoulders.

- The Mead Johnson nipple or nipple of choice (pigeon nipple, standard nipple, NUK nipple, etc.) can be used with the Mead Johnson flexible bottle.

- Use the nipple to touch the corner of the baby's lip to help stimulate mouth opening. When the baby's mouth opens, take care to place the nipple onto the body of the tongue, not in the space in front of the tongue.

- If the baby has a cleft lip and palate, allow the baby to try sucking the nipple first before beginning to use some gentle assistive squeezes of the bottle.

- Begin with one gentle squeeze of the bottle, watching the baby's reaction.

- Try to squeeze in a rhythmic manner in time to the baby's sucking.

- Try to avoid using a continuous squeezing motion as this will overwhelm the baby.

- Use regular squeezing at the beginning of the feeding when the baby is eating vigorously; slow the rate toward the middle and end of the feeding when the baby's sucking rate slows down.

Bottle Feeding Using the Haberman Feeder™

- The Haberman or Mini-Haberman Feeder™ has several parts: bottle, nipple, disc, collar, and valve membrane.

- Begin assembling the feeder by pressing the valve membrane onto the upper side of the disc (the stud should go through the center hole).

- Fill the bottle compartment with breast milk or formula. Put the valve membrane into the nipple, and then use the collar to put all the parts together onto the bottle. Squeeze the nipple compartment while the feeder is upright. Then turn the feeder upside down, releasing the nipple compartment. This will allow the formula to enter the nipple reservoir.

- Position the baby in a semi-upright position on your lap, holding the bottle in one hand and supporting the baby with your other arm/hand.

- Line up the shortest line (zero flow) on the nipple reservoir with the baby's nose.

- Touch the nipple to the corner of the baby's mouth, and when mouth opens, gently advance the nipple onto the baby's tongue.

- Try to position the nipple under any intact part of the palate.

- Allow the baby some time to begin sucking.

- Rotate the nipple until the medium line (medium flow) or longest line (maximum flow) is under the baby's nose—determine flow rate based upon baby's response.

- The nipple will release fluid as the baby compresses it with sucking.

- If needed, you may compress the reservoir to give extra assistance with fluid expression every second or third suck.

BOTTLE FEEDING USING THE PIGEON NIPPLE

- The pigeon nipple has a "Y"-shaped opening. Rub a soft clean cloth over the opening to loosen it before using.

- Use the nipple with a flexible bottle like the Mead Johnson.

- Find the "V" in the base of the nipple. This is the air vent that should be placed on the top of the nipple, under the infant's nose while feeding.

- Position the nipple on the infant's tongue. The infant's sucking motion will activate the flow.

FEEDING WITH THE MEDELA® SOFTCUP FEEDER

- The soft cup feeder has a silicone reservoir, one disc, one valve membrane, and a collar.

- The valve should be pressed onto the upper side of the disc so that the stud goes completely through the center hole.

- Slip the reservoir into the collar.

- Put the assembled valve into the reservoir, making sure that the valve and the high rim of the disc are facing the inside of the reservoir.

- Place the reservoir over the bottle and tighten the collar to make a good seal.

- Hold the feeder upright and squeeze below the pads of the reservoir.

- Keep squeezing and tip the feeder upside down.

- Release the pads and some fluid will flow into the reservoir; repeat until almost filled.

- Position the baby and present the soft cup to the lips; the baby's mouth will slightly open.

- Present small amounts of the fluid, allowing time for the baby to transfer and swallow each small amount given.

CHAPTER

6

DEVELOPMENTAL ASPECTS: LANGUAGE, COGNITION, AND PHONOLOGY

CHAPTER OUTLINE

INTRODUCTION

Children with a history of cleft palate are at risk for delays in the acquisition of speech skills and may be at risk for delays in early language development. It is obvious that children with a cleft palate will be behind their unaffected peers in the acquisition of early developmental phonemes because of the open palate. This delay will persist until the palate is repaired, and usually for some time postoperatively.

The articulation problems secondary to velopharyngeal insufficiency/incompetence (VPI) have been well documented in the literature. There is a good understanding of how the abnormal structure and function of the velopharyngeal valve affect speech by causing obligatory and compensatory errors (Trost-Cardamone, 1997). How the presence of orofacial anomalies can affect language and cognitive development is less clear. Of course, significant difficulties with speech production may cause expressive language skills to appear delayed due to the difficulty with production. However, there are many more subtle factors that may affect development in this population.

Children with craniofacial syndromes are at greatest risk for speech and language disorders. This is due not only to the orofacial anomalies, but also to neurological disorders and mental retardation that commonly occur with craniofacial syndromes.

This chapter outlines what is known about development of children with clefts and craniofacial conditions, particularly in the area of language. It is hoped that the reader will learn to be attentive to all aspects of development, including language and learning, when evaluating a child from one of these populations. Developmental delays are particularly important to recognize and remediate during the critical period of brain development in order for the child to reach his or her full potential.

FACTORS THAT CAN AFFECT DEVELOPMENT

Unlike other primates, humans have the innate ability to learn to communicate through spoken or verbal language. The ability to learn is the key factor and is dependent on the individual's cognitive abilities, or cognition. (Cognition is the ability to engage in conscious intellectual activities that are important for learning.) Although cognition is important for language learning, the development of language further enhances the development of cognitive skills (Dowling, 2004).

Language and cognitive development are dependent on some basic prerequisites, including intelligence, environmental stimulation, hearing, motivation, and attending skills. Normal anatomy and physiology of the speech mechanism are also important for expressive language production. When one considers the basic prerequisites for normal learning and speech production, it is easy to understand why some children with orofacial anomalies are at risk for delayed development.

This section describes these basic prerequisites and how these areas may be affected by the occurrence of a cleft or craniofacial condition.

Intelligence and Brain Structure

The most important requirement for speech and language learning is intelligence because intelligence affects the ability to learn. Since language skills must be learned indirectly through exposure to the environment, the child must have the intellectual ability to perceive, comprehend, assimilate, analyze, categorize, imitate, and then generate language.

Intelligence and brain development have a direct impact on the rate of acquisition of all developmental milestones. When intelligence is significantly below normal, there are usually generalized developmental delays that affect function in all aspects of development, including language and speech. Intelligence and cognitive function are totally dependent on the structure of the brain and the function of the central nervous system. Therefore, normal brain structure and function are necessary requirements for the development of both speech and language.

With respect to individuals with nonsyndromic clefts of the lip and/or palate, Nopoulos and colleagues (Nopoulos et al., 2001; Nopoulos et al., 2005; Nopoulos, Berg, Canady et al., 2002; Nopoulos, Berg, Van Demark et al., 2002), have found, using magnetic resonance imaging (MRI) technology, structural abnormalities in brain morphology of affected men. These authors reported finding midline anomalies, enlarged regions of the cerebrum, decreased volumes of the posterior cerebrum and cerebellum, and abnormalities in the frontal lobe. These findings suggest that there may be a relationship between facial development and brain development. It should be cautioned, however, that this research is new, and has not been replicated by others at this point.

Despite the aforementioned studies, research has not shown a marked difference in intellectual function between children with a history of nonsyndromic cleft and those with no congenital anomaly. Although some studies have shown minor differences in the early years of development (Fox, Lynch, & Brookshire, 1978; Kapp-Simon & Krueckeberg, 2000; Nieman & Savage, 1997; Snyder & Scherer, 2004; Speltz et al., 2000; Starr, Chinski, Canter, & Meier, 1977), this "intellectual depression" (McWilliams, 1970) may be due to other factors. This theory is supported by the fact that these early deficits tend to disappear with age, resolution of middle ear disease, and other treatment (McWilliams, 1970; McWilliams, Morris, & Shelton, 1990; Musgrave, McWilliams, & Matthews, 1975; Nieman & Savage, 1979). Therefore, children with nonsyndromic clefts do not appear to be at particular risk for intellectual impairment.

In contrast, children with a history of cleft palate only (CPO), especially those who have other congenital anomalies, are at risk for developmental and intellectual deficits (Broder, Richman, & Matheson, 1998; Goodstein, 1961; Lewis, 1961; Richman, 1980; Richman, Eliason, & Lindgren, 1988; Strauss & Broder, 1993). This is due to the fact that isolated cleft palate often occurs as part of a syndrome, which may include mental retardation as a phenotypic feature. In addition, these children are more likely to exhibit neurological dysfunction, sensorineural hearing loss, velopharyngeal dysfunction, other craniofacial anomalies, malocclusion, attention deficits, frequent hospitalizations, and even social isolation (Elfenbein, Waziri, & Morris, 1981; Peterson, 1973). McWilliams and Matthews (1979) found that in a population of 108 children with history of isolated cleft palate and other anomalies, 51% had a full-scale IQ of 89 or below and 37% had IQs of 69 or below.

There are many craniofacial syndromes, some that include clefts and some that do not, that include mental retardation or neuro-linguistic deficits as a phenotypic feature. Shprintzen (1998) listed the following cranio-facial conditions that can include mental retardation: Apert syndrome, BBB (Opitz) syndrome, Beckwith-Wiedemann syndrome, Carpenter syndrome, CHARGE association, Down syndrome, Cornelia de Lange syn-drome, fetal alcohol syndrome, fetal hydantoin, holoprosencephaly sequence, Noonan syndrome, otopalatodigital syndrome, Rubinstein-Taybi syndrome, Shprintzen-Goldberg I syndrome, Shprintzen-Goldberg II syndrome (Shprintzen et al., 1978), velocardiofacial syndrome, Weaver syndrome, and Williams syndrome.

Language deficit is one of the most com-monly expressed phenotypic features of veloc-ardiofacial syndrome (VCFS, also known as 22q11.2 deletion syndrome) (D'Antonio, Scherer, Miller, Kalbfleisch, & Bartley, 2001; Golding-Kushner, Weller, & Shprintzen, 1985; Scherer, D'Antonio, & Kalbfleisch, 1999; Scherer, D'Antonio, & Rodgers, 2001). In addition, several authors have shown that patients with VCFS demonstrate significant neurological abnormalities, including reduced brain volume of both white and grey matter (Eliez, Antonarakis, Morris, Dahoun, & Reiss, 2001; Eliez, Schmitt, White, & Reiss, 2000; Eliez et al., 2001; Kates et al., 2001, 2004; van Amelsvoort et al., 2004), cerebellar hypoplasia (Devriendt, Van Thienen, Swillen, & Fryns, 1996; Eliez et al., 2001; Lynch et al., 1995; van Amelsvoort et al., 2004), larger corpus cal-losum area (Antshel, Conchelos, Lanzetta, Fremont, & Kates, 2005), and Chiari malformation (Hultman et al., 2000). These findings certainly have implications for cogni-tive, social, and language development in the VCFS population.

Some syndromes and conditions do not have mental retardation or neurological dys-function as typical phenotypic features, but have the potential for causing impairment in intellectual or neurological function. For exa-mple, in craniofrontonasal dysplasia, intellect is generally normal unless there are also midline defects of the brain. In Crouzon syndrome, hydrocephalus with increased intracranial pressure may occur due to the craniosynosto-sis. If left untreated, this can have a permanent effect on intelligence and cognitive function.

Environmental Stimulation

Environmental stimulation and environmental experience are important factors in language development. Children must be exposed to a great deal of language and they must have experiences with the environment before words about the environment are meaningful to them. Therefore, children who live in a language-rich environment are likely to develop language skills faster and have a more extensive vocabulary than children with little language stimulation. Language learning is easier under the age of 5 during the period of critical brain development (Dowling, 2004). Therefore, stimulation during this period of time is particularly important.

Children with a history of cleft or cranio-facial condition are usually not different from other children in the amount of stimulation that they receive from their environment. In one study, the language input of mothers of children with clefts was found to be similar to the input of mothers of noncleft children (Chapman & Hardin, 1991). In some cases, children with a cleft or craniofacial condition may actually have an advantage over their unaffected peers. This is due to the fact that most of these children are followed by a cleft palate or craniofacial anomaly team and the speech-language pathologist on the team will usually counsel the parents on methods of language stimulation in the home. Some parents are so concerned about the child's development due to the anomalies that they become particularly diligent in working on language stimulation. (See Appendix 6–1 for a sample home program for parents to use in stimulating language.) Another advantage these children may have is that many qualify for enrollment in an early intervention program, most of which are geared toward the development of language skills.

Although some affected children may have some advantages in early stimulation, others are not as fortunate. Children with significant anomalies and serious medical conditions may undergo many surgical procedures and frequent hospitalizations in the early years. Unfortunately, a hospital room is usually not a language-rich environment. Additionally, due to the compromised medical condition and possibly due to the child's appearance, the severely affected child may not have as many opportunities to interact with others as their unaffected or less affected peers. This social isolation can negatively affect language learning.

Hearing

It is through sensory perception that we learn about the world around us and develop a method for communicating with each other. The need for adequate auditory skills for normal speech and language development is fairly obvious.

Children with a history of cleft palate are at high risk for chronic middle-ear effusion and conductive hearing loss due to eustachian tube malfunction. In addition, many craniofacial syndromes include conductive or sensorineural hearing loss as a phenotypic feature. For example, a primary phenotypic feature of Waardenburg syndrome is congenital sensorineural hearing loss that is usually severe and bilateral. Sensorineural hearing loss can also be found in hemifacial microsomia (also known as Goldenhar syndrome, facioauriculovertebral malformation sequence, and oculoauriculovertebral dysplasia), CHARGE association, Stickler syndrome, Treacher Collins syndrome, Turner syndrome, and others.

Even a mild, fluctuating conductive hearing loss can temporarily affect the acquisition of oral language skills. Speech development can be affected by the inability to adequately perceive high-frequency, low-intensity sounds. Language development can be affected by the strain required for hearing. Making that constant effort to hear is exhausting, so the child may respond by not listening. Consequently, less language is heard, perceived, analyzed, and learned.

A severe hearing loss or deafness affects the child's ability to perceive and thus imitate speech sounds. A child with a severe hearing impairment will have difficulty learning all aspects of language. Even resonance is affected by the inability to monitor and therefore modulate velopharyngeal function. As a result, verbal communication is extremely difficult, if not impossible, to acquire without hearing.

Hearing loss may be the primary reason that children with history of cleft often score lower on verbal performance measures than their noncleft peers in the early years (Broen et al., 1998; Jocelyn, Penko, & Rode, 1996; Kritzinger, Louw, & Hugo, 1996; Lamb et al., 1973). Additional support for hearing loss as a factor in early measures of intelligence comes from the studies that show that these differences in intelligence disappear with age or with the insertion of pressure-equalizing (PE) tubes (Musgrave et al., 1975; Paradise, 1998).

Motivation

The next prerequisite for language development is motivation. Although a new skill can be learned passively, the skill will be acquired much more rapidly if there is a need and desire to learn the skill. This general principal holds true for language learning.

In most cases, young children are motivated to talk because this is the best way to communicate. However, if a caregiver or older sibling anticipates the child's needs and wants, there is little reason to learn to talk, particularly under the age of two when gestures are effective. If the child was born with a birth defect, some families respond by overprotecting the child. They feel sorry for the child, especially during times of surgery. As a result, they may react by catering to the child's every need. Although this may be understandable at times, it can have a detrimental effect on the child's need to communicate and therefore, it may delay expressive language development. It is only when the child wants to communicate something more than the "here and now" that this gestural system is no longer effective. With an increase in the need to communicate, there is a corresponding increase in the motivation to communicate. It is at this point that language development will pick up, assuming that everything else is normal.

For the most part, children with a history of cleft are no different from their unaffected peers in communicating their needs through gestures during the first year (Long & Dalston, 1982a). During the second year, the child begins to use verbal language and discontinues the use of gestures because verbal language is usually a more effective form of communication. However, if the child has difficulty with speech sound production and therefore speech intelligibility is poor, verbal language may be an ineffective means of communication (Grunwell & Russell, 1988). Therefore, the child may revert back to using gestures, at least to augment speech. In addition, the child may compensate by keeping utterance length short. On the surface, this may appear to be an expressive language disorder due to the telegraphic nature of the speech. Instead, it is a compensatory strategy because shorter utterances are easier to produce clearly and easier for the listeners to understand. If intelligibility continues to be poor as the child gets older, this can cause the child to be less assertive when engaging in conversational skills as compared with others (Chapman, Graham, Gooch, & Visconti, 1998; Frederickson, Chapman, & Hardin-Jones, 2006). As an adult, the individual may continue to use shorter utterances to improve intelligibility (Pannbacker, 1975).

Attention

Another prerequisite for language learning is the ability to attend to the environment. Attention difficulties are a primary characteristic of *attention deficit-hyperactivity disorder* (ADHD). ADHD refers to a cluster of behavioral characteristics that involve impaired attention, impulsivity, distractibility, and hyperactivity (American Psychiatric Association, 2004). It has been estimated that 3% to 5% of elementary school-aged children have this disorder, making it the most prevalent psychiatric disorder of childhood (American Psychiatric Association, 1994). ADHD is five to nine times more prevalent in boys than in girls (Sanberg, Rutter, & Taylor, 1980).

When a child has a significant attention deficit, distractibility, and a high activity level, the stimulation from the environment may not be adequately perceived or processed, and language learning will be affected as a result. In addition, the child with ADHD is less likely to participate in language-enriching activities, such as reading, listening to a story, or playing a game. Children with ADHD are often diagnosed with learning disabilities (Cantwell & Baker, 1991; Cherkes-Julkowski, 1998; Sidoti, Marsh, Marty-Grames, & Noetzel, 1996; Tirosh, Berger, Cohn-Ophir, Davidovitch, & Cohen, 1998) and language disorders (Cantwell & Baker, 1991; Cherkes-Julkowski, 1998; Damico, Damico, & Armstrong, 1999; Fergusson & Horwood, 1992; Love & Thompson, 1988; Purvis & Tannock, 1997; Tirosh et al., 1998; Tirosh & Cohen, 1998; Wright, 1982). One study found that 30% of children with speech and language impairments also had ADHD (Beitchman, Hood, Rochon, & Peterson, 1989).

Although ADHD is usually diagnosed in children with no identified neurological lesion, the same characteristics are commonly seen in individuals with documented brain damage or neurological deficits (Max et al., 1998; Niemann, Ruff, & Kramer, 1996). Children with craniofacial syndromes that include neurological dysfunction are at significant risk for difficulties with attention and concentration. As an example, attention deficits and difficulty with concentration are typical problems with velocardiofacial syndrome (Heineman-de Boer, Van Haelst, Cordia-de Haan, & Beemer, 1999; Swillen et al., 1997, 1999).

Anatomy and Physiology

There are many physical prerequisites that are important for speech production. There must be structural integrity of the entire vocal tract.

In addition, the physiology must be normal for respiration, phonation, resonance, articulation and neurological function. Clefts and craniofacial conditions may include a variety of structural abnormalities, including dental malocclusion and velopharyngeal dysfunction. The effects of these abnormalities on speech are covered in the next three chapters.

DEVELOPMENT OF CHILDREN WITH CLEFTS AND CRANIOFACIAL SYNDROMES

Language Development and Learning

The literature on the developmental status of children with a history of cleft is often contradictory and difficult to interpret. This is partly due to the fact that children with clefts and craniofacial anomalies are very heterogeneous populations. They can differ not only in the type and severity of the cleft, but also with respect to other medical conditions, such as chronic middle ear effusion and hearing loss; the number of hospitalizations; the type and effectiveness of the surgical repairs; parental attitudes and involvement; and even environmental factors. Therefore, it is difficult to determine what typical development is for these children.

Regardless, several authors have reported that children with clefts show some early deficits in cognitive development or prelanguage skills during the first 3 years of life (Fox, Lynch, & Brookshire, 1978; Kapp-Simon & Krueckeberg, 2000; Nieman & Savage, 1979; Snyder & Scherer, 2004; Speltz et al., 2000; Starr, Chinski, Canter, & Meier, 1977). In addition, some studies have found that children with clefts have lower scores in verbal performance than nonverbal performance on standardized tests (Broen, Devers, Doyle, Prouty, & Moller, 1998; Estes & Morris, 1970; Lamb, Wilson, & Leeper, 1973; Ruess, 1965; Wirls, 1971). However, other studies found no verbal-nonverbal differences in the cleft population (Leeper, Pannbacker, & Roginski, 1980; McWilliams & Matthews, 1979) and no differences in comprehension as compared with unaffected peers (Long & Dalston, 1983). Some studies have reported that children with a repaired cleft have immature syntactic development, short utterance length, and overall delays in expressive language as compared with their unaffected peers (Horn, 1972; Morris, 1962; Smith & McWilliams, 1968; Spriestersbach, Darley, & Morris, 1958; Whitcomb, Ochsner, & Wayte, 1976). Others have found the linguistic abilities of children with repaired clefts to be within the normal range (Buescher & Paynter, 1973; Saxman & Bless, 1973). One study found that children with a history of cleft who demonstrate compensatory articulation productions had a higher frequency of language delays than those without compensatory productions (Pamplona & Ysunza, 2000).

The overall message is that when there is a history of cleft, there may be delays in early language development, especially in expressive language because this is dependent on speech production. However, in most cases, these delays seem to disappear with time (Musgrave, McWilliams, & Matthews, 1975; Shames & Rubin, 1979; Zimmerman & Canfield, 1968). This may be due to the cleft palate repair, the resolution of middle ear disease that can cause fluctuant hearing loss, and/or the correction of articulation and resonance problems that may affect expressive language.

Although language problems may not be a major issue in children with nonsyndromic clefts, they are very common in children with a syndrome. Learning disabilities, which can further affect language, are also commonly found in individuals with craniofacial syndromes (Broder et al, 1998; Richman, Eliason, & Lindgren, 1988; Strauss & Broder, 1993). For example, language disorders and learning disabilities are phenotypic features of velo-cardiofacial syndrome (VCFS) (Glaser et al., 2002; Golding-Kushner, Weller, & Shprintzen, 1985; Kok & Solman, 1995; Motzkin, Marion, Goldberg, Shprintzen, & Saenger, 1993; Scherer, D'Antonio, & Kalbfleisch, 1999; Shprintzen, 1998; Shprintzen et al., 1978; Swillen et al., 1999; Vantrappen et al., 1999).

Phonological/Articulation Development

Early sound production, in the form of cooing and babbling, is an important part of normal speech development. By associating the physical movement of sound production with the auditory results through a tactile-kinesthetic-auditory feedback loop, infants are able to learn to produce sounds volitionally. Infants with cleft palate, however, have an inadequate sound production mechanism and they frequently have an impaired auditory system due to hearing loss. With these factors alone, they are at risk for delays in phonological development, even after the palate is repaired (Jones et al., 2003; O'Gara & Logemann, 1988).

Certainly, infants with unrepaired clefts will have less variety in speech sound production than their unaffected peers, and may even vocalize less, at least until the palate is repaired (Long & Dalston, 1982b). Infants with an unrepaired cleft palate demonstrate an alteration in the manner of production with a predominant use of nasal phonemes (/m/, /n/) for most oral sounds. This is an obligatory error due to oral-nasal cavity coupling. Additionally, compensatory productions can occur due to structural constraints that restrict phonemic development (Harding & Grunwell, 1996; O'Gara & Logemann, 1988). As a result, infants with an open cleft may begin to use glottal stops rather than the oral plosives (/p/, /b/, /t/, /d/, /k/, /g/) that are typical of a normal babbling pattern (Chapman, 1991).

The open palate can also affect the infant's place of articulation. Unaffected infants use anterior sounds in prespeech productions (Roug, Landberg, & Lundberg, 1989; Smith & Oller, 1981; Stoel-Gammon, 1985). In contrast, infants with clefts, regardless of type, babble with a predominance of posterior consonants, particularly glottals and velars (Hardin-Jones, Chapman, & Schulte, 2003; Lohmander-Agerskov, Soderpalm, Friede, Persson, & Lilja, 1994; Russell, 1991; Willadsen & Albrechtsen, 2006). One study showed better phonological development in children treated with infant orthopedics during the first year than in those who were not (Konst, Rietveld, Peters, & Kuijpers-Jagtman, 2003).

The infant's abnormal phonological development as a result of the open palate can persist into early speech (Estrem & Broen, 1989; Hardin, 1991; O'Gara, Logemann, & Rademaker, 1994). In addition, if the palate is unrepaired when the child begins to use single words, then he or she will be able to say "mama," but "dada" will be replaced with "nana" (Lynch, Fox, & Brookshire, 1983).

Although early articulatory patterns persist for some time after palate repair, several investigators have found that within the first few years, glottal productions gradually decrease and the oral productions increase. As a result, the speech of those with a successful palate repair may gradually become similar to noncleft peers by the age of 4 or 5

(Chapman, 1993; Chapman & Hardin, 1992; O'Gara & Logemann, 1988; O'Gara et al., 1994).

How quickly children with repaired clefts are able to acquire oral sounds and "catch up" with their unaffected peers after the palate repair has been a subject of several investigations. One factor that may affect the acquisition of articulation skills is the age of palate repair. Many authors have suggested that children who undergo early palate repair demonstrate better overall speech than those with a later repair (Dorf & Curtin, 1990; Grobbelaar, Hudson, Fernandes, & Lentin, 1995; McWilliams et al., 1990; O'Gara & Logemann, 1988; Peterson-Falzone, 1996). Considering the critical period for brain development for speech sound production (Dowling, 2004), it makes sense that the longer the palate remains unrepaired, the harder it is to correct the child's speech. Another factor is regular otologic care, which can prevent hearing loss and help mitigate the risk for delayed speech development. A final factor is the effect of early intervention. Through early intervention, speech-language pathologists can do a great deal to lessen the effects of the cleft on developing communication skills. In particular, working on the production of oral sounds and oral airflow can be helpful. Speech (and language) stimulation at this age is often best done by training the parents to do this at home.

Usually, once the palate is repaired, most children will have adequate structure for speech sound production at around 10 months of age. However, they will have missed the developmental stage (usually around 6 months) where plosives are usually produced and practiced through normal babbling. As a result, some of these infants continue to show deficits in the production of certain early developmental sounds for some time after the palate is repaired (Jones, Chapman, & Hardin-Jones, 2003).

If the child has significant VPI following palate repair, this limits the oral consonants that can be produced. As the child's expressive language increases, a wider range of consonants is needed for intelligibility. In this situation, many children with VPI decrease their language output, or increase their consonant repertoire by developing active, compensatory articulation productions, where articulation is primarily produced in the pharynx or larynx. Harding and Grunwell (1996) reported that around 30 months of age, the nasal fricative became prevalent in the speech of their patients with a repaired cleft. This may be due to the fact that at this point in phonological development, there is a need for a fricative-plosive contrast, and a normal fricative may be difficult to produce when there is VPI. Once acquired and habituated, compensatory productions usually persist, even after the VPI is corrected.

Although compensatory productions can usually be corrected with speech therapy, delays in correcting the structure can have a serious impact on the time it takes to correct the errors, and long delays can even affect the ultimate prognosis. Just as the ability to learn a new language after the age of 6 years is decreased—and after puberty is almost impossible without retaining an accent—the ability to correct faulty speech patterns is also reduced as the child passes the "critical period" for brain development and speech/language learning (Dowling, 2004).

Another factor that may affect the speech development of children with craniofacial syndromes is oral-motor dysfunction, particularly in the form of apraxia. Children with velocardiofacial syndrome often demonstrate mild to severe apraxia in addition to obligatory and compensatory productions due to VPI

(Kummer, Lee, Stutz, Maroney, & Brandt, in press).

SUMMARY

Based on the existing research, it appears that children with nonsyndromic clefts are at risk for mild delays in development during the first three years of life. These delays may be secondary to factors such as fluctuating conductive hearing loss or VPI (McWilliams et al., 1990). When they occur, these delays are usually mild, and tend to improve with early intervention and time. Ultimately, the child usually catches up with his or her noncleft peers.

The risk for developmental delay is greatest for children with a known craniofacial syndrome or those with history of cleft palate only (which is often indicative of a syndrome). The language deficits found in many craniofacial syndromes have more complex etiologies than those found in the cleft population. Therefore, these children should be carefully evaluated for at an early age so that intervention can be initiated as soon as possible if needed.

In considering phonological development, note that, due to the open palate, children with cleft palate necessarily acquire speech sounds differently than their unaffected peers. Once the palate is repaired, the rate of this development varies and is affected by the child's age at the time of the repair. Even though the prognosis for normal speech development is fairly good once the palate is repaired, the child remains at risk for persistent articulation errors, compensatory productions, and abnormal resonance due to malocclusion and VPI. Therefore, phonological development should be carefully monitored, particularly throughout preschool years. Information concerning language stimulation can be found in the appendices at the end of this chapter.

FOR REVIEW, DISCUSSION, AND CRITICAL THINKING

1. What populations of children with clefts are at particular risk for developmental delays? Why is this?

2. In what cases could there be a concern about brain structure when there is a cleft lip and/or palate?

3. What recent evidence could explain the language disorders and neurological dysfunction in children with velocardiofacial syndrome?

4. Why do you think some children with craniofacial conditions actually receive more language stimulation than unaffected children? Why do some affected children receive less language stimulation than the norm?

5. Why do you think that children with a history of cleft palate may seem delayed in development in the early years, but seem to catch up by the time they are in school? What do you think could be done to mitigate these initial delays?

6. What is the affect of an open palate on speech sound acquisition? Why do children still demonstrate abnormal speech after the palate is repaired?

7. How would you explain to a physician that early palate repair is better for speech development and ultimate speech outcome than later palate repair?

8. Describe how you would counsel the parent of an infant about speech and language stimulation. In addition to regular stimulation techniques, what additional instructions would you give to the parent of a child with a cleft? What should be done differently after the palate repair?

REFERENCES

American Psychiatric Association. (2004). *Diagnostic and statistical manual of mental disorders* (4th ed.). Washington, DC: Author.

Antshel, K., Conchelos, J., Lanzetta, G., Fremont, W., & Kates, W. R. (2005). Behavioral and corpus callosum morphology relationships in velocardiofacial syndrome (22q11.2 deletion syndrome). *Psychiatry Research, 138*, 235–245.

Beitchman, J. H., Hood, J., Rochon, J., & Peterson, M. (1989). Empirical classification of speech/language impairments in children: II. Behavioral characteristics. *Journal of the American Academy of Child and Adolescent Psychiatry, 28*, 118–123.

Broder, H. L., Richman, L. C., & Matheson, P. B. (1998). Learning disability, school achievement, and grade retention among children with cleft: A two-center study. *Cleft Palate-Craniofacial Journal, 35*(2), 127–131.

Broen, P. A., Devers, M. C., Doyle, S. S., Prouty, J. M., & Moller, K. T. (1998). Acquisition of linguistic and cognitive skills by children with cleft palate. *Journal of Speech, Language, and Hearing Research, 41*(3), 676–687.

Buescher, N., & Paynter, E. (1973). *Linguistic abilities of children with palatal clefts.* Paper presented at the Annual Meeting of the American Cleft Palate Association, Oklahoma City, OK.

Cantwell, D. P., & Baker, L. (1991). Association between attention deficit-hyperactivity disorder and learning disorders. *Journal of Learning Disabilities, 24*(2), 88–95.

Chapman, K. L. (1991). Vocalizations of toddlers with cleft lip and palate. *Cleft Palate-Craniofacial Journal, 28*(2), 172–178.

Chapman, K. L. (1993). Phonologic processes in children with cleft palate. *Cleft Palate-Craniofacial Journal, 30*(1), 64–72.

Chapman, K. L., Graham, K. T., Gooch, J., & Visconti, C. (1998). Conversational skills of preschool and school-age children with cleft lip and palate. *Cleft Palate-Craniofacial Journal, 35*(6), 503–516.

Chapman, K. L., & Hardin, M. A. (1991). Language input of mothers interacting with their young children with cleft lip and palate. *Cleft Palate-Craniofacial Journal, 28*(1), 78–85; Discussion 85–86.

Chapman, K. L., & Hardin, M. A. (1992). Phonetic and phonological skills of two-year-olds with cleft palate. *Cleft Palate-Craniofacial Journal, 29*(5), 435–443.

Cherkes-Julkowski, M. (1998). Learning disability, attention-deficit disorder, and language impairment as outcomes of prematurity: A longitudinal descriptive study. *Journal of Learning Disabilities, 31*(3), 294–306.

Damico, J. S., Damico, S. K., & Armstrong, M. B. (1999). Attention-deficit hyperactivity disorder and communication disorders: Issues and clinical practices. *Child and Adolescent Psychiatric Clinics of North America, 8*(1), 37–60.

D'Antonio, L. L., Scherer, N. J., Miller, L. L., Kalbfleisch, J. H., & Bartley, J. A. (2001). Analysis of speech characteristics in children with velocardiofacial syndrome (VCFS) and children with phenotypic overlap without VCFS. *Cleft Palate-Craniofacial Journal, 38*(5), 455–467.

Devriendt, K., Van Thienen, M., Swillen, A., & Fryns, J. (1996). Cerebellar hypoplasia in a patient with velocardiofacial syndrome. *Developmental Medicine and Neurology, 38*, 945–949.

Dorf, D. S., & Curtin, J. W. (1990). Early cleft repair and speech outcome: A ten-year experience. In J. Bardach & H. L. Morris (Eds.), *Multidisciplinary management of cleft lip and palate* (pp. 341–348). Philadelphia: W. B. Saunders.

Dowling, J. E. (2004). *The great brain debate: Nature or nuture?* Washington, DC: Joseph Henry Press.

Elfenbein, J. L., Waziri, M., & Morris, H. L. (1981). Verbal communication skills of six children with craniofacial anomalies. *Cleft Palate Journal, 18*(1), 59–64.

Eliez, S., Antonarakis, S. E., Morris, M. A., Dahoun, S. P., & Reiss, A. L. (2001). Parental origin of the deletion 22q11.2 and brain development in velocardiofacial syndrome: A preliminary study. *Archives of General Psychiatry, 58*, 64–68.

Eliez, S., Blasey, C. M., Schmitt, E. J., White, C. D., Hu, D., & Reiss, A. L. (2001). Velocardiofacial syndrome: Are structural changes in the temporal and mesial temporal regions related to schizophrenia? *American Journal of Psychiatry, 158*, 447–453.

Eliez, S., Schmitt, J. E., White, C. D., & Reiss, A. L. (2000). Children and Adolescents with velocardiofacial syndrome. *American Journal of Psychiatry, 157*, 409–415.

Estes, R. E., & Morris, H. L. (1970). Relationships among intelligence, speech proficiency, and hearing sensitivity in children with cleft palates. *Cleft Palate Journal, 7*, 763–773.

Estrem, T., & Broen, P. A. (1989). Early speech production of children with cleft palate. *Journal of Speech and Hearing Research, 32*(1), 12–23.

Fergusson, D. M., & Horwood, L. J. (1992). Attention deficit and reading achievement. *Journal of Child Psychology and Psychiatry and Allied Disciplines, 33*(2), 375–385.

Fox, D., Lynch, J., & Brookshire, B. (1978). Selected developmental factors of cleft palate children between two and thirty-three months of age. *Cleft Palate Journal, 15*(3), 239–245.

Frederickson, M. S., Chapman, K. L., & Hardin-Jones, M. (2006). Conversational skills of children with cleft lip and palate: A replication and extension. *Cleft Palate-Craniofacial Journal, 43*(2), 179–188.

Glaser, B., Mumme, D. L., Blasey, C., Morris, M. A., Dahoun, S. P., Antonarakis, S. E., et al. (2002). Language skills in children with velocardiofacial syndrome (deletion 22q11.2). *Journal of Pediatrics, 140*(6), 753–758.

Golding-Kushner, K. J., Weller, G., & Shprintzen, R. J. (1985). Velocardiofacial syndrome: Language and psychological profiles. *Journal of Craniofacial Genetics and Developmental Biology, 5*(3), 259–266.

Goodstein, L. D. (1961). Intellectual impairment in children with cleft palates. *Journal of Speech and Hearing Research, 4,* 287.

Grobbelaar, A. O., Hudson, D. A., Fernandes, D. B., & Lentin, R. (1995). Speech results after repair of the cleft soft palate. *Plastic and Reconstructive Surgery, 95*(7), 1150–1154.

Grunwell, P., & Russell, V. J. (1988). Phonological development in children with cleft palate. *Clinical Linguistics and Phonetics, 2,* 75–95.

Hardin, M. A. (1991). Cleft palate: Intervention. *Clinics in Communication Disorders, 1*(3), 12–18.

Harding, A., & Grunwell, P. (1996). Characteristics of cleft palate speech. *European Journal of Disorders of Communication, 31,* 331–357.

Hardin-Jones, M., Chapman, K. L., & Schulte, J. (2003). The impact of cleft type on early vocal development in babies with cleft palate. *Cleft Palate-Craniofacial Journal, 40*(5), 453–459.

Hardin-Jones, M., Chapman, K., & Scherer, N. J. (2006, June 13). Early intervention in children with cleft palate. *The ASHA Leader, 11*(8), 8–9, 32.

Heineman-de Boer, J. A., Van Haelst, M. J., Cordia-de Haan, M., & Beemer, F. A. (1999). Behavior problems and personality aspects of 40 children with velocardiofacial syndrome. *Genetic Counseling, 10*(1), 89–93.

Horn, L. (1972). Language development of the cleft palate child. *Journal of South African Speech and Hearing Association, 19*(1), 17–29.

Hultman, C. S., Riski, J. E., Cohen, S. R., Burstein, F. D., Boydston, W. R., Hudgins, R. J., et al. (2000). Chiari malformation, cervical spine anomalies, and neurologic deficits in velocardiofacial syndrome. *Plastic and Reconstructive Surgery, 106*(1), 16–24.

Jocelyn, L. J., Penko, M. A., & Rode, H. L. (1996). Cognition, communication, and hearing in young children with cleft lip and palate and in control children: A longitudinal study. *Pediatrics, 97*(4), 529–534.

Jones, C. E., Chapman, K. L., & Hardin-Jones, M. A. (2003). Speech development of children with cleft palate before and after palatal surgery. *Cleft Palate-Craniofacial Journal, 40*(1), 19–31.

Kapp-Simon, K. A., & Krueckeberg, S. (2000). Mental development in infants with cleft lip and/or palate. *Cleft Palate-Craniofacial Journal, 37*(1), 65–70.

Kates, W. R., Burnette, C. P., Bessette, B. A., Folley, B. S., Strunge, L., Jabs, E. W., et al. (2004). Frontal and caudate alterations in velocardiofacial syndrome (deletion at chromosome 22q11.2). *Journal of Child Neurology, 19*(5), 337–342.

Kates, W. R., Burnette, C. P., Jabs, E. W., Rutberg, J., Murphy, A. M., Grados, M., et al. (2001). Regional cortical white matter reductions in velocardiofacial syndrome: A volumetric MRI analysis. *Biological Psychiatry, 49*(8), 677–684.

Kok, L. L., & Solman, R. T. (1995). Velocardiofacial syndrome: Learning difficulties and intervention. *Journal of Medical Genetics, 32*(8), 612–618.

Konst, E. M., Rietveld, T., Peters, H. F., & Kuijpers-Jagtman, A. M. (2003). Language skills of young children with unilateral cleft lip and palate following infant orthopedics: A randomized clinical trial. *Cleft Palate-Craniofacial Journal, 40*(4), 356–362.

Kritzinger, A., Louw, B., & Hugo, R. (1996). Early communication functioning of infants with cleft lip and palate. *South African Journal of Communication Disorders–die Suid-Afrikaanse Tydskrif vir Kommunikasieafwykings, 43*, 77–84.

Kummer, A. W., Lee, L., Stutz, L., Maroney, A., & Brandt, J. W. (2007). The prevalence of apraxic characteristics in patients with velocardiofacial syndrome as compared to other populations. *Cleft Palate-Craniofacial Journal, 44*(2), 175–181.

Lamb, M., Wilson, F., & Leeper, H. (1973). The intellectual function of cleft palate children compared on the basis of cleft type and sex. *Cleft Palate Journal, 10*, 367.

Leeper, H. A., Jr., Pannbacker, M., & Roginski, J. (1980). Oral language characteristics of adult cleft-palate speakers compared on the basis of cleft type and sex. *Journal of Communication Disorders, 13*(2), 133–146.

Lewis, R. (1961, April). A survey of intelligence of cleft lip and cleft palate children in Ontario. Presented at the 19th Annual Meeting of the American Association of Cleft Palate Rehabilitation, Montreal, Canada.

Lohmander-Agerskov, A., Soderpalm, E., Friede, H., Persson, E. C., & Lilja, J. (1994). Pre-speech in children with cleft lip and palate or cleft palate only: Phonetic analysis related to morphologic and functional factors. *Cleft Palate-Craniofacial Journal, 31*(4), 271–279.

Long, N. V., & Dalston, R. M. (1982a). Gestural communication in twelve-month-old cleft lip and palate children. *Cleft Palate Journal, 19*(1), 57–61.

Long, N. V., & Dalston, R. M. (1982b). Paired gestural and vocal behavior in one-year-old cleft lip and palate children. *Journal of Speech and Hearing Disorders, 47*(4), 403–406.

Long, N. V., & Dalston, R. M. (1983). Comprehension abilities of one-year-old infants with cleft lip and palate. *Cleft Palate Journal, 20*(4), 303–306.

Love, A. J., & Thompson, M. G. (1988). Language disorders and attention deficit disorders in young children referred for psychiatric services: Analysis of prevalence and a conceptual synthesis. *American Journal of Orthopsychiatry, 58*(1), 52–64.

Lynch, D. R., McDonald-McGinn, D. M., Zackai, E. H., Emanuel, B. S., Driscoll, D. A., Whitaker, L. A., et al. (1995). Cerebellar atrophy in a patient with velocardiofacial syndrome. *Journal of Medical Genetics, 32*(7), 561–563.

Lynch, J. I., Fox, D. R., & Brookshire, B. L. (1983). Phonological proficiency of two cleft palate toddlers with school-age follow-up. *Journal of Speech & Hearing Disorders*, *48*(3), 274–285.

Max, J. E., Arndt, S., Castillo, C. S., Bokura, H., Robin, D. A., Lindgren, S. D., Smith, W. L., Jr., Sato, Y., & Mattheis, P. J. (1998). Attention-deficit hyperactivity symptomatology after traumatic brain injury: A prospective study. *Journal of the American Academy of Child Adolescent Psychiatry*, *37*(8), 841–847.

McWilliams, B. J. (1970). Psychosocial development and modification. *ASHA Reports*, *5*, 165.

McWilliams, B. J., & Matthews, H. P. (1979). A comparison of intelligence and social maturity in children with unilateral complete clefts and those with isolated cleft palates. *Cleft Palate Journal*, *16*, 363.

McWilliams, B. J., Morris, H. L., & Shelton, R. L. (1990). Language disorders. In B. J. McWilliams, H. L. Morris, & R. L. Shelton (Eds.), *Cleft palate speech* (*Vol. 2*, pp. 236–246). Philadelphia: B. C. Decker.

Morris, H. L. (1962). Communication skills of children with cleft lip and palate. *Journal of Speech and Hearing Research*, *5*, 79.

Motzkin, B., Marion, R., Goldberg, R., Shprintzen, R., & Saenger, P. (1993). Variable phenotypes in velocardiofacial syndrome with chromosomal deletion. *Journal of Pediatrics*, *123*(3), 406–410.

Musgrave, R. H., McWilliams, B. J., & Matthews, H. P. (1975). A review of the results of two different surgical procedures for the repair of clefts of the soft palate only. *Cleft Palate Journal*, *12*, 281–290.

Neiman, G. S., & Savage, H. E. (1997). Development of infants and toddlers with clefts from birth to three years of age. *Cleft Palate-Craniofacial Journal*, *34*(3), 218–225.

Niemann, H., Ruff, R. M., & Kramer, J. H. (1996). An attempt towards differentiating attentional deficits in traumatic brain injury. *Neuropsychological Review*, *6*(1), 11–46.

Nopoulos, P., Berg, S., Canady, J., Richman, L., Van Demark, D., & Andreasen, N. C. (2002). Structural brain abnormalities in adult males with clefts of the lip and/or palate. *Genetics in Medicine*, *4*(1), 1–9.

Nopoulos, P., Berg, S., Van Demark, D., Richman, L., Canady, J., & Andreasen, N. C. (2001). Increased incidence of a midline brain anomaly in patients with nonsyndromic clefts of the lip and/or palate. *Journal of Neuroimaging*, *11*(4), 418–424.

Nopoulos, P., Berg, S., Van Demark, D., Richman, L., Canady, J., & Andreasen, N. C. (2002). Cognitive dysfunction in adult males with nonsyndromic clefts of the lip and/or palate. *Neuropsychologia*, *40*(12), 2178–2184.

Nopoulos, P., Choe, I., Berg, S., Van Demark, D., Canady, J., & Richman, L. (2005). Ventral frontal cortex morphology in adult males with isolated orofacial clefts: Relationship to abnormalities in social function. *Cleft Palate-Craniofacial Journal*, *42*(2), 138–144.

O'Gara, M. M., & Logemann, J. A. (1988). Phonetic analyses of the speech development of babies with cleft palate. *Cleft Palate Journal*, *25*(2), 122–134.

O'Gara, M. M., Logemann, J. A., & Rademaker, A. W. (1994). Phonetic features by babies with unilateral cleft lip and palate. *Cleft Palate-Craniofacial Journal*, *31*(6), 446–451.

Pamplona, M. C., Ysunza, A., Gonzalez, M., Ramirez, E., & Patino, C. (2000). Linguistic development in cleft palate patients with and without compensatory articulation disorder. *International Journal of Pediatric Otorhinolaryngology, 54*(2–3), 81–89.

Pannbacker, M. (1975). Oral language skills of adult cleft palate speakers. *Cleft Palate Journal, 12*(1), 95–106.

Paradise, J. L. (1998). Otitis media and child development: Should we worry? *Pediatric Infectious Disease Journal, 17*(11), 1076–1083; Discussion 1099–1100.

Peterson, S. J. (1973). Speech pathology in craniofacial malformations other than cleft lip and palate. *ASHA Reports, 8,* 11–131.

Peterson-Falzone, S. J. (1996). The relationship between timing of cleft palate surgery and speech outcome: What have we learned, and where do we stand in the 1990s? *Seminars in Orthodontics, 2*(3), 185–191.

Purvis, K. L., & Tannock, R. (1997). Language abilities in children with attention deficit hyperactivity disorder, reading disabilities, and normal controls. *Journal of Abnormal Child Psychology, 25*(2), 133–144.

Richman, L. C. (1980). Cognitive patterns and learning disabilities of cleft palate children with verbal deficits. *Journal of Speech and Hearing Research, 23*(2), 447–456.

Richman, L. C., Eliason, M. J., & Lindgren, S. D. (1988). Reading disability in children with clefts. *Cleft Palate Journal, 25*(1), 21–25.

Roug, L., Landberg, I., & Lundberg, L. J. (1989). Phonetic development in early infancy: A study of four Swedish children during the first eighteen months of life. *Journal of Child Language, 16*(1), 19–40.

Ruess, A. L. (1965). A comparative study of cleft palate children and their siblings. *Journal of Clinical Psychology, 21,* 354.

Russell, V. J. (1991). *Speech development in children with cleft lip and palate.* Unpublished doctoral dissertation, Leicester Polytechnic, Leicester, UK.

Sanberg, S. T., Rutter, M., & Taylor, E. (1980). Hyperkinetic disorder and conduct problem children in primary school population: Some epidemiological considerations. *Journal of Child Psychology and Psychiatry, 21,* 293–311.

Saxman, J., & Bless, D. (1973, April). Patterns of language development in cleft palate children aged three to eight years. Paper presented at the Annual Meeting of the American Cleft Palate Association, Oklahoma City, OK.

Scherer, N. J., D'Antonio, L. L., & Kalbfleisch, J. H. (1999). Early speech and language development in children with velocardiofacial syndrome. *American Journal of Medical Genetics, 88*(6), 714–723.

Scherer, N. J., D'Antonio, L. L., & Rodgers, J. R. (2001). Profiles of communication disorder in children with velocardiofacial syndrome: Comparison to children with Down syndrome. *Genetics in Medicine, 3*(1), 72–78.

Shames, G., & Rubin, H. (1979). Psycholinguistic measures of language and speech. In K. R. Bzoch (Ed.), *Communicative disorders related to cleft lip and palate* (p. 202). Boston: Little, Brown.

Shprintzen, R. J. (1998). Complex craniofacial disorders. In S. E. Gerber (Ed.), *Etiology and prevention of communicative disorders* (*Vol. 2,* pp. 147–199). San Diego, CA: Singular Publishing Group.

Shprintzen, R. J., Goldberg, R. B., Lewin, M. L., Sidoti, E. J., Berkman, M. D., Argamaso, R. V., & Young, D. (1978). A new syndrome involving cleft palate, cardiac anomalies, typical facies, and learning disabilities: Velocardiofacial syndrome. *Cleft Palate Journal, 15*(1), 56–62.

Sidoti, E. J., Jr., Marsh, J. L., Marty-Grames, L., & Noetzel, M. J. (1996). Long-term studies of metopic synostosis: Frequency of cognitive impairment and behavioral disturbances. *Plastic and Reconstructive Surgery, 97*(2), 276–281.

Smith, R. M., & McWilliams, B. J. (1968). Psycholinguistic abilities of children with clefts. *Cleft Palate Journal, 5,* 238–249.

Smith, B. L., & Oller, D. K. (1981). A comparative study of premeaningful vocalizations produced by normally developing and Down's syndrome infants. *Journal of Speech & Hearing Disorders, 46*(1), 46–51.

Snyder, L. E., & Scherer, N. (2004). The development of symbolic play and language in toddlers with cleft palate. *American Journal of Speech-Language Pathology, 13*(1), 66–80.

Speltz, M. L., Endriga, M. C., Hill, S., Maris, C. L., Jones, K., & Omnell, M. L. (2000). Cognitive and psychomotor development of infants with orofacial clefts. *Journal of Pediatric Psychology, 25*(3), 185–190.

Spriestersbach, D. C., Darley, F., & Morris, H. L. (1958). Language skills in children with cleft palate. *Journal of Speech and Hearing Research, 1,* 279–285.

Starr, P., Chinski, R., Canter, H., & Meier, J. (1977). Mental, motor, and social behavior of infants with cleft lip and/or palate. *Cleft Palate Journal, 14,* 140.

Stoel-Gammon, C. (1985). Phonetic inventories, 15–24 months: A longitudinal study. *Journal of Speech & Hearing Research, 28*(4), 505–512.

Strauss, R. P., & Broder, H. (1993). Children with cleft lip/palate and mental retardation: A subpopulation of cleft-craniofacial team patients. *Cleft Palate-Craniofacial Journal, 30*(6), 548–556.

Swillen, A., Devriendt, K., Legius, E., Eyskens, B., Dumoulin, M., Gewillig, M., & Fryns, J. P. (1997). Intelligence and psychosocial adjustment in velocardiofacial syndrome: A study of 37 children and adolescents with VCFS. *Journal of Medical Genetics, 34*(6), 453–458.

Swillen, A., Devriendt, K., Legius, E., Prinzie, P., Vogels, A., Ghesquiere, P., & Fryns, J. P. (1999). The behavioural phenotype in velo-cardio-facial syndrome (VCFS): From infancy to adolescence. *Genetic Counseling, 10*(1), 79–88.

Tirosh, E., Berger, J., Cohen-Ophir, M., Davidovitch, M., & Cohen, A. (1998). Learning disabilities with and without attention-deficit hyperactivity disorder: Parents' and teachers' perspectives. *Journal of Child Neurology, 13*(6), 270–276.

Tirosh, E., & Cohen, A. (1998). Language deficit with attention-deficit disorder: A prevalent comorbidity. *Journal of Child Neurology, 13*(10), 493–497.

Trost-Cardamone, J. E. (1997). Diagnosis of specific cleft palate speech error patterns for planning therapy of physical management needs. In K. R. Bzoch (Ed.), *Communicative disorders related to cleft lip and palate* (Vol. 4, pp. 313–330). Austin, TX: Pro-Ed.

Van Amelsvoort, T., Daly, E., Henry, J., Robertson, D., Ng, V., Owen, M., Murphy, K. C., & Murphy, D. G. (2004). Brain anatomy in adults with velocardiofacial syndrome with and without schizophrenia: Preliminary results of a structural magnetic resonance imaging study. *Archives of General Psychiatry, 61,* 1085–1096.

Vantrappen, G., Devriendt, K., Swillen, A., Rommel, N., Vogels, A., Eyskens, B., Gewillig, M., Feenstra, L., & Fryns, J. P. (1999). Presenting symptoms and clinical features in 130 patients with the veloc-ardiofacial syndrome. The Leuven experience. *Genetic Counseling, 10*(1), 3–9.

Whitcomb, L., Ochsner, G., & Wayte, R. (1976). A comparison of expressive language skills of cleft-palate and non-cleft-palate children: A preliminary investigation. *Journal of the Oklahoma Speech and Hearing Association, 3,* 25–28.

Willadsen, E., & Albrechtsen, H. (2006). Phonetic description of babbling in Danish toddlers born with and without unilateral cleft lip and palate. *Cleft Palate-Craniofacial Journal, 43*(2), 189–200.

Wirls, C. J. (1971). Psychosocial aspects of cleft lip and palate. In W. C. Grabb, S. W. Rosenstein, & K. Bzoch (Eds.), *Cleft lip and palate* (p. 119). Boston: Little, Brown.

Wright, G. F. (1982). Attention deficit disorder. *Journal of School Health, 52*(2), 119–120.

Zimmerman, J., & Canfield, W. (1968). Language and speech development. In R. Stark (Ed.), *Cleft palate: A multidiscipline approach* (p. 220). New York: Harper and Row.

Appendix 6–1

Language Stimulation Information for Parents

By Ann W. Kummer, Ph.D.

When helping a child who is having difficulty in the development of speech and language, it is important to understand how children normally acquire these skills. In order to learn to communicate, children need to:

- have many varied experiences within the environment;

- hear the speech of others;

- have an opportunity to repeat or imitate words and short sentences that are heard; and

- have a need or desire to communicate.

These experiences and opportunities are especially important for a child who is delayed in the development of speech and language.

General Principles for Speech and Language Stimulation

- Avoid discussing your child's speech or language problem in front of him/her. If someone else brings it up, express confidence in your child with words such as "We're working on it and he's doing great."

- Reward your child's speech attempts to communicate by giving him/her your full attention and not interrupting. Smile and respond to your child, even if you don't understand every word.

- Discourage the use of gestures unless all else fails. For the child who communicates solely by gesturing and pointing, select one particular thing for which a sound must be used as well.

- Try not to anticipate your child's every need. Encourage your child to <u>tell</u> you what he/she wants.

- Speak to your child constantly, even if he/she does not respond. Talk about what you are doing or what he/she is doing, as it is being done.

- Be a model of good speech. Speak clearly and in sentences with simple, but correct, grammar. You should not use "baby talk."

- Give your child an opportunity to speak— and then wait for his/her response.

- Use the speech your child has and build on it. Take what he/she says and repeat it, but with a longer or expanded sentence.

- Don't punish your child's efforts to talk by correcting every mistake.

- Provide as many meaningful and pleasant language experiences for your child as you can, such as story time or talking games.

STIMULATING RECEPTIVE LANGUAGE

Encourage your child to listen to sounds in his/her environment, including household sounds, music, and speech. Give him/her a chance to hear a variety of sounds and noises. Help him/her find the source of the sound.

Increase your child's awareness of sound and his/her ability to discriminate sounds by saying, "Can you hear a noise? What is it?"

Talk to your child as much as possible. Obtain eye contact with your child and try to maintain his/her attention as long as possible.

Help him/her to recognize his name and the names of others by using these names frequently.

Use gestures occasionally when you are talking to help the child understand what you are saying. Gestures for "bye," "come here," and "up" are examples.

Do a lot of naming for your child. Try to increase his/her understanding of words. Name words in categories, such as the following: body parts, clothing, household objects, toys, furniture, food, animals, tools, names of people (farmer, doctor, teacher), forms of transportation, colors, names of buildings (church, barn, school), verbs (i.e., jumping, sitting, eating), descriptive words (i.e., big, little, clean, dirty), pronouns (i.e., I, me, you), and prepositions (i.e., in, on, under).

Use picture books that have objects in categories. Point to pictures and then name them. Then, encourage the child to point to objects in the book as you name them. You may say, "Show me the _____," or "Point to the _____."

Cut out pictures in a catalog and paste them on paper in categories to make a language book. Name the pictures as you are working on this.

As you are doing various activities, name things for your child. You can name:

- Body parts—as you dress or bathe your child

- Clothing—as you put items in and out of a drawer or closet, or as you fold laundry

- Fruits, vegetables, and other foods—as you are doing grocery shopping or cooking
- Furniture—as you walk around a room
- Silverware and dishware—as you eat or do the dishes

Help your child to understand prepositions by asking him/her to place an object on, under, in front of, beside, or behind something else.

Play a game of "categories." Have your child think of all the items that he/she can in a particular category (i.e., foods, animals, and clothing).

Play a game of "opposites." Ask him/her the opposite of "hot," "tall," "good," "dirty," etc.

Stimulate your child's language by talking to him/her about things that you are doing and about things that he/she is doing. Describe the things that you both see, hear, feel, and taste.

Speak clearly using primarily short, simple sentences at first. Again, do not use "baby talk."

Expose your child to a variety of experiences such as: going to the zoo, going to the park, baking, grocery shopping, helping with yard work, etc. Comment on the objects, actions, textures, colors, shapes, smells, etc. Books are great, but a child learns first by doing and by having first-hand experience.

Help the child to respond appropriately to simple commands and directions such as:

"Point to _____."

"Put on your coat."

"Find the _____."

"Open the door."

"Give me the _____."

"Close the door."

"Go get the"

"Put your finger on the _____."

If the child is unable to understand a question or command, show him/her with a gesture or lead him/her through the activity. Then repeat the question or request.

Work to improve the child's understanding of questions, such as those that begin with "what," "who," "where," or "when."

Develop an understanding of simple number concepts. For example:

"Give me one _____."

"Give me two _____."

"Give me all of the _____."

"Give me some of the _____."

Help the child to understand the concepts of one versus many. For example:

"Put the *car* in the box." "Put the *cars* in the box."

Increase the child's ability to identify pictures and objects when given the function, such as:

"Show me what you eat."

"Show me what you wear on your foot."

Help the child to respond appropriately to commands involving two objects, such as:

"Give me the ball and the shoe."

Help the child to respond to commands involving action words, such as:

"Find the car and give it to John."

Use commands involving multiple objects or multiple action words.

STIMULATING EXPRESSIVE LANGUAGE

Respond to all spontaneous sound-making or verbalization by giving the child your full and immediate attention, and by giving a positive reinforcement, such as a hug or smile.

Develop imitation skills by encouraging the imitation of motor activities, such as clapping hands, rolling a ball back and forth, playing patty-cake, or playing peek-a-boo.

Encourage your child to make a lot of different sounds, including vowels and consonants. This can be done by producing sounds yourself and encouraging the child to imitate.

Repeat sounds that the child produces spontaneously to encourage back-and-forth imitation (i.e., uh-oh, mama, dada, nana, gaga, hi, etc.).

Have the child imitate animal and motor sounds.

Encourage the child to imitate speech sounds and single words. Have him/her watch and occasionally feel your lips, face, and throat as you produce sounds and words.

Encourage your child to use greetings, such as "Hi" and "Bye."

Help your child to say his/her own name.

Help your child to respond to questions with "yes" or "no" as appropriate.

Encourage your child to name familiar objects and pictures by saying to him/her, "What's this?"

Encourage your child to use action words (verbs) by saying such things as "What is the boy doing?"

Encourage your child to tell you what he/she wants rather than allowing him/her to use gestures. Try not to give him/her objects without having him/her vocalize at least sounds for it. You can say to the child, "Tell me what you want. Do you want a cookie? Tell me 'cookie.' You say 'cookie.'" Be careful not to demand a verbal request for something that you will give him/her anyway (like his milk). Encourage him/her to say these words too, but make your demands for items that you don't have to give him/her (such as a cookie or a toy).

Have your child name items by category (as noted before) and use sentences with these words.

Give your child phrases and sentences to imitate. If he is incapable of imitating a long sentence, give him/her the correct form and then a small part of the total utterance. For example:

> Adult: "The boy drives the car. You say, 'Boy drives.'"
>
> Child: "Boy drives."
>
> Adult: "Good, the boy drives the car."

If the child does not say the word or sentence correctly, don't correct him/her each time. Instead, you can repeat what the child said, but with the correct form. For example:

> Child: "Him/her eat cookie."
>
> Adult: "Right, he eats a cookie."
>
> Child: "Him/her falled down and break him/her arm."
>
> Adult: "He fell down and broke his arm? That's too bad."

Encourage spontaneous speech from your child as well as imitated speech. Respond to all attempts at conversation by giving your child your full attention and interacting with the child.

Give your child many opportunities to play with other children. This situation can be very conducive to spontaneous speech.

CHAPTER

7

RESONANCE DISORDERS AND VELOPHARYNGEAL DYSFUNCTION (VPD)

INTRODUCTION

During normal speech production, sound is generated by the vocal folds in the larynx and then changes as it resonates in the cavities of the vocal tract. The laryngeal sound and the resonances of the vocal tract provide the quality and uniqueness of an individual's voice. It is important that sound, airflow, and air pressures within the vocal tract are directed to both the oral and nasal cavities as appropriate for normal speech, and that there is no obstruction in the vocal cavities. The velopharyngeal valve plays a key role in this because it directs sound energy and airflow into the oral and nasal cavities during speech production. Velopharyngeal dysfunction or obstruction in the vocal tract can have a significant effect on resonance, *articulation,* and other aspects of speech production.

The purpose of this chapter is to acquaint the reader with different types of resonance disorders and the speech characteristics of velopharyngeal dysfunction. The various types and causes of velopharyngeal dysfunction will also be described.

NORMAL RESONANCE AND VELOPHARYNGEAL FUNCTION

Resonance, as it relates to voiced speech, is the modification of the sound that is generated by the larynx through selective enhancement of certain frequencies. This is determined by the size and shape of the cavities of the vocal tract (pharynx, oral cavity, and nasal cavity) and the function of the velopharyngeal valve.

The size and shape of the cavities of the vocal tract have a significant impact on the individual's speech, resonance, and overall vocal quality. For example, vowels, which are resonant sounds, are differentiated by changing the shape of the oral cavity with the tongue position, thus changing the formant frequencies of the oral sound. In addition, the vocal tract, which extends upward from the glottis, is a three-dimensional resonating tube that is highly modifiable. It changes in shape and size during speech due to the action of the hyoid muscle group. Because the larynx, pharynx, mandible, tongue, and velum are all interconnected by this musculature, movement of one of these structures may result in movement of the others (Huntington, 1968). As a result, the height of the velum and the configuration of the pharynx are affected by tongue position during the production of different speech phonemes (Tom, Titze, Hoffman, & Story, 2001). This changes the resonating quality of the vocal tract and has an effect on how the sound is perceived.

The shape and size of the vocal tract also affect the perception of pitch. With higher pitches, for example, the larynx raises to shorten the pharynx and the lateral pharyngeal walls contract to create a very narrow pharyngeal tube (Yanagisawa, Estill, Mambrino, & Talkin, 1991). To understand this effect, one can imagine the sound that is produced when blowing across a bottle. If the bottle is mostly full, the resonating volume in the bottle is short and small, resulting in high formant frequencies or high pitch. As the bottle is emptied, the resonating cavity becomes longer and often wider. This causes the sound to be lower due to lower formant frequencies. The same principle applies to wind instruments. A shorter chamber results in a higher sound and a longer chamber results in a lower sound.

When considering the effect of vocal tract shape and size on pitch and resonance, it is easy to understand why children, who have a relatively short pharynx, have higher resonating formants during speech than adults who have a longer pharynx. In addition, it has been shown that adult males and females differ with respect to oral and pharyngeal cavity sizes, which affects the formant frequencies and perception of voice quality (Bennett, 1981).

Anything that changes the length or shape of the resonating cavities can affect the quality of the voice. This includes changes to the pharynx that can occur due to pharyngoplasty surgeries. If a pharyngeal flap or sphincter is too low in the pharynx, for example, this can effectively shorten the resonating tube, causing an unwanted change in resonance.

The function of the velopharyngeal valve is described in Chapter 1. As noted previously, the velopharyngeal valve is responsible for directing sound energy and airflow from the pharynx into the oral cavity for oral sounds and into the nasal cavity for nasal sounds. Because air pressure and sound travel in a superior direction from the lungs to the oropharynx, the velopharyngeal valve must close completely in order to redirect all sound energy and airflow anteriorly into the oral cavity. The valve must then open for the production of nasal sounds and for nasal breathing.

RESONANCE DISORDERS AND VELOPHARYNGEAL DYSFUNCTION

Resonance disorders, particularly hypernasality, are often labeled inappropriately as "voice disorders" (Riski & Verdolini, 1999). However, hypernasality and other resonance disorders are not laryngeal in origin. Therefore, classifying these abnormalities as "resonance disorders" is more appropriate.

The structure and relative balance of sound energy in the cavities of the vocal tract determine whether the quality of the speech and voice is perceived as normal or as deviant due to a type of "nasality" (Kummer, 2003). Anything that disrupts the transmission of sound in the cavities of the vocal tract will cause abnormal resonance. This can include any form of obstruction, oronasal fistula, or velopharyngeal dysfunction.

Velopharyngeal dysfunction (VPD) refers to a condition where the velopharyngeal valve does not close consistently and completely during the production of oral sounds (D'Antonio, Muntz, Province, & Marsh, 1988; Folkins, 1988; Jones, 1991; Loney & Bloem, 1987; Marsh, 1991; Morris, 1992; Netsell, 1988; Penfold, 1997; Witt et al., 1997). This term is also used when the velopharyngeal valve does not open consistently and completely during the production of nasal sounds due to apraxia. VPD is a general term that can be used when etiology is not specified.

Unfortunately, the literature is full of inconsistencies in the use of terminology for disorders of the velopharyngeal valve. Some authors and clinicians use the common terms velopharyngeal inadequacy, velopharyngeal impairment, velopharyngeal insufficiency, velopharyngeal incompetence, and velopharyngeal dysfunction interchangeably; whereas others use these terms in a specific way to suggest etiology (Loney & Bloem, 1987; Trost, 1981; Trost-Cardamone, 1981, 1989).

As suggested by Trost-Cardamone (1989), the term *velopharyngeal insufficiency (VPI)* ☉ is used in this text to describe an anatomical or structural defect that prevents adequate velopharyngeal closure. Velopharyngeal insufficiency is the most common type of VPD because it includes a short velum, which is common in children with a history of cleft palate after the palate repair (Figure 7–1). *Velopharyngeal incompetence (VPI)* ☉ is used to refer to a neuromotor or physiological disorder that results in poor movement of the velopharyngeal structures (Figure 7–2). Finally, *velopharyngeal mislearning* ☉ refers to inadequate velopharyngeal closure secondary to faulty development of appropriate articulation patterns. This degree of specificity in terminology is felt to be important because each of these categories of velopharyngeal dysfunction has a different underlying cause and therefore, the treatment is very different.

When etiology is not known or not specified, VPI (for velopharyngeal insufficiency or incom-

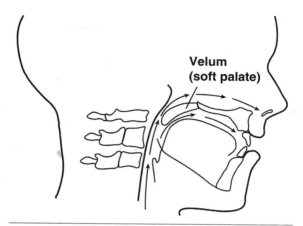

FIGURE 7–2 Velopharyngeal incompetence. In this case, the velum doesn't move well enough to achieve velopharyngeal closure during speech.

petence) is used for disorders that are medically based and not due to mislearning. *Velopharyngeal dysfunction* is used as a broad term that encompasses all disorders that affect the velopharyngeal valve.

There are various types of resonance disorders due to causes such as velopharyngeal dysfunction, oronasal fistula, or obstruction in the vocal tract. These disorders are described as follows.

Hypernasality

Hypernasality is a resonance disorder that occurs when there is abnormal *coupling* (sharing of acoustic energy) of the oral and nasal cavities during speech. In particular, it is abnormal nasal resonance during the production of nonnasal (oral) sounds. Hypernasality is often described as muffled or characterized by mumbling. This is due to the *damping* (sound absorption) effect as the sound goes through the turbinates of the nasal cavity (Buder, 2005). Audio samples of various degrees of hypernasality in children, men, and women can

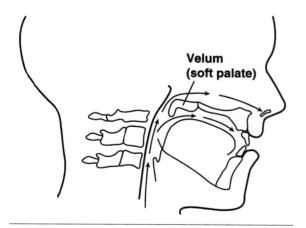

FIGURE 7–1 Velopharyngeal insufficiency. In this case, the velum is too short to achieve velopharyngeal closure during speech.

be found on the Web site of the American Cleft Palate-Craniofacial Association (2006).

Because hypernasality is due to abnormal resonance of sound, it is always associated with speech sounds that are phonated (Cassassolles et al., 1995). It is particularly perceptible on vowels, because they are relatively long in duration and are typically not substituted with a different placement. Hypernasality is more noted on high vowels than low vowels (Andrews & Rutherford, 1972). This is due to the high tongue position, which reduces oral resonance space and causes partial impedance of sound coming through the oral cavity. This causes an increase in sound pressure, which can result in increased transmission of sound through the velum. If the velum is thin, due to a submucous cleft for example, this can significantly add to the perception of hypernasality, even in the absence of velopharyngeal dysfunction.

When there is mild-to-moderate hypernasality, *nasalization of oral phonemes* is common. For example, it makes sense that when the velopharyngeal valve remains open during the attempted production of a voiced plosive, the acoustic product will be the nasal cognate of that sound (i.e., m/b, n/d, and ng/g). Nasalization can also occur on other oral sounds, and nasal sounds can even be substituted for voiceless sounds. As a result, there may be a predominate use of the nasal sounds (/m/, /n/, and /ng/) throughout connected speech. Hypernasality on vowels and nasalization of phonemes will often increase in connected speech due to the additional demands on the velopharyngeal mechanism and on the oral-motor system.

The cause of hypernasality is usually velopharyngeal insufficiency, but can also be due to velopharyngeal incompetence. In either case, hypernasality is most noted with larger velopharyngeal openings and is not usually

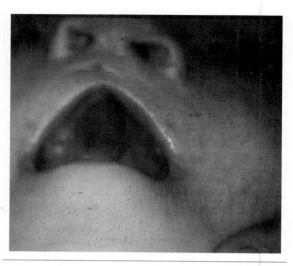

FIGURE 7–3   A very large palatal fistula that would cause significant hypernasality.

perceived with smaller openings. Hypernasality can also be due to an oronasal fistula that is fairly large (Figure 7–3). When hypernasality is caused by velopharyngeal mislearning, it is due to inappropriate placement of certain sounds (i.e., ng/l, ng/r, hypernasality only on high vowels, etc.). Therefore, this type of hypernasality is phoneme-specific.

Hypernasality should not be confused with a "nasal twang," which has been described as a characteristic of certain dialects. Although this quality may seem hypernasal to some, the nasal twang is not "nasal" at all. Instead, this quality has been found to occur with pharyngeal area narrowing and vocal tract shortening (Story, Titze, & Hoffman, 2001; Titze, Bergan, Hunter, & Story, 2003; Yanagisawa, Estill, Mambrino, & Talkin, 1991; Yanagisawa, Kmucha, & Estill, 1990).

Hyponasality and Denasality

Hyponasality occurs when there is a reduction in normal nasal resonance during speech due to blockage in the nasopharynx or nasal cavity.

The overall perceptual feature is that the individual sounds "stuffed up." The term *denasality* is typically used to refer to total nasal airway obstruction and the resultant effect on resonance. Because it is impossible to know if there is total blockage of the nasal cavity through a perceptual assessment alone, the term hyponasality is more commonly used.

Hyponasality particularly affects the production of the nasal consonants (/m/, /n/, /ng/). When nasal resonance is reduced, nasal consonants sound similar to their oral phoneme cognates (b/m, d/n, g/ng). Hyponasality can also affect the quality of vowels if it is severe. This is due to the fact that all vowels, particularly high vowels, have some nasal resonance due to transmission of sound through the velum.

The cause of hyponasality is almost always obstruction somewhere in the nasopharynx or nasal cavity. Anything that reduces the size of the nasopharynx can result in hyponasality, as well as in other signs of upper airway obstruction, including a chronic open mouth posture, mouth breathing, loud snoring, and sleep apnea. Common causes of nasal obstruction in a general population include swelling of the nasal passages secondary to allergic rhinitis or the common cold, adenoid hypertrophy, or even hypertrophic tonsils that intrude into the pharynx (Kummer et al., 1993). In these cases, medical or surgical intervention is needed. The only exception is when characteristics of hyponasality occur due to apraxia of speech. In this case, the cause is difficulty coordinating velopharyngeal movements with anterior articulation. As a result, the velum may not lower rapidly enough for nasal phonemes once it is in a raised position for oral sounds.

Hyponasality is very common in individuals with a history of cleft palate, and it may actually be more common than hypernasality in adolescents and adults in this population. One reason for this is that VPI is usually corrected in the preschool or early school years so that hypernasality is no longer present as the individual gets older. However, because the surgical procedures that are designed to correct VPI narrow or reduce the size of the nasopharyngeal space, hyponasality is a common complication of the surgery (de Serres et al., 1999; Hall, Golding-Kushner, Argamaso, & Strauch, 1991; Thurston, Larson, Shanks, Bennett, & Parsons, 1980; Witt, Myckatyn, & Marsh, 1998). Other common causes of hyponasality in individuals with a history of cleft palate or craniofacial conditions include a deviated septum (particularly with unilateral clefts), choanal stenosis or atresia, a stenotic naris, or maxillary retrusion which restricts the pharyngeal and nasal cavity space (Riski, 1995). Maxillary retrusion with midface deficiency is common in individuals with a history of cleft lip and palate and it is also a phenotypic feature of several craniofacial syndromes, such as Crouzon syndrome, Apert syndrome, and Pfeiffer syndrome. Maxillary advancement can often decrease hyponasality and improve characteristics of airway obstruction (Dalston, 1996; Maegawa et al., 1998; McCarthy et al., 1979).

Because the cause of hyponasality is almost always obstruction somewhere in the nasal cavity or pharynx, further evaluation and treatment should be done by a physician. Speech therapy is indicated only if the hyponasality is inconsistent and is due to timing errors as a result of apraxia of speech.

Cul-de-Sac Resonance

Cul-de-sac resonance, like hyponasality, is due to obstruction. It occurs when the transmission of acoustic energy is blocked—and therefore, the sound is trapped in a blind pouch with only one entrance and no other outlet. The speech is perceived as muffled and has been described as "potato-in-the-mouth" speech (Finkelstein, Bar-Ziv, Nachmani, Berger, & Ophir, 1993). This is actually a great description because if the speaker did have a potato in the mouth, the sound would be blocked by the potato so that much of it would remain in the pharynx. In addition, the potato would absorb some of the sound.

One cause of cul-de-sac resonance is very large tonsils that block the entrance to the oral cavity (like a potato!) (Kummer et al., 1993; Shprintzen et al., 1987). As a result of this blockage, the sound energy is trapped and vibration occurs primarily in the oropharynx. The sound quality is low intensity and "muffled" because it is partially absorbed by the pharyngeal tissues. Cul-de-sac resonance can even occur due to a scar or obstruction on the pharyngeal wall in the hypopharynx (Figure 7–4).

Cul-de-sac resonance is common in children with a history of cleft palate because it can be due to a combination of VPI and blockage of the nasal cavity (as with a deviated septum). This can be simulated by producing a series of nasal phonemes (i.e., ma, ma, ma, ma, ma) or simulating hypernasality while pinching the nose. Because sound energy cannot be released through the nose, it will be "trapped" in the nasal cavity. (It

should be noted that pinching the nose during simulation of hypernasality does not result in oral resonance. This is because the blockage is at the front of the nasal cavity and not in the area of the velopharyngeal valve.) With this type of cul-de-sac resonance, the blockage could be due to a deviated septum, nasal polyps, or stenotic nares.

Cul-de-sac resonance is always due to a structural abnormality, particularly a blockage of one of the resonating cavities. Therefore, this type of resonance disorder requires medical or surgical intervention to eliminate the cause.

Mixed Resonance

Mixed resonance is a combination of any of the above types of resonance. Although hypernasality and hyponasality cannot occur simultaneously, they can occur at different times in the connected speech of the same individual. Mixed resonance is common in individuals with apraxia due to inappropriate timing of the upward movement of the velum on nasal sounds and the downward movement of the velum on oral sounds (Netsell, 1969).

If there is velopharyngeal insufficiency in addition to blockage in the nasal cavity, the predominate characteristic of connected speech may be hypernasality, with hyponasality during the production of nasal consonants. If the blockage is lower in the pharynx and fairly large however, the most notable characteristic may be hyponasality.

In addition to mixed resonance, some individuals demonstrate hyponasality and nasal air emission, which has the same cause as hypernasality (Dalston, Warren, & Dalston, 1991). Again, this does not occur simultaneously, but on different speech sounds. A common cause for this combination is enlarged, yet irregular adenoid tissue. During the production of oral sounds, the velum closes against the adenoid pad, but a tight velopharyngeal seal

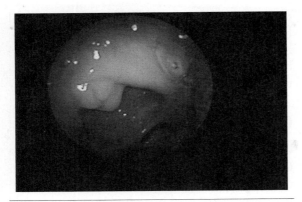

FIGURE 7–4 Scar band on the posterior pharyngeal wall. This can impede the transmission of sound energy through the pharynx, thus causing cul-de-sac resonance.

cannot be obtained due to the irregular tissue. As a result, there is nasal air emission. On the other hand, when the velum goes down for the production of nasal sounds, the adenoid pad is large enough that it obstructs the transmission of sound into the nasal cavity, thus causing hyponasality.

OTHER EFFECTS OF VELOPHARYNGEAL DYSFUNCTION ON SPEECH

In addition to hypernasality, velopharyngeal dysfunction (or even an oronasal fistula) can affect speech in many other ways. These are described further in the following sections.

Nasal Air Emission

Nasal air emission occurs when there is an attempt to build up intraoral air pressure for the production of consonants in the presence of a leak in the system (velopharyngeal valve or oronasal fistula). Some of the airflow is released through the nose, causing a disruption in the aerodynamic process of speech. It is most noted on *pressure-sensitive phonemes* (plosives, fricatives, and affricates). It does not occur during the production of vowels or semivowels because there is no need to build up air pressure for these phonemes. Nasal emission often occurs with hypernasality, but can also occur with normal resonance.

Nasal emission can be very loud and distracting, very soft and barely audible, or it can be inaudible. This has to do with the size of the opening. When there is a fairly large opening, there is little resistance to the flow. Although there is significant loss of air pressure through the nose, this type of nasal emission is not very audible due to the minimal amount of friction produced with

the sound. When there is a smaller velopharyngeal opening, there is greater resistance to the flow. This causes the nasal emission to be more audible. When the opening is very small, the resistance causes the airflow to become turbulent as it passes through the valve. The air is released on the nasal side of the opening with a great deal of pressure, which causes bubbling of the nasal secretions. This can be seen easily through nasopharyngoscopy, but even through videofluoroscopy when there is a coating of barium. This type of nasal emission has been called *nasal turbulence*. However, the sound that is heard is primarily due to bubbling of secretions, and therefore, some prefer to use the term *nasal rustle* (Kummer et al., 1989, 1992; Mason & Grandstaff, 1971). Nasal congestion can increase nasal airway resistance and make this distortion even more noticeable (Kummer, 2003; Warren, Wood, & Bradley, 1969).

A nasal rustle can be very loud and distracting and can mask the sound of the consonant, thus affecting the quality and intelligibility of speech. Voiceless fricatives are more often distorted by nasal emission or a nasal rustle because they are associated with more air pressure than their voiced counterparts where the adduction of the vocal folds attenuates the air pressure somewhat.

Nasal emission due to VPI usually occurs on all pressure-sensitive sounds. If the nasal occurs only on sibilant sounds (/s/, /z/, /sh/, /zh/, /ch/, /j/), particularly /s/, it is probably due to faulty articulation (velopharyngeal mislearning) rather than VPI because complete closure is obtained on the other sounds. Phoneme-specific nasal air emission (PSNAE) occurs most commonly when the individual uses a posterior nasal fricative as a substitution for sibilants (see "Posterior Nasal Fricative" in this chapter.) In this case, changing articulatory placement will result in elimination of the nasal emission.

Nasal Grimace

A nasal grimace often accompanies significant nasal emission (Figure 7–5). It can be seen as a muscle contraction just above the nasal bridge or at the side of the nares. Just as muscle contractions can be noted in the face when a person is trying to lift something heavy, the nasal grimace seems to be an overflow muscle reaction that occurs with extreme effort to achieve velopharyngeal closure. Once velopharyngeal function is corrected, this contraction during speech usually disappears spontaneously.

Weak or Omitted Consonants

When air flows through the velopharyngeal valve or an oronasal fistula, it reduces the amount of air pressure that is available in the oral cavity for the production of consonants. This causes the consonants to be weak in intensity and pressure, or causes them to be omitted completely (Baken, 1987; McWilliams et al., 1990b). There is usually a direct inverse relationship between the amount of nasal air emission and the pressure for production of oral consonants. Therefore, the greater the nasal air

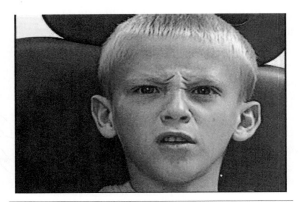

FIGURE 7–5 Nasal grimace during speech. Note the contraction above the nose and at the side of the nose. This is due to the extra effort of trying to achieve velopharyngeal closure.

emission, the weaker the consonants will tend to be.

Weak consonants are expected primarily with the unobstructed form of nasal emission, because there is more airflow through the nasal cavity with this form. The weak consonants, in addition to the nasal emission or hypernasality, cause the speech to sound muffled and indistinct.

Short Utterance Length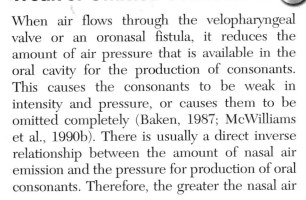

When there is significant nasal emission due to an unobstructed opening, this reduces the oral air pressure available for connected speech. Therefore, more frequent breaths are required during speech for replacing the air pressure (Kummer et al., 2003). This causes utterance length to be shortened and connected speech to be choppy.

It has been shown that individuals with a large velopharyngeal opening attempt to raise intraoral pressure by increasing airflow rate during consonant production. As a result, they may produce respiratory volumes that are twice that of normal speakers (Warren et al., 1969). This increased effort makes speech physically difficult and can cause the individual to become fatigued during speech.

Altered Rate and Speech Segment Durations

Speech segment durations have been shown to be abnormal in individuals with VPI (Forner, 1983). Using spectrograms to measure segment durations, Forner found that the utterances produced by children with a history of cleft palate and VPI were longer than those of unaffected peers. In addition, subjects with hypernasality had longer voice onset times than those with normal or less disordered speech. These findings may be due, at least in part, to the need to increase respiratory effort and to take more frequent breaths to compensate for the rapid loss of air pressure through the nose. Certainly, these findings suggest that coordinating speech production in the presence of a malfunctioning velopharyngeal valve is very difficult and thus affects the overall rate of speech.

Compensatory and Obligatory Articulation Productions

Speech characteristics, such as hypernasality, nasal air emission, weak consonants, and short utterance length are the direct result of a velopharyngeal or palatal opening. Therefore, these characteristics have been described as *passive speech characteristics* (Harding & Grunwell, 1996, 1998) or *obligatory errors* (Trost-Cardamone, 1990) because they are the product of structural abnormality rather than learned abnormal articulation behaviors.

In contrast, articulation productions that are not the direct result of velopharyngeal dysfunction, but rather are the individual's response to this dysfunction, are considered *active speech characteristics* (Harding & Grunwell, 1996, 1998) or *compensatory errors* (Trost-Cardamone, 1990). Compensatory articulation productions are often developed by the individual as a response to inadequate intraoral air pressure for normal articulation. When the compensatory productions are used, the manner of production is usually maintained. However, the place of articulation is altered and moved posteriorly to the pharynx or larynx. This allows the individual to take advantage of the air pressure that is available in the pharynx before it is reduced because of the velopharyngeal opening.

A distinction between obligatory errors and compensatory errors is important to make because the compensatory characteristics are under the patient's control and can therefore

be modified with speech therapy. Obligatory errors are purely the result of abnormal structure and require surgical or prosthetic intervention for correction.

The various types of obligatory and compensatory articulation productions are described further in the following sections. For an excellent tutorial on the various types of compensatory productions, please refer to the 1987 videotape made by Trost-Cardamone (see references).

Middorsum Palatal Stop (Palatal-Dorsal Production)

The *middorsum palatal stop*, also called a *palatal-dorsal production*, is a stop consonant that is produced with the dorsum of the tongue against the middle of the hard palate (Trost, 1981) (Figure 7–6). This production is substituted for the lingual-alveolar sounds (/t/, /d/, /n/, /l/) and

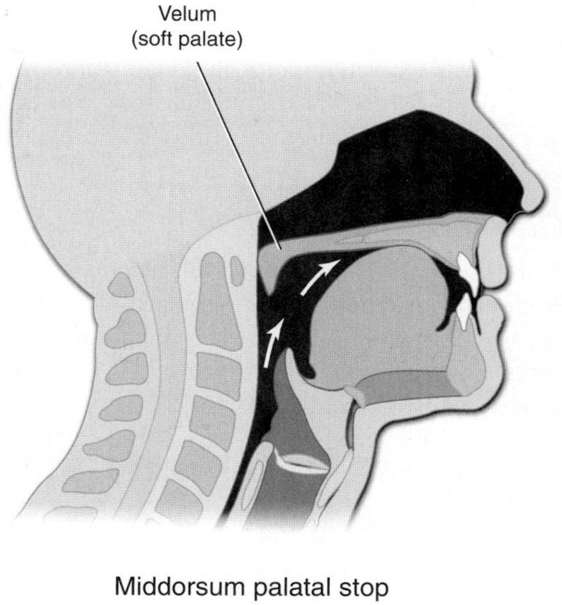

Velum
(soft palate)

Middorsum palatal stop

FIGURE 7–6 Diagram of the tongue position for a middorsum palatal stop (palatal dorsal production).

often for the velar sounds (/k/, /g/). Because the place of production is between that for lingual-alveolars and velars, the boundaries for distinguishing the two placements are lost and the acoustic product sounds like a cross between the two placements. In some cases, a palatal-dorsal placement will also be used for the production of sibilant sounds (/s/, /z/, /sh/, /zh/, /ch/, and /j/). This results in a lateral lisp (Gibbon & Crampin, 2001).

The middorsum palatal stop can be an obligatory error, but it is usually compensatory as a result of anterior oral cavity crowding. If the individual has a Class III malocclusion or anterior crossbite, the maxillary teeth are positioned behind the mandibular teeth. As a result, the alveolar ridge is well behind the position of the tongue tip. The individual compensates for the relative anterior position of the tongue by pulling it back. As the tongue retracts and goes down, the dorsum goes up to articulate against the alveolar ridge or palate. This error is common in individuals with a history of cleft palate, but can also be seen in individuals with macroglossia. When there is a midpalatal fistula, the individual may use this placement to occlude the fistula, thus preventing nasal emission through the opening.

Generalized Backing

Some individuals with VPI will articulate with posterior articulation for other oral sounds (Trost-Cardamone, 1997). This includes using velar sounds as a substitution for anterior sounds (Ainoda, Yamashita, & Tsukada, 1985; Powers, 1962). In some cases, the anterior sounds (lingual-alveolars and bilabials) are actually *coarticulated* with the velars, where the plosive is actually produced (Gibbon, Ellis, & Crampin, 2004). Backing of phonemes occurs for several reasons. Posterior articulation allows the individual to impound air pressure in the back of the oral cavity. In addition, the back of

the tongue can help to push the velum upward to assist with closure as a compensatory strategy for VPI (Brooks, Shelton, & Youngstrom, 1965; McWilliams et al., 1990b).

Velar Fricative

The *velar fricative* is produced with the back of the tongue in the same position as for the production of a /y/ sound (Figure 7–7). With the back of the tongue elevated and positioned under the velum, a small space is created. The velar fricative is produced as air is forced through that small opening. The velar fricative may be substituted for any fricative sound, but is most commonly substituted for sibilants. It can be voiced or voiceless. This production is sometimes difficult to distinguish from a pharyngeal fricative, but with good diagnostic technique, the source of the friction sound can be located.

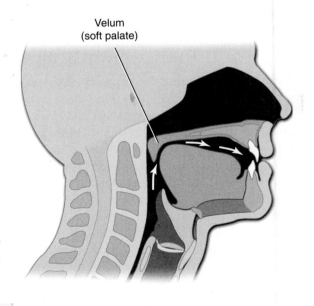

Velum
(soft palate)

Velar fricative

FIGURE 7–7 Diagram of the tongue position for a velar fricative.

Nasalization of Oral Consonants

The *nasalization of oral phonemes* is an obligatory error due to an open velopharyngeal valve. For example, when the velopharyngeal valve remains open during production of voiced plosives, the acoustic product will sound like their nasal cognates (m/b, n/d, and ng/g). In this case, placement of the phoneme is preserved, but manner is necessarily changed from oral to nasal due to the open velopharyngeal port. Nasalized phonemes are usually associated with the presence of hypernasality and are the result of a large velopharyngeal opening.

Nasalization of Vowels

High vowels normally have more nasal resonance than low vowels. This is due to the fact that the high tongue position causes more acoustic impedance than the open oral cavity of a low vowel (Jones, 2005). In addition, due to the constriction, there is increased pressure above the high point of the vowel. As such, there is likely more transpalatal transmission of sound energy through the velum (Gildersleeve-Neumann & Dalston, 2001). Some children with a history of cleft raise the back of the tongue too high so that it actually articulates very close to or against the velum (Gibbon, Smeaton-Ewins, & Crampin, 2005) (Figure 7–8). This blocks the sound from entering the oral cavity and forces it to travel through the nasal cavity, causing nasalization. Even individuals without a history of cleft can demonstrate phoneme-specific hypernasality due to a high tongue position on high vowels. Although velopharyngeal closure may be normal during the production of consonants on nasopharyngoscopy, the resonance may be perceived as hypernasal due to the increase in oral impedance on high vowels (Karnell, Schultz, & Canady, 2001).

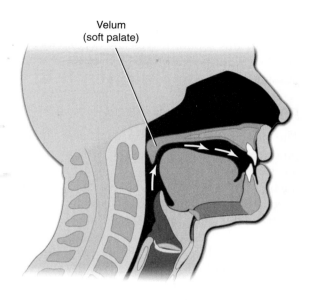

Velum
(soft palate)

Nasalized vowels

FIGURE 7–8 Diagram of the tongue position for nasalized vowels.

Nasal Snort

The nasal snort is produced by a forcible emission of air pressure through the nose that results in a noisy, sneeze-like sound. The *nasal snort* is typically associated with the production of /s/ blends. It often occurs concurrently with a nasal grimace. The nasal snort may be an obligatory error and occur with nasal emission, a compensatory error due to VPI, or an articulation error due to mislearning.

Nasal Sniff

The *nasal sniff* is not a common compensatory articulation production, but it does occur. In this case, the phoneme is produced by a forcible inspiration through the nose. In a sense, this is the opposite of nasal emission. The nasal sniff is usually substituted for sibilant sounds, particularly the /s/. Due to the difficulty in coordinating the inspiration and expiration during articulation with this sound, it typically occurs only in the final word position, rather than in all word positions.

Pharyngeal Plosive

The *pharyngeal plosive* is a consonant that is produced with the back of the tongue against the pharyngeal wall (Figure 7–9). During production of this sound, the dorsum of the tongue is convex in configuration and low in the oral cavity tongue. The entire tongue moves posteriorly in order to articulate against the posterior pharyngeal wall and uses the air pressure that can be established in the pharynx. An increase in pharyngeal activity can often be noted by observing the throat area. Due to the difficulty of producing this phoneme, there is often a longer duration between the consonant and the following vowel than is typically noted with other consonant placements. Pharyngeal plosives can be voiced or unvoiced. Although they can be substituted for other consonants, they are typically substituted only for the velar plosives (/k/, /g/). It is more common for glottal stops to be substituted for other sounds, probably because glottal stops are much easier to produce and can be coarticulated.

Pharyngeal Fricative

A pharyngeal fricative is another consonant that uses the back of the tongue and pharynx (Figure 7–10). It is produced when the tongue is retracted so that the base of the tongue approximates, but does not touch, the pharyngeal wall. A friction sound occurs as the air pressure is forced through the narrow opening that is created between the base of the tongue and pharyngeal wall. Pharyngeal fricatives can be substituted for fricatives and affricates, and

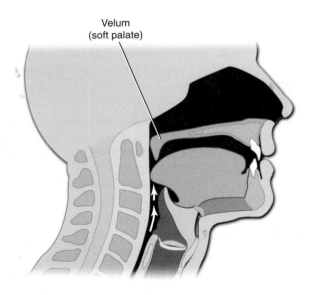

Velum
(soft palate)

Pharyngeal plosive

FIGURE 7–9 Diagram of the tongue position for a pharyngeal plosive.

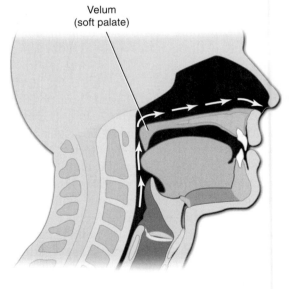

Velum
(soft palate)

Pharyngeal fricative

FIGURE 7–10 Diagram of the tongue position for a pharyngeal fricative.

are usually substituted for the sibilant sounds (/s/, /z/, /sh/, /zh/, /ch/, and /j/). Pharyngeal fricatives can be voiced or unvoiced, although the unvoiced version is most commonly noted. A pharyngeal fricative can sound similar to a lateral lisp, particularly to an inexperienced listener. It is important to make the right judgment as to which sound is being produced because this judgment will have a significant impact on the recommendations for treatment (see Chapter 12).

Pharyngeal Affricate

A *pharyngeal affricate* has the same initial placement as a pharyngeal plosive and pharyngeal fricative. A pharyngeal affricate can sometimes be difficult to distinguish from a pharyngeal fricative, especially in connected speech. However, as with other affricates, this sound combines the manner of a plosive and a fricative. Therefore, the pharyngeal affricate is the combination of either a pharyngeal plosive or a glottal stop and a pharyngeal fricative. As with the other pharyngeal compensatory productions, an increase in pharyngeal activity can be noted in the throat area during speech. Pharyngeal affricates typically are substituted for the other affricates (/ch/ and /j/), although they can be substituted for the other sibilant sounds (/s/, /z/, /sh/, and /zh/). They can be unvoiced or voiced.

Posterior Nasal Fricative

The *posterior nasal fricative* is a misarticulation characterized by audible nasal emission and friction in the posterior nasal pharynx (Trost, 1981). During production, the back of the tongue is often up and articulating against the velum as in an /ng/ placement. Because the tongue blocks the entrance into the oral cavity, air is forced through the velopharyngeal valve (Figure 7–11). A posterior nasal fricative can

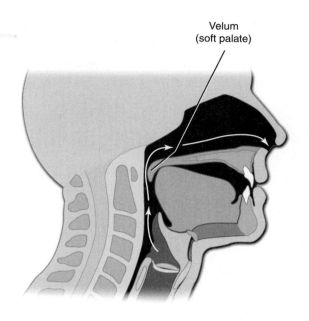

Velum (soft palate)

Posterior nasal fricative

FIGURE 7–11 Diagram of the tongue position for a posterior nasal fricative.

be seen on videofluoroscopy or through nasopharyngoscopy as incomplete closure of the velopharyngeal valve. The nasal emission is perceived as a nasal rustle. The posterior nasal fricative can be a compensatory articulation production as a result of VPI or it can be a learned misarticulation that results in phoneme-specific nasal emission. The posterior nasal fricative may be used as a substitution for any of the pressure-sensitive phonemes, but it is typically used for sibilants, particularly /s/.

Glottal Stop

A glottal stop is a plosive sound that is produced with a forceful adduction of the vocal folds and ventricular folds (often called the false vocal folds) (Figure 7–12). There is a build-up of subglottic air pressure and then sudden separation of the true and false vocal

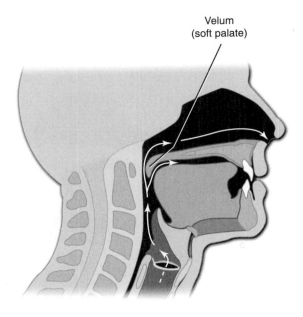

Velum
(soft palate)

Glottal stop with coarticulated
/t/ placement

FIGURE 7–12 Diagram of the tongue position for a glottal stop with a coarticulated /t/.

folds to release the air pressure and create airflow. The perceptual produce is essentially a grunt sound. This can often be seen by increased laryngeal activity in the throat area. Glottal stops are typically substituted for plosive sounds, but they may also be substituted for fricatives and affricates, especially if the individual has not yet developed the fricative manner in his or her phonemic repertoire. A glottal stop is usually perceived as a voiced phoneme because this production results in rapid voice onset for the vowel. Unlike other compensatory productions, glottal stops can be coarticulated with other phonemes. This coarticulation is characterized by one manner of production with simultaneous valving at two places of production (Trost-Cardamone, 1997). Visually, it appears as if the

individual is producing the sound correctly with appropriate oral placement, even though the plosive production is actually produced at the glottis. Because air pressure is released at the glottis, there is no need for velopharyngeal closure, so glottal stops often appear to be associated with a significant velopharyngeal opening (Henningsson & Isberg, 1986). It is important to note, however, that this does not reflect the individual's ability to achieve velopharyngeal closure when oral phonemes are attempted.

Substitution of /h/ for Voiceless Plosives

Voiceless plosives require a build-up of intra-oral air pressure and sudden release for production. If there is significantly reduced oral air pressure during production, the oral sound will not be heard. Instead, the airflow through the vocal folds will be the only perceptible distinctive feature, resulting in the acoustic product of /h/ (Harding & Grunwell, 1998). This may be obligatory or compensatory as part of a pattern of glottal and pharyngeal articulation.

Breathiness

A breathy vocal quality may be used as a strategy to compensate for VPI. With lower subglottic pressure, this compensatory strategy can reduce the amount of nasal air emission. In addition, a breathy voice can mask the perception of hypernasality because there is less sound intensity in the nasal cavity.

Dysphonia

Dysphonia is characterized by breathiness, hoarseness, low intensity, and/or glottal fry during phonation. Children with a history of congenital anomalies or VPI have an increased risk for dysphonia for several reasons (D'Antonio et al.,

1988; Hess, 1959; McWilliams, Bluestone, & Musgrave, 1969; McWilliams, Lavorato, & Bluestone, 1973; McWilliams, Morris, & Shelton, 1990a).

A common finding in individuals with mildly impaired velopharyngeal valving is a hyperfunctional voice disorder. This is due to increased respiratory and muscular effort, including hyperadduction of the vocal folds, with attempts to close the velopharyngeal port. Initially, this behavior may cause thickening and edema of the vocal folds, ultimately leading to the formation of vocal nodules (Boone & McFarlane, 1988). *Vocal nodules* may also develop secondary to the use of glottal stops as a compensatory articulation strategy (Figure 7–13). Since glottal stops are produced by quickly and forcibly abducting the vocal folds after full adduction, damage to the vocal fold edges is not surprising. Speech

therapy to increase oral airflow when there is VPI is not only ineffective, but it can also cause or exacerbate vocal-fold pathology (McWilliams et al., 1990b).

Other causes of voice disorders in these populations include laryngeal anomalies, particularly in those individuals with congenital malformation syndromes. When there is VPI, the lack of adequate oral acoustic energy in combination with the absorption of sound energy by the pharyngeal tissues results in a damping effect, causing the voice to be low in intensity (Bernthal & Beukelman, 1977). Finally, low intensity and breathiness may occur as a compensatory strategy to mask the hypernasality and nasal air emission, as previously noted.

FACTORS THAT IMPACT SPEECH CHARACTERISTICS AND SEVERITY

The severity of VPI can vary from a very small pinhole-sized opening to a very large opening that includes the entire velopharyngeal port. However, the size of the velopharyngeal opening does not correlate well with the severity of the speech disorder and the effect on intelligibility (Jones, 2005; Warren et al., 1969). The lack of a one-to-one correlation is due to several factors, including the separate effects of gap size on acoustics versus aerodynamics, the consistency of closure, and the confounding effects of altered articulation and phonation.

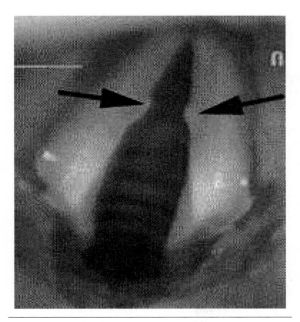

FIGURE 7–13   Bilateral vocal nodules as seen through endoscopy.

Size of the Velopharyngeal Opening

If the effects of articulation and phonation are factored out or if both are normal, there still would be a poor correlation between the size of the velopharyngeal opening and the severity of the speech. However, specific speech characteristics can be predictors of the approximate size of the opening (Table 7–1). This has to do with basic principles of physics and the acoustic effects of forcing air and sound through various sized openings.

One basic law of physics is that any type of flow (water, air, or sound) will continue in the same direction unless it is blocked by another force. In normal speech, airflow and sound energy move in a superior direction from the glottis through the pharynx. With closure of the velopharyngeal valve, the flow is redirected anteriorly into the oral cavity. When there is a velopharyngeal opening during speech, the flow is only partially redirected anteriorly. Because the airflow is perpendicular to the opening, even a very small opening will result in some form of nasal escape (Kummer, Briggs, & Lee, 2003; Kummer, Curtis, Wiggs, Lee, & Strife, 1992).

If the velopharyngeal opening is large, air and sound will go through the opening without much resistance. The movement of air is unobstructed, turbulence is low, and nasal emission is not very audible. Instead, hypernasality is most noticeable. Oral sounds may be "nasalized" in that they will sound similar to nasal phonemes at the same placement (i.e., /m/ for bilabials, /n/ for lingual-alveolars, and /ng/ for velars). Oral sounds may also be substituted by compensatory productions (pharyngeal phonemes or glottal stops) due to the lack of sufficient intraoral air pressure. Because there is a significant amount of nasal air emission (although not very audible), any attempted oral consonants will be very weak in intensity and pressure. In addition, utterance length will be short due to the need to take more frequent breaths to compensate for the loss of air pressure.

If the velopharyngeal opening is moderate in size, there will be similar characteristics as for a large opening. However, hypernasality will be less severe and nasal emission will be more audible. This is because with a smaller opening, there is more resistance to the flow of

TABLE 7–1 Perceptual Characteristics of Speech as a Prediction of Velopharyngeal Gap Size

Perceptual Characteristics	Predict	Relative Gap Size
Severe hypernasality Weak consonants Short utterance length	⇒	(large oval)
Moderate hypernasality Audible nasal emission Weak consonants Short utterance length	⇒	(medium oval)
Mild hypernasality Audible nasal emission	⇒	(small oval)
Nasal rustle (turbulence)	⇒	(smallest oval)

air as it comes through the valve, causing a turbulence sound. Also, there is more intraoral air pressure, so consonants are stronger and utterance length is less affected than with a larger opening.

Small openings are typically characterized by normal speech and resonance. However, as noted before, a small opening usually causes a very loud and distracting nasal rustle (Kummer et al., 1992, 2003). The nasal rustle can be loud enough to mask the oral sound that is being articulated, which also affects the intelligibility of speech. Therefore, the speech quality from a small opening may be judged to be more severely affected than the speech quality from a larger opening.

Individuals who demonstrate a small, yet consistent velopharyngeal gap have been termed the *almost-but-not-quite* (ABNQ) group by Morris (1984). These individuals are generally not stimulable for improvement through auditory discrimination training or articulation therapy. This is because an underlying structural or physiological disorder precludes complete velopharyngeal closure. Therefore, surgical or prosthetic management is more appropriate. Correction is definitely indicated, even though the opening is small, because this size of opening often results in more severely affected speech than a larger opening.

Inconsistency of Velopharyngeal Closure

If velopharyngeal closure is inconsistent, the quality of speech may also be variable. Inconsistent velopharyngeal closure is most common in individuals who have a small velopharyngeal opening. Morris (1984) termed this subgroup of individuals the *sometimes-but-not-always* (SBNA) group. Individuals in this group may

be able to achieve total closure with effort. However, just as it is difficult to carry a 50-pound weight for long, it is difficult for these individuals to continue to exert enough effort to maintain that closure for a prolonged period of time. Closure may be complete for single words or short utterances, but may break down with the motoric demands of connected speech. Speech may be best at the beginning of the day, but become noticeably worse as the day goes on and the individual becomes fatigued. Velopharyngeal closure may also be inconsistent due to apraxia of speech. Inconsistencies in velopharyngeal closure can result in significant variations in the quality of speech and perception of resonance.

Abnormal Articulation and Phonation

Another factor that affects the intelligibility of speech and judgments of severity is the status of articulation. If the individual has developed good articulation skills and has preserved the appropriate place of articulation, the overall intelligibility of speech will be better than that of a person with the same opening who has poor articulation skills. If the individual compensates for VPI by *backing of phonemes*, or if the person has articulation errors related to malocclusion, oral-motor dysfunction, or delayed acquisition, these errors will affect the overall intelligibility of speech and the judgment of severity.

The quality of phonation is a final factor that affects judgments of severity. The use of a breathy voice may reduce the perception of nasal emission and hypernasality. In addition, increased vocal effort may temporarily increase velopharyngeal function and decrease gap size for improved resonance (McHenry, 1997). On the other hand, low volume and other dysphonic characteristics, such as hoarseness and glottal fry, can have a negative effect on the overall intelligibility of the speech.

CAUSES OF VELOPHARYNGEAL DYSFUNCTION

Velopharyngeal Insufficiency (VPI)

As noted above, velopharyngeal insufficiency (VPI) refers to a structural defect that causes the velum to be too short to close against the posterior pharyngeal wall. For velopharyngeal contact to be made, the velum must be of sufficient length and width, once elevation and stretching have occurred, to span the depth of the velopharynx and achieve firm contact. There are many causes of discrepancies between the length of the velum and the needed length for firm velopharyngeal contact. These causes will be described.

History of Cleft Palate

Velopharyngeal insufficiency occurs most commonly in individuals with a history of cleft palate. Although surgeons attempt to achieve as much velar length during the cleft palate repair as possible, approximately 20% of patients with a history of cleft palate will demonstrate velopharyngeal insufficiency following the cleft repair. Even scar tissue in a repaired cleft palate may increase, dampen, or in some way alter transpalatal acoustic transmission (Gildersleeve-Neumann & Dalston, 2001).

Submucous Cleft Palate

The characteristics of a submucous cleft are described in Chapter 2. Although the vast majority of individuals with submucous cleft

will have normal speech, even through adulthood (Chen, Wu, & Noordhoff, 1994; McWilliams, 1991), some will have characteristics of velopharyngeal insufficiency. This can be due to a hypoplastic musculus uvulae muscle, or a more obvious defect on the nasal surface of the velum. Because the defect in the velum is typically in the midline, this is usually where the velopharyngeal gap will be as well.

One characteristic of a submucous cleft is a zona pellucida, which is an area of thin mucosa and little, if any, muscle. Because the velum is thin, there is more transpalatal transmission of sound energy through it to the nasal cavity. Therefore, even if the velopharyngeal valve is functioning normally, there may be hypernasality due to this defect.

Short Velum or Deep Pharynx

Velopharyngeal insufficiency is sometimes noted when, despite normal velar morphology, the velum appears short relative to the posterior pharyngeal wall (Figure 7–1). When the velum cannot stretch enough to meet the posterior pharyngeal wall during speech, complete velopharyngeal closure cannot be achieved. In some cases, this is due to a congenitally short velum. In other cases, it is due to a deep pharynx secondary to cranial base abnormalities (Haapanen, Heliovaara, & Ranta, 1991; Peterson-Falzone, 1985). As noted in Chapter 13, the relative length of the velum and depth of the pharynx cannot be determined by an intraoral examination since velopharyngeal contact occurs above the level of view.

Adenoid Atrophy

Individuals with a repaired cleft palate or with a submucous cleft may demonstrate normal speech and resonance during the preschool and early school years, but experience gradual deterioration in velopharyngeal closure when they reach adolescence. With the onset of puberty, there is often significant, and sometimes sudden, atrophy of the adenoid tissue. As a result, there is an increase in the distance between the velum and posterior pharyngeal wall. If the velum is normal with no scarring from a cleft repair or no submucous cleft, it eventually stretches to accommodate the difference in the depth of the pharynx. Therefore, normal velopharyngeal closure is maintained. However, if there is a history of cleft or there is a submucous cleft, the velum may not be capable of stretching and lengthening. As a result, the involution of the adenoid tissue causes a gradual loss of velopharyngeal competence (Handelman & Osborne, 1976; Mason & Warren, 1980; Morris, Wroblewski, Brown, & Van Demark, 1990; Shapiro, 1980; Siegel-Sadewitz & Shprintzen, 1986). When this occurs, parents often report that their child "mumbles," doesn't speak loud enough, or has become "lazy" with speech.

Irregular Adenoids

Although it is not commonly recognized, irregular adenoids can cause velopharyngeal insufficiency in some cases (Ren, Isberg, & Henningsson, 1995). Even when the adenoid pad is large, velopharyngeal insufficiency can occur if the tissue is "bumpy" or irregular due to either indentations (Figure 7–14A) or projections on the surface. In this case, as the velum closes against the adenoid for speech, it does not achieve a tight seal. This results in a small velopharyngeal (actually veloadenoidal) opening (Figure 7–14B). Since the opening is usually small, it rarely causes hypernasality. In fact, there may be hyponasality if the adenoid tissue is large. However, this opening will cause nasal air emission. Ironically, irregular adenoids

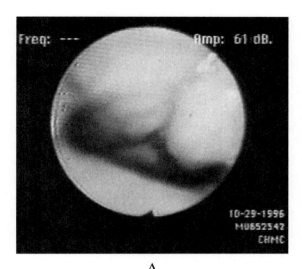

A

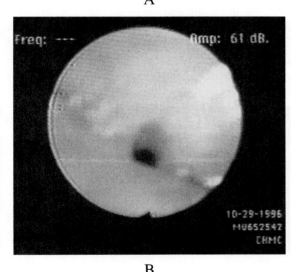

B

FIGURE 7–14 (A and B) A. A deep cleft in the surface of the adenoid pad. B. As a result of adenoid irregularity, the velum is unable to achieve a tight seal against the adenoid, resulting in nasal air emission.

commonly occur after adenoidectomy. Since the entire adenoid capsule cannot be removed during adenoidectomy, some regrowth of the tissue often occurs. As it regrows, irregularities in the surface are often found.

Hypertrophic Tonsils

The tonsils are located in the oral cavity between the anterior and posterior faucial pillars (see Chapter 8). As such, they usually do not have any effect on velopharyngeal function because they normally sit well below and anterior to the velopharyngeal valve. On rare occasions, however, hypertrophic tonsils can cause mechanical interference with the function of the velopharyngeal valve. If one tonsil is much larger than the other, it will often push the velum upward on that side. Due to the pulling and stretching of the velum on that side, the uvula will deviate and appear to point to the large tonsil. Large tonsils can restrict the medial movement of the lateral pharyngeal walls, thus affecting velopharyngeal closure. Large tonsils can force the tongue to move down and forward during speech. This can interfere with the articulation of velar sounds (/k/, /g/) and even

affect velopharyngeal activity for these sounds (Henningsson & Isberg, 1988).

The most dramatic effect of hypertrophic tonsils on velopharyngeal function occurs when a tonsil is so large that its upper pole projects into the pharynx (Figure 7–15A). If it is positioned between the velum and posterior pharyngeal wall, it prevents the velum from achieving an adequate velopharyngeal seal during speech (Figure 7–15B) (Kummer et al., 1993; MacKenzie-Stepner, Witzel, Stringer, & Laskin, 1987; Misra, Gill, & Lal, 1981; Peterson-Falzone, 1985; Shprintzen, Sher, & Croft, 1987). This results in a small velopharyngeal gap, which usually causes nasal air emission. The tonsil in the pharynx can also obstruct sound transmission into both the oral and nasal cavities, causing a mixture of hyponasality and cul-de-sac resonance. Tonsillectomy is obviously indicated to eliminate these characteristics.

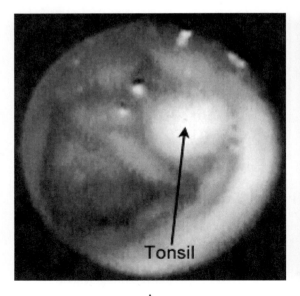

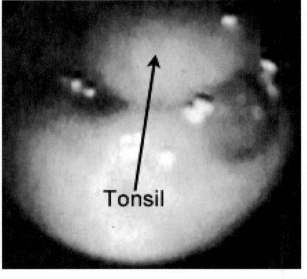

A

B

FIGURE 7–15 (A and B) A. Large tonsil on the right that can be seen in the nasopharynx from above through nasopharyngoscopy. B. Tonsil can be seen between the velum and posterior pharyngeal wall during velopharyngeal closure. During closure, a small opening remains, just to the left of the tonsil. There is a bubble in this area due to nasal air emission.

CASE REPORT

Enlarged Tonsils

Ellen was a 9-year-old child with a history of normal speech and language development. She had never had speech therapy. However, her speech had gradually become "nasal" and hard to understand over about a two-year period. The parents reported that Ellen had also begun to snore loudly at night.

Upon examination, Ellen was noted to have an open mouth posture with an anterior tongue position at rest. An evaluation of speech revealed normal articulation, but nasal emission during the production of pressure-sensitive phonemes. Resonance was characterized by hyponasality and a cul-de-sac quality.

An intra-oral examination revealed the cause of the speech characteristics. The right tonsil was very large and extended medially beyond the point of the midline of the oropharynx. The left tonsil was of normal size. A nasopharyngoscopy assessment showed the tonsil to be in the nasopharynx and between the velum and posterior pharyngeal wall during velopharyngeal closure. Because of the position of the tonsil, complete velopharyngeal closure could not be achieved, resulting in nasal air emission. The large tonsil in the pharynx interfered with the transmission of sound energy into the nasal cavity during the production of nasal sounds, thus causing hyponasality. The size of the tonsils also blocked the sound energy from entering the oral cavity during the production of oral sounds. This was the cause of the cul-de-sac resonance.

Given these findings, the obvious treatment was a tonsillectomy. Once this was done, resonance returned to normal and nasal air emission was no longer noted. Ellen was able to maintain a closed mouth posture and snoring was no longer noted at night.

Velopharyngeal Insufficiency (VPI) Posttreatment

Adenoidectomy

A well-known and well-documented risk of an adenoidectomy is postoperative velopharyngeal insufficiency (Andreassen, Leeper, & MacRae, 1991; Blum & Neel, 1983; Croft, Shprintzen, & Ruben, 1981; Donnelly, 1994; Eufinger, Eggeling, & Immenkamp, 1994; Fernandes, Grobbelaar, Hudson, & Lentin, 1996; Kummer, Myer, Smith, & Shott, 1993; Parton & Jones, 1998; Ren, Isberg, & Henningsson, 1995; Robinson, 1992; Seid, 1990; Witzel, Rich, Margar-Bacal, & Cox, 1986). This is due to the fact that young children with a prominent adenoid pad usually achieve veloadenoidal closure rather than velopharyngeal closure (Figure 7–16). Removal of the

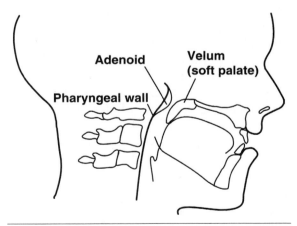

FIGURE 7–16   Position of the adenoid in the pharynx. The adenoid pad can help with closure in many cases. In many young children, there is veloadenoidal closure rather than velopharyngeal closure.

adenoids results in a deeper nasopharynx and a greater distance for the velum to stretch in order to achieve closure. (For more information regarding adenoids, please see Chapter 8.)

Hypernasality or nasal emission following adenoidectomy can occur in individuals with no velar defect. However, this is typically short lived, lasting from a few hours to no more than six weeks. Certain compensations occur in the velopharyngeal mechanism to adapt to the changes in the pharyngeal dimension. These compensations include an increase in velar mobility, an increase in velar height during closure, an increase in velar stretch, and increased movement of the pharyngeal walls (Neiman & Simpson, 1975). Therefore, in most cases, the speech returns to normal once these adaptations are made.

Permanent velopharyngeal insufficiency following adenoidectomy occurs in approximately 1 out of 1500 procedures (Donnelly, 1994). This problem is more likely to occur if there is an underlying congenital abnormality of the velum. Although obvious velar abnormalities are usually ruled out by oral inspection prior to performing an adenoidectomy, many patients with velopharyngeal insufficiency following adenoidectomy are found through nasopharyngoscopy to have an occult submucous cleft after the fact (Parton & Jones, 1998; Schmaman, Jordaan, & Jammine, 1998). Certainly, individuals with a history of cleft palate are at much greater risk for velopharyngeal insufficiency following adenoidectomy due to possible tenuous velopharyngeal closure preoperatively, scarring of the velum, and the lack of reserve muscle mass to stretch postoperatively (Parton & Jones, 1998). Therefore, adenoidectomy is usually contraindicated for these individuals. If, however, the adenoid pad is so large that it causes airway obstruction or blocks the opening to the eustachian tube on one or both sides, a conservative adenoidectomy can be done. In this case, only a small portion of the adenoid pad is removed.

Tonsillectomy

As noted previously, the tonsils reside in the oral cavity (not in the nasopharynx, where the adenoids are located). Therefore, unlike adenoidectomy, tonsillectomy is highly unlikely to cause problems with speech. There are two possible exceptions, however. First, it has been hypothesized that significant scarring of the posterior faucial pillar postoperatively could potentially affect lateral pharyngeal wall movement. There may be a particular concern for individuals who are prone to forming *keloids*, which is excessive scar tissue formed during healing.

Another cause, although it is rare, is a learned protection response after the surgery. Tonsillectomy can result in significant pain for a week or 10 days after the procedure. Opening and closing the velopharyngeal valve for swallowing and speech can exacerbate the pain. Postoperative avoidance of velopharyngeal closure can become habituated in some patients, resulting in severe velopharyngeal dysfunction following the surgery (Gibb & Stewart, 1975). This is treated as a learned compensatory strategy.

Maxillary Advancement

Individuals with midface retrusion and Class III malocclusion can often benefit from maxillary advancement. This can be done through either *orthognathic surgery* or maxillary distraction (see Chapter 20). The purpose of maxillary advancement is to correct midface deficiency in order to normalize the occlusion and the facial profile. Maxillary advancement results in a dramatic improvement in facial aesthetics. In addition, the normalization of occlusion often results in improved articulation, particularly of sibilant sounds (Kummer, Strife, Grau, Creaghead, & Lee, 1989; McCarthy, Coccaro, & Schwartz, 1979). If there is nasal obstruction or hyponasality due to nasal airway resistance, maxillary

CASE REPORT

Velopharyngeal Dysfunction following Tonsillectomy

Ashley was a 12-year-old with a history of mouth breathing and loud snoring at night. She had had an adenoidectomy at the age of 5 with no effect on speech.

A tonsillectomy was done with no complications. However, Ashley refused to swallow for several days postoperatively. As a result, she was kept in the hospital for three days on IV fluids. She did not speak much for 9–10 days after the surgery.

Once she began to speak, her speech was severely hypernasal. In addition, she experienced significant nasal regurgitation of fluids if her head was turned down even slightly. Nasopharyngoscopy showed very little velopharyngeal movement during speech or with swallowing. In addition, the tongue base was being held in an anterior position. It was hypothesized that this occurred initially to avoid pain during velopharyngeal movement, and then became habituated after the pain resolved.

Ashley was seen for speech therapy for six sessions in four weeks. As a result of the therapy, speech and swallowing returned to normal. A lesson to be learned from this case is that, even when severe velopharyngeal incompetence is noted perceptually and through nasopharyngoscopy, it reflects only what the individual is currently doing with the velopharyngeal mechanism. It does not reflect what the individual is capable of doing.

advancement can reduce or eliminate these problems by increasing the nasal cavity space (Dalston & Vig, 1984). Although maxillary advancement can improve aesthetics, articulation, the nasal airway, and hyponasality, it can have a negative effect on velopharyngeal function. With this procedure, the anterior movement of the maxilla results in movement of the posterior border of the hard palate, with its soft palate attachments. This results in an increase in the pharyngeal depth. If there is only tenuous velopharyngeal closure preoperatively or if the velum is scarred due to a previous velar repair, it may not be able to stretch adequately following the surgery to span the entire pharyngeal depth.

The exact risk of velopharyngeal insufficiency following maxillary advancement is not known, but it is not a common occurrence in individuals who have no history of cleft palate or velar abnormality. In fact, the velopharyngeal mechanism normally makes the same types of

adaptations following maxillary advancement as it does following normal adenoid atrophy or adenoidectomy (Kummer et al., 1989). Therefore, most individuals will not experience a long-term problem with velopharyngeal function postoperatively. Those at greatest risk for hypernasality following maxillary advancement are the individuals who often can benefit the most from the procedure, particularly patients with a history of cleft palate (Haapanen, Kalland, Heliovaara, Hukki, & Ranta, 1997; Kummer et al., 1989; Maegawa, Sells, & David, 1998; Mason, Turvey, & Waren, 1980; McCarthy et al., 1979; Okazaki et al., 1993; Watzke, Turvey, Warren, & Dalston, 1990). The risk appears to be somewhat related to the amount of advancement, so that those with the greatest maxillary movement are at greatest risk for velopharyngeal dysfunction postoperatively (Maegawa et al., 1998). If speech and velopharyngeal function deteriorate after maxillary advancement, secondary surgery for speech is usually done (Maegawa et al., 1998) (see Chapter 18).

Oral Cavity Tumors

Oral cavity tumors occur in both children and in adults. In children, the most common tumor is an *hemangioma*, which is a congenital anomaly in which a proliferation of blood vessels results in a large mass. In adults, malignant tumors of the oral cavity are more commonly seen. When a tumor or growth interferes with function or becomes life-threatening, it is usually resected. Resections of areas of the oral cavity can affect the integrity of the separation of the nasal and oral cavities and the function of the velopharyngeal valve (Bodin, Lind, & Arnander, 1994; Brown, Zuydam, Jones, Rogers, & Vaughan, 1997; Fee, Gilmer, & Goffinet, 1988; Myers & Aramany, 1977; Rintala, 1987; Yoshida, Michi, Yamashita, & Ohno, 1993). This is particularly a concern if tissue is taken from the hard palate, velum, or pharyngeal walls. The use of radiation for oral or pharyngeal tumors can also affect the function of the velopharyngeal valve. It can cause shrinkage of not just the tumor, but also of the adjacent structures, including the velum and pharyngeal walls. When this occurs, surgical correction is often not possible due to the tissue damage.

Velopharyngeal Incompetence (VPI)

Velopharyngeal incompetence refers to a physiological deficiency that results in poor movement of the velopharyngeal structures. Velopharyngeal incompetence is characterized by poor elevation and inadequate "knee action" of the velum during speech (Figure 7–2). On lateral videofluoroscopy, the velum will often appear to be below the level of the hard palate during speech and the *velar eminence* (high

point of the velum as it bends) will not be significant when there is velopharyngeal incompetence. Lateral pharyngeal wall motion may also be very poor so that there is minimal medial movement to assist with closure. There are many causes of velopharyngeal incompetence, as will be further discussed.

Abnormal Muscle Insertion

Velopharyngeal incompetence can occur following a cleft palate repair due to poor muscle function. Even though the surgeon may attempt to dissect the levator veli palatini muscle and repair its orientation, it does not guarantee that this muscle will function normally for speech. If there is a submucous cleft palate that extends through the velum, the levator veli palatini muscle inserts into the hard palate (refer to Figure 2–14 in Chapter 2), rendering it useless in elevating the velum for speech.

Hypotonia and Poor Pharyngeal Wall Movement

Generalized hypotonia can affect the movement of the entire velopharyngeal valve, including the pharyngeal walls. It should be noted, however, that extensive lateral wall motion is normally noted only in the sagittal pattern of closure, which is the least common pattern found in both normal and abnormal speakers (Witzel & Posnick, 1989). Therefore, when lateral wall motion is limited, it may not be the result of a physiological defect. Instead, this may be a normal finding, particularly if the primary pattern of closure is the coronal pattern (Finkelstein, Talmi, Nachmani, Hauben, & Zohar, 1992; Shprintzen, Rakof, Skolnick, & Lavorato, 1977; Siegel-Sadewitz & Shprintzen, 1982; Skolnick, Shprintzen, McCall, & Rakoff, 1975; Witzel & Posnick, 1989). In addition, posterior pharyngeal wall motion is limited, even in normal speakers. Therefore, the observation of a lack of lateral or posterior pharyngeal wall motion in an abnormal speaker is not particularly significant.

Dysarthria

Dysarthria is a form of oral-motor dysfunction that affects all the subsystems of speech, including respiration, phonation, resonance, and articulation. It is characterized by abnormalities of strength, range of motion, speed, accuracy, and tonicity of the speech muscles due to central and/or peripheral nervous system impairment. As a result, speech is very slow, slurred, and characterized by inaccurate movement of the articulators. Hypernasality secondary to velopharyngeal incompetence is one of the primary characteristics of dysarthria (Yorkston, Beukelman, & Traynor, 1988). Other common characteristics of velopharyngeal incompetence due to dysarthria include weak consonants and short utterance length due to the nasal air emission.

Dysarthria with hypernasality has been associated with a variety of neurological causes. It can be secondary to either upper or lower motor neuron lesions. Some of the causes include cerebral palsy (Ansel & Kent, 1992; Neilson & O'Dwyer, 1981; Platt, Andrews, & Howie, 1980; Platt, Andrews, Young, & Quinn, 1980), myasthenia gravis (Hagstrom, Parsons, Landa, & Robson, 1979; Wolski, 1967), myotonic dystrophy (Hillarp, Ekberg, Jacobsson, Nylander, & Aberg, 1994; Salomonson, Kawamoto, & Wilson, 1988), neurofibromatosis (Pollack & Shprintzen, 1981), and cerebral or brainstem tumors (Lefaivre, Cohen, Riski, & Burstein, 1997; Van Mourik, Catsman-Berrevoets, Yousef-Bak, Paquier, & van Dongen, 1998). Dysarthria with hypernasality has been associated with mental retardation or developmental delay (Bradley, 1979; Heller, Gens, Moe, & Lewin, 1974; Kline & Hutchinson, 1980; Peterson-Falzone, 1985) and it can also occur secondary to acquired neurological damage due to traumatic brain injury (TBI) (Theodoros, Murdoch, Stokes, & Chenery, 1993; Upton & Berger, 1995; Workinger & Netsell, 1992) or cerebral vascular accident (CVA) (Thompson & Murdoch, 1995). Any disorder that causes cerebral, cerebellar, or brainstem damage can cause dysarthria with hypernasality.

Apraxia

Apraxia of speech, also called *verbal apraxia*, *dyspraxia*, *developmental apraxia*, or just *apraxia*, is another oral-motor disorder that can cause velopharyngeal incompetence. Apraxia is characterized by difficulty executing volitional oral movements, and sequencing oral movements for connected speech. Although we typically think of apraxia as affecting the anterior articulators (lips, tongue, and jaws), it can also affect the posterior articulators (velopharyngeal valve) and other subsystems of speech (respiration and phonation) (Bradley, 1997; McWilliams, Morris, & Shelton, 1990b; Trost-Cardamone, 1989). Due to the difficulty in coordinating and sequencing velopharyngeal movement during speech, the velum may go down inappropriately for oral sounds, causing hypernasality, and go up inappropriately for nasal sounds, causing hyponasality. The timing of closure may be affected so that closure does not occur until after the initiation of phonation, when it is too late (Warren, Dalston, & Mayo, 1993; Warren, Dalston, Trier, & Holder, 1985). The velum may drop down inappropriately due to a difficulty in maintaining closure, or it may appear to pulse up and down during connected speech, rather than staying up throughout the production of oral sounds. Velopharyngeal incompetence as a result of apraxia is usually very inconsistent. The speaker may produce both correct and incorrect productions of each phoneme, even within

CASE REPORT

Hypernasality Secondary to Dysarthria

Brandon was a 20-year-old college student when he had a cerebral hemorrhage secondary to an arterial venous (AV) malformation. This affected his speech, swallowing, the movement of the right side of the body, his walking, and vision. Fortunately, there was no cognitive loss. Brandon had received speech therapy for characteristics of dysarthria.

Brandon was referred to our VPI clinic since one of the primary concerns was hypernasality. He had already tried a prosthetic device, but this was not effective and caused other problems. At the time of the evaluation, Brandon was found to have normal articulatory placement, but characteristics of dysarthria including slow rate, imprecise movements, difficulty with initiation of movements for sound production, and labored movement. Articulation was affected by weak consonants due to significant nasal air emission. In addition, there was poor breath support, short utterance length, glottal fry, aphonia at the ends of utterances, and severe hypernasality.

Nasopharyngoscopy (an nasal endoscopic procedure) showed inconsistent velar elevation, with occasional touch closure of the velum against the posterior pharyngeal wall at midline. The velum was noted to tire easily, however, and drop down inappropriately. There was also poor lateral pharyngeal wall motion.

Since prosthetic treatment had been tried unsuccessfully, it was decided to try surgical intervention (specifically a pharyngeal flap). The goals of the surgery were to improve the quality and clarity of speech while decreasing the effort to produce speech.

Brandon was seen six weeks postoperatively for a reassessment. At that time, he demonstrated significantly improved speech. The hypernasality was reduced to a mild degree and the nasal air emission was only slight. Of most significance was the increase in oral pressure and thus, speech sound clarity. In addition, utterance length was longer and Brandon no longer needed to take frequent breaths to replenish breath support since there was less loss of air pressure for speech. In fact, Brandon was able to count to 23 on one breath rather than to 4 as he had preoperatively.

Although the pharyngeal flap did not result in a total correction of speech, it did result in significant improvement in the quality and clarity of speech. It also made speech less effortful. Brandon and his family were very pleased with the result.

---

a single utterance. All errors, including those of resonance, will tend to increase in severity, with an increase in utterance length and phonemic complexity. Although there will be mixed resonance, the predominant feature, particularly in longer utterances, is hypernasality.

Cranial Nerve Defects

Individuals with either congenital or acquired lower motor neuron damage may demonstrate specific velopharyngeal paralysis or paresis (weakness) of the velum or pharyngeal musculature (Rousseaux, Lesoin, & Quint, 1987). This can occur with involvement of the glossopharyngeal nerve (CN IX), the vagus nerve (CN X), or the hypoglossal nerve (CN XII). The paralysis or paresis is usually unilateral and can occur in the absence of other oral-motor deficits. When the vagus nerve (CN X) is involved, there may also be unilateral involvement of the larynx and vocal fold on the same side. With unilateral paralysis or paresis, one side of the velum will elevate normally during speech and may achieve closure. On the affected side, however, the velum will hang down during speech and a velopharyngeal opening will occur on that side of the midline. When this is observed from an intraoral perspective, the velum can be seen to droop on the affected side and the uvula will point to the side with better movement. Unilateral paralysis or paresis of the velum is commonly observed in individuals with hemifacial microsomia (Luce, McGibbon, & Hoopes, 1977).

Velar Fatigue and Stress Incompetence

Playing a wind instrument requires more intraoral air pressure and more velopharyngeal strength and stamina than speech. As a result, velopharyngeal incompetence secondary to stress on the mechanism has been reported in wind instrument musicians who do not have characteristics of velopharyngeal dysfunction in speech (Dibbell, Ewanowski, & Carter, 1979; Gordon, Astrachan, & Yanagisawa, 1994; Peterson-Falzone, 1985; Shanks, 1990). When velar fatigue occurs suddenly or only in certain circumstances, such as when playing a wind instrument, the person should be monitored over a period of time because this may be the first symptom of a progressive neurological disorder.

Velopharyngeal Mislearning

Velopharyngeal mislearning can cause abnormal resonance and nasal air emission with speech. Although the speech characteristics may sound just like those of individuals with velopharyngeal insufficiency or incompetence, individuals with velopharyngeal mislearning are not candidates for surgical or prosthetic

intervention. Instead, speech therapy is usually successful in correcting their functional speech characteristics.

Faulty Articulation

During normal articulation development, some children, including those with normal structures, learn to produce certain speech sounds incorrectly, resulting in an articulation/phonological disorder. Some misarticulations cause the velopharyngeal valve to open. This results in nasal resonance on certain oral sounds or nasal emission on selected consonants. Although this is *phoneme-specific* and does not occur on all sounds, connected speech will be perceived as "nasal."

A common misarticulation is the substitution of a *pharyngeal fricative* or a *posterior nasal fricative* for sibilant sounds (/s/, /z/, /sh/, /zh/, /ch/, /j/), particularly /s/ and /z/. Due to the way these sounds are produced, there is nasal emission with production. This is called *phoneme-specific nasal air emission* (PSNAE) because it only occurs on certain speech sounds and is the result of faulty articulation rather than an anatomical defect or physiological disorder. In addition, children with severe articulation disorders will often use glottal stops as a consonant placeholder. This is the same sound that is used as a compensatory production by children who have inadequate intraoral air pressure, so this can be confused with VPI.

Substitutions such as ng/l or ng/r will result in an overall perception of hypernasality in connected speech because /ng/ is a nasal sound. The /i/ vowel (as in the word "tea") has a tongue position that is just below that of /ng/. Some individuals will nasalize the vowel /i/ due to an abnormally high tongue position that restricts sound from entering the oral cavity (Falk & Kopp, 1968; McDonald & Baker, 1951; McWilliams et al., 1990b).

The back of the tongue may even articulate against the velum during /i/, further restricting oral resonance. 🔊 Limited mouth opening can have a similar effect because of the restriction on oral resonance.

Finally, generalized oral inactivity can cause characteristics of velopharyngeal dysfunction. This is due to the fact that when there is poor movement of the anterior articulators, it usually results in poor movement of the posterior articulators, which are the velopharyngeal structures.

Habituated Speech Patterns

Characteristics of VPI can continue, even after surgical correction of the cause. This is because the individual has already learned and habituated speech patterns of articulation prior to correction of the structures. In addition, the individual's auditory feedback loop that monitors resonance can cause hypernasality to persist, because it was the "normal" sound of the speech before surgical correction.

Since changing structure does not change function, speech therapy is usually required to change those patterns once the structural defects have been corrected. Postoperative speech therapy is important to help the individual to learn to make the best use of the new anatomical structure and to correct compensatory articulation errors that occurred as a result of the VPI.

Lack of Auditory Feedback

Consonants are produced with both auditory and articulation feedback. The accuracy of vowel production, however, depends primarily on auditory feedback. Because there is no tactile-kinesthetic feedback with vowels or with velopharyngeal movements, vowels (which primarily determine resonance) can be greatly affected by hearing loss. Individuals with severe hearing loss or deafness usually demonstrate abnormal resonance due to the inability to monitor resonance. The velopharyngeal valve may close inappropriately on nasal phonemes and open on oral phonemes, causing hypernasality, hyponasality, or mixed resonance (Abdullah, 1988; Fletcher & Daly, 1976; Ysunza & Vazquez, 1993). In addition, cul-de-sac resonance is common in individuals who are deaf (Subtelny, Whitehead, & Samar, 1992). This is due to retraction of the tongue and deflection of the epiglottis towards the pharyngeal wall, thus altering the characteristics of the vocal tract.

SUMMARY

The quality of voiced sounds is determined by the vibration of sound energy in the cavities of the vocal tract (pharynx, oral cavity, and nasal cavity). Resonance depends on the size and shape of these cavities and the function of the velopharyngeal valve. Resonance disorders can be due to abnormal coupling of the oral and the nasal cavity (hypernasality) or blockage in the vocal tract (hyponasality or cul-de-sac resonance). Although these disorders are not always treated by the speech-language pathologist, they should be correctly diagnosed by the speech-language pathologist so that recommendations for appropriate treatment can be made.

The velopharyngeal valve is responsible for directing sound energy from the pharynx into the oral cavity during speech. Velopharyngeal dysfunction can cause a variety of abnormal speech characteristics, including hypernasality, which is related to the acoustic aspect of speech, and nasal emission, which is related to the aerodynamic aspect of speech. Nasal emission can also cause weak or omitted consonants, short utterance length, and compensatory articulation productions. Dysphonia also occurs commonly with velopharyngeal dysfunction. Velopharyngeal dysfunction can be caused by structural abnormalities (velopharyngeal insufficiency), physiological disorders (velopharyngeal incompetence), or articulation errors (velopharyngeal mislearning).

The speech-language pathologist needs to be knowledgeable about the effects of velopharyngeal dysfunction on speech so that these problems can be managed appropriately.

FOR REVIEW, DISCUSSION, AND CRITICAL THINKING

1. What is resonance as it relates to speech? Discuss factors relating to the vocal tract that can alter resonance. Why is resonance primarily associated with vowels rather than consonants?

2. How is a resonance disorder similar to a voice disorder? How is it different?

3. How are velopharyngeal insufficiency, velopharyngeal incompetence, and velopharyngeal mislearning similar? How are they different? Why do you think making a distinction between these types of velopharyngeal dysfunctions is an important part of an evaluation of abnormal resonance?

4. Describe the basic characteristics of hyponasality, hypernasality, cul-de-sac resonance, and mixed resonance. What are the possible causes of each? Try to imitate each type of abnormal resonance.

5. Describe the difference between hypernasality and nasal air emission with speech. What other speech characteristics can occur with significant nasal emission and why? Try to imitate these characteristics.

6. What is the difference between an obligatory articulation error and a compensatory articulation error? Give examples of each. Why do you think it is important to make a distinction between the two types of errors?

7. What are some of the causes of dysphonia in children with either a history of cleft palate or another craniofacial condition?

8. How does the size of the velopharyngeal gap affect speech characteristics? Why do you think it is important to understand this relationship? Why do you think the relationship between the size of the gap and the speech characteristics is not always the same when comparing different individuals?

9. List some of the causes of velopharyngeal insufficiency, velopharyngeal incompetence, and velopharyngeal mislearning. How do you think some of these causes could be treated?

REFERENCES

Abdullah, S. (1988). A study of the results of speech language and hearing assessment of three groups of repaired cleft palate children and adults. *Annals of the Academy of Medicine of Singapore, 17*(3), 388–391.

Ainoda, N., Yamashita, K., & Tsukada, S. (1985). Articulation at age 4 in children with early repair of cleft palate. *Annals of Plastic Surgery, 15*(5), 415–422.

American Cleft Palate-Craniofacial Association (2006). [Speech samples]. Retrieved May 2, 2006 from http://www.acpa-cpf.org / EducMeetings/speechSamples/index.htm

Andreassen, M. L., Leeper, H. A., & MacRae, D. L. (1991). Changes in vocal resonance and nasalization following adenoidectomy in normal children: Preliminary findings. *Journal of Otolaryngology, 20*(4), 237–242.

Andrews, J. R., & Rutherford, D. (1972). Contribution of nasally emitted sound to the perception of hypernasality of vowels. *Cleft Palate Journal*, 9, 147–156.

Ansel, B. M., & Kent, R. D. (1992). Acoustic-phonetic contrasts and intelligibility in the dysarthria associated with mixed cerebral palsy. *Journal of Speech and Hearing Research*, 35(2), 296–308.

Baken, R. J. (1987). *Clinical measurement of speech and voice*. Boston: College-Hill Press.

Bennett, S. (1981). Vowel formant frequency characteristics of preadolescent males and females. *Journal of the Acoustical Society of America*, 69(1), 231–238.

Bernthal, J. E., & Beukelman, D. R. (1977). The effect of changes in velopharyngeal orifice area on vowel intensity. *Cleft Palate Journal*, 14(1), 63–77.

Blum, D. J., & Neel, H. B. D. (1983). Current thinking on tonsillectomy and adenoidectomy. *Comprehensive Therapy*, 9(12), 48–56.

Bodin, I. K., Lind, M. G., & Arnander, C. (1994). Free radial forearm flap reconstruction in surgery of the oral cavity and pharynx: Surgical complications, impairment of speech and swallowing. *Clinics in Otolaryngology*, 19(1), 28–34.

Boone, D. R., & McFarlane, S. (1988). *The voice and voice therapy* (4th ed.). Englewood Cliffs, NJ: Prentice-Hall.

Bradley, D. P. (1979). Congenital and acquired palatopharyngeal insufficiency. In K. R. Bzoch (Ed.), *Communicative disorders related to cleft lip and palate* (Vol. 2, pp. 77–89). Boston: Little, Brown and Company.

Bradley, D. P. (1997). Congenital and acquired velopharyngeal inadequacy. In K. R. Bzoch (Ed.), *Communicative disorders related to cleft lip and palate* (Vol. 4, pp. 23–243). Austin, TX: Pro-Ed.

Brooks, A. R., Shelton, R. L., & Youngstrom, K. A. (1965). Compensatory tongue-palate-posterior pharyngeal wall relationships in cleft palate. *Journal of Speech and Hearing Disorders*, 30, 166.

Brown, J. S., Zuydam, A. C., Jones, D. C., Rogers, S. N., & Vaughan, E. D. (1997). Functional outcome in soft palate reconstruction using a radial forearm free flap in conjunction with a superiorly based pharyngeal flap. *Head & Neck*, 19(6), 524–534.

Buder, E. H. (2005). The acoustics of nasality: Steps towards a bridge to source literature. *Perspectives on Speech Science and Orofacial Disorders*, 15(1), 9–14.

Cassassolles, S., Paulus, C., Ajacques, J. C., Berger-Vachon, C., Laurent, M., & Perrin, E. (1995). Acoustic characterization of velar insufficiency in young children. *Revue de Stomatologie et de Chirurgie Maxillofaciale*, 96(1), 13–20.

Chen, K. T., Wu, J., & Noordhoff, S. M. (1994). Submucous cleft palate. *Chang Keng I Hsueh*, 17(2), 131–137.

Croft, C. B., Shprintzen, R. J., & Ruben, R. J. (1981). Hypernasal speech following adenotonsillectomy. *Otolaryngology—Head & Neck Surgery*, 89(2), 179–188.

Dalston, R. M. (1996). Velopharyngeal impairment in the orthodontic population. *Seminars in Orthodontics*, 2(3), 220–227.

Dalston, R. M., & Vig, P. S. (1984). Effects of orthognathic surgery on speech: A prospective study. *American Journal of Orthodontics*, 86(4), 291–298.

Dalston, R. M., Warren, D. W., & Dalston, E. T. (1991). A preliminary investigation concerning the use of nasometry in identifying patients with hyponasality and/or nasal airway impairment. *Journal of Speech and Hearing Research*, 34(1), 11–18.

D'Antonio, L. L., Muntz, H. R., Province, M. A., & Marsh, J. L. (1988). Laryngeal/voice findings in patients with velopharyngeal dysfunction. *Laryngoscope, 98*(4), 432–438.

De Serres, L. M., Deleyiannis, F. W., Eblen, L. E., Gruss, J. S., Richardson, M. A., & Sie, K. C. (1999). Results with sphincter pharyngoplasty and pharyngeal flap. *International Journal of Pediatratic Otorhinolaryngology, 48*(1), 17–25.

Dibbell, D. G., Ewanowski, S., & Carter, W. L. (1979). Successful correction of velopharyngeal stress incompetence in musicians playing wind instruments. *Plastic and Reconstructive Surgery, 64*(5), 662–664.

Donnelly, M. J. (1994). Hypernasality following adenoid removal. *Irish Journal of Medical Science, 163*(5), 225–227.

Eufinger, H., Eggeling, V., & Immenkamp, E. (1994). Velopharyngoplasty with or without tonsillectomy and/or adenotomy—A retrospective evaluation of speech characteristics in 143 patients. *Journal of Craniomaxillofacial Surgery, 22*(1), 37–42.

Falk, M. L., & Kopp, G. A. (1968). Tongue position and hypernasality in cleft palate speech. *Cleft Palate Journal, 5*(3), 228–237.

Fee, W. E., Jr., Gilmer, P. A., & Goffinet, D. R. (1988). Surgical management of recurrent nasopharyngeal carcinoma after radiation failure at the primary site. *Laryngoscope, 98*(11), 1220–1226.

Fernandes, D. B., Grobbelaar, A. O., Hudson, D. A., & Lentin, R. (1996). Velopharyngeal incompetence after adenotonsillectomy in noncleft patients. *British Journal of Oral and Maxillofacial Surgery, 34*(5), 364–367.

Finkelstein, Y., Bar-Ziv, J., Nachmani, A., Berger, G., & Ophir, D. (1993). Peritonsillar abscess as a cause of transient velopharyngeal insufficiency. *Cleft Palate-Craniofacial Journal, 30*(4), 421–428.

Finkelstein, Y., Talmi, Y. P., Nachmani, A., Hauben, D. J., & Zohar, Y. (1992). On the variability of velopharyngeal valve anatomy and function: A combined peroral and nasendoscopic study. *Plastic and Reconstructive Surgery, 89*(4), 631–639.

Fletcher, S. G., & Daly, D. A. (1976). Nasalance in utterances of hearing-impaired speakers. *Journal of Communication Disorders, 9*(1), 63–73.

Folkins, J. W. (1988). Velopharyngeal nomenclature: Incompetence, inadequacy, insufficiency, and dysfunction. *Cleft Palate Journal, 25*(4), 413–416.

Forner, L. L. (1983). Speech segment durations produced by five- and six-year-old speakers with and without cleft palates. *Cleft Palate Journal, 20*(3), 185–198.

Gibb, A. G., & Stewart, I. A. (1975). Hypernasality following tonsil dissection—Hysterical aetiology. *Journal of Laryngology and Otology, 89*(7), 779–781.

Gildersleeve-Neumann, C. E., & Dalston, R. M. (2001). Nasalance scores in noncleft individuals: Why not zero? *Cleft Palate-Craniofacial Journal, 38*(2), 106–111.

Gordon, N. A., Astrachan, D., & Yanagisawa, E. (1994). Videoendoscopic diagnosis and correction of velopharyngeal stress incompetence in a bassoonist. *Annals of Otology, Rhinology, and Laryngology, 103*(8, Pt. 1), 595–600.

Haapanen, M. L., Heliovaara, A., & Ranta, R. (1991). Hypernasality and the nasopharyngeal space. A cephalometric study. *Journal of Craniomaxillofacial Surgery, 19*(2), 77–80.

Haapanen, M. L., Kalland, M., Heliovaara, A., Hukki, J., & Ranta, R. (1997). Velopharyngeal function in cleft patients undergoing maxillary advancement. *Folia Phoniatrica et Logopedica, 49*(1), 42–47.

Hagstrom, W. J., Parsons, R. W., Landa, S. J., & Robson, M. C. (1979). Familial velopharyngeal incompetence caused by myasthenia gravis. *Annals of Plastic Surgery*, 3(6), 555–557.

Hall, C. D., Golding-Kushner, K. J., Argamaso, R. V., & Strauch, B. (1991). Pharyngeal flap surgery in adults. *Cleft Palate-Craniofacial Journal*, 28(2), 179–182; Discussion 182–183.

Handelman, C. S., & Osborne, G. (1976). Growth of the nasopharynx and adenoid development from one to eighteeen years. *Angle Orthodontist*, 46(3), 243–259.

Harding, A., & Grunwell, P. (1996). Characteristics of cleft palate speech. *European Journal of Disorders of Communication*, 31(4), 331–357.

Harding, A., & Grunwell, P. (1998). Active versus passive cleft-type speech characteristics. *International Journal of Language and Communication Disorders*, 33(3), 329–352.

Heller, J. C., Gens, G. W., Moe, D. G., & Lewin, M. L. (1974). Velopharyngeal insufficiency in patients with neurologic, emotional, and mental disorders. *Journal of Speech and Hearing Disorders*, 39(3), 350–359.

Henningsson, G. E., & Isberg, A. M. (1986). Velopharyngeal movement patterns in patients alternating between oral and glottal articulation: A clinical and cineradiographical study. *Cleft Palate Journal*, 23(1), 1–9.

Henningsson, G., & Isberg, A. (1988). Influence of tonsils on velopharyngeal movements in children with craniofacial anomalies and hypernasality. *American Journal of Orthodontics and Dentofacial Orthopedics*, 94(3), 253–261.

Hess, D. A. (1959). Pitch, intensity and cleft palate voice quality. *Journal of Speech and Hearing Research*, 2, 113.

Hillarp, B., Ekberg, O., Jacobsson, S., Nylander, G., & Aberg, M. (1994). Myotonic dystrophy revealed at videoradiography of deglutition and speech in adult patients with velopharyngeal insufficiency: Presentation of four cases. *Cleft Palate-Craniofacial Journal*, 31(2), 125–133.

Huntington, D. A. (1968). Anatomical and physiological bases for speech. In D. C. Spriestersbach & C. Sherman (Eds.), *Cleft palate and communication* (pp. 1–25). New York: Academic Press.

Jones, D. L. (1991). Velopharyngeal function and dysfunction. *Clinics in Communication Disorders*, 1(3), 19–25.

Jones, D. L. (2005). Perceptual aspects of nasality. *Perspectives on Speech Science and Orofacial Disorders*, 15(1), 9–14.

Karnell, M. P., Schultz, K., & Canady, J. (2001). Investigations of a pressure-sensitive theory of marginal velopharyngeal inadequacy. *Cleft Palate-Craniofacial Journal*, 38(4), 346–357.

Kline, L. S., & Hutchinson, J. M. (1980). Acoustic and perceptual evaluation of hypernasality of mentally retarded persons. *American Journal of Mental Deficiency*, 85(2), 153–160.

Kummer, A. W., Briggs, M., & Lee, L. (2003). The relationship between the characteristics of speech and velopharyngeal gap size. *Cleft Palate-Craniofacial Journal*, 40(6), 590–596.

Kummer, A. W., Curtis, C., Wiggs, M., Lee, L., & Strife, J. L. (1992). Comparison of velopharyngeal gap size in patients with hypernasality, hypernasality and nasal emission, or nasal turbulence (rustle) as the primary speech characteristic. *Cleft Palate-Craniofacial Journal*, 29(2), 152–156.

Kummer, A. W., Myer, C. M. I., Smith, M. E., & Shott, S. R. (1993). Changes in nasal resonance secondary to adenotonsillectomy.

American Journal of Otolaryngology, *14*(4), 285–290.

Kummer, A. W., Strife, J. L., Grau, W. H., Creaghead, N. A., & Lee, L. (1989). The effects of Le Fort I osteotomy with maxillary movement on articulation, resonance, and velopharyngeal function. *Cleft Palate Journal*, *26*(3), 193–199; Discussion 199–200.

Lefaivre, J. F., Cohen, S. R., Riski, J. E., & Burstein, F. D. (1997). Velopharyngeal incompetence as the presenting symptom of malignant brainstem tumor. *Cleft Palate-Craniofacial Journal*, *34*(2), 154–158.

Loney, R. W., & Bloem, T. J. (1987). Velopharyngeal dysfunction: Recommendations for use of nomenclature. *Cleft Palate Journal*, *24*(4), 334–335.

Luce, E. A., McGibbon, B., & Hoopes, J. E. (1977). Velopharyngeal insufficiency in hemifacial microsomia. *Plastic and Reconstructive Surgery*, *60*(4), 602–606.

MacKenzie-Stepner, K., Witzel, M. A., Stringer, D. A., & Laskin, R. (1987). Velopharyngeal insufficiency due to hypertrophic tonsils. A report of two cases. *International Journal of Pediatric Otorhinolaryngology*, *14*(1), 57–63.

Maegawa, J., Sells, R. K., & David, D. J. (1998). Speech changes after maxillary advancement in 40 cleft lip and palate patients. *Journal of Craniofacial Surgery*, *9*(2), 177–182; Discussion 183–184.

Marsh, J. L. (1991). Cleft palate and velopharyngeal dysfunction. *Clinics in Communication Disorders*, *1*(3), 29–34.

Mason, R. M., & Grandstaff, H. L. (1971). Evaluating the velopharyngeal mechanism in hypernasal speakers. *Language, Speech, and Hearing Services in the Schools*, *2*(4), 53–61.

Mason, R., Turvey, T. A., & Warren, D. W. (1980). Speech considerations with maxillary advancement procedures. *Journal of Oral Surgery*, *38*(10), 752–758.

Mason, R. M., & Warren, D. W. (1980). Adenoid involution and developing hypernasality in cleft palate. *Journal of Speech and Hearing Disorders*, *45*(4), 469–480.

McCarthy, J. G., Coccaro, P. J., & Schwartz, M. D. (1979). Velopharyngeal function following maxillary advancement. *Plastic and Reconstructive Surgery*, *64*(2), 180–189.

McDonald, E. T., & Baker H. (1951). Cleft palate speech: An integration of research and clinical observation. *Journal of Speech and Hearing Disorders*, *16*, 9–20.

McHenry, M. A. (1997). The effect of increased vocal effort on estimated velopharyngeal orifice area. *American Journal of Speech-Language Pathology*, *6*(4), 55–61.

McWilliams, B. J. (1991). Submucous clefts of the palate: How likely are they to be symptomatic? *Cleft Palate-Craniofacial Journal*, *28*(3), 247–249; Discussion 250–251.

McWilliams, B. J., Bluestone, C. D., & Musgrave, R. H. (1969). Diagnostic implications of vocal cord nodules in children with cleft palate. *Laryngoscope*, *79*(12), 2072–2080.

McWilliams, B. J., Lavorato, A. S., & Bluestone, C. D. (1973). Vocal cord abnormalities in children with velopharyngeal valving problems. *Laryngoscope*, *83*, 1745.

McWilliams, B. J., Morris, H. L., & Shelton, R. L. (1990a). Disorders of phonation and resonance. In B. J. McWilliams, H. L. Morris, & R. L. Shelton (Eds.), *Cleft palate speech* (Vol. 2, pp. 247–268). Philadelphia: B. C. Decker.

McWilliams, B. J., Morris, H. L., & Shelton, R. L. (1990b). The nature of the velopharyngeal mechanism. In B. J. McWilliams, H. L. Morris, & R. L. Shelton (Eds.), *Cleft palate speech* (Vol. 2, pp. 197–235). Philadelphia: B.C. Decker.

Misra, U. C., Gill, R. S., & Lal, M. (1981). Tonsil transposition into posterior pharyngeal wall in palato-pharyngeal incompetence. *Journal of Laryngology and Otology, 95*(7), 713–716.

Morris, H. L. (1984). Types of velopharyngeal incompetence. In H. Winitz (Ed.), *Treating articulation disorders: For clinicians by clinicians* (p. 211). Baltimore: University Park Press.

Morris, H. L. (1992). Some questions and answers about velopharyngeal dysfunction during speech. *American Journal of Speech-Language Pathology, 1*(3), 26–28.

Morris, H. L., Wroblewski, S. K., Brown, C. K., & Van Demark, D. R. (1990). Velarpharyngeal status in cleft palate patients with expected adenoidal involution. *Annals of Otology, Rhinology, and Laryngology, 99*(6, Pt. 1), 432–437.

Myers, E. N., & Aramany, M. A. (1977). Rehabilitation of the oral cavity following resection of the hard and soft palate. *Transactions of the American Academy of Ophthalmology and Otolaryngology, 84*(5), 941–951.

Neilson, P. D., & O'Dwyer, N. J. (1981). Pathophysiology of dysarthria in cerebral palsy. *Journal of Neurolology, Neurosurgery, and Psychiatry, 44*(11), 1013–1019.

Neiman, G. S., & Simpson, R. K. (1975). A roentgencephalometric investigation of the effect of adenoid removal upon selected measures of velopharyngeal function. *Cleft Palate Journal, 12*, 377–389.

Netsell, R. (1969). Evaluation of velopharyngeal function in dysarthria. *Journal of Speech and Hearing Disorders, 34*(2), 113–122.

Netsell, R. (1988). Velopharyngeal dysfunction. In D. Yoder & R. Kent (Eds.), *Decision-making in speech-language pathology* (pp. 150–151). Toronto: B. C. Decker.

Okazaki, K., Satoh, K., Kato, M., Iwanami, M., Ohokubo, F., & Kobayashi, K. (1993). Speech and velopharyngeal function following maxillary advancement in patients with cleft lip and palate. *Annals of Plastic Surgery, 30*(4), 304–311.

Parton, M. J., & Jones, A. S. (1998). Hypernasality following adenoidectomy: A significant and avoidable complication. *Clinical Otolaryngology, 23*(1), 18–19.

Penfold, C. N. (1997). Management of velopharyngeal dysfunction [Letter; comment]. *British Journal of Oral and Maxillofacial Surgery, 35*(6), 454.

Peterson-Falzone, S. J. (1985). Velopharyngeal inadequacy in the absence of overt cleft palate. *Journal of Craniofacial Genetics and Developmental Biology Supplement, 1*, 97–124.

Platt, L. J., Andrews, G., & Howie, P. M. (1980). Dysarthria of adult cerebral palsy: II. Phonemic analysis of articulation errors. *Journal of Speech and Hearing Research, 23*(1), 41–55.

Platt, L. J., Andrews, G., Young, M., & Quinn, P. T. (1980). Dysarthria of adult cerebral palsy: I. Intelligibility and articulatory impairment. *Journal of Speech and Hearing Research, 23*(1), 28–40.

Pollack, M. A., & Shprintzen, R. J. (1981). Velopharyngeal insufficiency in neurofibromatosis. *International Journal of Pediatric Otorhinolaryngology, 3*(3), 257–262.

Powers, G. R. (1962). Cinefluorographic investigation of articulatory movements of selected individuals with cleft palates. *Journal of Speech and Hearing Research, 5*, 59.

Ren, Y. F., Isberg, A., & Henningsson, G. (1995). Velopharyngeal incompetence and persistent hypernasality after adenoidectomy in children without palatal defect. *Cleft Palate Craniofacial-Journal, 32*(6), 476–482.

Rintala, A. E. (1987). Solitary metastatic melanoma of the soft palate. *Annals of Plastic Surgery, 19*(5), 463–465.

Riski, J. E. (1995). Speech assessment of adolescents. *Cleft Palate-Craniofacial Journal, 32*(2), 109–113.

Riski, J. E., & Verdolini, K. (1999). Is hypernasality a voice disorder? *ASHA, 41*(1), 10–11.

Robinson, J. H. (1992). Association between adenoidectomy, velopharyngeal incompetence, and submucous cleft [Letter]. *Cleft Palate-Craniofacial Journal, 29*(4), 385.

Rousseaux, M., Lesoin, F., & Quint, S. (1987). Unilateral pseudobulbar syndrome with limited capsulothalamic infarction. *European Neurology, 27*(4), 227–230.

Salomonson, J., Kawamoto, H., & Wilson, L. (1988). Velopharyngeal incompetence as the presenting symptom of myotonic dystrophy. *Cleft Palate Journal, 25*(3), 296–300.

Schmaman, L., Jordaan, H., & Jammine, G. H. (1998). Risk factors for permanent hypernasality after adenoidectomy. *South African Medical Journal, 88*(3), 266–269.

Seid, A. B. (1990). Velopharyngeal insufficiency versus adenoidectomy for obstructive apnea: A quandary [Clinical conference]. *Cleft Palate Journal, 27*(2), 200–202.

Shanks, J. C. (1990). Velopharyngeal incompetence manifested initially in playing a musical instrument. *Journal of Voice, 4*(2), 169–171.

Shapiro, R. S. (1980). Velopharyngeal insufficiency starting at puberty without adenoidectomy. *International Journal of Pediatric Otorhinolaryngology, 2*(3), 255–260.

Shprintzen, R. J., Rakof, S. J., Skolnick, M. L., & Lavorato, A. S. (1977). Incongruous movements of the velum and lateral pharyngeal walls. *Cleft Palate Journal, 14*(2), 148–157.

Shprintzen, R. J., Sher, A. E., & Croft, C. B. (1987). Hypernasal speech caused by tonsillar hypertrophy. *International Journal of Pediatric Otorhinolaryngology, 14*(1), 45–56.

Siegel-Sadewitz, V. L., & Shprintzen, R. J. (1982). Nasopharyngoscopy of the normal velopharyngeal sphincter: An experiment of biofeedback. *Cleft Palate Journal, 19*(3), 194–200.

Siegel-Sadewitz, V. L., & Shprintzen, R. J. (1986). Changes in velopharyngeal valving with age. *International Journal of Pediatric Otorhinolaryngology, 11*(2), 171–182.

Skolnick, M. L., Shprintzen, R. J., McCall, G. N., & Rakoff, S. (1975). Patterns of velopharyngeal closure in subjects with repaired cleft palate and normal speech: A multi-view videofluoroscopic analysis. *Cleft Palate Journal, 12,* 369–376.

Story, B. H., Titze, I. R., & Hoffman, E. A. (2001). The relationship of vocal tract shape to three voice qualities. *Journal of the Acoustical Society of America, 109*(4), 1651–1667.

Subtelny, J. D., Whitehead, R. L., & Samar, V. J. (1992). Spectral study of deviant resonance in the speech of women who are deaf. *Journal of Speech & Hearing Research, 35*(3), 574–579.

Theodoros, D., Murdoch, B. E., Stokes, P. D., & Chenery, H. J. (1993). Hypernasality in dysarthric speakers following severe closed head injury: A perceptual and instrumental analysis. *Brain Injury, 7*(1), 59–69.

Thompson, E. C., & Murdoch, B. E. (1995). Disorders of nasality in subjects with upper motor neuron type dysarthria following cerebrovascular accident. *Journal of Communication Disorders, 28*(3), 261–276.

Thurston, J. B., Larson, D. L., Shanks, J. C., Bennett, J. E., & Parsons, R. W. (1980). Nasal obstruction as a complication of pharyngeal flap surgery. *Cleft Palate Journal*, *17*(2), 148–154.

Titze, I. R., Bergan, C. C., Hunter, E. J., & Story, B. (2003). Source and filter adjustments affecting the perception of the vocal qualities twang and yawn. *Logopedics, Phoniatrics, Vocology*, *28*(4), 147–155.

Tom, K., Titze, I. R., Hoffman, E. A., & Story, B. H. (2001). Three-dimensional vocal tract imaging and formant structure: Varying vocal register, pitch, and loudness. *Journal of the Acoustical Society of America*, *109*(2), 742–747.

Trost, J. E. (1981). Articulatory additions to the classical description of the speech of persons with cleft palate. *Cleft Palate Journal*, *18*(3), 193–203.

Trost-Cardamone, J. E. (1987). Cleft palate misarticulations: A teaching tape [Videotape]. California State University, Northridge, CA: Instructional Media Center.

Trost-Cardamone, J. E. (1989). Coming to terms with VPI: A response to Loney and Bloem. *Cleft Palate Journal*, *26*(1), 68–70.

Trost-Cardamone, J. E. (1990). Speech in the first year of life: A perspective on early acquisition. In D. E. Kernahan & S. W. Rosenstein (Eds.), *Cleft lip and palate: A system of management* (pp. 91–103). Baltimore: Williams & Wilkins.

Trost-Cardamone, J. E. (1997). Diagnosis of specific cleft palate speech error patterns for planning therapy of physical management needs. In K. R. Bzoch (Ed.), *Communicative disorders related to cleft lip and palate* (Vol. 4, pp. 313–330). Austin, TX: Pro-Ed.

Upton, L. G., & Berger, M. K. (1995). Use of pharyngoplasty to improve resonance in adult closed-head injury patients: Report of cases [see Comments]. *Journal of Oral and Maxillofacial Surgery*, *53*(6), 717–719.

Van Mourik, M., Catsman-Berrevoets, C. E., Yousef-Bak, E., Paquier, P. F., & van Dongen, H. R. (1998). Dysarthria in children with cerebellar or brainstem tumors. *Pediatric Neurology*, *18*(5), 411–414.

Warren, D. W., Dalston, R. M., & Mayo, R. (1993). Hypernasality in the presence of "adequate" velopharyngeal closure. *Cleft Palate-Craniofacial Journal*, *30*(2), 150–154.

Warren, D. W., Dalston, R. M., Trier, W. C., & Holder, M. B. (1985). A pressure-flow technique for quantifying temporal patterns of palatopharyngeal closure. *Cleft Palate Journal*, *22*(1), 11–19.

Warren, D. W., Wood, M. T., & Bradley, D. P. (1969). Respiratory volumes in normal and cleft palate speech. *Cleft Palate Journal*, *6*, 449–460.

Watzke, I., Turvey, T. A., Warren, D. W., & Dalston, R. (1990). Alterations in velopharyngeal function after maxillary advancement in cleft palate patients. *Journal of Oral and Maxillofacial Surgery*, *48*(7), 685–689.

Witt, P. D., Myckatyn, T., & Marsh, J. L. (1998). Salvaging the failed pharyngoplasty: Intervention outcome. *Cleft Palate-Craniofacial Journal*, *35*(5), 447–453.

Witt, P. D., O'Daniel, T. G., Marsh, J. L., Grames, L. M., Muntz, H. R., & Pilgram, T. K. (1997). Surgical management of velopharyngeal dysfunction: Outcome analysis of autogenous posterior pharyngeal wall augmentation. *Plastic and Reconstructive Surgery*, *99*(5), 1287–1296; Discussion 1297–1300.

Witzel, M. A., & Posnick, J. C. (1989). Patterns and location of velopharyngeal valving problems: Atypical findings on video nasopharyngoscopy. *Cleft Palate Journal*, *26*(1), 63–67.

Witzel, M. A., Rich, R. H., Margar-Bacal, F., & Cox, C. (1986). Velopharyngeal insufficiency after adenoidectomy: An 8-year review. *International Journal of Pediatric Otorhinolaryngology*, *11*(1), 15–20.

Wolski, W. (1967). Hypernasality as the presenting symptom of myasthenia gravis. *Journal of Speech and Hearing Disorders*, *32*(1), 36–38.

Workinger, M. S., & Netsell, R. (1992). Restoration of intelligible speech 13 years post–head injury. *Brain Injury*, *6*(2), 183–187.

Yanagisawa, E., Estill, J., Mambrino, L., & Talkin, D. (1991). Supraglottic contributions to pitch raising. Videoendoscopic study with spectroanalysis. *Annals of Otology, Rhinology, and Laryngology*, *100*(1), 19–30.

Yanagisawa, E., Kmucha, S. T., & Estill, J. (1990). Role of the soft palate in laryngeal functions and selected voice qualities. Simultaneous velolaryngeal videoendoscopy

[Published erratum appears in *Annals of Otology, Rhinology, and Laryngology*, *99*(6, Pt. 1), 431] [see Comments]. *Annals of Otology, Rhinology, and Laryngology*, *99*(1), 18–28.

Yorkston, K. M., Beukelman, D. R., & Traynor, C. D. (1988). Articulatory adequacy in dysarthric speakers: A comparison of judging formats. *Journal of Communication Disorders*, *21*(4), 351–361.

Yoshida, H., Michi, K., Yamashita, Y., & Ohno, K. (1993). A comparison of surgical and prosthetic treatment for speech disorders attributable to surgically acquired soft palate defects. *Journal of Oral and Maxillofacial Surgery*, *51*(4), 361–365.

Ysunza, A., & Vazquez, M. C. (1993). Velopharyngeal sphincter physiology in deaf individuals. *Cleft Palate-Craniofacial Journal*, *30*(2), 141–143.

CHAPTER

8

EAR, NOSE, AND THROAT ANOMALIES: EFFECTS ON SPEECH AND RESONANCE

J. PAUL WILLGING, M.D.

ANN W. KUMMER, PH.D.

CHAPTER OUTLINE

INTRODUCTION

Craniofacial disorders can have a great impact on the function of head and neck structures. In addition, the typical disease processes that exist in the general population are often found with an increased prevalence in this specific group of patients.

   The purpose of this chapter is to review the anatomy of the ear, nose, and throat. Congenital anomalies and acquired disorders of these structures are also described. Because the ear, nose, and throat are particularly important for speech production, abnormalities of these structures can have a significant effect on the quality and intelligibility of speech.

THE EAR

Patients born with craniofacial anomalies may have associated malformations of the external or middle ear. Abnormalities of the inner ear are less commonly encountered, but can occur. These malformations can affect aesthetics and can cause hearing loss that ultimately affects the ability to communicate.

Anatomy of the Ear

The *external ear* is comprised of the pinna and the external auditory canal. The *pinna* is the delicate cartilaginous framework surrounding the *external auditory canal* (Figure 8–1A). It functions to direct sound energy into the auditory canal, which is a skin-lined canal leading to the eardrum.

   The *middle ear* is a hollow space within the temporal bone. The *mastoid cavity* connects to the middle ear space posteriorly and is comprised of a collection of air cells within the temporal bone. Both the middle ear and *mastoid cavities* are lined with a mucous membrane. The *tympanic membrane*, also called the *eardrum*, is considered part of the middle ear. The tympanic membrane transmits sound energy through the ossicles to the inner ear. The three tiny bones in the middle ear are called the *ossicles* and they include the malleus, incus, and stapes.

The *malleus* (hammer) is firmly attached to the tympanic membrane. The *incus* (anvil) has an articulation with the malleus and the stapes. The

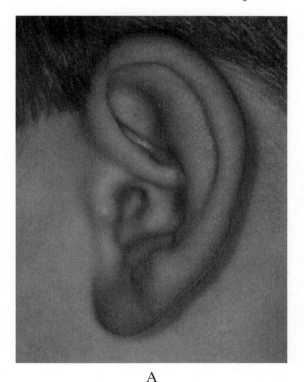

A

FIGURE 8–1 (A and B)   A. A normal pinna. The pinna is composed of fibroelastic cartilage covered by a thin layer of skin. The delicate folding of the cartilage provides the normal shape of the ear. (*continues*)

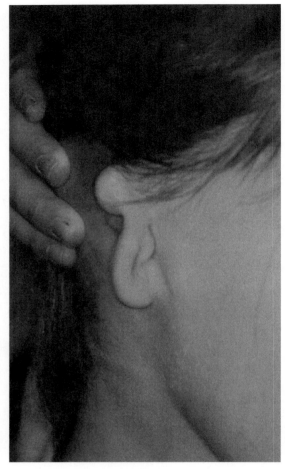

B

FIGURE 8–1 (A and B) *(continued)* B. A case of microtia. Microtia is the result of abnormal development of the external ear. The more severe the external deformity, the more likely it is that the middle ear cannot be reconstructed, despite the fact that the external ear and middle ear develop from different sites of origin.

stapes acts as a piston to create pressure waves within the fluid-filled cochlea. The tympanic membrane and ossicles act to amplify the sound energy and efficiently introduce this energy into the liquid environment of the cochlea.

The *inner ear* consists of the cochlea and semicircular canals. The *cochlea* is composed of a bony spiral tube that is shaped as a snail's shell. Within this bony tube are delicate membranes separating the canal into three separate fluid-filled spaces. The *organ of corti* is the site where mechanical energy introduced into the cochlea is converted into electrical stimulation conducted by the auditory nerves to the auditory cortex, which provides an awareness of sound. Inner and outer *hair cells* (sensory cells with hairlike properties) of the cochlea may be damaged by a variety of mechanisms leading to sensorineural hearing loss.

A second function of the inner ear is balance. The *semicircular canals* are the loop-shaped tubular parts of the inner ear that provide a sense of spatial orientation. They are oriented in three planes at right angles to one another. They provide a sense of spatial orientation. The *saccule* and *utricle* are additional sensory organs within the inner ear that provide a sensation of acceleration. Hair cells within these organs have small calcium carbonate granules that respond to gravity and acceleration forces to create the sense of motion.

Malformations of the External Ear

Patients with craniofacial anomalies, especially those with syndromes, often have *microtia*, which is a malformation of the pinna (Brent, 1999) (Figure 8–1B). The more severely malformed the pinna is, the greater the chances are for significant problems within the middle ear or involving the ossicles (Kountakis, Helidonis, & Jahrsdoerfer, 1995). When there is microtia of the external ear, it is not uncommon to also find aural atresia. *Aural atresia*, also called *auditory atresia*, refers to the congenital abnormality of closure of the external auditory canal. The external auditory canal and tympanic membrane may be very small, or may fail to develop entirely, as in Treacher Collins syndrome, hemifacial microsomia, or Nager syndrome. This results in a *conductive hearing loss* because the sound energy cannot travel directly through the external auditory canal to the tympanic membrane and therefore, cannot reach the inner ear.

Children with bilateral aural atresia require bone-conducting hearing aids. These may be conventional aids that make contact with the skull by means of a headband, or may be bone-anchored hearing aids that are implanted into the skull where they are osseointegrated for a rigid attachment. Bone conduction hearing aids directly vibrate the end organ within the cochlea. Children with unilateral aural atresia generally do not require a hearing aid if their hearing is normal in the unaffected ear. It is of interest that children with aural atresia rarely experience ear infections. The explanation for this is not known.

Reconstruction of the auditory canal, tympanic membrane, and ossicular chain can be done in the early school years. Patients with bilateral aural atresia benefit from reconstruction with an improvement in hearing. Patients with unilateral atresia are often reconstructed, but the benefits are less easily quantifiable. The risk of this surgical procedure lies in the potential damage to the CN VII (Jahrsdoerfer & Lambert, 1998), which is the facial nerve. This is the main nerve that controls motion on each side of the face. Damage to the nerve can cause paralysis of one side of the face. The paralysis may be complete or partial, temporary or permanent, depending on the degree of injury to the nerve. Computed tomography (CT) scans of the temporal bone can be used in predicting the course of the facial nerve in atretic ears, but these scans are not always of value. A rating scale has been developed to predict the outcome of the surgical correction of the external auditory canal and tympanic membrane. It is based on the overall development of the middle ear space, the size and

position of the ossicles, the presence of the stapes, and the position of the facial nerve.

Malformations of the Middle Ear

When malformations are found in the external ear, there are often malformations or anomalies of the middle ear structures as well. This may include abnormal formation of the ossicles, as can be found in Crouzon, Apert, and Goldenhar syndromes. In some cases, there is fusion of the ossicles to the surrounding bone. When the ossicles are abnormally formed or fused, this affects the transmission of the sound to the inner ear, causing a conductive hearing loss.

In many cases, surgical correction is possible for abnormalities of the external auditory canal, the tympanic membrane, or the ossicles (Jahrsdoerfer, Yeakley, Aguilar, Cole, & Gray, 1992). In addition, hearing aids allow correction of most kinds of conductive hearing loss.

Eustachian Tube Dysfunction and Middle Ear Disease

The middle ear and mastoid cavities must have the air that is within them replenished at regular intervals to prevent problems from developing. This is accomplished by the function of the eustachian tube.

Otitis Media

The *eustachian tube* connects the middle ear with the nasopharynx. This tube is closed at rest, and opens when the tensor veli palatini muscle, which is attached directly to the cartilage of the eustachian tube, contracts in the act of swallowing. As the eustachian tube opens, it allows for middle ear ventilation and the equalization of middle ear pressure with the pressure of the environment. When the eustachian tube fails to function normally, fluids tend to develop within the middle ear space due to the negative pressure, resulting in *middle ear effusion*. If the eustachian tube begins to function, the fluids will be absorbed by the lymphatics in the middle ear mucosa, and the normal condition will be restored. If the eustachian tube continues to malfunction, however, the middle ear effusion will persist. Bacteria can ascend the eustachian tube and grow in this effusion, leading to an ear infection called *acute otitis media* (Figure 8–2).

Causes of Eustachian Tube Dysfunction

All young children, even those without ear anomalies, are at risk for middle ear disease. This is due to the fact that in children, the eustachian tubes are oriented in such a way that the tensor veli palatini muscles, which open the tube, are directed at an unfavorable angle for this function. In addition, the eustachian tubes lie in a horizontal plane between the nasopharynx and the middle ear, which impairs middle ear drainage and allows for reflux of secretions from the pharynx into the tube. Both of these anatomic relationships predispose children to an

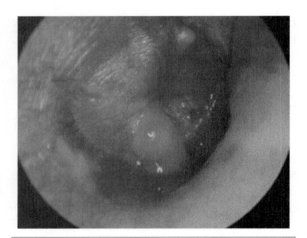

FIGURE 8–2 Acute otitis media treated with a myringotomy. The infected middle ear fluid can be seen exuding from the hole created in the eardrum.

increased tendency for ear infections. As growth and development occur, the skull base flexes upon itself, moving the origin of the eustachian tube musculature into a more favorable orientation for the opening of the tube. The palate also drops over time in relation to the ear, resulting in a 45° angulation of the eustachian tube up to the middle ear. This angulation prevents some of the reflux of nasopharyngeal secretions into the eustachian tube and thereby minimizes the incidence of infections (Figure 8–3).

In addition to the normal risk for middle ear disease in the early years, patients with cleft palate or other craniofacial anomalies are at increased risk for recurrent otitis media or persistent middle ear effusions (Sheahan, Miller, Earley, Sheahan, & Blayney, 2004). A cleft palate or any abnormality that affects the soft palate, and therefore the tensor veli palatini muscle, may have an adverse affect on eustachian tube function, and therefore the middle ear. Patients with a cleft palate also have abnormally shaped eustachian tube cartilages with abnormal attachment to the tensor veli palatini muscle (Bluestone, Beery, Cantekin, & Paradise, 1975; Bluestone, Paradise, Beery, & Wittel, 1972; Doyle, Cantekin, & Bluestone, 1980; Durr & Shapiro, 1989; Heller, Gens, Croft, & Moe, 1978; Paradise, 1976; Paradise et al., 1974; Paradise & Bluestone, 1974; Trujillo, 1994).

Effects and Complications of Otitis Media

Acute otitis media is a common disease process in children. Half of children under the age of 3 have had at least one episode of otitis. The children frequently have high fever and severe ear pain. As a result, they are often inconsolable. Occasionally, the tympanic membrane ruptures due to both the increased pressure produced by the inflammatory process in the middle ear and the toxic effect of the bacterial infection.

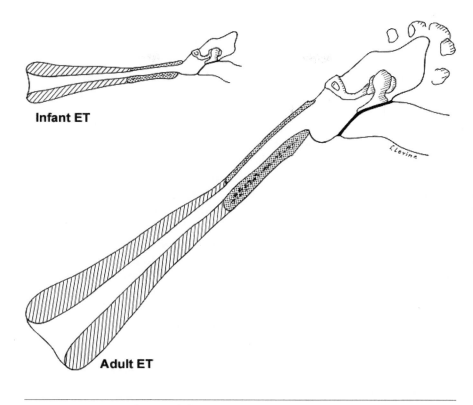

FIGURE 8–3 Angulation of the eustachian tube in an infant and an adult. The angulation of the eustachian tube changes with growth and development. In the young child, the eustachian tube ascends up to the middle ear at a 10-degree angle. In the adult, this angle changes to 45 degrees. The orientation of the musculature around the eustachian tube also changes over time, improving the ability to ventilate the middle ear with age.

In addition to causing discomfort and pain, otitis media causes a conductive hearing loss because of the diminished mobility of the tympanic membrane in vibrating against the ossicles in the middle ear. The extent of the conductive hearing loss is variable, ranging from 5–55 decibels according to the physical nature of the effusion. It is unlikely that mild hearing loss will cause speech and language difficulties, but it is likely that diminished hearing can aggravate an underlying tendency for the development of articulation errors and can disrupt speech and language acquisition (Hubbard, Paradise, McWilliams, Elster, & Taylor, 1985). Auditory stimulation is particularly important during the first year of life. During this time, the neurons in the auditory brainstem are maturing, and the neural connections are being formed (Sininger, Doyle, & Moore, 1999). If sensory input to the auditory nervous system is interrupted during early development, this can have a detrimental effect on speech and language learning (Rvachew, Slawinski, Williams, & Green, 1999). Hearing must always be evaluated in the presence of speech and language difficulties to ensure normal auditory function prior to initiation of therapeutic intervention for speech and language disorders.

One serious potential complication of otitis media is *mastoiditis*, which is an infection within the temporal bone that begins to erode bone, leading to potentially life-threatening complications. Mastoiditis is essentially a closed-space abscess that has the ability to erode bone. The infection often extends laterally behind the ear, causing the ear to protrude from the side of the head. It could also erode medially, causing meningitis or brain abscess.

Another potential serious complication of repeated ear infections is sensorineural hearing loss. The toxins produced by the bacteria may enter the cochlea through the delicate membranes in the middle ear. With repeated exposure to these toxins, the hair cells of the cochlea may be damaged, leading to a permanent hearing loss.

Treatment of Otitis Media

Acute otitis media is treated with oral antibiotics that will sterilize the middle ear effusion and result in rapid resolution of the child's ear symptoms. Antibiotics treat the infection, but will not make the fluid resolve. The middle ear fluid will persist in children after the infection has been resolved for about one month in 40% of patients, up to two months in 20% of patients, and about three months in 5% of patients (Teele, Klein, & Rosner, 1980). With fluid present in the middle ear, antibiotics may help prevent additional infections from developing but will have no effect in speeding the resolution of the effusion.

The treatment for recurrent acute otitis media often includes multiple courses of antibiotics. However, the potential for the development of antibiotic-resistant bacteria increases with the number of antibiotics prescribed and the total duration of antibiotic treatment.

Chronic antibiotic use in the treatment of *noninfected* middle ear effusion has been one of the major factors in the development of antibiotic-resistant bacteria.

While the fluid is in the middle ear space, a mild conductive hearing loss will be present. Once the eustachian tube begins to function normally, allowing a return to normal middle ear pressure and normal aeration function, the fluid in the middle ear will be absorbed.

Surgical intervention is recommended if the child has had six or more episodes of otitis, or the child has had a middle ear effusion that persists for three months or longer and is associated with a conductive hearing loss. Recurrent acute otitis media and persistent middle ear effusions are treated with a myringotomy and insertion of ventilation tubes (American Academy of Family Physicians, American Academy of Otolaryngology Head and Neck Surgery, & American Academy of Pediatrics Subcommittee on Otitis Media With Effusion, 2004; Rosenfeld et al., 2004). A *myringotomy* is a small, surgical incision that is made in the tympanic membrane to allow for drainage of middle ear fluid. *Ventilation tubes*, also called *pressure-equalizing (PE) tubes* (Figure 8–4), are surgically inserted in the eardrum to provide an alternate route for air to enter the middle ear if the eustachian tube is nonfunctional. Ventilation tubes do not correct the underlying problems related to recurrent

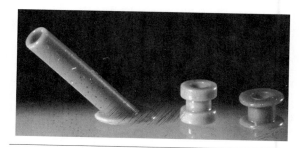

FIGURE 8–4   Examples of types of pressure-equalizing (PE) tubes.

otitis media. Instead, they bypass the eustachian tube function until growth and development have progressed to the point where normal eustachian tube function can be achieved. If normal pressures can be established in the middle ear, the effusion will resolve and not recur, and the irritative effect of the effusion on the mucosa will reverse, leading to a normal middle ear system. The conductive hearing loss due to the effusion will also disappear, returning hearing to normal.

Ventilation tubes typically remain in the eardrum for a length of time determined by their size. The longer the flanges of the tube, the longer their retention will be. The tubes will generally extrude within one to two years. As the tube is expelled, the tympanic membrane heals. Ventilation tubes are generally required only once in the majority (80%) of patients requiring their placement. If recurring ear infections are again encountered after the ventilation tubes have extruded, another set of tubes can be inserted.

An adenoidectomy is often considered in conjunction with the second set of tubes. The eustachian tubes open on either side of the nasopharynx with the adenoid lying between these openings. If the adenoid is enlarged, or if the adenoid is frequently infected, mucosal edema or the adenoid tissue itself may obstruct the eustachian tube openings, contributing to continued middle ear pathology (Nguyen, Manoukian, Yoskovitch, & Al-Sebeih, 2004). An adenoidectomy may be beneficial in establishing improved eustachian tube function (Gates, Avery, Prihoda, & Cooper, 1987).

A particularly aggressive approach to the management of recurrent ear infections is required for patients with craniofacial anomalies, given their increased risk. This includes early insertion of ventilation tubes. In fact, those children who have a cleft lip and palate often have PE tubes inserted prophylactically at the time of the palate repair. Children with craniofacial anomalies should have their hearing tested by 6 months of age, and have repeat testing performed as necessary.

Following palatoplasty, eustachian tube function usually improves and the incidence of ear infections decreases. Ventilation tube insertion prior to palate repair is associated with a high incidence of drainage through the tube, creating a nuisance condition. The incidence rates of recurrent otitis media among children with a history of a cleft palate never reach that of a child born with a normal palate, but approach it over time.

Malformations of the Inner Ear

Structural malformations of the inner ear arise from abnormal development of the otic capsule within the temporal bone. Abnormalities of the inner ear are uncommon, but may be associated with craniofacial anomalies, especially with certain syndromes (Stickler, Treacher Collins, hemifacial microsomia, etc.). Inner ear abnormalities typically cause a *sensorineural hearing loss*, which is a problem with the creation of nerve impulses within the inner ear or the transmission of the nerve impulse through the brainstem to the auditory cortex. Cochlear implants are offered as a means to treat sensorineural hearing loss in patients who derive no benefit from conventional hearing aids (Moores, 2005).

THE NOSE

Anatomy of the Nose

The function of the nose is threefold. It filters inspired air of gross contaminants, it warms the air, and it humidifies the air to the saturation point. These functions are enhanced by the turbulent airflow created as the inspired air impacts the intranasal structures. The nasal septum separates the nasal cavity into two halves. It lies in the midline and is cartilaginous anteriorly and bony posteriorly. The turbinates are bones that are covered with mucosa and are attached to the lateral walls of the nasal cavity. The turbinates create small eddies of air currents, which maximize contact of the inspired air with the nasal mucosa. The nasal mucosa demonstrates a period of vascular engorgement followed by a period of decongestion. The engorgement of the nasal lining promotes humidification and warming of the inspired air. The mucous blanket covering the nasal mucosa traps particulate contaminants. This nasal cycle alternates between sides every 90 minutes. The sinuses are air-filled spaces that are found in the cheeks and between the eyes. These structures are shown in Figure 8–5 as they would be seen through computed tomography.

Malformations of the Nose

Anomalies of the nose range from severe external deformities (facial clefting) to abnormalities of the nasal base (cleft lip and palate) to internal derangement (deviated nasal septum). A deviated nasal septum may occur as a result of a cleft palate where there is inadequate structural support for the cartilaginous septum to remain in the midline. The septum generally deflects into the cleft side of the nose. A deviated septum may also occur as a result of birth trauma, when the nose of the neonate is forced against the pelvis during delivery, causing the septum to slip off the maxillary crest.

In addition to obstructing the airflow through the nasal passages, a significantly deviated septum may affect nasal resonance during speech. Hyponasality may result due to the decreased transmission of sound energy through the nasal cavity. Cul-de-sac resonance may result in severe cases if the sound energy vibrates in a completely obstructed nasal cavity.

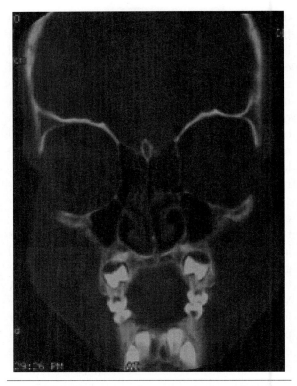

FIGURE 8–5 Computed tomography scan of the nose and paranasal sinuses. This scan shows the nasal cavities separated by the nasal septum. The turbinates are the small bones arising from the lateral aspect of the nasal cavity. The sinuses are air-filled spaces that are found in the cheeks and between the eyes.

Anomalies can also be noted in the front and back openings of the nasal cavity. The nasal cavity opens anteriorly through the nares and posteriorly through the choanae. The choanal openings communicate with the nasopharynx. The anterior nasal openings can be narrowed by overgrowth of the maxilla, an anomaly known as *pyriform aperture stenosis* (Brown, Myer, & Manning, 1989). The posterior choanae may be narrowed in a condition known as *choanal stenosis*, or completely blocked, as in *choanal atresia*. These abnormalities can be either unilateral or bilateral.

Neonates are obligate nasal breathers. Neonates with bilateral choanal atresia will attempt nasal respiration, and when it is unsuccessful, they become fussy and eventually begin to cry. The infants breathe well while crying, but as they settle down, they again attempt nasal respiration unsuccessfully, only to repeat the process. Without early surgical intervention, this cyclical cyanosis can lead to death from exhaustion. Choanal atresia occurs more commonly in females and has an incidence of 1:8000 births (Kubba, Bennett, & Bailey, 2004). It is associated with other congenital abnormalities in 50% of patients.

FACIAL STRUCTURES

Maxilla

Maxillary retrusion (also known as *midface deficiency*) is a common anomaly, especially in individuals with repaired cleft lip and palate. It is characterized by a small upper jaw (maxilla) relative to the lower jaw (mandible). This is due to the inherent deficiency in the maxilla from the cleft and the possible restriction in maxillary growth with the surgical repair. With maxillary retrusion, there is usually at least an anterior crossbite and often a *Class III malocclusion*, where the maxilla is retrusive relative to the mandible (see Chapter 9).

In normal occlusion, the maxillary teeth overlap the mandibular teeth and the tongue remains within the mandibular arch. The tongue tip has sufficient room for movement, including elevation, within the oral cavity. When there is maxillary retrusion, however, the tongue tip may be anterior to the alveolar ridge and anterior to the maxillary teeth. When this is the case, the production of anterior sounds, such as sibilants (/s/, /z/, /sh/, /ch/, and /j/), lingual-alveolar sounds (/t/, /d/, /n/, /l/), labiodental sounds (/f/ and /v/), and even bilabial sounds (/p/, /b/, /m/) can be affected. See Chapter 9 for more information regarding the effects of occlusion on speech.

Facial Nerve

Facial paralysis may occur as a result of an injury (surgical or traumatic), infection (as in *Bell's palsy*) (Chen & Wong, 2005; Peitersen, 1992), or due to congenital abnormalities of the nerve or associated muscles. The paralysis may be partial, as in hemifacial microsomia, or may be complete and bilateral, as in Moebius syndrome. Bilateral facial paralysis can result in mask-like facies. A lack of facial expression can inhibit lip movement for feeding and speech (Goldberg, DeLorie, Zuker, & Manktelow, 2003; Meyerson & Foushee, 1978). Facial paralysis can affect the ability to produce bilabial and even labiodental sounds. The individual may learn to compensate by producing these sounds with the tongue tip. Some individuals become very adept in producing the sound in a way that is acoustically similar to the labial sound.

THE ORAL CAVITY

The oral cavity extends from the lips anteriorly to the faucial pillars posteriorly. Anomalies of the oral cavity are common and can have a significant effect on speech. Dental anomalies are discussed in Chapter 9 and are therefore not covered in this chapter.

Lips

The lips are paired structures. They function in articulation, eating, and preventing *sialorrhea* (drooling). A common problem following a cleft lip repair is a short upper lip. The lip is deficient in tissue because of the cleft, and also secondary to the contractile effects of the scar from the cleft lip repair. If the premaxilla is protrusive, the relative shortening of the lip is further increased, resulting in the appearance of a protrusive lower lip. Even if the upper lip is of normal length, a protrusive premaxilla may make it appear to be short and can interfere with normal bilabial closure.

When the upper lip is short, there may be difficulties in the production of bilabial sounds, because total lip closure is difficult to accomplish. As a result, the individual may compensate by producing bilabial sounds with a labiodental placement. This can result in a remarkably similar sound to the bilabial sound so that most listeners do not notice a distortion. However, this production looks different and can be distracting to the listener.

There may be additional anomalies of the upper lip following repair of a cleft lip. There may be a mismatch of the vermilion border, asymmetry of the lip, or a flattening of Cupid's bow. The obicularis oris muscle must be approximated during the lip repair, or a discontinuity of these muscle bundles may be apparent over time. These anomalies are cosmetic and do not affect speech.

Mouth

Congenital abnormalities of the size and shape of the mouth can occur, especially with some syndromes. The suffix "*stomia*" is used for the word "mouth." This is not to be confused with the suffix "*somia*," which refers to body. *Macrostomia* refers to an excessively large mouth opening. When this occurs, one corner of the mouth may extend into the cheek, making the mouth opening on that particular side large and distorted in appearance. This is particularly common with hemifacial microsomia. On the other hand, *microstomia* refers to a small mouth opening. Microstomia more often results from acquired injuries, such as electrical burns sustained after a child chews on an electrical cord. Severe contractures of the mouth are possible secondary to scarring.

Macrostomia does not usually cause speech problems. On the other hand, if the microstomia is severe enough to affect mouth opening, it can affect articulation and cause cul-de-sac resonance.

Tongue

Abnormalities of the tongue are associated with certain syndromes. The tongue may be very large in a condition called *macroglossia*. This is one of the main characteristics of Beckwith-Wiedemann syndrome (Figure 8–6). When this occurs, the tongue does not fit the oral cavity space, and therefore, it protrudes past the alveolar ridge. This often results in an open-mouth posture. As the dentition develops, an anterior open bite may occur due to the position of the tongue in the area where the teeth should be. The chronic open-mouth posture can also contribute to excessive drooling. Macroglossia can affect the production of tongue tip sounds and can cause either a frontal or lateral distortion of sibilants (Van Borsel, Van Snick, & Leroy, 1999). It can also contribute to the use of palatal-dorsal articulation, especially if the tongue tip rests anterior to the alveolar ridge.

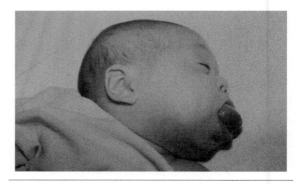

FIGURE 8–6 Macroglossia secondary to Beckwith-Wiedemann syndrome. Beckwith-Wiedemann syndrome is a congenital disorder characterized by macroglossia, omphalocele, hypoglycemia, and abnormalities of the kidneys, pancreas, and adrenal cortex. This photo demonstrates macroglossia with severe discrepancy between the size of the oral cavity and the size of the tongue.

The opposite problem of macroglossia is *microglossia*, which is a small tongue, especially in relation to the oral cavity space. This may cause difficulty with tongue tip sounds, but it often has no detrimental effect on speech.

Other lingual (tongue) anomalies include a *lobulated tongue* (refer to Figure 13–20 in Chapter 13). In this case, the tongue may appear to have multiple lobes, with fissures between each lobe. This is common in orofaciodigital (OFD) syndrome. A lobulated tongue may or may not affect lingual mobility. However, if mobility is affected, speech will be affected as well.

Finally, a discussion of lingual anomalies would not be complete without a mention of ankyloglossia. *Ankyloglossia*, commonly referred to as "*tongue-tie*," is a condition where the lingual frenulum is congenitally short and attaches to the anterior tongue tip (Figure 8–7). The attachment may be right at the tip of the tongue, rather than a third of the way back, as is normally seen. Ankylosis of the tongue can also occur after radical oral surgery, causing the same limitations in tongue tip movement.

When there is ankylosis of the tongue, tongue tip protrusion results in an indentation in the tip of the tongue, making a heart-shaped notch. The lingual frenulum is frequently short in newborns, but it tends to correct itself as the child grows (Garcia Pola, Gonzalez Garcia, Garcia Martin, Gallas, & Seoane Leston, 2002). With ankyloglossia, lingual movement can be somewhat restricted, particularly for eating (Kern, 1991). This can affect the person's ability to move a bolus in the mouth in preparation for swallowing, particularly if the bolus is in the *buccal sulcus* (area between the teeth and cheeks).

Ankyloglossia has less effect on speech, because very little tongue tip excursion is needed for normal speech production (Kummer, 2005; Moller, 1994). In fact, the farthest that the tongue needs to protrude is against the back of the maxillary incisors for a /th/ sound, and the most it has to elevate is to the alveolar ridge for the /l/ sound. Since ankyloglossia rarely causes problems with speech, unless there is also oral-motor dysfunction, frenulectomy is usually not indicated for speech purposes. However, it may be indicated for feeding purposes and to improve aesthetics.

Palate

Palatal arch anomalies are common, particularly in individuals with a history of cleft palate, and also in patients with other craniofacial syndromes. These anomalies include abnormalities in the height, width, and configuration of the palatal arch. The palatal vault may be low and flat due to collapsed lateral palatal segments or it may be very high and narrow, causing crowding of the teeth and tongue. A narrow, high-arched palate is often seen in children who have had an endotracheal tube at birth.

Whenever the palatal arch is low, flat, or narrow, it restricts the oral cavity space, which may cause the tongue to protrude. As the tongue protrudes, the tongue tip is in an abnormal position for tongue tip articulation. As a result,

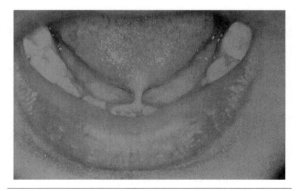

FIGURE 8–7 Ankyloglossia. Ankyloglossia is a condition describing the attachment of the lingual frenulum to the anterior tongue tip. It may impede normal tongue mobility, but rarely requires intervention for speech purposes.

distortion of speech is inevitable. The obligatory error would be a frontal lisp or fronting of anterior sounds. The compensatory error would be a palatal-dorsal placement due to the articulation of the dorsum of the tongue against the palate as the tongue is retracted. When this placement is used for sibilant sounds, it typically results in a lateral distortion or lateral lisp.

A *palatal fistula*, also called an *oronasal fistula*, is a hole or opening in the palate that goes all the way through to the nasal cavity. It is important to make a distinction between a fistula that is "intentional" versus one that is "unintentional" (Folk, D'Antonio, & Hardesty, 1997). A fistula can occur as an unintentional postoperative complication of a cleft repair due to a lack of adequate healing. The most common site for a breakdown of the mucoperiosteum that results in an unintentional fistula is at the junction of the hard and soft palate. On the other hand, an anterior fistula in the alveolus or in the area of the incisive foramen is often left open intentionally by the surgeon, especially when there was a bilateral cleft lip and palate. The fistula is later closed with an alveolar bone graft.

Depending on its size and location, a fistula can cause nasal air emission and even hypernasality. A small fistula is usually not symptomatic for speech because during speech, the airflow courses parallel to rather than perpendicular to the fistula opening. A small fistula that is asymptomatic can become symptomatic, however, with maxillary expansion because this can make it larger. If the fistula is above the tongue tip, there may be nasal air emission on lingual-alveolar sounds as the tongue tip elevates, thus pushing the airstream into the fistula. A moderate-sized fistula can cause consistent nasal air emission on all sounds, particularly anterior sounds. Only a very large fistula will cause hypernasality. A fistula can result in nasal regurgitation of fluids and can even cause

food to become stuck in the opening and in the nasal cavity.

If the fistula is symptomatic for speech, it should be covered prosthetically or should be surgically closed. If a patient demonstrates inadequate velopharyngeal movement and a symptomatic fistula, the fistula should be covered prior to considering intervention for the velopharyngeal dysfunction. Research has shown that an open fistula can affect levator veli palatini muscle movement, and thus velopharyngeal function (Isberg & Henningsson, 1987; Tachimura, Hara, Koh, & Wada, 1997). The only way to determine the potential for velopharyngeal function is to close the fistula and thus the anterior leak in the system. If velopharyngeal dysfunction persists after closure of the fistula, surgical correction of the velopharyngeal dysfunction will also be needed to normalize the speech and resonance.

Tonsils and Adenoids

The tonsils surround the opening to the oropharynx. The *faucial tonsils* are located on either side of the mouth between the anterior and posterior faucial pillars. The *lingual tonsils* are located at the base of the tongue. The *pharyngeal tonsil*, also know as the adenoid, is located in the nasopharynx. This collection of lymphoid tissue is known as *Waldeyer's ring*.

This lymphoid tissue is most important during the first two years of life. Foreign materials entering the body through the nose and mouth pass over this specialized tissue. Antigens adhere to the specialized lining of this tissue where it is incorporated into the substance of the tonsil to be presented to the immune system. This is one of the body's surveillance systems whereby antibodies can be developed to ward off infections (Brodsky, Moore, Stanievich, & Ogra, 1988). Over time, the tonsil and adenoid tissue tends to atrophy. Generally, by the age of 16, the tissue persists as only small remnants. By that age, there is much redundancy in the system—so that if surgical intervention is required to remove adenotonsillar tissue, no alteration in immunity would be expected after their removal. The entire gastrointestinal tract is lined with the same types of tissue as the tonsils and adenoid, and a similar function is maintained through this system.

CAUSES OF UPPER AIRWAY OBSTRUCTION

Adenotonsillar Hypertrophy

Adenotonsillar hypertrophy is the enlargement of both the tonsil and adenoid tissue to the point where there is interference with the airway. Upper airway obstruction, and its related characteristics, is a major concern with adenotonsillar hypertrophy. The etiology for this overgrowth of tissue is unknown, but is thought to be secondary to chronic stimulation from infection or allergic sources.

Adenotonsillar hypertrophy may be relative in that it can occur with normal-sized tonsils and adenoid tissue, but with relatively small adjacent structures. For example, patients with midface hypoplasia, as in Crouzon, Apert, and Down syndromes, may have an adenoid pad situated in a relatively small nasopharynx, creating the obstructive symptoms. A similar problem may occur in patients with retrognathia (as is common in Treacher Collins syndrome or Pierre Robin sequence), where normal adenoid tissue combined with a narrow oropharyngeal inlet and glossoptosis can create obstruction.

Tonsillar Hypertrophy

The size of the pharyngeal tonsils is graded on a four-point scale. Tonsils that are 1+ in size are contained within the tonsillar pillars; tonsils

that are 2+ extend minimally beyond the tonsillar pillars; tonsils that are 3+ obstruct the oropharyngeal inlet to a moderated degree; and finally, tonsils that are 4+ in size touch in the midline (Figure 8–8A). Occasionally, one tonsil will be significantly larger than the other (Figure 8–8B). This abnormal growth pattern can be a cause for concern.

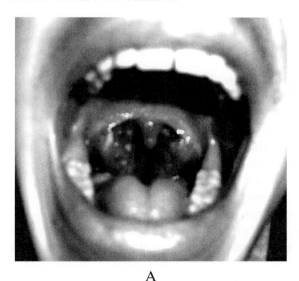

A

B

FIGURE 8–8 (A and B) A. Large (grade 4+) tonsils bilaterally. B. A large tonsil on the patient's left side. Asymmetric tonsils are a cause for concern, as a tumor may be causing the abnormal growth pattern. In this example, the left tonsil is a grade 4, whereas the right tonsil is a grade 1.

If one or both of the tonsils are excessively large (grade 3+ or larger), they fill the oropharynx and can actually intrude into the nasopharynx. This blockage of the entrance to the oral cavity can cause cul-de-sac resonance, and the blockage of sound transmission into the nasal cavity can cause hyponasality. If the tonsil is large enough to intrude into the area of the velopharyngeal port, it can prevent a tight seal during velopharyngeal closure, resulting in velopharyngeal insufficiency and causing nasal air emission (see Figure 7–15A and Figure 7–15B in Chapter 7) (Kummer, Billmire, & Myer, 1993; MacKenzie-Stepner, Witzel, Stringer, & Laskin, 1987; Shprintzen, Sher, & Croft, 1987). With large tonsils, it is possible for a single patient to demonstrate a mixture of hyponasality, cul-de-sac resonance, and nasal air emission (Finkelstein, Bar-Ziv, Nachmani, Berger, & Ophir, 1993). (See Chapter 7 for more information.)

Hypertrophic tonsils can indirectly affect articulation. If there is airway obstruction, the tongue will often compensate by moving down and forward in order to open the airway. When the tongue is always in an anterior position, this can cause fronting of sibilants and even fronting of lingual-alveolar sounds.

Lingual Tonsil Hypertrophy

Lingual tonsil hypertrophy occurs infrequently but may cause airway obstruction (Figure 8–9). This may be a particular problem in children with Down syndrome (Donnelly, Shott, LaRose, Chini, & Amin, 2004). If the airway is affected, the tongue may be forced into an anterior position, causing fronting of anterior consonants during speech. The lingual tonsil may also block transmission of sound energy into the oral cavity, causing cul-de-sac resonance. The lingual tonsils, however, are rarely large enough to require removal.

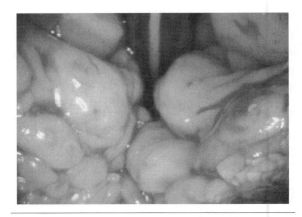

FIGURE 8–9 Lingual tonsils. Lingual tonsils are located in the base of the tongue. The can enlarge to the point that the airway is partially obstructed, leading to breathing difficulties. The larynx cannot be seen in this photograph due to the enlargement of the lingual tonsils. The valleculla is completely filled with lingual tonsil tissue.

Adenoid Hypertrophy

Enlarged adenoids can obstruct the nasopharyngeal airway or even the choanal opening into the nose (Figure 8–10). This can potentially

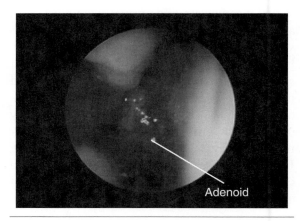

Adenoid

FIGURE 8–10 Adenoid tissue blocking the choana. The adenoid is a collection of lymphoid tissue in the nasopharynx. It has the capacity to enlarge and block nasal respiration. At times the adenoid tissue can grow into the posterior aspect of the nose, completely blocking the posterior choanae.

affect both hearing and speech. As noted above, hypertrophic adenoids can obstruct the opening to the eustachian tube and disrupt middle ear function. During speech, they can interfere with sound transmission into the nasal cavity, thus causing hyponasality. If the adenoid pad is irregular in configuration, this can affect the firmness of the veloadenoidal seal during speech, thus causing nasal air emission. See Chapter 7 for more information about the effects on speech.

Airway obstruction due to adenoid hypertrophy may be characterized by *stertorous* (a heavy snoring sound) respiration, chronic mouth breathing, loud snoring, and even sleep apnea. With sleep apnea, the child appears to be very restless during sleep and is constantly tossing and turning to find a position where breathing can occur with decreased effort. The marginal airway is compromised further by the generalized hypotonia associated with deep sleep. This hypotonia causes collapse of the hypopharyngeal structures. The tongue base also retrodisplaces, causing further compromise of the airway. An *obstructive sleep apnea* (OSA) event is a period where the child is exerting muscular forces to inspire but is unsuccessful in moving air into the lungs. When observed in children, this is significant and requires attention. *Polysomnography* (a sleep study) may be beneficial if questions arise regarding the extent of the sleep disturbances. Information from polysomnography can help to determine appropriate treatment.

Evidence of airway obstruction due to enlarged adenoids may be visible in the child's face. The typical *adenoid facies* is characterized by an open-mouth posture, anterior tongue position, the forward and downward position of the mandible, facial elongation, suborbital coloring (black eyes) and puffy eyes, and the appearance of pinched nostrils.

TREATMENT OF UPPER AIRWAY OBSTRUCTION

Tonsillectomy

If the hypertrophic tonsils cause upper airway obstruction, recurrent tonsillitis, or peritonsillar abscess, tonsillectomy is indicated. When a tonsillectomy is done, the tonsils are removed in their entirety, including the capsule deep to the tonsil. This can result in alteration of oropharyngeal anatomy. Despite this change, tonsillectomy usually either has no effect on speech or has a positive effect by eliminating a source of blockage at the entry to the oral cavity. Tonsillectomy is not contraindicated in patients with risk for velopharyngeal insufficiency since they do not contribute to velopharyngeal function (D'Antonio, Snyder, & Samadani, 1996).

Although it occurs very rarely, hypernasality has been reported following tonsillectomy (Gibb & Stewart, 1975; Haapanen, Ignatius, Rihkanen, & Ertama, 1994). This can be due to either abnormal scarring of the faucial pillars, which can restrict movement, or it can be due to a protection response secondary to the pain of the procedure. This protection response inhibits velopharyngeal movement for both swallowing and speech and remains after the pain is no longer present. Fortunately, this is easy to correct with only a few speech therapy sessions in most cases.

Adenoidectomy

The indications for adenoidectomy include airway obstruction and in some cases, intractable middle ear effusion (Darrow & Siemens, 2002). With adenoidectomy, the capsule deep to the adenoid pad is left in place, as it is protecting the underlying bone of the skull base. Because the capsule is left in place, it is possible to have some regrowth of the adenoid over time. When it occurs, this regrowth can be very irregular tissue. During speech, this can affect the firmness of the veloadenoidal seal, causing nasal air escape.

Hypernasality following adenoidectomy is always a risk (Donnelly, 1994; Fernandes, Grobbelaar, Hudson, & Lentin, 1996; Kavanagh & Beckford, 1988; Parton & Jones, 1998; Pulkkinen, Ranta, Heliovaara, & Haapanen, 2002; Ren, Isberg, & Henningsson, 1995; Saunders, Hartley, Sell, & Sommerlad, 2004; Schmaman, Jordann, & Jammine, 1998; Witzel, Rich, Margar-Bacal, & Cox, 1986), although the risk is minimal and has been estimated to be between 1:1500 and at 1:3000. Frequently, patients who have hypernasality after adenoidectomy are later found to have an occult submucous cleft (Saunders et al., 2004). There are several risk factors for hypernasality due to velopharyngeal insufficiency following adenoidectomy. These include a family history of hypernasality or palatal clefting, a repaired cleft palate, a submucous cleft, and a history of nasal regurgitation or sucking difficulties as an infant. In addition, individuals with oral-motor dysfunction or other neuromuscular problems can also be considered at risk with this procedure. If the patient has upper airway obstruction due to enlarged adenoids, yet is at risk for hypernasality postoperatively, a conservative superior half-adenoidectomy can be performed (Finkelstein, Wexler, Nachmani, & Ophir, 2002). With this procedure, the airway obstruction can be relieved while maintaining adequate tissue inferiorly for the velum to impact and create an adequate seal.

Temporary velopharyngeal insufficiency during the first week or two following adenoidectomy is very common. Due to their location in the pharynx, the adenoid pads assist in velopharyngeal closure in young children so that preschool children usually have veloadenoidal closure rather than velopharyngeal closure (Maryn, Van Lierde, De Bodt, & Van Cauwenberge, 2004) (Figure 8–11). When this tissue is suddenly removed, the soft palate must extend farther posteriorly, or the lateral walls must extend farther medially, to achieve closure. Most patients are able to accomplish this adjustment in velopharyngeal function within a few days or weeks. If the hypernasality or nasal emission persists beyond six to eight weeks, it is unlikely to resolve spontaneously. Surgical repair would then be required to correct the velopharyngeal insufficiency.

Tracheostomy

A *tracheostomy* is a surgical procedure that is done to relieve conditions that cause life-threatening airway obstruction. The tracheostomy

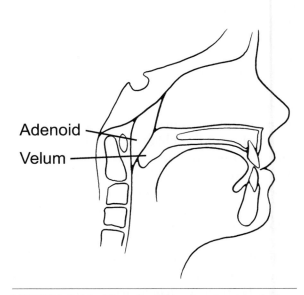

FIGURE 8–11 The adenoid pad assists in velopharyngeal closure in children. The sudden removal of adenoid tissue during adenoidectomy requires compensation of soft palate motion to maintain proper velopharyngeal closure. If any abnormality exists in the architecture or neurological function of the palate, this compensation may not be successful, which leads to nasal air escape.

procedure is done by making a vertical incision in the midline of the neck overlying the trachea. The trachea is incised vertically, usually through the third and fourth rings, creating an opening in the anterior wall of the trachea. A tracheostomy tube is then inserted into the tracheal opening, and the edges of the opening are sutured to the skin in the neck. The stoma is the opening through which the patient can breathe.

Tracheostomy is often indicated for certain congenital anomalies, such as subglottic stenosis, tracheal stenosis, or laryngeal web. Infants born with Pierre Robin sequence are often candidates for tracheostomy due to the airway problems that occur as a result of the small mandible and glossoptosis (Figure 8–12). Tracheostomy is also indicated for patients who cannot adequately raise their secretions from their airway and, therefore, need frequent suctioning. This includes patients who are unconscious, those with a paralysis that precludes coughing, and

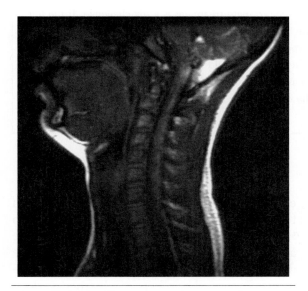

FIGURE 8–12 Glossoptosis. The tongue base is too far back in the pharynx, causing significant airway obstruction.

those with significant chest pain, which inhibits coughing.

Uvulopalatopharyngoplasty (UPPP)

In the pediatric population, upper airway obstruction is primarily caused by adenotonsillar hypertrophy. Therefore, *adenotonsillectomy* is the obvious choice for treatment. In teenagers and adults, however, the tonsils and adenoids are very small and therefore are not likely to cause obstruction. When older patients demonstrate obstructive sleep apnea, it is often secondary to redundant mucosa of the soft palate and posterior pharyngeal wall that is causing the oropharyngeal inlet to be small. In these cases, the treatment of the obstruction is a surgical procedure called a *uvulopalatopharyngoplasty* (UPPP) (Blythe, Henrich, & Pillsbury, 1995; Croft & Golding-Wood, 1990; Fairbanks, 1990; Isberg & Henningsson, 1987; Kavey, Whyte, Blitzer, & Gidro-Frank, 1990; Yanagisawa & Weaver, 1997).

As part of the UPPP, the remaining tonsil tissue is removed and the anterior and posterior tonsillar pillars are sewn together to open the oropharyngeal inlet. The free margin of the soft palate is resected along with the uvula, and the soft palate is oversewn. Although snoring is usually markedly improved as a result of this procedure, the overall effect on the sleep apnea is often disappointing. Fortunately, if done properly, this procedure does not seem to have a negative effect on resonance (Rihkanen & Soini, 1992; Salas-Provance & Kuehn, 1990).

Other surgical procedures are also done for obstructive sleep apnea including procedures that advance the tongue base anteriorly, reduce the size of the tongue base, or reposition the tongue along with the mandible and maxilla.

CASE REPORT

Upper Airway Obstruction, Hypernasality, and CPAP

Tam was a Vietnamese male born with bilateral complete cleft lip and palate. The cleft lip was closed in Vietnam, but the palate was left unrepaired. When Tam entered the United States at the age of 21, the palate was still open and he did not speak any English. Soon after arriving in this country, the palate was repaired and a pharyngeal flap (to correct velopharyngeal dysfunction) was done. Although the prognosis for correcting speech is guarded when the palate is closed that late, Tam exceeded all expectations. He received several months of speech therapy following his surgery and he quickly developed oral production of speech sounds and also learned English.

Tam was seen for an evaluation in VPI clinic several years later at the age of 27. At that time, articulation was normal for the production of all speech sounds. However, Tam's accent had a negative effect on the intelligibility of his speech. Resonance was found to be mildly hypernasal, but very acceptable. There was barely audible nasal air emission during the production of pressure-sensitive phonemes. At the same time, Tam reported difficulty with nasal breathing and significant snoring at night, which was the primary reason for his return.

A nasopharyngoscopy (endoscopy) assessment showed the cause of these symptoms. Although the pharyngeal flap was an appropriate width and in good position, the lateral ports (for breathing on either side of the flap) were small for normal nasal breathing. During speech, the right port closed completely, but the left port remained partially open. Therefore, it was determined that the narrow ports restricted nasal breathing, particularly during sleep, but the open left port caused the hypernasality during speech.

With this combination of symptoms, determining the appropriate treatment is a big challenge. If the left port was narrowed further for speech, it would increase the airway problems. On the other hand, opening the ports to improve nasal breathing would increase the hypernasality. Therefore, it was decided that the current balance of the needs for speech and breathing was the best that could be achieved. However, since nasal obstruction was a concern at night, a sleep study was done. This confirmed sleep apnea so CPAP was recommended to be used at night. With this option, the flap could be left intact for speech, yet the airway was forced open at night for sleep.

Continuous Positive Airway Pressure (CPAP)

Frequently, *continuous positive airway pressure (CPAP)* is required for long-term resolution of the obstructive apnea. The CPAP equipment consists of a face mask and an air pressure generator. The patient wears the mask over the nose during sleep, and a certain level of continuous positive air pressure, usually in the range of 6 to 20 cm H_2O, is delivered to the pharynx through the nose. This forces the airway open and prevents pharyngeal collapse during respiration. Although CPAP is effective in overcoming the effects of obstructive sleep apnea, long-term nightly use of the machine leads to a high degree of noncompliance over time.

SUMMARY

The ears, the nose, and the oral cavity are essential organs for verbal communication. Congenital anomalies of these structures can therefore interfere with the development of articulation and language and the production of normal speech and resonance. Speech-language pathologists, whether working directly with craniofacial anomalies or not, need to form a partnership with otolaryngologists to adequately diagnose these disorders and treat them appropriately.

FOR REVIEW, DISCUSSION, AND CRITICAL THINKING

1. Describe both the normal structures of the ear and the potential malformations in patients that have craniofacial anomalies.

2. What is the purpose of eustachian tube function? Describe normal eustachian tube function, including the action of the muscle. What happens if the eustachian tube does not function normally?

3. Why are young children more prone to otitis media than adults? Why are children with a history of cleft palate particularly at risk for chronic middle ear effusion and otitis media? What can be done prophylactically for children who are at particular risk?

4. Describe potential malformations of the nose. How could these malformations affect resonance? If there is abnormal resonance, is the individual a candidate for speech therapy? Why or why not?

5. Describe the purpose and location of the tonsils and adenoids.

6. What are the potential effects of tonsillar hypertrophy? What are the potential effects of adenoid hypertrophy?

7. Describe the potential risks and benefits of adenoidectomy. Describe the potential risks and benefits of tonsillectomy.

8. Why is it important to discuss the tonsils and adenoids separately? Why do you think people confuse the risk and benefits of tonsillectomy versus adenoidectomy?

9. What are treatment options for upper airway obstruction? What would you recommend for a child who has airway obstruction that immediately follows placement of a pharyngeal flap?

REFERENCES

American Academy of Family Physicians, American Academy of Otolaryngology Head and Neck Surgery, & American Academy of Pediatrics Subcommittee on Otitis Media With Effusion. (2004). Otitis media with effusion. *Pediatrics*, *113*(5), 1412–1429.

Bluestone, C. D., Beery, Q. C., Cantekin, E. I., & Paradise, J. L. (1975). Eustachian tube ventilatory function in relation to cleft palate. *Annals of Otology, Rhinology, and Laryngology*, *84*(3, Pt. 1), 333–338.

Bluestone, C. D., Paradise, J. L., Beery, Q. C., & Wittel, R. (1972). Certain effects of cleft palate repair on eustachian tube function. *Cleft Palate Journal*, *9*, 183–193.

Blythe, W. R., Henrich, D. E., & Pillsbury, H. C. (1995). Outpatient uvuloplasty: An inexpensive, single-staged procedure for the relief of symptomatic snoring.

Otolaryngology—Head & Neck Surgery, *113*(1), 1–4.

Brent, B. (1999). The pediatrician's role in caring for patients with congenital microtia and atresia. *Pediatric Annals*, *28*(2), 374–383.

Brodsky, L., Moore, L., Stanievich, J., & Ogra, P. (1988). The immunology of tonsils in children: The effect of bacterial load on the presence of B- and T-cell subsets. *Laryngoscope*, *98*(1), 93–98.

Brown, O. E., Myer, C. M., III, & Manning, S. C. (1989). Congenital nasal pyriform aperture stenosis. *Laryngoscope*, *99*(1), 86–91.

Chen, W. X., & Wong, V. (2005). Prognosis of Bell's palsy in children—Analysis of 29 cases. *Brain & Development*, *27*(7), 504–508.

Croft, C. B., & Golding-Wood, D. G. (1990). Uses and complications of uvulopalatopharyngoplasty. *Journal of Laryngology and Otology*, *104*(11), 871–875.

D'Antonio, L. L., Snyder, L. S., & Samadani, S. (1996). Tonsillectomy in children with or at risk for velopharyngeal insufficiency: Effects on speech. *Otolaryngology—Head & Neck Surgery*, *115*(4), 319–323.

Darrow, D. H., & Siemens, C. (2002). Indications for tonsillectomy and adenoidectomy. *Laryngoscope*, *112*(8, Suppl. 100, Pt. 2), 6–10.

Donnelly, L. F., Shott, S. R., LaRose, C. R., Chini, B. A., & Amin, R. S. (2004). Causes of persistent obstructive sleep apnea despite previous tonsillectomy and adenoidectomy in children with Down syndrome as depicted on static and dynamic cine MRI. *American Journal of Roentgenology*, *183*(1), 175–181.

Donnelly, M. J. (1994). Hypernasality following adenoid removal. *Irish Journal of Medical Science*, *163*(5), 225–227.

Doyle, W. J., Cantekin, E. I., & Bluestone, C. D. (1980). Eustachian tube function in cleft palate children. *Annals of Otology, Rhinology,* *and Laryngology Supplement*, *89*(3, Pt. 2), 34–40.

Durr, D. G., & Shapiro, R. S. (1989). Otologic manifestations in congenital velopharyngeal insufficiency. *American Journal of Diseases of Children*, *143*(1), 75–77.

Fairbanks, D. N. (1990). Uvulopalatopharyngoplasty complications and avoidance strategies. *Otolaryngology—Head & Neck Surgery*, *102*(3), 239–245.

Fernandes, D. B., Grobbelaar, A. O., Hudson, D. A., & Lentin, R. (1996). Velopharyngeal incompetence after adenotonsillectomy in noncleft patients. *British Journal of Oral and Maxillofacial Surgery*, *34*(5), 364–367.

Finkelstein, Y., Bar-Ziv, J., Nachmani, A., Berger, G., & Ophir, D. (1993). Peritonsillar abscess as a cause of transient velopharyngeal insufficiency. *Cleft Palate-Craniofacial Journal*, *30*(4), 421–428.

Finkelstein, Y., Wexler, D. B., Nachmani, A., & Ophir, D. (2002). Endoscopic partial adenoidectomy for children with submucous cleft palate. *Cleft Palate-Craniofacial Journal*, *39*(5), 479–486.

Folk, S. N., D' Antonio, L. L., & Hardesty, R. A. (1997). Secondary cleft deformities. *Clinics in Plastic Surgery*, *24*(3), 599–611.

Garcia Pola, M. J., Gonzalez Garcia, M., Garcia Martin, J. M., Gallas, M., & Seoane Leston, J. (2002). A study of pathology associated with short lingual frenum. *Journal of Dentistry for Children*, *69*(1), 59–62.

Gates, G., Avery, C., Prihoda, T., & Cooper, J. J. (1987, December 3). Effectiveness of adenoidectomy and tympanostomy tubes in the treatment of chronic otitis media with effusion. *New England Journal of Medicine*, *317*, 1444–1451.

Gibb, A. G., & Stewart, I. A. (1975). Hypernasality following tonsil dissection—Hysterical aetiology. *Journal of Laryngology and Otology*, 89(7), 779–781.

Goldberg, C., DeLorie, R., Zuker, R. M., & Manktelow, R. T. (2003). The effects of gracilis muscle transplantation on speech in children with Moebius syndrome. *Journal of Craniofacial Surgery*, 14(5), 687–690.

Haapanen, M. L., Ignatius, J., Rihkanen, H., & Ertama, L. (1994). Velopharyngeal insufficiency following palatine tonsillectomy. *European Archives of Oto-Rhino-Laryngology*, 251(3), 186–189.

Heller, J. C., Gens, G. W., Croft, C. B., & Moe, D. G. (1978). Conductive hearing loss in patients with velopharyngeal insufficiency. *Cleft Palate Journal*, 15(3), 246–253.

Hubbard, T. W., Paradise, J. L., McWilliams, B. J., Elster, B. A., & Taylor, F. H. (1985). Consequences of unremitting middle ear disease in early life: Otologic, audiologic, and developmental findings in children with cleft palate. *New England Journal of Medicine*, 312(24), 1529–1534.

Isberg, A., & Henningsson, G. (1987). Influence of palatal fistulas on velopharyngeal movements: A cineradiographic study. *Plastic and Reconstructive Surgery*, 79(4), 525–1530.

Jahrsdoerfer, R., & Lambert, P. (1998, May). Facial nerve injury in congenital aural atresia surgery. *American Journal of Otology*, 19, 283–287.

Jahrsdoerfer, R., Yeakley, J., Aguilar, E., Cole, R., & Gray, L. (1992). Grading system for the selection of patients with congenital aural atresia. *American Journal of Otology*, 13(1), 6–12.

Kavanagh, K. T., & Beckford, N. S. (1988). Adenotonsillectomy in children: Indications and contraindications. *Southern Medical Journal*, 81(4), 507–514.

Kavey, N. B., Whyte, J., Blitzer, A., & Gidro-Frank, S. (1990). Postsurgical evaluation of uvulopalatopharyngoplasty: Two case reports. *Sleep*, 13(1), 79–84.

Kern, I. (1991, July 1). Tongue tie. *Medical Journal of Australia*, 155, 33–34.

Kountakis, S., Helidonis, E., & Jahrsdoerfer, R. (1995). Microtia grade as an indicator of middle ear development in aural atresia. *Archives of Otolaryngology—Head & Neck Surgery*, 121(8), 885–886.

Kubba, H., Bennett, A., & Bailey, C. M. (2004). An update on choanal atresia surgery at Great Ormond Street Hospital for Children: Preliminary results with Mitomycin C and the KTP laser. *International Journal of Pediatric Otorhinolaryngology*, 68(7), 939–945.

Kummer, A. W. (2005, Dec. 27). To clip or not to clip? That's the question. *The ASHA Leader*, 10(17), 6–7, 30.

Kummer, A. W., Billmire, D. A., & Myer, C. M. D. (1993). Hypertrophic tonsils: The effect on resonance and velopharyngeal closure. *Plastic and Reconstructive Surgery*, 91(4), 608–611.

MacKenzie-Stepner, K., Witzel, M. A., Stringer, D. A., & Laskin, R. (1987). Velopharyngeal insufficiency due to hypertrophic tonsils. A report of two cases. *International Journal of Pediatric Otorhinolaryngology*, 14(1), 57–63.

Maryn, Y., Van Lierde, K., De Bodt, M., & Van Cauwenberge, P. (2004). The effects of adenoidectomy and tonsillectomy on speech and nasal resonance. *Folia Phoniatrica et Logopedica*, 56(3), 182–191.

Meyerson, M. D., & Foushee, D. R. (1978). Speech, language and hearing in Moebius syndrome: A study of 22 patients. *Developmental Medicine & Child Neurology*, 20(3), 357–365.

Moller, K. T. (1994). Dental-occlusal and other oral conditions and speech. In J. E. Bernthal & N. W. Bankson (Eds.), *Child phonology: Characteristics, assessment, and intervention with special populations* (pp. 3–28). New York: Thieme Medical Publishers, Inc.

Moores, D. F. (2005). Cochlear implants: An update. *American Annals of the Deaf, 150*(4), 327–328.

Nguyen, L. H., Manoukian, J. J., Yoskovitch, A., & Al-Sebeih, K. H. (2004). Adenoidectomy: Selection criteria for surgical cases of otitis media. *Laryngoscope, 114*(5), 863–866.

Paradise, J. L. (1976). Management of middle ear effusions in infants with cleft palate. *Annals of Otology, Rhinology, and Laryngology, 85*(2, Suppl. 25, Pt. 2), 285–288.

Paradise, J. L., & Bluestone, C. D. (1974). Early treatment of the universal otitis media of infants with cleft palate. *Pediatrics, 53*(1), 48–54.

Paradise, J. L., Alberti, P. W., Bluestone, C. D., Cheek, D. B., Lis, E. F., & Stool, S. E. (1974). Pediatric and otologic aspects of clinical research in cleft palate. *Clinics in Pediatrics (Phila), 13*(7), 587–593.

Parton, M. J., & Jones, A. S. (1998). Hypernasality following adenoidectomy: A significant and avoidable complication. *Clinics in Otolaryngology, 23*(1), 18–19.

Peitersen, E. (1992). Natural history of Bell's palsy. *Acta Oto-Laryngologica. 492*(Suppl.), 122–124.

Pulkkinen, J., Ranta, R., Heliovaara, A., & Haapanen, M. L. (2002). Craniofacial characteristics and velopharyngeal function in cleft lip/palate children with and without adenoidectomy. *European Archives of Oto-Rhino-Laryngology, 259*(2), 100–104.

Ren, Y. F., Isberg, A., & Henningsson, G. (1995). Velopharyngeal incompetence and persistent hypernasality after adenoidectomy in children without palatal defect. *Cleft Palate-Craniofacial Journal, 32*(6), 476–482.

Rihkanen, H., & Soini, I. (1992). Changes in voice characteristics after uvulopalatopharyngoplasty. *European Archives of Otorhinolaryngology, 249*(6), 322–324.

Rosenfeld, R. M., Culpepper, L., Doyle, K. J., Grundfast, K. M., Hoberman, A., Kenna, M. A., et al. (2004). Clinical practice guideline: Otitis media with effusion. *Otolaryngology—Head & Neck Surgery, 130*(5, Suppl.), 95–118.

Rvachew, S., Slawinski, E., Williams, M., & Green, C. (1999). The impact of early onset otitis media on babbling and early language development. *Journal of the Acoustical Society of America, 105*(1), 467–475.

Salas-Provance, M. B., & Kuehn, D. P. (1990). Speech status following uvulopalatopharyngoplasty [see Comments]. *Chest, 97*(1), 111–117.

Saunders, N. C., Hartley, B. E., Sell, D., & Sommerlad, B. (2004). Velopharyngeal insufficiency following adenoidectomy. *Clinical Otolaryngology & Allied Sciences, 29*(6), 686–688.

Schmaman, L., Jordaan, H., & Jammine, G. H. (1998). Risk factors for permanent hypernasality after adenoidectomy. *South Africa Medical Journal, 88*(3), 266–269.

Sheahan, P., Miller, I., Earley, M. J., Sheahan, J. N., & Blayney, A. W. (2004). Middle ear disease in children with congenital velopharyngeal insufficiency. *Cleft Palate-Craniofacial Journal, 41*(4), 364–367.

Shprintzen, R. J., Sher, A. E., & Croft, C. B. (1987). Hypernasal speech caused by tonsillar hypertrophy. *International Journal of*

Pediatric Otorhinolaryngology, *14*(1), 45–56.

Sininger, Y., Doyle, K., & Moore, J. (1999). The case for early identification of hearing loss in children: Auditory system development, experimental auditory deprivation, and development of speech perception and hearing. *Pediatric Clinics of North America*, *46*(2), 1–14.

Tachimura, T., Hara, H., Koh, H., & Wada, T. (1997). Effect of temporary closure of oronasal fistulae on levator veli palatini muscle activity. *Cleft Palate-Craniofacial Journal*, *34*(6), 505–511.

Teele, D., Klein, J., & Rosner, B. (1980). Epidemiology of otitis media in children. *Annals of Otology, Rhinology, and Laryngology*, *89*(3, Suppl.), 5–6.

Trujillo, L. (1994). Prevention of conductive hearing loss in cleft palate patients. *Folia Phoniatrica et Logopedica*, *46*(3), 123–126.

Van Borsel, J., Van Snick, K., & Leroy, J. (1999). Macroglossia and speech in Beckwith-Wiedemann syndrome: A sample survey study. *International Journal of Language & Communication Disorders*, *34*(2), 209–221.

Witzel, M. A., Rich, R. H., Margar-Bacal, F., & Cox, C. (1986). Velopharyngeal insufficiency after adenoidectomy: An 8-year review. *International Journal of Pediatric Otorhinolaryngology*, *11*(1), 15–20.

Yanagisawa, E., & Weaver, E. M. (1997). An unusual appearance of velopharyngeal closure in a post-uvulopalatopharyngoplasty patient. *Ear Nose and Throat Journal*, *76*(1), 14–15.

CHAPTER
9

DENTAL ANOMALIES ASSOCIATED WITH CLEFT LIP/PALATE: EFFECTS ON SPEECH

RICHARD CAMPBELL, D.M.D., M.S.

MURRAY DOCK, D.D.S., M.S.D.

WITH CONTRIBUTIONS FROM ANN W. KUMMER, PH.D.

CHAPTER OUTLINE

INTRODUCTION

Dental problems in children with cleft lip and palate or craniofacial syndromes can be quite complex. These problems frequently require dental specialists to coordinate treatment with other health care providers in order to properly manage the patient (Kirschner & LaRossa, 2000; Kuijpers-Jagtman, Borstlap-Engels, Spauwen, & Borstlap, 2000; Mouradian, Omnell, & Williams, 1999). The specialists involved usually include a pediatric dentist, an orthodontist, an oral maxillofacial surgeon, and a prosthodontist (Strong, 2002; Turvey, Vig, & Fonseca, 1996; Vasan, 1999). Together, they monitor and treat problems of the developing dentition, occlusion, and facial growth of the cleft lip/palate patient (Strauss, 1998, 1999). As dental professionals reconstruct the oral environment, the speech-language pathologist can correct functional modifications in speech that may have developed due to abnormal structure. Close cooperation between the dental specialists and the speech-language pathologist leads to a more holistic management of the structural and functional effects of dental and speech abnormalities.

A brief review of the dentition and its effect on speech production follows. Oral anatomy was covered in Chapter 1 and will not be repeated in this chapter.

NORMAL DENTITION

The dentition can be visualized as two arches of teeth, a maxillary and a mandibular arch. Each arch consists of a right and left half, so that the teeth in the arch are paired, one of each on either side (Figure 9–1).

There are two sets of teeth. The first set is known as the primary or *deciduous* teeth (Figure 9–2). They are sometimes referred to as deciduous because they are shed and replaced by the second set of teeth. The second set is known as the secondary, permanent, or *succedaneous* teeth. To be strictly correct, the permanent molars have no primary precursors and so they are not truly succedaneous.

Many terms are used to describe the positions of the teeth in the arch (Figure 9–1). The dental midline is at the apex of the arch where the left and right halves join. The direction toward the midline is *mesial*. The direction away from the midline is *distal*.

The outer part of the arch that touches the lip is *labial*. The part of the arch that is posterior to the canine teeth is frequently referred to as *buccal*, for the buccinator muscle that moves the cheeks. The inner part of the upper and lower arch that is in contact with the tongue is referred to as *lingual*. Many clinicians refer to the inner part of the upper arch as *palatal*, because of its proximity to the surface of the hard palate.

Number and Types of Teeth

In the deciduous dentition there are 20 teeth, 10 in each arch. In one arch, starting from the midline and moving distally, the pairs are the central incisors, the lateral incisors, the canines (cuspids), the primary first molars, and the primary second molars (Figure 9–2).

In the permanent dentition there are 32 teeth, 16 in each arch (see Figure 9–1). In one arch, starting from the midline and proceeding

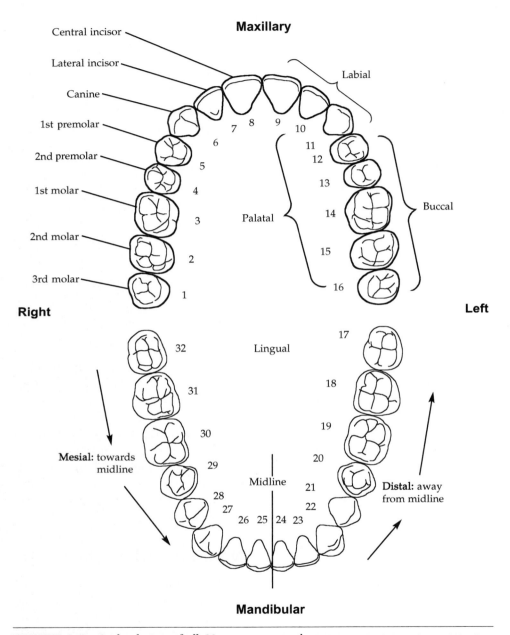

FIGURE 9–1   Occlusal view of all 32 permanent teeth. (Modified and printed with permission from LifeART Super Anatomy 6 Collection. Baltimore, MD: Lippincott Williams & Wilkins.)

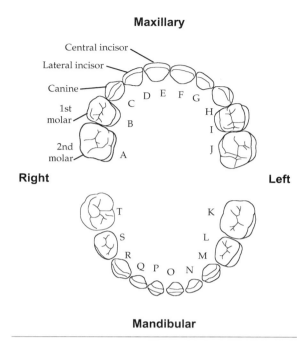

FIGURE 9–2 Occlusal view of all 20 primary teeth. (Modified and printed with permission from LifeART Super Anatomy 6 Collection. Baltimore, MD: Lippincott Williams & Wilkins.)

to the distal, the pairs are the central incisors, the lateral incisors, the canines (cuspids), the first premolars (first bicuspids), the second premolars (second bicuspids), the first molars (6-year molars), the second molars (12-year molars) and lastly, the third molars (wisdom teeth). In addition to these anatomical names, the primary teeth are often lettered A through T, and the permanent teeth are numbered 1 through 32.

The incisor teeth are somewhat shovel shaped and their biting surfaces are thin, knifelike edges. The remaining teeth have rounded points for chewing. The points are known as cusps. Canines have one point or cusp. Premolars typically have two cusps, although they may sometimes have three. Cusps are arranged in rows, one to the outside (buccal or labial) and one to the inside (palatal or lingual). Upper molars have four cusps, two buccal and two palatal (or lingual). Lower molars have four or five cusps, two or three buccal and two lingual. This buccal cusp to lingual cusp arrangement creates a valley between the cusps, called the *central fossa*. Variations in the shapes of teeth and the number of cusps do occur, but are usually of only academic interest to the clinician.

Occlusion and Molar Relationship

Dental occlusion is the manner in which the teeth fit together, or the bite. In normal occlusion, the upper arch overlaps the lower arch, so that the cusps of one arch fit into the fossae of the opposing arch (Figure 9–3).

The anterior-posterior relationship of the mesiobuccal cusp of the upper molar to the buccal groove of the lower molar is used to classify the type of occlusion. First described by Angle, the *Angle Classification System* differentiates normal occlusion and three types of malocclusion. Brilliant in its simplicity, it remains in widespread use today (Table 9–1) (Katz, 1992; Proffit & Fields, 2000).

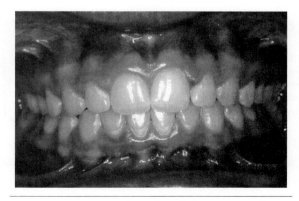

FIGURE 9–3 Normal overlap of the upper teeth over the lower teeth.

TABLE 9–1   Angle's Classification of Occlusion and Skeletal Relationships

Classification	Example	Skeletal Classification	Diagram
Class I occlusion The *mesiobuccal* cusp of the upper molar occludes in the buccal groove of the lower molar; the remaining teeth are arranged upon a smoothly curving line.	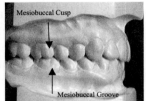	Class I—Normal	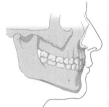
Class I malocclusion Normal relationship of the molars, but line of occlusion incorrect because of malposed teeth, rotations, or other causes.	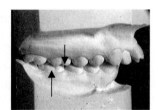	Class I—Normal	(same as above)
Class II malocclusion Lower molar distally positioned relative to upper molar; line of occlusion not specified.	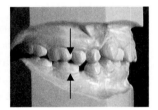	Class II—Mandibular retrusion and/or maxillary protrusion	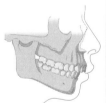
Class III malocclusion Lower molar mesially positioned relative to upper molar; line of occlusion not specified.	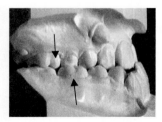	Class III—Mandibular protrusion and/or maxillary retrusion	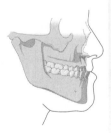

Mesiobuccal Cusp

Mesiobuccal Groove

Skeletal Relationships

The Angle classification applies only to tooth relationships. It does not account for the influence of the relationship of the upper jaw to the lower jaw on tooth position or facial profile. Consequently, the Angle system must be supplemented to describe skeletal relationships. Angle's concept of the upper molar to lower molar relationship has been applied to describe the upper jaw to lower jaw relationship. The jaw relationships may be referred to as Class I, Class II, and Class III (see Table 9–1). Often the jaw relationship mirrors the dental relationship.

Cephalometric radiographs are lateral skull films, taken with the patient's head held in a standardized position (Figure 9–4). *Cephalometric analyses* are used to measure the jaw relationship and the soft tissue profile of the forehead, nose, lips, and chin (Figure 9–5). An abnormal skeletal relationship may result from the upper jaw, the lower jaw, or both being out of normal position relative to the base of the skull.

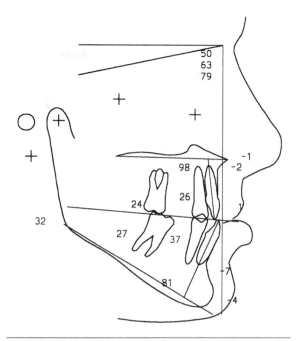

FIGURE 9–5 Cephalometric tracing. A tracing of a cephalometric X-ray is made so that measurement can be drawn without damaging the film. A set of measurements is called an analysis, and is frequently named after its founder, i.e., the Steiner Analysis, or the McNamara Analysis. This particular depiction is the COGS Analysis or Cephalometric Analysis for Orthognathic Surgery devised by Burstone. The image was generated by Dentofacial Planner.

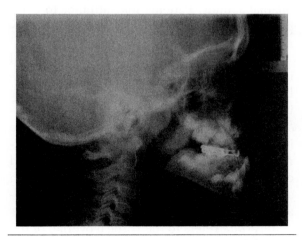

FIGURE 9–4 Cephalometric X-ray. A cephalometric X-ray is a lateral skull film made with a cephalostat, a device with ear rods and a nasal bridge rest to allow reproducible head positioning. This allows comparisons of X-rays of the patient taken at different times for use in longitudinal growth studies.

DENTAL ANOMALIES AND SPEECH

With normal occlusion, the tongue rests in the mandible behind the mandibular incisors. The maxillary teeth overlap the mandibular teeth. This leaves plenty of room for the tongue tip to articulate freely in the oral cavity against and under the alveolar ridge. In addition, the upper and lower lips are approximated, making bilabial and labiodental sounds easy to produce.

When there are dental or occlusal anomalies, however, this can inhibit the function of the tongue and lips, causing speech problems (Shprintzen et al., 1985). Many speech sounds can be affected because most consonants are produced in the front of the oral cavity near the anterior dental arch (Shprintzen, Siegel-Sadewitz, Amato, & Goldberg, 1985).

Abnormalities of the dentition can cause either obligatory or compensatory errors (Trost-Cardamone, 1997). Obligatory errors occur when the labial or lingual position is correct, but the structural abnormalities interfere with movement during speech, resulting in distortion. Compensatory errors occur when there are structural abnormalities, and the labial or lingual position is altered in order to compensate for these abnormalities, resulting in substitution errors.

The sounds that are most commonly affected are sibilant phonemes (/s/, /z/, /sh/, /zh/, /ch/, /j/), because these sounds are produced partly by the teeth. Dental abnormalities may also affect labiodental phonemes (/f/, /v/), lingual-alveolar phonemes (/t/, /d/, /n/, /l/), and bilabial sounds (/p/, /b/, /m/). There does not appear to be a direct relationship between the severity of the malocclusion and the severity of the misarticulation, however. Instead, the individual's ability to adapt to structural abnormalities plays a significant role in the amount of distortion that results in speech (Johnson & Sandy, 1999).

Dental anomalies have the greatest effect on speech if they are present before or during speech development. The learned sound pattern may reflect a means to compensate for the structural restraints of the abnormality. These abnormalities have the least effect on speech if they occur after the development of normal speech, which is why speech is only minimally affected when individuals lose teeth in the adult years. Even edentulous people are usually able to articulate clearly. In addition, when there is premature loss of the deciduous incisors due to decay, this does not tend to affect speech unless there is also maxillary crowding (Gable, Kummer, Lee, Creaghead, & Moore, 1995).

Incisor Relationship

Overjet is the horizontal relationship of the upper to the lower incisors (Figure 9–6). It is typically measured in millimeters from the labial surface of the lower incisor to the labial surface of the upper incisor, with the teeth in occlusion. A normal amount of overjet is about 2 mm, with upper incisors and lower incisors in light contact. If the upper incisors are displaced anteriorly, with overjet greater than 2 mm, then labioversion is said to occur. Maxillary incisors that are labioverted protrude out toward the lips and in severe cases may prevent lip closure.

Labioversion affects speech by interfering with lip closure. This may alter the production of bilabial sounds. Patients may attempt to compensate for this by using a labiodental placement as a substitute for bilabial articulation.

Underjet refers to a reversal of the normal incisor position, so that the upper incisors are lingual to the lower incisors (Figure 9–7). This is also called *linguoversion* or *anterior crossbite*, and implies that most of the incisors are involved. Underjet can be measured in millimeters. Maxillary incisors that are linguoverted can interfere with tongue-tip movement, which alters the production of sibilants and lingual-alveolar sounds.

Overbite refers to the vertical overlap of the upper and lower incisors (Figure 9–8). It also may be measured in millimeters, though it is often reported as a percentage of coverage of the lower incisors by the upper incisors. Normal overbite is approximately 2 mm or

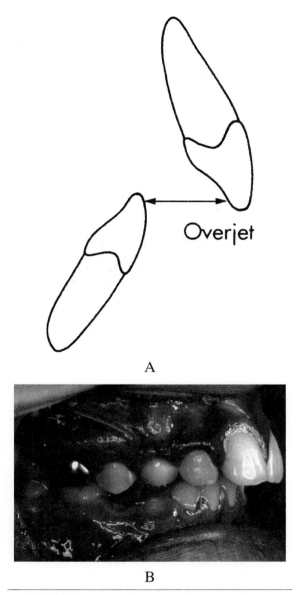

A

B

FIGURE 9–6 (A and B) Normal overjet. A. Overjet is the horizontal overlap of the incisors. B. Normal values average 2 mm. Larger values indicate increased overjet, usually from incisor protrusion. (Modified from *Contemporary Orthodontics*, 3rd ed., by W. R. Proffit and H. W. Fields, Jr., 2000. St. Louis, MO: Mosby-Yearbook, Inc. Copyright Mosby-Yearbook, Inc., 2000. Reprinted with permission.)

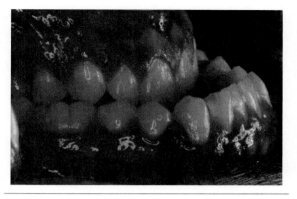

FIGURE 9–7 Underjet. Underjet is when the upper incisors are lingual to the lower incisors, as seen in this case of severe underjet.

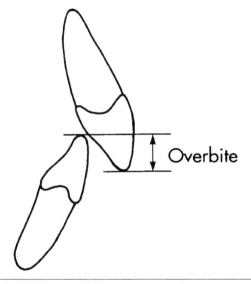

FIGURE 9–8 Overbite. An overbite is measured as the vertical overlap of the incisors from the incisal edges. Often expressed as a percentage of overbite, in this instance the upper incisor overlaps the lower incisor by approximately 50%, which may be expressed as a 50% overbite. (Modified from *Contemporary Orthodontics*, 3rd ed., by W. R. Proffit and H. W. Fields, Jr., 2000. St. Louis, MO: Mosby-Yearbook, Inc. Copyright Mosby-Yearbook, Inc. 2000. Reprinted with permission.)

about 25%. Greater amounts of overbite are associated with deep overbite, or *deepbite*. In some instances, the upper teeth completely overlap the lower, which is 100% overbite. If the lower incisors are in contact with the palate, this too is considered a 100% overbite. Deep overbite is usually associated with crowding and restricted tongue movement, which may alter the production of sibilants and lingual-alveolar sounds.

Diastema

A *diastema* is a space or opening between the teeth, usually the upper central incisors. A diastema usually does not affect speech (Figure 9–9).

Dental Anomalies with Clefts

Anomalies of the teeth and jaws are common in children with either repaired cleft of the lip and alveolus (primary palate) or craniofacial anomalies. These anomalies include missing teeth, supernumerary teeth, rotated teeth, crowding, crossbite, Class III malocclusion, open bite, and protruding premaxilla. Each of these anomalies has the potential to cause a

distortion of speech as noted in the following sections.

Missing Teeth

Congenitally missing teeth are a frequent finding in patients with history of cleft of the primary palate (Figure 9–10 A and B). Even children with a history of submucous cleft have an increased frequency of missing teeth or other dental abnormalities (Heliovaara, Ranta,

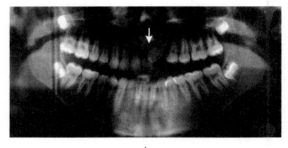

A

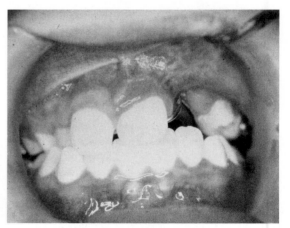

B

FIGURE 9–10 (A and B) Missing teeth from cleft site. A. A panoramic X-ray demonstrating a permanent tooth missing from the cleft site. The upper left lateral incisor (tooth #10) is frequently missing, as it is in this case (see the arrow), and the upper left canine has moved into its place. B. Missing teeth in the line of the cleft. The lateral incisor and canine are both missing.

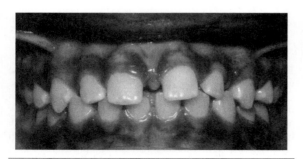

FIGURE 9–9 Diastema. A diastema is a space or opening between any of the teeth. Clinicians commonly use the term diastema to indicate the space between the maxillary central incisors, as seen in this case.

& Rautio, 2004). Most frequently, the missing teeth include the maxillary lateral incisor or the canine because these are the teeth that border the incisive suture lines or the cleft. Even when present, teeth in the area of the cleft may be smaller than normal, misshapen, or malformed.

The effect of missing teeth on speech depends on the size of the oral cavity. If oral cavity size is normal, there may be no effect on speech (Moller, 1994). If there is oral cavity crowding, however, due to a low, flat, or narrow maxillary arch, or maxillary retrusion or macroglossia, then the tongue will tend to seek an opening. This can be done by either opening the dental arch completely, or by seeking an opening in the dental arch where there are missing teeth. If the opening is in the line of the cleft and the tongue deviates to that opening, this will result in a lateral lisp because the air stream is redirected to the opposite side of the opening. A similar thing occurs if the maxillary central incisors are missing and there is oral cavity crowding. When this occurs, the tongue may protrude through the anterior opening during speech, producing a frontal lisp on sibilants and in some cases, lingual-alveolar sounds.

Rotated Teeth

Rotated teeth are common in individuals who have had a cleft of the primary palate (see Figure 9–11). Central incisors and lateral incisors, if present, are most often affected. The incisors may also be fused at the roots. Fortunately, this is more commonly found in the primary than in the permanent dentition. Rotated or malformed teeth affect speech by interfering with tongue-tip movement and diverting the air stream laterally, causing a lateral lisp. Patients who attempt to compensate for the interference of a rotated tooth by

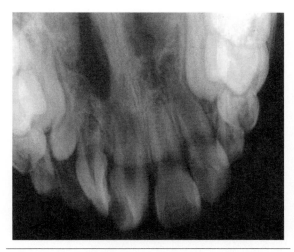

FIGURE 9–11 Rotated teeth in the cleft site. An occlusal X-ray demonstrates that teeth in the line of the cleft are frequently malpositioned or rotated about the long axis of the roots. In this view the maxillary right central and lateral incisors arrows are rotated approximately 90 degrees each, so that the lingual surfaces of their crowns are facing each other. By comparison, the maxillary left central and lateral incisors are nearly normal with almost no rotation (the right side of this view). Note that there is also a supernumerary tooth distal to the rotated incisors.

retracting the tongue will also have a lateral distortion because this causes the dorsum to be elevated and in the way of the airstream.

Supernumerary or Ectopic Teeth

Instead of missing teeth, *supernumerary teeth* (extra teeth) (Figure 9–12A) or *ectopic teeth* (teeth that erupt in an abnormal position) (Figure 9–12B) may occur in the line of the cleft. These often remain unerupted, although they will occasionally erupt partially or even completely. If erupted, a supernumerary tooth may be displaced palatally or labially. A similar problem occurs with an ectopic tooth, which is a normal tooth that erupts into an abnormal position.

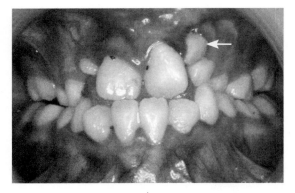

A

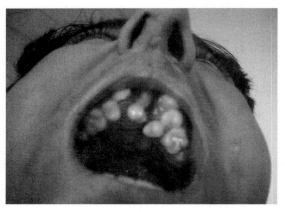

B

FIGURE 9–12 (A and B) Supernumerary and ectopic teeth. A. An extra tooth may occur in the line of the cleft, as in this case of a supernumerary primary incisor, distal and superior to the patient's maxillary left central incisor (arrow). B. Multiple ectopic teeth in the area of lingual movement for speech.

Depending on its placement, the ectopic or supernumerary tooth may interfere with tongue movement, causing distortion of lingual-alveolar sounds or even interdental sounds. Sibilants can be affected by the diversion of the airstream laterally, causing a lateral lisp. If the tooth is in the area of the alveolar ridge, the patient may learn to compensate by using the dorsum of the tongue for articulation, resulting in distortion of tongue-tip sounds.

Crossbite

Crossbite is a common dental abnormality in children with a history of cleft lip and palate. In crossbite, the normal overlap of the upper teeth to the lower teeth is reversed, so that the lower teeth overlap the upper teeth buccally. A crossbite may involve only one upper and one lower tooth, called a *single-tooth crossbite* (Figure 9–13). When multitooth crossbites occur, they are described by their position in the dental arch as either anterior or posterior.

An *anterior crossbite* may involve any or all of the anterior teeth: the central incisors, lateral incisors, or canines (Figure 9–14). *Anterior crossbites*, characterized by the maxillary incisors positioned inside the mandibular incisors, are commonly seen in patients with dental or skeletal Class III malocclusion. *Posterior crossbite* involves any combination of teeth distal (posterior) to the canines and usually occurs because the maxilla is too narrow. Often, a multiple-tooth crossbite involves a combination of anterior as well as posterior teeth. When a posterior crossbite is limited to one side of the arch, the

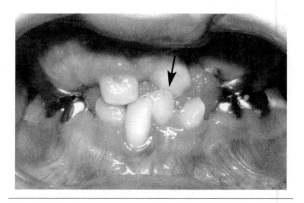

FIGURE 9–13 Single-tooth crossbite. A crossbite involving only one tooth may be referred to as a single-tooth crossbite. Often a maxillary central or lateral incisor is involved, as in this case of the upper left central incisor being displaced lingually to the lower left central incisor (see the arrow).

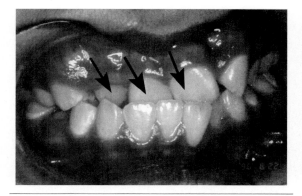

FIGURE 9–14 Anterior crossbite. When most of the incisors are involved in crossbite, an anterior crossbite is said to have occurred, as in this patient with anterior crossbite of both of the maxillary central incisors and the maxillary right cuspid (arrows).

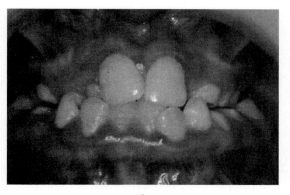

A

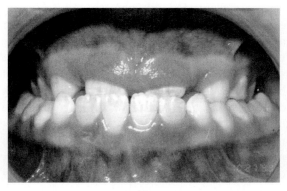

B

FIGURE 9–16 (A and B) Bilateral crossbite. A. The maxillary posterior teeth on both sides are lingual to the mandibular teeth. B. When all the maxillary teeth fit inside the mandibular teeth, a total crossbite exists.

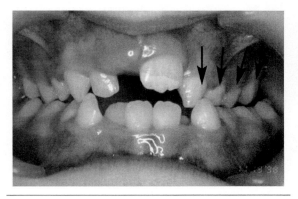

FIGURE 9–15 Unilateral posterior crossbite. The posterior teeth of the patient's maxillary left side are lingual to the mandibular teeth (arrows). This is referred to as a posterior crossbite. It may also be called a unilateral posterior crossbite.

crossbite is referred to as being unilateral (Figure 9–15). When both the right and left posterior sides are involved, the crossbite is referred to as being bilateral (Figure 9–16A). When mild, a bilateral crossbite may produce a shift of the mandible to one side, which gives the clinical appearance of a unilateral crossbite. A more severe bilateral posterior crossbite rarely produces such a shift of the mandible. Careful examination of the patient's occlusion as the teeth first contact during closure helps to distinguish bilateral crossbite with mandibular shift from a true unilateral crossbite. A *buccal crossbite* occurs when one or more maxillary teeth are positioned buccally such that the maxillary lingual cusps reside buccal to the mandibular cusps. The relatively rare *Brodie crossbite* occurs when the lingual cusps of all the maxillary posterior teeth are buccal to the mandibular teeth (Figure 9–16B).

A crossbite can affect speech in several ways. An anterior crossbite, especially with Class III malocclusion, may cause distortion of sibilants or lingual-alveolar sounds due interference of the maxillary incisors (Kummer, Strife, Grau, Creaghead, & Lee, 1989; Moller, 1994; Taher, 1997). If the tongue remains in normal position in the mandible despite the anterior crossbite, this may cause a frontal lisp as an obligatory error. If the tongue retracts to compensate for crowding of the anterior part of the oral cavity, this can cause the dorsum to elevate and articulate with the palate, resulting in a middorsum palatal placement (palatal-dorsal production), a lateral lisp on sibilants (/s/, /z/, /zh/, /sh/, /ch/, /j/), and even a lateral distortion on lingual-alveolar sounds (/t/, /d/, /n/, /l/). An anterior crossbite may interfere with labiodental placement sounds (/f/, /v/) because it is difficult to retract the bottom lip far enough back to the position of the maxillary incisors. As a result, the individual may use a reverse labiodental placement so that the upper lip articulates with the mandibular incisors (Moller, 1994). A posterior crossbite can restrict oral cavity size, resulting in a distortion of speech because the teeth will often open during articulation to compensate. Complete crossbite can result in the distortion of many sounds, particularly tongue-tip sounds, due to the very limited space for normal tongue movement.

Protruding Premaxilla

Infants affected by bilateral cleft lip and palate often have a protruding premaxilla at birth. This condition has been attributed to an overgrowth of the premaxilla, which is untethered by the lateral palatal segments. Past treatment included surgical removal of the premaxilla (Figure 9–17A), but this had deleterious effects on midfacial growth (Proffit, White, & Sarver, 2003). Fortunately, the procedure has been abandoned. The lateral

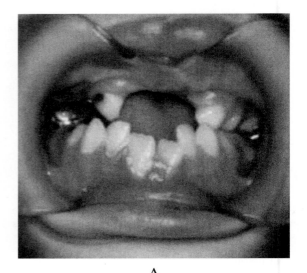

A

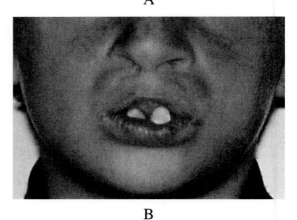

B

FIGURE 9–17 (A and B) A. Missing maxillary incisors due to excision of the premaxilla. Fortunately, this procedure is no longer done. B. Protruding premaxilla.

segments, lacking sufficient palatal shelf resistance, are displaced medially so that there is no room for the premaxilla to fit in its normal position. Untreated, the premaxilla remains protrusive due to lack of space (Figure 9–17B).

When the premaxilla is in an anterior position, the position of the alveolar ridge relative to the tongue tip may be altered, causing a mild distortion of sibilants. A protruding premaxilla can particularly interfere with lip closure and therefore the production of bilabial sounds (/p/, /b/, /m/). Labiodental placement may be used as a substitute. This results in little distortion in speech, but it may be visually distracting because of abnormal lip placement.

Open Bite

Open bite occurs when one or more maxillary teeth fail to occlude with the opposing mandibular teeth (Figure 9–18). Open bites primarily affect the anterior dentition (anterior open bite) and less commonly the posterior dentition (lateral open bite). Causes of open bite include missing teeth, digit or pacifier sucking habits, and skeletal discrepancies. Open bites will be sealed by the tongue on swallowing, which is often confused as tongue thrust (Proffit & Fields, 2000).

An open bite has the same potential effect on speech production as missing teeth, but the effect is usually more pronounced. An anterior open bite is most likely to affect the production of sibilant sounds, particularly the fricatives (/s/, /z/, /sh/, /zh/), but often the affricates (/ch/, /j/) as well. With an anterior open bite, there is a tendency for the tongue to seek the opening, particularly if there is oral cavity crowding. As a result, sounds are produced interdentally, resulting in a frontal lisp. Even if the tongue remains in the normal position, the acoustic product may lack appropriate sibilance. A lateral open bite is less likely to affect speech because it is away from the tongue tip and is lateral to the direction of the airstream. If the tongue tip moves toward the open bite, however, it will divert the airstream to the contralateral side and result in a lateral distortion of sibilants.

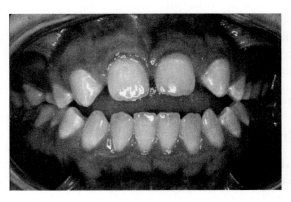

B

FIGURE 9–18 (A and B) Open bite. A. The anterior teeth are not in contact. B. Open bite is often attributed to tongue thrust, but little evidence exists to support that assumption. Open bite is difficult to treat, often in-volving orthognathic surgery in conjunction with orthodontics. (Figure A is from *Contemporary Orthodontics*, 3rd ed., by W. R. Proffit and H. W. Fields, Jr., 2000. St. Louis, MO: Mosby-Yearbook, Inc. Copyright Mosby-Yearbook, Inc. 2000. Reprinted with permission.)

↕ Open bite

A

TABLE 9–2   Stages of Dental Development and Treatment in Cleft Lip and Palate

Infant stage	0–12 months	Maxillary orthopedics, lip repair, palate repair
Primary dentition	1 to 6 years	Correction of crossbites affecting mandibular posture
Early mixed dentition	6 to 9 years	Maxillary expansion for bone graft as indicated
Late mixed dentition	9 to 12 years	Incisor alignment and maxillary expansion for bone graft if not done earlier
Adolescent dentition	12 to 18 years	Orthodontics, orthognathic surgery often required, prosthodontics if needed

DENTAL DEVELOPMENT AND STAGES OF CLEFT TREATMENT

Treatment of dental problems in children with a history of cleft lip and palate is timed to follow the normal stages of dental development. For instance, maxillary expansion to correct crossbite may be coordinated with the eruption of specific teeth, because it also serves to prepare the patient for secondary alveolar bone grafting (Table 9–2). Some interventions may be done to coincide with growth spurts as in mixed dentition treatment. Others may be delayed until the completion of growth, such as combined orthodontic and orthognathic surgical treatment (Posnick & Ricalde, 2004; Vig & Turvey, 1985).

Infant Stage

Most infants are born without any erupted teeth. The infant stage, therefore, involves the eruption of the primary teeth and lasts until 12 months of age. Occasionally a tooth may be present at birth and should be examined by a pediatric dentist to evaluate its stability in the arch. Most often, these teeth are not supernumerary and every attempt should be made to retain them when possible.

The eruption sequence for the primary teeth, as well as for the permanent teeth, is fairly predictable (Table 9–3); however, there

TABLE 9–3   Tooth Eruption for Primary and Permanent Dentitions

Primary Tooth	Maxillary	Mandibular
Central	10 mo.	8 mo.
Lateral	11 mo.	13 mo.
Canine	19 mo.	20 mo.
1st Molar	16 mo.	16 mo.
2nd Molar	29 mo.	27 mo.
Permanent Tooth		
Central	7.25 yr.	6.25 yr.
Lateral	8.25 yr.	7.5 yr.
Canine	11.5 yr.	10.5 yr.
1st Premolar	10.25 yr.	10.5 yr.
2nd Premolar	11 yr.	11.25 yr.
1st Molar	6.25 yr.	6 yr.
2nd Molar	12.5 yr.	12 yr.
3rd Molar	20 yr.	20 yr.

Source: Adapted from Profit and Field, 2000.

is considerable variation from one individual to another with regard to chronological timing. For primary teeth, a variation in eruption of 6 months on either side of the expected eruption is no cause for alarm. The lower primary incisors are usually the first teeth to erupt, at around 8 months of age. The remaining incisors are close behind, completing their eruption by 10 to 13 months of age. The canines erupt between 19 and 20 months, followed by the first molars at 16 months, and finally the second molars by 27 to 29 months (Proffit & Fields, 2000).

Treatment for an infant with a cleft lip and palate typically consists of two stages: lip closure and then palate closure. In the first stage, at about 12 weeks of age, the surgeon closes the lip. This facilitates feeding and the improvement in the infant's appearance helps with the parents' psychosocial adjustment. At the second stage, between 9 to 12 months of age, the cleft of the palate is closed.

The surgeon and dentist may need to adjust their treatment approach according to the size of the cleft and whether the cleft is unilateral or bilateral. In the case of a small unilateral or bilateral cleft of the lip, the lip can be closed without any need for manipulation of the alveolar segments. In the case of a large unilateral cleft (Figure 9–19), many surgeons prefer to have the interalveolar gap reduced prior to lip closure. Bilateral clefts of the lip and palate are more challenging (Figure 9–20). Not only are there two clefts to deal with but

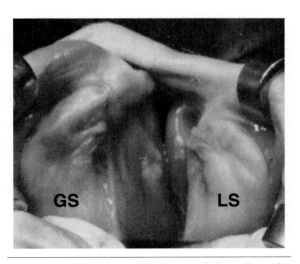

FIGURE 9–19 The occlusal view of the palate of a newborn with unilateral cleft lip and palate. The greater segment (GS) is on the left in the photograph and the lesser segment (LS) is on the right.

there is often a protruding premaxillary segment (Bitter, 2001; Liao, Huang, Liou, Lin, & Ko, 1998). Additionally, the posterior alveolar segments often will be narrow. Treatment is usually directed at retracting the protruding premaxillary segment while widening the narrow lateral segments.

There are numerous ways to accomplish alignment of the alveolar segments in both unilateral and bilateral clefts of the palate. Regardless of which technique is chosen, the process is referred to as *palatal orthopedics* or infant oral *orthopedics* (Figure 9–21, A–D). The techniques include, from least invasive to most invasive: taping of the lip (Figure 9–22, A–C); elastic straps over the lip and attached to a bonnet; passive molding appliances with or without taping; lip adhesion (temporary surgical closure) prior to lip repair; and pin-retained active intraoral appliances (Cho, 2001; Oosterkamp et al., 2005). Each method has advantages and disadvantages (Table 9–4). The choice of one method over another will vary, depending on the individual needs of the patient, the experience of the practitioners, and the overall philosophy regarding palatal orthopedics at a particular treatment center. Palatal orthopedic methods are controversial and remain a lively topic of debate among practitioners. Indeed, some authors disparage any repositioning of the palatal segments. These authors also suggest that these procedures may result in decreased midfacial growth (Berkowitz, Mejia, & Bystrik, 2004; Bongaarts, Kuijpers-Jagtman, van't Hof, & Prahl-Andersen, 2004). Hopefully, further research will elucidate the appropriate application of each method (Berkowitz et al., 2005; Braumann, Keilig, Bourauel, & Jager, 2002; Chan, Hayes, Shusterman, Mulliken, & Will, 2003; Millard, Latham, Huifen, Spiro, & Morovic, 1999; Prahl, Kuijpers-Jagtman, van't Hof, & Prahl-Andersen, 2003, 2005).

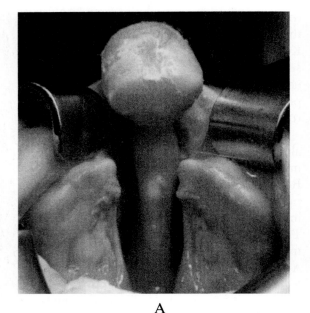

A

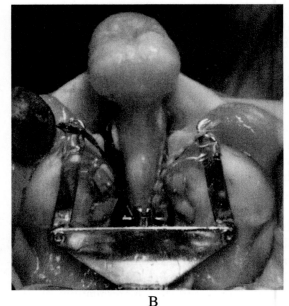

B

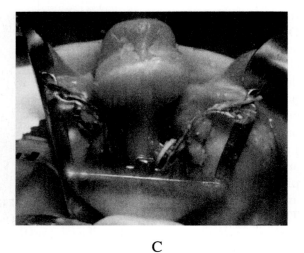

C

FIGURE 9–20 (A–C) A. The occlusal view of the palate of an infant with bilateral cleft lip and palate. The premaxillary segment is at the top middle of the photograph and the two lateral segments are on either side, left or right and posterior to the premaxillary segment in the photograph. B. A pin-retained appliance used to reposition the segments. C. The maxillary segment is retracted and the lateral segment is widened.

The cleft condition affects not only the lip and alveolus, but the nose as well. For infants with complete cleft lip, *nasal molding* is often done to reposition the deformed nasal cartilage and lengthen the deficient columella. The technique involves applying pressure to the tip of the affected nostril from an intraoral or extraoral approach and can be done in combination with alveolar molding of cleft palatal segments (Cutting et al., 1998; Da Silveira et al., 2003). The nasal molding appliance is worn from early infancy for a period of several months after the lip is closed (Doruk & Kilic, 2005). In bilateral clefts, attempts are made to lengthen the columella of the nose, again with an intraoral/nasal appliance and various struts of wire or acrylic. Quite often,

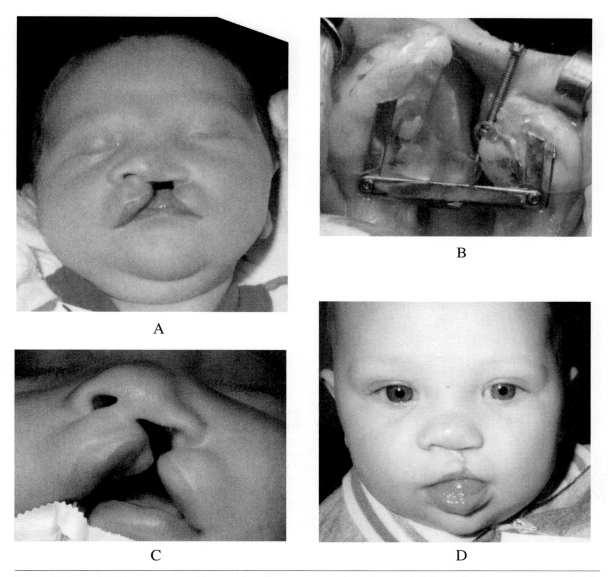

FIGURE 9–21 (A–D) Pin-retained intraoral appliance. A. A wide unilateral cleft lip and palate. B. In cases of wide clefts, some surgeons prefer to have the width of the cleft between greater and lesser segments reduced with an appliance. C. The appliance gives a closer approximation of the lip segments. D. The close approximation of the segments allows for lip closure with less tension than by other means.

taping is required (Grayson & Cutting, 2001; Grayson & Maull, 2004).

Some centers also perform primary *alveolar bone grafting* in the infant stage. An attempt to

bridge the gap between the bony segments of the alveolus is made by placing bone formation-inducing material, such as split thickness rib or cancellous bone from the hip, into the cleft site

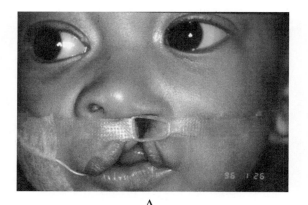

A

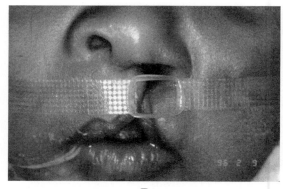

B

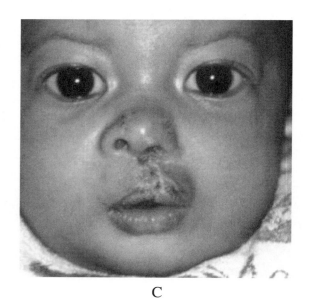

C

FIGURE 9–22 (A–C) Taping of the lip. Narrow separations of the lip may be approximated by extraoral taping, in this case with an additional elastic, making surgical closure less difficult. A. Beginning of taping. This shows separation of lip. B. After a few weeks the lip segments are approximated. C. In this view, taken very shortly after lip closure, one can appreciate that there is little tension across the now joined lip segments.

(Hathaway, Eppley, Hennon, Nelson, & Sadove, 1999; Hathaway, Eppley, Nelson, & Sadove, 1999; Rosenstein, Dado, Kernahan, Griffith, & Grasseschi, 1991). The goal is to unify the alveolar segments into a continuous arch, thus consolidating the maxilla into one piece. Primary grafting is intended to stabilize the arch, thereby preventing future crossbite, as well as to create bone, which will provide a path for the eruption of teeth near the cleft (Lee, Grayson, Cutting, Brecht, & Lin, 2004).

Unfortunately, results are mixed; some infants will gain the desired arch unity and sufficient bone for tooth eruption, but many do not. Markedly decreased growth of the midface is another undesirable effect that has been associated with primary alveolar bone grafting. Centers debate differences in surgical technique and timing as it relates to success or failure (Pfeifer, Grayson, & Cutting, 2002; Sachs, 2002). In particular, much attention has been focused on the amount of gingival, nasal,

TABLE 9–4 Methods of Unilateral Cleft Lip and Palate Closure

Method	Advantages	Disadvantages
Surgical only	Quick, no pre-op manipulations required.	Limited to smaller clefts, no control of segment position post-op.
Taping	Noninvasive, no dental impressions required.	Parent cooperation essential, skin irritation common, no control of segments.
Passive molding plates with or without taping	Allows some repositioning of segments. Serves as retainers, aids feeding.	Dental impressions required. Parents' cooperation a must. Denture adhesives often used.
Lip adhesion	Decreases size of intra-alveolar gap, allows tension-free closure.	Requires additional surgery. Surgeon must perform final closure through scar tissue. No post-op segment control.
Pin-retained active appliance	Greater control of segments. Effective at reducing wide clefts. Allows tension-free lip closure.	Requires dental impressions or visit for placement, parent cooperation. Long-term effects on maxillary growth unknown.

and oral mucosa that is manipulated by the surgeon in closing the infant alveolar cleft. This procedure is often called *gingivoperiosteoplasty*, particularly in reference to closing the cleft of the alveolus with raised gingival flaps at the same time that the palatal closure is performed (Millard et al., 1999). Success rates are low and secondary alveolar bone grafting procedures may be required (Millard et al., 1999; Renkielska, Wojtaszek-Slominska, & Dobke, 2005). After the lip and palate are closed, the infant enjoys a reprieve from dental and surgical intervention for a few years until the primary dentition erupts.

Primary Dentition (1–6 Years)

The primary dentition is usually complete by 24 to 30 months of age with 10 teeth in the upper arch and 10 in the lower arch. Ideally, there should be spacing between all of the primary teeth. This may be upsetting to some parents, but spacing of the primary teeth is necessary so that there is room for the larger permanent teeth that will replace them. Thus,

a child with little or no spacing between the primary teeth is at risk for significant crowding of the permanent teeth (Ngan, Alkire, & Fields, 1999). Children with repaired cleft lip and palate often demonstrate maxillary retrusion, attributed to surgical scarring, as well as a maxilla that is smaller than normal in every dimension. Therefore, it is not unusual to see crowding associated with the primary teeth in this population (DiBiase, DiBiase, Hay, & Sommerlad, 2002; Garrahy, Millett, & Ayoub, 2005).

There may be several dental abnormalities in the primary dentition at this stage. The area of the cleft may be missing a primary lateral incisor. Conversely, a *supernumerary tooth* (extra tooth) may be located near the cleft site. They may appear either palatally or labially, but are not often directly in the cleft due to its deficit of tissue. Malformations of these teeth are common (Chapple & Nunn, 2001; Maciel, Costa, & Gomide, 2005; Malanczuk, Opitz, & Retzlaff, 1999). Also, natal or neonatal teeth are a common finding in children with either unilateral or bilateral clefting (Cabete,

Gomide, & Costa, 2000). Crossbite in the cleft area is also very common due to the altered anatomy of the palate. The maxilla in unilateral clefts consists of two segments, a *lesser segment* on the cleft side (cleft segment) and a *greater segment* on the noncleft side (noncleft segment) (see Figure 9–19). The greater and lesser segments are not joined at the site of the cleft, and as a result, they can be displaced by lip pressure; thus, it is common to find crossbite on the affected side. In bilateral clefts, there are three maxillary segments, one premaxillary segment, and two lateral segments. The lateral segments may be displaced medially, which frequently results in a bilateral crossbite. The premaxillary segment may be protrusive (see Figure 9–20).

Clinicians have long been aware that children with a repaired cleft lip and palate frequently appear to have relatively normal upper to lower jaw relationships in the primary dentition (Figure 9–23A); this, however, does not last into adolescence (Figure 9–23B) (Grayson, Bookstein, McCarthy, & Mueeddin, 1987). Although the cleft maxilla is smaller than those of unaffected children, the mandible also is normally smaller at this stage of development. Thus, maxillary position may appear to be relatively normal in the primary dentition stage because mandibular growth has not yet begun. During the adolescent growth spurt, however, the mandible increases to its normal size. Unfortunately, as the mandible grows, the maxilla appears more and more retrusive, thereby exposing its deficiency (Lisson, Hanke, & Trankmann, 2004; Scheuer, Holtje, Hasund, & Pfeifer, 2001; Veleminska, Smahel, & Mullerova, 2003).

Children with clefts are at risk for periodontal disease localized to teeth near the cleft; therefore, every effort to establish proper oral hygiene measures at home should be made (Chapple & Nunn, 2001; Dewinter et al.,

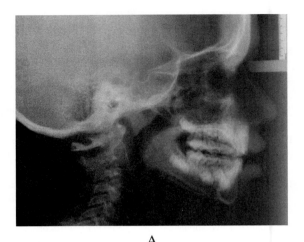

A

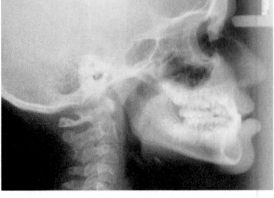

B

FIGURE 9–23 (A and B) Normal occlusion in early dentition that changes in adolescence. A. The jaw and dental relationships are good in the early mixed dentition cephalogram of a patient with unilateral cleft lip and palate. This patient exhibits a nearly Class I occlusion and midfacial retrusion is not obvious. B. Unfortunately, because of the mandibular growth spurt of adolescence, the relationships have changed for the worse. The patient now has a dental and skeletal Class III malocclusion with underbite and underjet, manifestations of the lack of midfacial growth often seen in patients with cleft lip and palate.

2003; Gaggl, Schultes, Karcher, & Mossbock, 1999; Kirchberg, Treide, & Hemprich, 2004; Schultes, Gaggl, & Karcher, 1999; Quirynen et al., 2003). Few conditions require orthodontic intervention in the primary dentition. However, any crossbite that causes a functional shift of the mandible—that is, a reposturing of the mandible to achieve a more comfortable bite—will need to be addressed as soon as feasible. Left untreated, such posturing may cause overgrowth of one *condyle* (jaw joint), resulting in an asymmetry of the mandible. This will appear as a chin that is deviated to the nonaffected side (Proffit & Fields, 2000). In children with clefts, a significant narrowing of the maxillary segments is sometimes addressed in the primary dentition, especially if a crossbite or crowding of the primary teeth occurs.

Treatment for crossbite in the primary dentition usually involves some form of maxillary expansion. Maxillary expansion may be started at 4 to 5 years of age in a cooperative child. Either one of two appliances is usually chosen for maxillary expansion. One appliance, the quad helix, consists of orthodontic bands on the most posterior molars, and frequently the primary canines as well (Figure 9–24A) (Kirchberg, Treide, & Hemprich, 2004). The bands are connected by a palatal spring that has two posterior loops, each adjacent to a molar, and two anterior loops. These four loops or helices give the quad helix its name. Some clinicians prefer to not include the helices and the resulting W-shaped palatal spring is called a *W-arch*. The other appliance frequently used to correct crossbite is a *rapid palatal expander*, or RPE. It consists of two or four orthodontic bands connected by a jackscrew in the middle of the palate (Figure 9–24B). Turning the screw creates the necessary force to widen the arch. The rapid palatal expander is capable of delivering very heavy forces so it must be used with caution in the primary dentition. The goal for either the *quad helix* or the rapid palatal expander is to create adequate width of the maxilla. Because children with clefts may also have an anterior crossbite, some clinicians may

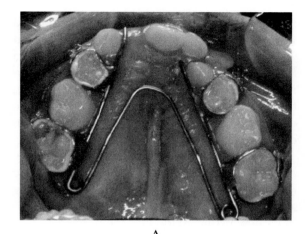

A

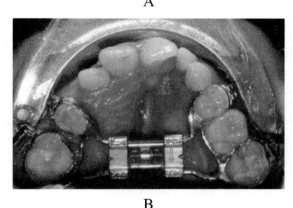

B

FIGURE 9–24 (A and B) Appliances used for maxillary expansion. A. The quad helix consists of a palatal spring that has four helices. B. The rapid palatal expander (RPE) consists of a jackscrew mechanism that is activated with a key by the parents. Both appliances are versatile in that they can be modified to fit the individual needs of the patient. For instance, the quad helix actually has only two helices. The anterior helices were not used in this case due to the constricted space of the anterior palate. Both appliances are bulky and may interfere with articulation while in use.

wish to correct incisor position at this time (Sakamoto, Sakamoto, Harazaki, Isshiki, & Yamaguchi, 2002). This is rarely necessary with primary incisors and should be reserved for the permanent incisors and then preferably at a stage of nearly completed root development.

Maxillary expansion can be accomplished within a few months in most cases. Children with repaired palatal clefts must have a fixed lingual upper arch wire to maintain the maxillary expansion. Without proper retention, the scar tissue of the repaired cleft palate exerts a strong tendency toward relapse into crossbite.

In children with repaired cleft palate, maxillary expansion may achieve crossbite correction but often at the expense of widening any preexisting oronasal fistula, or even opening a new fistula. Widening the narrow arch of the cleft palate separates the greater and lesser segments, resulting in tightly stretched tissue over the deficient or absent bone of the palate. Without proper bony support, palatal tissue necrosis may occur, which causes the fistula to manifest. These fistulae may be temporarily obturated with acrylic added to arch wires or with removable acrylic plates. Definitive repair is usually accomplished later with an alveolar bone graft (Proffit, White, & Sarver, 2003).

Early Mixed Dentition (6–9 Years)

Malpositioned permanent incisors are often the most noticeable sign that children with a repaired cleft lip and palate are entering the early mixed dentition stage. The permanent lower central incisors usually erupt first, followed by the upper central incisors and lower lateral incisors, and finally the upper lateral incisors. The permanent first molars usually erupt shortly after the lower central incisors, but it is not uncommon for them to erupt first.

In children who have had unilateral or bilateral clefts, it is common for the now erupting upper incisors to be misaligned. Figure 9–25 A–D shows some examples of misaligned maxillary teeth secondary to a cleft. Although unaesthetic, these crowded incisors should not be corrected with orthodontics at this stage. The crowns of these teeth may be visible but the root formation remains very much incomplete. As a general rule, it takes at least three years after crown eruption before root formation is complete. The pressure from orthodontic appliances at this stage can damage forming roots, frequently resulting in roots of less than half their normal length. Consequently, correcting anterior misalignment is not advised until after completion of root formation to avoid a poor long-term prognosis for these teeth (Reisberg, 2000; Rivkin, Keith, Crawford, & Hathorn, 2000a, 2000b).

During the mixed dentition stage, the interosseous sutures of the maxilla are beginning to fuse together but the mandible is beginning its growth spurt. The incidence of crossbite increases as the jaw discrepancy increases. If the patient requires maxillary advancement, a *reverse pull headgear* may be an option (Figure 9–26 A–C). This is also an excellent time to correct any crossbite that may exist, using the crossbite appliance as anchorage for the face mask (Kawakami, Yagi, & Takada, 2002; Sakamoto et al., 2002). A typical quad helix, or *rapid palatal expander,* with labial hooks for facemask attachment is used. Treatment is usually timed before the age of 8 to take advantage of remaining maxillary growth before suture fusion begins. Face-mask treatment requires 12 to 14 hours of wear per day to show midface improvement (Ahn, Figueroa, Braun, & Polley, 1999). Some clinicians report success with the addition of a chin cup appliance (Ishikawa, Kitazawa, Iwasaki, & Nakamura, 2000).

Another consideration of the early mixed dentition is the eruption of the lateral incisor, if present, and the need for an alveolar bone graft

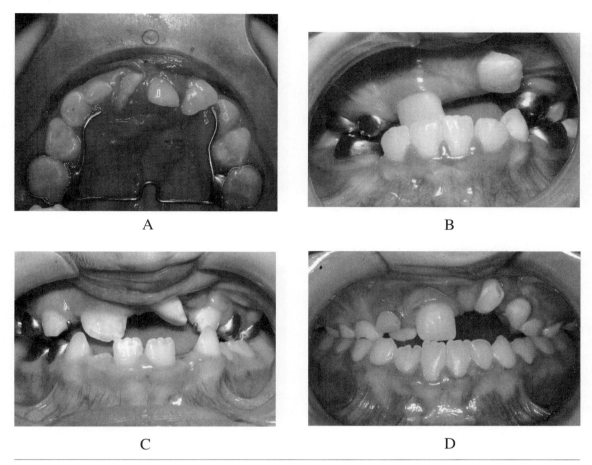

FIGURE 9–25 (A–D)   The erupting upper incisors are often misaligned in children who have had a unilateral or bilateral cleft. Figures A–D show various examples of misaligned maxillary incisors as the result of a cleft.

(Figure 9–27 A–C). As with primary bone grafting, a secondary alveolar bone graft is meant to introduce bone-matrix-inducing material into the alveolar cleft site. The introduced bone stimulates new bone formation in the cleft site. When successful, the introduced bone replaces the missing alveolar ridge, which provides bone for normal eruption of the permanent teeth and also serves as the missing nasal floor and piriform (nasal) rim (De Riu, Lai, Congiu, & Tullio, 2004; Hynes & Earley,

2003). Frequently, illiac crestal (hip) bone is used, although other sources of bone such as the tibia, cranium, anterior chin, freeze-dried cadaver bone, and artificial substitutes, such as hydroxy apatite, have been used (Bohman, Yamashita, Baek, & Yen, 2004; Chin, Ng, Tom, & Carstens, 2005; Enemark, Jensen, & Bosch, 2001; Hughes & Revington, 2002; Kalaaji, Lilja, Elander, & Friede, 2001; Nwoku, Al Atel, Al Shlash, Oluyadi, & Ismail, 2005; Sivarajasingam, Pell, Morse, & Shepherd,

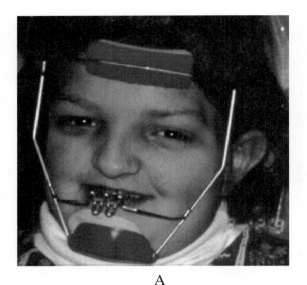

A

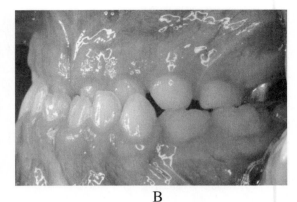

B

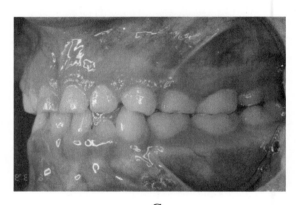

C

FIGURE 9–26 (A–C) A patient with reverse-pull headgear. A. Removable reverse-pull headgear, also known as a Delaire facial mask, can be used in cooperative children to correct midfacial retrusion. An appliance attached to the teeth engages the elastic bands on the facemask to generate an anterior force on the teeth that is transmitted to the maxilla and its surrounding interosseous sutures. B. Underbite due to maxillary deficiency, as shown in this photograph, is an indication for this device before treatment. C. The correction achievable with the facial mask is readily apparent in this patient.

2001). Secondary alveolar bone grafting is highly predictable in unilateral clefts when the greater and lesser segments are stabilized properly, and approaches a 95% success rate (Arctander, Kolbenstvedt, Aalokken, Abyholm, & Froslie, 2005; Bajaj, Wongworawat, & Punjabi, 2003; Hynes & Earley, 2003; Kindelan & Roberts-Harry, 1999; Williams, Semb, Bearn, Shaw, & Sandy, 2003). In repairing bilateral clefts, many clinicians prefer to graft one side at a time. Success rates with this technique approach 90% (Bohman et al., 2004; Kamakura, Yamaguchi, Kochi, Sato, & Motegi, 2003).

Simultaneous grafting of the bilateral cleft has a greater chance for failure, with success rates dropping to 70% (Mao, Ma, & Li, 2000; Shashua & Omnell, 2000).

It is important for the clinician to note whether the lateral incisor is well formed and suitable for use as a fully functioning tooth (Shashua & Omnell, 2000; Solis, Figueroa, Cohen, Polley, & Evans, 1998). As a tooth erupts, it carries its periodontal ligament and bony attachment with it. Without adequate bone, the erupting tooth will have a periodontal defect. This compromises not only the

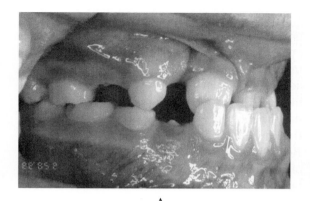

A

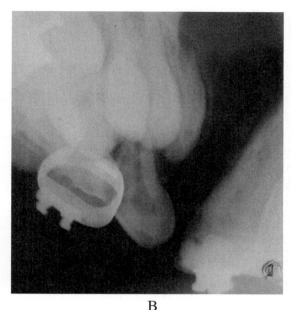

B

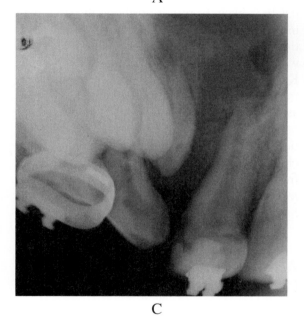

C

FIGURE 9–27 (A–C) A patient needing an alveor bone graft. A. One can see the notching of the alveolus between the primary canine and the permanent lateral incisor. B. In the occlusal radiograph one can see the developing lateral incisor and the deficiency of alveolar bone. This is an indication for alveolar bone grafting. The anterior crossbite and narrowness of the maxilla will be corrected orthodontically prior to the bone graft. This gives the surgeon better access to the cleft and allows the lateral incisor to erupt through normal bone, thereby avoiding periodontal defects. C. In this example of a larger defect, one can appreciate the deficiency of bone.

lateral incisor but other teeth adjacent to the defect as well. If the lateral incisor is usable it is best for it to erupt through bone. Thus, when the lateral incisor is beginning to reach one-half to two-thirds of normal root length, the maxilla should be prepared for secondary alveolar bone grafting (Hogan, Shand, Heggie, & Kilpatrick, 2003; Matsui, Echigo, Kimizuka, Takahashi, & Chiba, 2005; Murthy & Lehman, 2005). Maxillary expansion will usually be required, if

it hasn't already been accomplished earlier. In cases in which the maxillary lateral incisor is missing or unusable, many clinicians prefer to delay bone grafting until the maxillary canine is ready to erupt, usually at around age 11 to 13 (Da Silva Filho, Teles, Ozawa, & Filho, 2000). Delaying expansion, when possible, has the benefit of not overwhelming the child with constant orthodontic treatment. Some clinicians argue, however, that delaying the bone graft until the time of canine eruption creates a defect around the central incisor. More studies are needed to evaluate the long-term outcome of periodontal health as it relates to early versus late grafting (De Moor, De Vree, Cornelis, & De Boever, 2002; Dempf, Teltzrow, Kramer, & Hausamen, 2002; Kolbenstvedt, Aalokken, Arctander, & Johannessen, 2002; Schultze-Mosgau, Nkenke, Schlegel, Hirschfelder, & Wiltfang, 2003; Witherow, Cox, Jones, Carr, & Waterhouse, 2002).

Late Mixed Dentition (9–12 Years)

Once the permanent incisors and first molars have erupted, visible changes in the dentition are not noticeable for two to three years. Midface retrusion, if present, may become more noticeable during this stage (see Figure 9–23). Late mixed dentition treatment may involve maxillary expansion for alveolar bone grafting, if it hasn't been done earlier, and is now timed around the eruption of the maxillary canine. Root formation of the incisors may have progressed to the point that they may now be aligned orthodontically. This may be begun one to three months (Vig, 1999) after bone grafting, which provides sufficient bone into which to move the incisors, especially in bilateral clefts (Cavassan Ade, de Albuquerque, & Filho, 2004; Semb & Ramstad, 1999). Missing teeth may be replaced by adding artificial teeth to the orthodontic appliances, at least as a temporary measure.

Late mixed dentition treatment may also involve problems common to children without clefts. These may include space maintenance for prematurely lost primary teeth, the need to control moderate to severe crowding problems through selective tooth extraction, or correction of jaw position with dentofacial orthopedic measures, such as headgear or functional appliances. The limitation of decreased maxillary growth in children with repaired clefts must be considered when prescribing any of these treatment modalities. Most clinicians will attempt to accomplish interceptive orthodontic treatment in a 12- to 18-month period, so that the child may have a rest from orthodontic treatment until the permanent dentition completely erupts. Realistic assessment of the risks and benefits of treatment in the late mixed dentition needs to be considered before initiating treatment (Proffit, & Fields, 2000). The child with cleft lip and palate is likely to require orthodontic treatment in the permanent dentition and it is well known that tooth eruption is frequently delayed patients with clefts (McNamara, Foley, Garvey, & Kavanagh, 1999). Every attempt should be made to delay or combine treatment as much as possible to avoid "orthodontic fatigue" in the patient (Kapp-Simon, 2004). Much of orthodontic treatment depends on the cooperation of the child, and cooperation will not be forthcoming from the child who is "burned out" or simply tired of orthodontic treatment (Proffit, White, & Sarver, 2003).

Adolescent Dentition (12–18 Years)

Hopefully, by the time of eruption of the permanent dentition, crossbites have been corrected, alveolar bony defects are repaired, the incisors are well aligned, crowding has been managed, and the child has experienced good maxillary growth. Unfortunately, this is not always the case (Veleminska et al., 2003). For many children with clefts, the maxilla remains hypoplastic in all dimensions: vertical, sagittal, and transverse (Gaggl, Schultes, & Karcher, 1999). The adolescent growth spurt may have made these deficits more noticeable due to both the mandible's relatively normal growth as well as the growth of the nose (Scheuer et al., 2001). This discrepancy, an underdeveloped maxilla and normal mandible, often leads to one of two possible jaw relationships, a Class III with deep underbite or a Class I with anterior openbite.

When facial growth is complete, replacement of missing teeth with dental prostheses, such as bridgework or dental implants, may be necessary. Dental implants are cylindrical pieces of titanium that can take the place of a missing tooth's root and are able to support crowns (Kearns, Perrott, Sharma, Kaban, & Vargervik, 1997). The coordinated involvement of the surgeon, orthodontist, and prosthodontist is required for a successful outcome (Vig & Turvey, 1985).

If a severe anterior crossbite persists during growth, the mandibular incisors may overerupt, causing a deep underbite. Because the maxilla is smaller than normal, the middle portion of the face is simply not as long as ideal, and thus the mandible may be overclosed, further contributing to deep underbite. Conversely, in some patients with relatively normal occlusion, mandibular growth may have been directed inferiorly and posteriorly. This allows the teeth to remain in a more normal occlusion but results in a longer facial profile and possible open bite (Lisson, Hanke, & Trankmann, 2004). Fortunately, these two phenomena appear to be occurring less often now, because improvements in surgical techniques have led to fewer detrimental effects on maxillary growth. Thus, adolescent treatment in about 80% of children with a repaired cleft may involve orthodontics alone (Figure 9–28 A–D). The remaining 20% often require orthodontics as well as orthognathic surgery to align the dental arches (see Figure 9–21) (Figueroa et al., 1993; Proffit,, White, & Sarver, 2003). These percentages vary from one treatment center to another.

Orthognathic surgery, which is surgery of the bones of the jaws, frequently involves a maxillary Le Fort I osteotomy to reposition the maxilla anteriorly (Figure 9–29 A–D and see Figure 19–4) (Heliovaara, Ranta, Hukki, & Rintala, 2002). (See Chapter 19 for more information.) Orthodontic treatment, in preparation for surgery, intentionally worsens the discrepancy between the upper and lower teeth in order to create sufficient space for maximum jaw repositioning. When facial growth is complete, replacement of missing teeth with dental prostheses, such as bridgework or *dental implants*, may be necessary. Dental implants are cylindrical pieces of titanium that can take the place of a missing tooth's root and are able to support crowns (Fukuda, Takahashi, & Iino, 2003; Isono et al., 2002). The coordinated involvement of the surgeon, orthodontist, and prosthodontist is required for a successful outcome (Kawakami, Yokozeki, Horiuchi, & Moriyama, 2004; Kramer et al., 2005; Laine, Vahatalo, Peltola, Tammisalo, & Happonen, 2002).

A recent development in orthognathic surgical treatment is *distraction osteogenesis* (Figure 9–30 A–C). This involves making a *corticotomy* (cut in bone) in the middle of a bone, then slowly distracting the cut ends apart with a mechanical device. New osteoid is able to regenerate between the cut ends and in time becomes normal bone, obviating the need for bone grafts (Kusnoto, Figueroa, & Polley, 2001). Pioneered in mandibular applications by Molina and Monasterio in Mexico and McCarthy in the United States, this is a very effective treatment option when indicated (Albert, 2000; Kita, Kochi, Imai, Yamada, & Yamaguchi, 2005; McCarthy, Katzen, Hopper, & Grayson, 2002). Distraction osteogenesis is especially effective in correcting severe discrepancies that are not amenable to standard surgical techniques. Rigid external distraction osteogenesis for the midface was introduced by

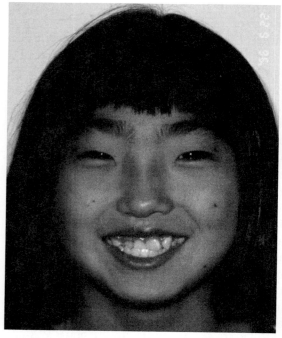

A

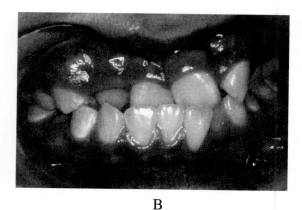

B

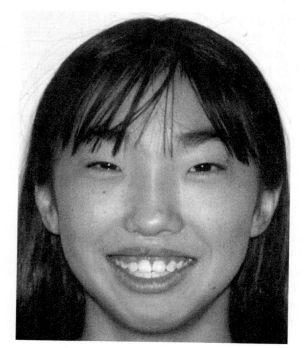

C

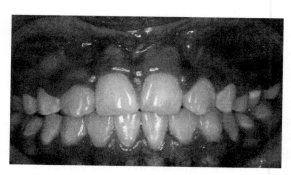

D

FIGURE 9–28 (A–D)   Adolescent treatment with orthodontics only. A. This patient with right unilateral cleft lip and palate exhibits only mild midfacial retrusion. B. The anterior crossbite of this patient was judged to be amenable to orthodontic treatment alone. Orthognathic surgery was not considered to be necessary. C. After adolescent growth and orthodontic treatment the facial proportions remain well balanced. D. The post treatment occlusal result was excellent. One lateral incisor was missing, the remaining lateral incisor was extracted and the canines were substituted for the lateral incisors.

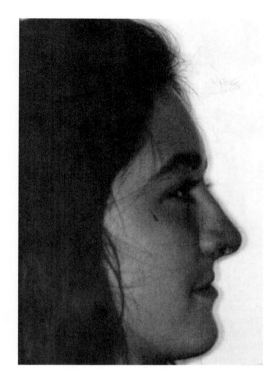

A

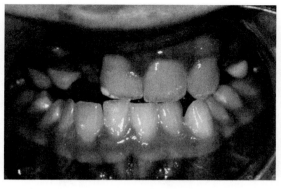

B

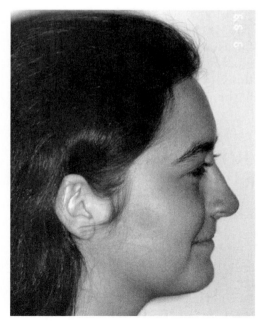

C

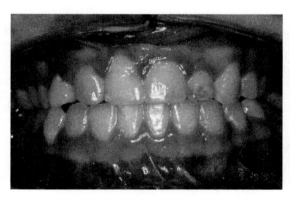

D

FIGURE 9–29 (A–D) Adolescent dentition treatment orthodontics and orthognathic surgery. A. This patient with unilateral right cleft lip and palate was judged to need orthodontics and orthognathic surgery to correct her moderate midfacial retrusion. B. This shows her malocclusion with anterior and posterior crossbite and missing right lateral incisor. C. After orthodontic preparation, she underwent a Le Fort I maxillary osteotomy to advance the upper jaw and teeth, as well as malar implants to augment the cheeks. As a result, she has an improved profile and upper lip position. D. Postoperative occlusion is greatly improved as well. Extraction of multiple teeth to correct her malocclusion only (without maxillary advancement surgery) would have lessened her lip support and given her an "aged" or edentulous appearance.

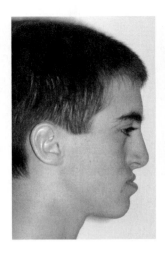 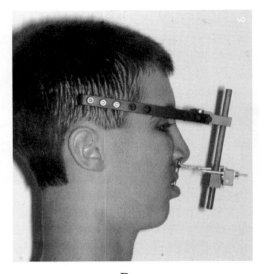 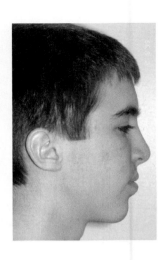

A   B   C

FIGURE 9–30 (A–C) Rigid external distraction osteogenesis. A. This patient with bilateral cleft lip and palate exhibits midfacial retrusion that is far outside the limits of conventional orthognathic surgery. B. He elected to undergo the rigid external distraction proceedure of Polley and Figueroa. Following maxillary Le Fort I osteotomy, the rigid framework is attached to the skull with scalp pins and the maxilla is pulled forward or "distracted" with a screw mechanism over about an eight-week period. C. Following stabilization, the headframe is removed, and the improvement in facial profile can be readily seen.

Polley and Figueroa (Figueroa & Polley, 1999; Figueroa, Polley, & Ko, 1999; Guyette, Polley, Figueroa, & Smith, 2001; Polley & Figueroa, 2000), although internal appliances are appearing as well (Cohen, 1999). Orthodontists and surgeons work closely together to determine the final occlusion with these techniques (Motohashi & Kuroda, 1999). The field is rapidly changing; indications and treatment timing are still being developed (Swennen, Figueroa, Schierle, Polley, & Malevez, 2000), and new devices and their variants are being introduced at a rapid pace. At present, distraction osteogenesis is primarily being used to reduce or correct severe facial deformities (Figueroa, Polley, Friede, & Ko, 2004; Liou & Tsai, 2005; Mitsugi, Ito, & Alcalde, 2005; Wang et al., 2005; Yen et al., 2005; Zwahlen & Butow, 2004).

Lastly, an adolescent who has had orthodontics and orthognathic surgery is likely to require prosthodontic replacement of missing teeth. This is frequently accomplished with fixed crowns and bridges, dental implants, or less commonly with removable prostheses such as dentures or partials (Moore & McCord, 2004; Reisberg, 2004). (See Chapter 20.)

THE ROLE OF SPEECH THERAPY

Speech-language pathologists and dental professionals must work closely together to correct problems of speech related to the dentition in the child with a history of cleft lip and palate (Pinsky & Goldberg, 1977; Shprintzen et al., 1985). The role of the speech-language pathologist is to first determine if the speech errors are related to dentition, and if so, if they are obligatory or compensatory. Speech therapy is not appropriate for *obligatory errors* (Shprintzen, 1991). Instead, correction of the structural problem, or dentition, is required. If all of the speech errors are obligatory as a result of the faulty structure, then correcting the structure will correct the speech without the need for speech therapy (Kummer et al., 1989; Wakumoto et al., 1996). On the other hand, if there are *compensatory errors* as a result of the structural abnormality, then speech therapy will be required, preferably after correction of the dentition. Speech-language pathologists and dentists should coordinate their interventions to coincide with the stages of dental development, as outlined in the preceding sections (Shprintzen, McCall, & Skolnick, 1975). Coordination of treatment timing, sequencing, and follow-up are important for the efficient use of resources and for ensuring the best overall outcome (Shprintzen, 1982).

SUMMARY

Children with cleft lip and palate or other craniofacial anomalies are at risk for dental and occlusal abnormalities that include missing teeth, supernumerary teeth, rotated teeth, crowding, anterior crossbite, Class III malocclusion, open bite, and protruding premaxilla. All of these abnormalities can affect speech by affecting the movement of the tongue tip or lips. Crowding of the oral cavity, particularly anterior crowding, can cause lisps and a palatal placement for tongue-tip and sibilant sounds.

Because so many children with craniofacial anomalies have dental and speech problems, it is important for dental professionals and speech-language pathologists to work closely together. Interdisciplinary communication and coordination will help to determine the appropriate form of treatment needed to achieve a maximal outcome in aesthetics, mastication, and speech.

FOR REVIEW, DISCUSSION, AND CRITICAL THINKING

1. Discuss the number and type of teeth in a normal maxillary and mandibular arch of a 6-year-old. How is adult dentition different?

2. What is the Angle Classification System? Define Class I, Class II, and Class III occlusion. Which type of malocclusion is commonly seen in individuals with a history of cleft lip and palate? Why do you think that is?

3. What types of dental anomalies have the potential to affect speech? List the category of phonemes that are most likely to be affected by dental anomalies, and list other categories of phonemes that can be affected.

4. What types of compensatory articulation errors might you expect with an anterior crossbite and Class III malocclusion? What is the appropriate treatment?

5. What types of obligatory errors might you expect with an anterior crossbite and Class III malocclusion? What is the appropriate treatment?

6. Describe the dental concerns and usual dental or orthodontic treatment during the following stages: infant stage, primary dentition (1–6 years), early mixed dentition (6–9 years), late mixed dentition (9–12 years), and adolescent dentition (12–18 years).

REFERENCES

Ahn, J. G., Figueroa, A. A., Braun, S., & Polley, J. W. (1999). Biomechanical considerations in distraction of the osteotomized dento-maxillary complex. *American Journal of Orthodontics & Dentofacial Orthopedics, 116*(3), 264–270.

Albert, T. W. (2000). Oral and maxillofacial surgery: Considerations in cleft nasal deformities. *Facial Plastic Surgery, 16*(1), 79–84.

Arctander, K., Kolbenstvedt, A., Aalokken, T. M., Abyholm, F., & Froslie, K. F. (2005). Computed tomography of alveolar bone grafts 20 years after repair of unilateral cleft lip and palate. *Scandinavian Journal of Plastic & Reconstructive Surgery & Hand Surgery, 39*(1), 11–14.

Bajaj, A. K., Wongworawat, A. A., & Punjabi, A. (2003). Management of alveolar clefts. *Journal of Craniofacial Surgery, 14*(6), 840–846.

Berkowitz, S., Duncan, R., Evans, C., Friede, H., Kuijpers-Jagtman, A. M., Prahl-Anderson, B., et al. (2005). Timing of cleft palate closure should be based on the ratio of the area of the cleft to that of the palatal segments and not on age alone. *Plastic and Reconstructive Surgery, 115*(6), 1483–1499.

Berkowitz, S., Mejia, M., & Bystrik, A. (2004). A comparison of the effects of the Latham-Millard procedure with those of a conservative treatment approach for dental occlusion and facial aesthetics in unilateral and bilateral complete cleft lip and palate: Part I. Dental occlusion. *Plastic and Reconstructive Surgery, 113*(1), 1–18.

Bitter, K. (2001). Repair of bilateral clefts of lip, alveolus and palate. Part 1: A refined method for the lip-adhesion in bilateral cleft lip and palate patients. *Journal of Craniomaxillofacial Surgery, 29*(1), 39–43.

Bohman, P., Yamashita, D. D., Baek, S. H., & Yen, S. L. (2004). Stabilization of an edentulous premaxilla for an alveolar bone graft: Case report. *Cleft Palate-Craniofacial Journal, 41*(2), 214–217.

Bongaarts, C. A., Kuijpers-Jagtman, A. M., van 't Hof, M. A., & Prahl-Andersen, B. (2004). The effect of infant orthopedics on the occlusion of the deciduous dentition in children with complete unilateral cleft lip and palate (Dutchcleft). *Cleft Palate-Craniofacial Journal 41*(6), 633–641.

Braumann, B., Keilig, L., Bourauel, C., & Jager, A. (2002). Three-dimensional analysis of morphological changes in the maxilla of patients with cleft lip and palate. *Cleft Palate-Craniofacial Journal, 39*(1), 1–11.

Cabete, H. F., Gomide, M. R., & Costa, B. (2000). Evaluation of primary dentition in cleft lip and palate children with and without natal/neonatal teeth. *Cleft Palate-Craniofacial Journal, 37*(4), 406–409.

Cavassan Ade, O., de Albuquerque, M. D., & Filho, L. C. (2004). Rapid maxillary expansion after secondary alveolar bone graft in a patient with bilateral cleft lip and palate. *Cleft Palate-Craniofacial Journal, 41*(3), 332–339.

Chan, K. T., Hayes, C., Shusterman, S., Mulliken, J. B., & Will, L. A. (2003). The effects of active infant orthopedics on occlusal relationships in unilateral complete cleft lip and palate. *Cleft Palate-Craniofacial Journal, 40*(5), 511–517.

Chapple, J. R., & Nunn, J. H. (2001). The oral health of children with clefts of the lip, palate, or both. *Cleft Palate-Craniofacial Journal, 38*(5), 525–528.

Chin, M., Ng, T., Tom, W. K., & Carstens, M. (2005). Repair of alveolar clefts with recombinant human bone morphogenetic protein (rhBMP-2) in patients with clefts. *Journal of Craniofacial Surgery, 16*(5), 778–789.

Cho, B. (2001). Unilateral complete cleft lip and palate repair using lip adhesion and passive alveolar molding appliance. *Journal of Craniofacial Surgery, 12*(2), 148–156.

Cohen, S. R. (1999). Midface distraction. *Seminars in Orthodontics, 5*(1), 52–58.

Cutting, C., Grayson, B., Brecht, L., Santiago, P., Wood, R., & Kwon, S. (1998). Presurgical columellar elongation and primary retrograde nasal reconstruction in one-stage bilateral cleft lip and nose repair. *Plastic and Reconstructive Surgery, 101*(3), 630–639.

Da Silva Filho, O. G., Teles, S. G., Ozawa, T. O., & Filho, L. C. (2000). Secondary bone graft and eruption of the permanent canine in patients with alveolar clefts: Literature review and case report. *Angle Orthodontist, 70*(2), 174–178.

Da Silveira, A. C., Oliveira, N., Gonzalez, S., Shahani, M., Reisberg, D., Daw, J. L., Jr., et al. (2003). Modified nasal alveolar molding appliance for management of cleft lip defect. *Journal of Craniofacial Surgery, 14*(5), 700–703.

De Moor, R. J., De Vree, H. M., Cornelis, C., & De Boever, J. A. (2002). Cervical root resorption in two patients with unilateral complete cleft of the lip and palate. *Cleft Palate-Craniofacial Journal, 39*(5), 541–545.

De Riu, G., Lai, V., Congiu, M., & Tullio, A. (2004). Secondary bone grafting of alveolar cleft. *Minerva Stomatologica, 53*(10), 571–579.

Dempf, R., Teltzrow, T., Kramer, F. J., & Hausamen, J. E. (2002). Alveolar bone grafting in patients with complete clefts: A comparative study between secondary and tertiary bone grafting. *Cleft Palate-Craniofacial Journal, 39*(1), 18–25.

Dewinter, G., Quirynen, M., Heidbuchel, K., Verdonck, A., Willems, G., & Carels, C. (2003). Dental abnormalities, bone graft quality, and periodontal conditions in patients with unilateral cleft lip and palate at different phases of orthodontic treatment. *Cleft Palate-Craniofacial Journal, 40*(4), 343–350.

DiBiase, A. T., DiBiase, D. D., Hay, N. J., & Sommerlad, B. C. (2002). The relationship between arch dimensions and the 5-year index in the primary dentition of patients with complete UCLP. *Cleft Palate-Craniofacial Journal, 39*(6), 635–640.

Doruk, C., & Kilic, B. (2005). Extraoral nasal molding in a newborn with unilateral cleft lip and palate: A case report. *Cleft Palate-Craniofacial Journal, 42*(6), 699–702.

Enemark, H., Jensen, J., & Bosch, C. (2001). Mandibular bone graft material for reconstruction of alveolar cleft defects: Long-term results. *Cleft Palate-Craniofacial Journal, 38*(2), 155–163.

Figueroa, A. A., & Polley, J. W. (1999). Management of severe cleft maxillary deficiency with distraction osteogenesis: Procedure and results. *American Journal of Orthodontic and Dentofacial Orthopedics, 115*(1), 1–12.

Figueroa, A. A., Polley, J. W., & Ko, E. W. (1999). Maxillary distraction for the management of cleft maxillary hypoplasia with a rigid external distraction system. *Seminars in Orthodontics, 5*(1), 46–51.

Figueroa, A. A., Polley, J. W., Friede, H., & Ko, E. W. (2004). Long-term skeletal stability after maxillary advancement with distraction osteogenesis using a rigid external distraction device in cleft maxillary deformities. *Plastic and Reconstructive Surgery, 114*(6), 1382–1392; Discussion 1393–1384.

Fukuda, M., Takahashi, T., & Iino, M. (2003). Dentoalveolar reconstruction of a missing premaxilla using bone graft and endosteal implants. *Journal of Oral Rehabilitation*, 30(1), 87–90.

Gable, T. O., Kummer, A. W., Lee, L., Creaghead, N. A., & Moore, L. J. (1995). Premature loss of the maxillary primary incisors: Effect on speech production. *Journal of Dentistry for Children*, 62(3), 173–9.

Gaggl, A., Schultes, G., & Karcher, H. (1999). Aesthetic and functional outcome of surgical and orthodontic correction of bilateral clefts of lip, palate, and alveolus. *Cleft Palate-Craniofacial Journal*, 36(5), 407–412.

Gaggl, A., Schultes, G., Karcher, H., & Mossbock, R. (1999). Periodontal disease in patients with cleft palate and patients with unilateral and bilateral clefts of lip, palate, and alveolus. *Journal of Periodontology*, 70(2), 171–178.

Garrahy, A., Millett, D. T., & Ayoub, A. F. (2005). Early assessment of dental arch development in repaired unilateral cleft lip and unilateral cleft lip and palate versus controls. *Cleft Palate-Craniofacial Journal*, 42(4), 385–391.

Grayson, B. H., Bookstein, F. L., McCarthy, J. G., & Mueeddin, T. (1987). Mean tensor cephalometric analysis of a patient population with clefts of the palate and lip. *Cleft Palate Journal*, 24(4), 267–277.

Grayson, B. H., & Cutting, C. B. (2001). Presurgical nasoalveolar orthopedic molding in primary correction of the nose, lip, and alveolus of infants born with unilateral and bilateral clefts. *Cleft Palate-Craniofacial Journal*, 38(3), 193–198.

Grayson, B. H., & Maull, D. (2004). Nasoalveolar molding for infants born with clefts of the lip, alveolus, and palate. *Clinics in Plastic Surgery*, 31(2), 149–158, vii.

Guyette, T. W., Polley, J. W., Figueroa, A., & Smith, B. E. (2001). Changes in speech following maxillary distraction osteogenesis. *Cleft Palate-Craniofacial Journal*, 38(3), 199–205.

Hathaway, R. R., Eppley, B. L., Hennon, D. K., Nelson, C. L., & Sadove, A. M. (1999). Primary alveolar cleft bone grafting in unilateral cleft lip and palate: Arch dimensions at age 8. *Journal of Craniofacial Surgery*, 10(1), 58–67.

Hathaway, R. R., Eppley, B. L., Nelson, C. L., & Sadove, A. M. (1999). Primary alveolar cleft bone grafting in unilateral cleft lip and palate: Craniofacial form at age 8. *Journal of Craniofacial Surgery*, 10(1), 68–72.

Heliovaara, A., Ranta, R., Hukki, J., & Rintala, A. (2002). Skeletal stability of Le Fort I osteotomy in patients with isolated cleft palate and bilateral cleft lip and palate. *International Journal of Oral & Maxillofacial Surgery*, 31(4), 358–363.

Heliovaara, A., Ranta, R., & Rautio, J. (2004). Dental abnormalities in permanent dentition in children with submucous cleft palate. Acta Odontologica Scandinavica, 62(3), 129–31.

Hogan, L., Shand, J. M., Heggie, A. A., & Kilpatrick, N. (2003). Canine eruption into grafted alveolar clefts: A retrospective study. *Australian Dental Journal*, 48(2), 119–124.

Hughes, C. W., & Revington, P. J. (2002). The proximal tibia donor site in cleft alveolar bone grafting: Experience of 75 consecutive cases. *Journal of Craniomaxillofacial Surgery*, 30(1), 12–16; Discussion 17.

Hynes, P. J., & Earley, M. J. (2003). Assessment of secondary alveolar bone grafting using a modification of the Bergland grading system. *British Journal of Plastic Surgery*, 56(7), 630–636.

Ishikawa, H., Kitazawa, S., Iwasaki, H., & Nakamura, S. (2000). Effects of maxillary protraction combined with chin-cap therapy in unilateral cleft lip and palate patients. *Cleft Palate-Craniofacial Journal*, 37(1), 92–97.

Isono, H., Kaida, K., Hamada, Y., Kokubo, Y., Ishihara, M., Hirashita, A., et al. (2002). The reconstruction of bilateral clefts using endosseous implants after bone grafting. *American Journal of Orthodontics & Dentofacial Orthopedics*, 121(4), 403–410.

Johnson, N. C. L., & Sandy, J. R. (1999). Tooth position and speech—Is there a relationship? *The Angle Orthodontist*, 69(4), 306–310.

Kalaaji, A., Lilja, J., Elander, A., & Friede, H. (2001). Tibia as donor site for alveolar bone grafting in patients with cleft lip and palate: Long-term experience. *Scandinavian Journal of Plastic & Reconstructive Surgery & Hand Surgery*, 35(1), 35–42.

Kamakura, S., Yamaguchi, T., Kochi, S., Sato, A., & Motegi, K. (2003). Preliminary report of two-stage secondary alveolar bone grafting for patients with bilateral cleft lip and palate. *Cleft Palate-Craniofacial Journal*, 40(5), 449–452.

Kapp-Simon, K. A. (2004). Psychological issues in cleft lip and palate. *Clinics in Plastic Surgery*, 31(2), 347–352.

Katz, M. I. (1992). Angle classification revisited 2: A modified Angle classification [see Comments]. *American Journal of Orthodontic and Dentofacial Orthopedics*, 102(3), 277–284.

Kawakami, M., Yagi, T., & Takada, K. (2002). Maxillary expansion and protraction in correction of midface retrusion in a complete unilateral cleft lip and palate patient. *Angle Orthodontist*, 72(4), 355–361.

Kawakami, S., Yokozeki, M., Horiuchi, S., & Moriyama, K. (2004). Oral rehabilitation of an orthodontic patient with cleft lip and palate and hypodontia using secondary bone grafting, osseo-integrated implants, and prosthetic treatment. *Cleft Palate-Craniofacial Journal*, 41(3), 279–284.

Kearns, G., Perrott, D. H., Sharma, A., Kaban, L. B., & Vargervik, K. (1997). Placement of endosseous implants in grafted alveolar clefts. *Cleft Palate-Craniofacial Journal*, 34(6), 520–525.

Kindelan, J., & Roberts-Harry, D. (1999). A 5-year post-operative review of secondary alveolar bone grafting in the Yorkshire region. *British Journal of Orthodontics*, 26(3), 211–217.

Kirchberg, A., Treide, A., & Hemprich, A. (2004). Investigation of caries prevalence in children with cleft lip, alveolus, and palate. *Journal of Craniomaxillofacial Surgery*, 32(4), 216–219.

Kirschner, R. E., & LaRossa, D. (2000). Cleft lip and palate. *Otolaryngologic Clinics of North America*, 33(6), 1191–1215, v–vi.

Kita, H., Kochi, S., Imai, Y., Yamada, A., & Yamaguchi, T. (2005). Rigid external distraction using skeletal anchorage to cleft maxilla united with alveolar bone grafting. *Cleft Palate-Craniofacial Journal*, 42(3), 318–327.

Kolbenstvedt, A., Aalokken, T. M., Arctander, K., & Johannessen, S. (2002). CT appearances of unilateral cleft palate 20 years after bone graft surgery. *Acta Radiologica*, 43(6), 567–570.

Kramer, F. J., Baethge, C., Swennen, G., Bremer, B., Schwestka-Polly, R., & Dempf, R. (2005). Dental implants in patients with orofacial clefts: A long-term follow-up study. *International Journal of Oral & Maxillofacial Surgery*, 34(7), 715–721.

Kuijpers-Jagtman, A. M., Borstlap-Engels, V. M., Spauwen, P. H., & Borstlap, W. A. (2000). Team management of orofacial clefts. *Nederlands Tijdschrift voor Tandheelkunde, 107*(11), 447–451.

Kummer, A. W., Strife, J. L., Grau, W. H., Creaghead, N. A., & Lee, L. (1989). The effects of Le Fort I osteotomy with maxillary movement on articulation, resonance, and velopharyngeal function. *Cleft Palate Journal, 26*(3), 193–199; Discussion 199–200.

Kusnoto, B., Figueroa, A. A., & Polley, J. W. (2001). Radiographic evaluation of bone formation in the pterygoid region after maxillary distraction with a rigid external distraction (RED) device. *Journal of Craniofacial Surgery 12*(2), 109–117; Discussion 118.

Laine, J., Vahatalo, K., Peltola, J., Tammisalo, T., & Happonen, R. P. (2002). Rehabilitation of patients with congenital unrepaired cleft palate defects using free iliac crest bone grafts and dental implants. *International Journal of Oral Maxillofacial Implants, 17*(4), 573–580.

Latham, R. A. (1980). Orthopedic advancement of the cleft maxillary segment: A preliminary report. *Cleft Palate Journal, 17*(3), 227–233.

Latham, R. A., Kusy, R. P., & Georgiade, N. G. (1976). An extraorally activated expansion appliance for cleft palate infants. *Cleft Palate Journal, 13*, 253–261.

Lee, C. T., Grayson, B. H., Cutting, C. B., Brecht, L. E., & Lin, W. Y. (2004). Prepubertal midface growth in unilateral cleft lip and palate following alveolar molding and gingivoperiosteoplasty. *Cleft Palate-Craniofacial Journal, 41*(4), 375–380.

Liao, Y. F., Huang, C. S., Liou, J. W., Lin, W. Y., & Ko, W. C. (1998). Premaxillary size and craniofacial growth in patients with cleft lip and palate. *Chang-Keng I Hsueh Tsa Chih (Tai-Pei), 21*(4), 391–396.

Liou, E. J., & Tsai, W. C. (2005). A new protocol for maxillary protraction in cleft patients: Repetitive weekly protocol of alternate rapid maxillary expansions and constrictions. *Cleft Palate-Craniofacial Journal, 42*(2), 121–127.

Lisson, J. A., Hanke, I., & Trankmann, J. (2004). Vertical changes in patients with complete unilateral and bilateral cleft lip, alveolus and palate. *Journal of Orofacial Orthopedics, 65*(3), 246–258.

Maciel, S. P., Costa, B., & Gomide, M. R. (2005). Difference in the prevalence of enamel alterations affecting central incisors of children with complete unilateral cleft lip and palate. *Cleft Palate-Craniofacial Journal, 42*(4), 392–395.

Malanczuk, T., Opitz, C., & Retzlaff, R. (1999). Structural changes of dental enamel in both dentitions of cleft lip and palate patients. *Journal of Orofacial Orthopedics, 60*(4), 259–268.

Mao, C., Ma, L., & Li, X. (2000). A retrospective study of bilateral alveolar bone grafting. *Chinese Medical Sciences Journal, 15*(1), 49–51.

Matsui, K., Echigo, S., Kimizuka, S., Takahashi, M., & Chiba, M. (2005). Clinical study on eruption of permanent canines after secondary alveolar bone grafting. *Cleft Palate-Craniofacial Journal, 42*(3), 309–313.

McCarthy, J. G., Katzen, J. T., Hopper, R., & Grayson, B. H. (2002). The first decade of mandibular distraction: Lessons we have learned. *Plastic and Reconstructive Surgery, 110*(7), 1704–1713.

McNamara, C. M., Foley, T. F., Garvey, M. T., & Kavanagh, P. T. (1999). Premature dental eruption: Report of case. *Journal of Dentistry for Children, 66*(1), 70–72.

Millard, D. R., Latham, R., Huifen, X., Spiro, S., & Morovic, C. (1999). Cleft lip and palate treated by presurgical orthopedics, gingivoperiosteoplasty, and lip adhesion (POPLA) compared with previous lip adhesion method: A preliminary study of serial dental casts. *Plastic and Reconstructive Surgery, 103*(6), 1630–1644.

Mitsugi, M., Ito, O., & Alcalde, R. E. (2005). Maxillary bone transportation in alveolar cleft-transport distraction osteogenesis for treatment of alveolar cleft repair. *British Journal of Plastic Surgery, 58*(5), 619–625.

Moller, K. T. (1994). Dental-occlusal and other oral conditions and speech. In J. E. Bernthal & N. W. Bankson (Eds.), *Child phonology: Characteristics, assessment, and intervention with special populations* (pp. 3–28). New York: Thieme Medical Publishers, Inc.

Moore, D., & McCord, J. F. (2004). Prosthetic dentistry and the unilateral cleft lip and palate patient. The last 30 years. A review of the prosthodontic literature in respect of treatment options. *European Journal of Prosthodontics & Restorative Dentistry, 12*(2), 70–74.

Motohashi, N., & Kuroda, T. (1999). A 3-D computer-aided design system applied to diagnosis and treatment planning in orthodontics and orthognathic surgery. European *Journal of Orthodontics, 21*(3), 263–274.

Mouradian, W. E., Omnell, M. L., & Williams, B. (1999). Ethics for orthodontists. *Angle Orthodontist, 69*(4), 295–299.

Murthy, A. S., & Lehman, J. A. (2005). Evaluation of alveolar bone grafting: A survey of ACPA teams. *Cleft Palate-Craniofacial Journal, 42*(1), 99–101.

Ngan, P., Alkire, R. G., & Fields, H., Jr. (1999). Management of space problems in the primary and mixed dentitions. *Journal of the American Dental Association, 130*(9), 1330–1339.

Nwoku, A. L., Al Atel, A., Al Shlash, S., Oluyadi, B. A., & Ismail, S. (2005). Retrospective analysis of secondary alveolar cleft grafts using iliac of chin bone. *Journal of Craniofacial Surgery 16*(5), 864–868.

Oosterkamp, B. C., Van Oort, R. P., Dijkstra, P. U., Stellingsma, K., Bierman, M. W., & de Bont, L. G. (2005). Effect of an intraoral retrusion plate on maxillary arch dimensions in complete bilateral cleft lip and palate patients. *Cleft Palate-Craniofacial Journal, 42*(3), 239–244.

Pfeifer, T. M., Grayson, B. H., & Cutting, C. B. (2002). Nasoalveolar molding and gingivoperiosteoplasty versus alveolar bone graft: An outcome analysis of costs in the treatment of unilateral cleft alveolus. *Cleft Palate-Craniofacial Journal, 39*(1), 26–29.

Pinsky, T. M., & Goldberg, H. J. (1977). Potential for clinical cooperation between dentistry and speech pathology. *International Dental Journal, 27*(4), 363–369.

Polley, J., & Figueroa, A. (2000). Re: Maxillary distraction osteogenesis: A method with skeletal anchorage. *Journal of Craniofacial Surgery 11*(3), 295.

Posnick, J. C., & Ricalde, P. (2004). Cleft-orthognathic surgery. *Clinics in Plastic Surgery, 31*(2), 315–330.

Prahl, C., Kuijpers-Jagtman, A. M., van't Hof, M. A., & Prahl-Andersen, B. (2003). A randomized prospective clinical trial of the effect of infant orthopedics in unilateral cleft lip and palate: Prevention of collapse of the alveolar segments (Dutchcleft). *Cleft Palate-Craniofacial Journal, 40*(4), 337–342.

Prahl, C., Kuijpers-Jagtman, A. M., van't Hof, M. A., & Prahl-Andersen, B. (2005). Infant orthopedics in UCLP: Effect on feeding, weight, and length: A randomized clinical trial (Dutchcleft). *Cleft Palate-Craniofacial Journal, 42*(2), 171–177.

Proffit, W. R., & Fields, H. W., Jr. (2000). *Contemporary Orthodontics* (3rd ed.). St. Louis, MO: Mosby.

Proffit, W. R., White, R. P., & Sarver, D. M. (2003). *Contemporary treatment of dentofacial deformity*. St. Louis, MO: Mosby.

Quirynen, M., Dewinter, G., Avontroodt, P., Heidbuchel, K., Verdonck, A., & Carels, C. (2003). A split-mouth study on periodontal and microbial parameters in children with complete unilateral cleft lip and palate. *Journal of Clinical Periodontology, 30*(1), 49–56.

Reisberg, D. J. (2000). Dental and prosthodontic care for patients with cleft or craniofacial conditions. *Cleft Palate-Craniofacial Journal, 37*(6), 534–537.

Reisberg, D. J. (2004). Prosthetic habilitation of patients with clefts. *Clinics in Plastic Surgery, 31*(2), 353–360.

Renkielska, A., Wojtaszek-Slominska, A., & Dobke, M. (2005). Early cleft lip repair in children with unilateral complete cleft lip and palate: A case against primary alveolar repair. *Annals of Plastic Surgery, 54*(6), 595–597; Discussion 598–599.

Rivkin, C. J., Keith, O., Crawford, P. J., & Hathorn, I. S. (2000a). Dental care for the patient with a cleft lip and palate. Part 1: From birth to the mixed dentition stage. *British Dental Journal, 188*(2), 78–83.

Rivkin, C. J., Keith, O., Crawford, P. J., & Hathorn, I. S. (2000b). Dental care for the patient with a cleft lip and palate. Part 2: The mixed dentition stage through to adolescence and young adulthood. *British Dental Journal, 188*(3), 131–134.

Rosenstein, S., Dado, D. V., Kernahan, D., Griffith, B. H., & Grasseschi, M. (1991). The case for early bone grafting in cleft lip and palate: A second report. *Plastic and Reconstructive Surgery, 87*(4), 644–654; Discussion 655–656.

Sachs, S. A. (2002). Nasoalveolar molding and gingivoperiosteoplasty verses alveolar bone graft: An outcome analysis of costs in the treatment of unilateral cleft alveolus. *Cleft Palate-Craniofacial Journal, 39*(5), 570; Author reply 570–571.

Sakamoto, T., Sakamoto, S., Harazaki, M., Isshiki, Y., & Yamaguchi, H. (2002). Orthodontic treatment for jaw deformities in cleft lip and palate patients with the combined use of an external-expansion arch and a facial mask. *Bulletin of Tokyo Dental College, 43*(4), 223–229.

Scheuer, H. A., Holtje, W. J., Hasund, A., & Pfeifer, G. (2001). Prognosis of facial growth in patients with unilateral complete clefts of the lip, alveolus and palate. *Journal of Craniomaxillofacial Surgery, 29*(4), 198–204.

Schultes, G., Gaggl, A., & Karcher, H. (1999). Comparison of periodontal disease in patients with clefts of palate and patients with unilateral clefts of lip, palate, and alveolus. *Cleft Palate-Craniofacial Journal, 36*(4), 322–327.

Schultze-Mosgau, S., Nkenke, E., Schlegel, A. K., Hirschfelder, U., & Wiltfang, J. (2003). Analysis of bone resorption after secondary alveolar cleft bone grafts before and after canine eruption in connection with orthodontic gap closure or prosthodontic treatment. *Journal of Oral & Maxillofacial Surgery, 61*(11), 1245–1248.

Semb, G., & Ramstad, T. (1999). The influence of alveolar bone grafting on the orthodontic and prosthodontic treatment of patients with cleft lip and palate. *Dental Update, 26*(2), 60–64.

Shashua, D., & Omnell, M. L. (2000). Radiographic determination of the position of the maxillary lateral incisor in the cleft alveolus and parameters for assessing its habilitation prospects. *Cleft Palate-Craniofacial Journal, 37*(1), 21–25.

Shprintzen, R. J. (1982). Palatal and pharyngeal anomalies in craniofacial syndromes. *Birth Defects Original Article Series, 18*(1), 53–78.

Shprintzen, R. J. (1991). Fallibility of clinical research. *Cleft Palate-Craniofacial Journal, 28*(2), 136–140.

Shprintzen, R. J., McCall, G. N., & Skolnick, M. L. (1975). A new therapeutic technique for the treatment of velopharyngeal incompetence. *Journal of Speech and Hearing Disorders, 40*(1), 69–83.

Shprintzen, R. J., Siegel-Sadewitz, V. L., Amato, J., & Goldberg, R. B. (1985). Anomalies associated with cleft lip, cleft palate, or both. *American Journal of Medical Genetics, 20*(4), 585–595.

Sivarajasingam, V., Pell, G., Morse, M., & Shepherd, J. P. (2001). Secondary bone grafting of alveolar clefts: A densitometric comparison of iliac crest and tibial bone grafts. *Cleft Palate-Craniofacial Journal, 38*(1), 11–14.

Solis, A., Figueroa, A. A., Cohen, M., Polley, J. W., & Evans, C. A. (1998). Maxillary dental development in complete unilateral alveolar clefts. *Cleft Palate-Craniofacial Journal, 35*(4), 320–328.

Strauss, R. P. (1998). Cleft palate and craniofacial teams in the United States and Canada: A national survey of team organization and standards of care. The American Cleft Palate-Craniofacial Association (ACPA) Team Standards Committee. *Cleft Palate-Craniofacial Journal, 35*(6), 473–480.

Strauss, R. P. (1999). The organization and delivery of craniofacial health services: The state of the art. *Cleft Palate-Craniofacial Journal, 36*(3), 189–195.

Strong, S. M. (2002). Adolescent dentistry: Multidisciplinary treatment for the cleft lip/palate patient. *Practical Procedures & Aesthetic Dentistry, 14*(4), 333–338; Quiz 340, 342.

Swennen, G., Figueroa, A. A., Schierle, H., Polley, J. W., & Malevez, C. (2000). Maxillary distraction osteogenesis: A two-dimensional mathematical model. *Journal of Craniofacial Surgery 11*(4), 312–317.

Taher, A. (1997). Speech defect associated with Class III jaw relationship. *Plastic and Reconstructive Surgery, 99*(4), 1200.

Trost-Cardamone, J. E. (1997). Diagnosis of specific cleft palate speech error patterns for planning therapy of physical management needs. In K. R. Bzoch (Ed.), *Communicative disorders related to cleft lip and palate* (Vol. 4, pp. 313–330). Austin, TX: Pro-Ed.

Turvey, T. A., Vig, K. W. L., & Fonseca, R. J. (1996). *Facial clefts and craniosynostosis, principles and management.* Chapel Hill, NC: W. B. Saunders.

Vasan, N. (1999). Management of children with clefts of the lip or palate: An overview. *New Zealand Dental Journal, 95*(419), 14–20.

Vargervik, K. (1981). Orthodontic management of unilateral cleft lip and palate. *Cleft Palate Journal, 18*(4), 256–270.

Veleminska, J., Smahel, Z., & Mullerova, Z. (2003). Facial growth and development during the pubertal period in patients with complete unilateral cleft of lip and palate. *Acta Chirurgiae Plasticae, 45*(1), 22–31.

Vig, K. W. (1999). Alveolar bone grafts: The surgical/orthodontic management of the cleft maxilla. *Annals of the Academy of Medicine, Singapore, 28*(5), 721–727.

Vig, K. W., & Turvey, T. A. (1985). Orthodontic-surgical interaction in the management of cleft lip and palate. *Clinics in Plastic Surgery, 12*(4), 735–748.

Wakumoto, M., Isaacson, K. G., Friel, S., Suzuki, N., Gibbon, F., Nixon, F., Hardcastle, W. J., & Mishi, K. (1996). Preliminary study of the articulatory reorganization of fricative consonants following osteotomy. *Folia Phoniatrica et Logopedica, 48*(6), 275–89.

Wang, X. X., Wang, X., Yi, B., Li, Z. L., Liang, C., & Lin, Y. (2005). Internal midface distraction in correction of severe maxillary hypoplasia secondary to cleft lip and palate. *Plastic and Reconstructive Surgery, 116*(1), 51–60.

Williams, A., Semb, G., Bearn, D., Shaw, W., & Sandy, J. (2003). Prediction of outcomes of secondary alveolar bone grafting in children born with unilateral cleft lip and palate. *European Journal of Orthodontics, 25*(2), 205–211.

Witherow, H., Cox, S., Jones, E., Carr, R., & Waterhouse, N. (2002). A new scale to assess radiographic success of secondary alveolar bone grafts. *Cleft Palate-Craniofacial Journal, 39*(3), 255–260.

Yen, S. L., Yamashita, D. D., Gross, J., Meara, J. G., Yamazaki, K., Kim, T. H., et al. (2005). Combining orthodontic tooth movement with distraction osteogenesis to close cleft spaces and improve maxillary arch form in cleft lip and palate patients. *American Journal of Orthodontics & Dentofacial Orthopedics, 127*(2), 224–232.

Zwahlen, R. A., & Butow, K. W. (2004). Maxillary distraction resulting in facial advancement at Le Fort III level in cleft lip and palate patients: A report of two cases. *Oral Surgery, Oral Medicine, Oral Pathology, Oral Radiology & Endodontics, 98*(5), 541–545.

CHAPTER

10

PSYCHOSOCIAL ASPECTS OF CLEFT LIP/PALATE AND CRANIOFACIAL ANOMALIES

JANET R. SCHULTZ, PH.D., ABPP

CHAPTER OUTLINE

INTRODUCTION

When a baby is born, the infant is not just born to his parents. The child is born into a family, a social network, and society. These layers of context into which the child is born are also forces that impact on the child's development. At the same time, the child brings into the world his or her genetic endowment and the characteristics developed during intrauterine life. Among these are temperament, certain instinctual behaviors, and physical appearance. For some children, one aspect is a cleft lip and/or palate. The child's genetic contribution interacts with the complex context into which he or she is born so that the developing individual is both affected by and affecting that environment.

FAMILY ISSUES

Initial Shock and Adjustment

The birth of a child is typically a happy event. Parents' first questions almost always include, "Is the baby all right?" When a baby is born with a cleft lip and/or palate, there is typically immediate knowledge of the cleft and, therefore, distress. When an infant is born with a cleft of the velum or a submucous cleft however, hours (or longer) may elapse before the parents are informed that there is a problem.

When something is wrong with the baby, there is often a period of shock and sadness. For many families, there is also a period of mourning the anticipated child and adjusting to the situation in which they find themselves (van Staden & Gerhardt, 1995). Usually, resolution of these feelings comes after the beginning of the whirlwind demand of medical concerns that characterize early infancy for many children with a cleft. Many parents of babies with clefts have never heard of clefts before their child's birth (Middleton, Lass, Starr, & Pannbacker, 1986). They have never seen a cleft before the repair and know little about the problem other than what they are told at the time of the baby's birth. The parents' adjustment is affected by the extent of the deformity, visibility of the cleft, elapsed time before seeing the baby, their coping style, and the social support they receive.

Family support has been found to be a significant factor in overall adjustment (Bradbury & Hewison, 1994; Sank, Berk, Cooper, & Marazita, 2003). Low levels of social support appear to be one predictor of depression in mothers, with higher levels of education and fewer children being seen as protective (Sank, Berk, Cooper, & Marazita, 2003). Strong feelings of love, hurt, fear, disappointment, betrayal, resentment, protectiveness, and guilt are often present. However, these negative feelings tend to subside fairly rapidly without impairing the parent-child relationship on a long-term basis (Clifford, 1969, 1971). One reason for this relatively rapid resolution is the "fixable" quality of clefts at this point in history. On the other hand, there are some mixed findings that mothers may be less responsive to and interactive with infants with clefts than they are with babies without anomalies. Children with any kind of physical anomalies appear to be more at risk of physical abuse than children without anomalies.

For a few families, the birth of a child with a cleft is a serious disruption, but for most, it is a difficult but manageable time. Mothers of babies with clefts reported higher levels of stress and more concerns about their competence as parents than mothers of healthy babies (Speltz, Armsden, & Clarren, 1990). The same mothers also reported a higher degree of marital conflict. There is little evidence, however, that the divorce rate is higher in these families. In several studies, about 10% of parents reported that their marriage was adversely affected, while a quarter to a third reported that the birth of a child with a cleft brought the parents closer together. Reproductive plans generally were unaltered by the birth of child with a cleft (Andrews-Casal et al., 1998). A study in Germany found that mothers of children over the age of one reported the same levels of quality of life, depression, and anxiety as a normative sample (Weigl, Rudolph, Eysholdt, & Rosanowski, 2005).

Feeding problems, discussion of surgery and appliances, and the question of how to talk to other people about the baby's anomaly color the experience of the first few weeks of their baby's life. Parents may find themselves supporting grandparents or other relatives rather than receiving support themselves. Sometimes families pull together, but other times there are questions or, worse, accusations about the reason for the cleft, perhaps with finger pointing at the other side of the family. Parents of infants with visible differences are likely to experience the staring of other adults and some children when they take their babies out in public. These experiences may serve to confirm the fears of social rejection, which tend to rise rapidly in the minds of parents at their first contact with the baby. These challenges may actually help to create strong, protective bonds to the babies,

however. Coy, Speltz, and Jones (2002) found that babies with cleft lip and palate were more securely attached to their parents than those who had cleft palate only.

Parents may also have other children to attend to during this time. Parents often find it difficult to explain to siblings that the baby looks different and has something wrong, even when they reassure them that the doctors are going to fix it. Whenever there is a new baby, parents also have to balance the time required for taking care of the baby with the needs of the other children. That can be a more daunting task if the baby requires a longer time to feed, has frequent ear infections, or requires surgery and other medical visits. Parents' stress correlates with adjustment problems in the child's life. Therefore, intervening with parents who are experiencing considerable stress may help to prevent adjustment problems for the child later in life.

Health care professionals, generally nurses or pediatricians, can be important sources of support and information for parents in the early months. Focusing more on what is "right" with the baby than what is "wrong" is often helpful, as is consistent availability. Parents also want to talk, to show their feelings, and to check out their fears. In addition, many parents want contact with other parents of children with clefts (Strauss, Sharp, Lorch, & Kachalia, 1995). It is comforting to talk to people who have been through the same experiences. Parents seem less afraid to "look stupid" in the eyes of sympathetic veterans of the process and may voice more of their fears and questions with them.

A number of hospitals have systems in place to help parents of newborns with clefts link with veteran parents of somewhat older children. Parents compare experiences and solutions to problems and daily care challenges. A common activity is sharing pictures, which the newer parents often use as a peek into the future of their own child.

Cleft Palate as a Chronic Medical Condition

Dealing with the medical system is a common event in the lives of parents of babies with clefts. Visits to physicians may be experienced as reminders of the baby's anomaly or as an evaluation of their efficacy as parents. Charting the infant's growth is important but may be more threatening when feeding has been a major challenge. Contacts with health professionals also raise the possibility, regardless of actual probability, of hearing more bad news. It is very important to parents that health care professionals relate to their child as a person, and not as an assortment of physical problems.

The first surgery is often a stressful and frightening time for family members. Having a helpless little baby taken from their arms for surgery reawakens many of the sad, frightened, and protective feelings that may have quieted since the birth. Moreover, it places the parents and other family members in direct confrontation with their powerlessness to fix the baby's problems themselves. For many of the normal challenges of growing up, parents and grandparents have the ability to "make it all better" for their children. This role is impossible when surgery is required. Parents have to trust the surgeon and all of the professionals involved and let go, often leaving them feeling out of control of the situation. There is always at least a bit of concern that something may go wrong and that the baby could die. The decision for parents as to whether surgery is worth the risk only becomes more complicated as the child grows older and the emphasis is more on appearance.

Additionally, children with a history of cleft have been found to show negative mood and behavior changes following surgery. In one of the rare longitudinal studies of children with a history of cleft who have had surgery, Koomen and Hoeksma (1993) found changes in behavior that primarily had to do with the increased desire of the infants to be in the presence of or in contact with their mothers. They interpreted their findings as suggesting that attachment to parents may be impaired by cleft repair and the child's subsequent hospitalization. On the other hand, these findings were inconsistent and their significance outside the laboratory of some question.

Helping parents recognize that they hold a unique role with their children that no health professional can assume is often important, especially in the case of prolonged hospitalizations. Practical advice about staying with the infant during the entire hospitalization, preparing siblings for the event and the baby's changed appearance, and caring for the baby after surgery can increase a parent's sense of being able to contribute to the child's wellbeing. For the baby, having a parent or other familiar adult available during the entire time he or she is in the hospital for surgery is important for security and comfort.

Some aspects of dealing with the medical system will continue to be problematic for parents for years. Even when there are positive relationships between health care professionals and parents, the medical system is still often quite overwhelming. The demands of the system in terms of paperwork and insurance approval, the expense involved, the complexity of the layout of many hospitals, and the experience of seeing their child as others, especially plastic surgeons, see their child can lead to a variety of negative feelings. Frustration with the system can be directed as anger toward important professionals and even lead to noncompliance to the medical regimen.

The intensity of the family members' negative feelings about the child's cleft and the associated stresses usually diminishes over time, with resurgent peaks at times of surgery, social rejection, or the child's own distress. Parents often experience some fatigue during the whole process and are eager for everything to be done. Disagreement between the parents regarding medical decisions is not unusual. As the child grows older, this disagreement can even be between parents and the child, especially during the teen years. Parental fears may be reawakened when the teenager or adult child moves into a serious relationship where reproductive and, hence, genetic issues are important.

When the parent also has a history of cleft, these issues have an added dimension. It usually answers the question of why the child was born with a cleft. Although the parent is in an unusually good position to be knowledgeable about and understanding of the child's situation, there is also the risk that unresolved negative experiences from the parent's past may color his or her response to the challenges facing the child. Sometimes parents make decisions that reflect an attempt to "get it right this time." It is particularly important to help the parent see differences between his or her situation and that of the child's. An important factor here is the advancement of surgical techniques since the parent's own repair.

Although having a child with a cleft is stressful, there is no evidence that it leads to a higher frequency of psychiatric symptoms in parents. An older study (Goodstein, 1960) compared the personality profiles of parents of children with a history of cleft to those of parents of children with no known abnormalities. Using the *Minnesota Multiphasic Personality Inventory* (MMPI), the researchers found no significant differences between the groups and no unique patterns emerged. Similarly, a large interview study found that parents of children with a history of cleft reported the same kinds of social life, recreation, and entertainment as the group of parents of unaffected children.

School Issues

Knowledge and Expectation of Teachers

Teachers have reported not knowing very much about cleft lip and palate (like most of the population). They often have little information, and some of it may be incorrect. Teachers as a group have also been found to underestimate the intelligence of children with a history of cleft, especially when either appearance or speech is quite impaired (Richman, 1978). They also may expect less from the children who look different than those who appear normal (Richman & Eliason, 1982). These underestimates shape their expectations for the children and may result in lower performance and less positive evaluations of the children's academic performance. Several studies have found that children with clefts do not achieve the level that would be predicted by their intelligence alone.

Learning Ability and School Performance

Intelligence, as measured by formal IQ tests, seems to be in the average range for children with a history of clefts but who have no other identified syndromes. By contrast, children with various syndromes that may include clefts tend to score lower on intelligence tests. Children with a history of nonsyndromic cleft, however, generally score lower on test sections that require verbal skills, especially oral responses, than they do on more performance-based sections. Moreover, many have specific learning disabilities, which may be misdiagnosed as attention deficit/hyperactivity disorder if language-learning characteristics are not taken into account (Richman, Ryan, Wilgenbusch, & Millard, 2004).

Children with cleft lip and palate who have reading disabilities have been shown to have specific deficits in rapid naming and verbal expression. Their problem does not appear to be phonemic awareness despite some early attempts to link reading problems to articulation difficulties (Richman & Ryan, 2003). Children with cleft palate only show more speech and language disorders than both nonaffected peers and those with cleft lip and palate (Broen, Devers, Doyle, Prouty, & Moller, 1998; Estes & Morris, 1970; Goodstein, 1961; Lamb, Wilson, & Leeper, 1973). They are also more likely to have serious reading disabilities, often evident in the primary grades (Richman & Millard, 1997). Some studies have found that over half of children with cleft palate only show significant reading problems in first- and second-grade years. A full third still show reading problems at age 13. Girls are less often affected than boys (Broder, Richman, & Matheson, 1998). Other studies have found that children with a history of cleft and speech problems often lack self-confidence in reading aloud, which may influence the teacher's evaluation of their abilities. However, many of the supporting studies are older and may not have differentiated children with syndromes, such as velocardiofacial syndrome, confounding the results. Teenagers with a history of cleft do not show a greater dropout rate than their unaffected peers. As a group they attain the same educational levels as other young adults. In fact, one study in Europe found persons with a history of cleft had a lower rate of dropping out than their peers (Ramstad, Ottem, & Shaw 1995b).

Social Interaction

In the early years of a child's life, the negative social implications of the cleft are primarily experienced by the parents. They are the ones who note the stares or answer the questions about the child's condition. By the preschool years, however, the child starts to be asked directly about what happened to his or her lip. Sometimes the question comes from well-meaning adults who believe the child's scar to be from a fall or a minor accident. Other times, it comes from curious peers who notice a difference in the child's appearance. While preschool children prefer attractive children as friends, they are rarely cruel or tease their peers. They notice differences in appearance, speech, and behavior, but unless the differences interfere, they are not generally important in play relationships. One of the advantages of enrolling children with a history of cleft in good preschool or day care programs is the opportunity for the child to build social skills and confidence without parents being present, and at a time when teasing and rudeness is rare.

By school age, a significant number of children with a history of cleft do not have as many friendships as other children their age. This situation appears to be a result of the interaction of several factors. First, children with a history of cleft, especially girls, seem to be more socially inhibited than their peers. They are sometimes reluctant to risk new friendships; other times, they have difficulty in initiating and maintaining new friendships. Second, the lack of friends may relate to the interaction challenges associated with hearing impairment and speech difficulties. Third, appearance may be a contributor as well. Joyce Tobiasen (1988, 1989) showed pictures of children to second- through fourth-graders. Some of the children in the pictures had no cleft, some had a unilateral cleft, and some had a bilateral cleft visible in the photographs. The viewers rated the pictured children on personal qualities. Children rated those with a bilateral cleft as having fewer positive attributes than those with a unilateral cleft, and both cleft groups fared worse than the children without a visible cleft. The younger viewers were harsher in their ratings than the somewhat older ones. The degree of facial impairment is strongly correlated with perceptions of attractiveness and social desirability. On the other hand, an individual child's social relationships cannot be accurately predicted on the basis of facial attractiveness alone. The child's temperament, family support, social skills, and coping strategies also make a difference in that regard. Interestingly, children with a history of cleft tend to describe having more friends than their peers acknowledge. This may reflect misjudgment of what constitutes friendship or perhaps lower expectations about what constitutes a friend.

In most studies, older children and teenagers reported significant concerns about interpersonal relationships. The trend toward overinhibition and shyness continues into adolescence. Slifer and his colleagues videotaped interactions of 8–15 year olds with and without clefts, finding that those with clefts responded less often to questions from peers and made fewer choices during interactions (Slifer, Amari, Diver, Hilley, Beck, Kane, & McDonnell, 2004). Their parents rated them as less socially competent as well. Those young people with clefts who rated themselves as more socially acceptable were more likely to look their peers

in the face. In another study, adult Japanese women with clefts showed fewer physical signs of interest in conversations and smiled less frequently than their counterparts who had no clefts (Adachi, Kochi, & Yamaguchi, 2003).

These differences in nonverbal behavior could reflect their conversational experiences growing up or might indicate that those with clefts have other, perhaps neurologic, differences which are expressed in part through social skills. The latter was supported by the findings of Nopoulos, Choe, Berg, Van Demark, Canady, and Richman (2005). Their findings from MRI of men with nonsyndromic clefts and normal controls indicated that there were morphologic abnormalities in the part of the brain known to govern social functioning and that the larger the abnormality, the more problems in socializing. It may be that differences in social skills and interaction styles are attributable to neuropsychological differences which are just being identified.

How these differences may relate to romantic outcomes is not yet known. Although the frequency of dating relationships among young people with a history of cleft relative to their peers has not been studied, it appears that teens with a history of cleft show more self-doubts and have lower expectations for relationships than their peers. Adults with a history of cleft have been found to marry later than their peers and siblings. In studies in other countries, adults have been seen as generally showing good psychological adjustment, but fewer were in long-term relationships or married. Women, in particular, worried about their appearance.

Teasing

Teasing is one social problem that parents worry about starting in the early years. Most children, regardless of cleft status, are teased at least occasionally by peers. On the other hand, longstanding, cruel teasing which results in ostracism is not a common childhood occurrence. Although the conclusion is not as solid as some, it appears that children with a history of cleft are teased more often than typical peers (Broder, Smith, & Strauss, 2001). It seems at least to be influenced by physical appearance and speech differences because children tend to report less teasing after surgeries that address those problems.

Other factors that affect teasing appear to be the child's personality and social standing, response to teasing, and adult response to peer teasing. Children who laugh off teasing or respond in kind appear to be teased less than those who respond with distress or helpless anger. Use of humor seems to be particularly helpful. Similarly, attributing teasing to a flaw in the person who does the teasing rather than to him- or herself is protective of the child's self-esteem. Recognizing that cruel comments about a cleft reflect ignorance about a topic well understood by the child as well as a lack of either compassion or kindness puts the blame squarely on the person making the comments, rather than the person commented upon.

Adult response, especially at school, influences the likelihood of teasing. Helping the child to present information about the cleft and the various surgeries can reduce teasing, especially among children in lower grades. It reduces the uncertainty of peers, activates empathy in some of the children, and generally reduces the status of the cleft as a sensitive spot to hit when teasing. Children of any age reduce the frequency of teasing when school officials take an active role in demonstrating that respect for all students is expected. On the other hand, when teasing is viewed as an inevitable behavior of children ("Kids will be cruel, there's not much we can do about it"), teasing is more likely to continue or increase.

By high school, for all adolescents, teasing tends to diminish or take on a friendlier tone, including for those with a history of cleft. There is a greater understanding of clefts and a generally greater acceptance of differences. When unpleasant teasing does continue, however, it can take on a cruel edge and even a group rejection that may result in social withdrawal. Some social scientists see this kind of teasing as having the same power and domination quality as more general "bullying." Most adults report that teasing and social intimidation are not part of their lives.

Self-Perception

Children develop a concept of themselves over time and part of that concept is their self-worth. Because children have not developed a clear sense of self at early ages, most studies begin at school age. Children with a history of cleft have been consistently found to have more negative self-concepts compared to their unaffected peers (Broder & Strauss, 1989; Kapp-Simon, 1986; Slifer, Beck, Amari, Diver, Hilley, Kane, & McDonnell, 2003; Strauss & Fenson, 2005). They see themselves as less acceptable to their peers, less socially competent, less satisfied with their facial appearance, and more often report that they are sad or angry. Broder and Strauss (1989) found that children with both cleft lip and palate scored lower than those with an "invisible" cleft palate only, but children with a history of any type of cleft rated themselves less well than unaffected children. Higher levels of acceptance of the cleft were associated with better self-concepts. In school-age children with a history of cleft, greater physical attractiveness correlated with better overall adjustment (Pillemer & Cook, 1989). Similarly, satisfaction with their own appearance was related to the adjustment and older teens and young adults were more satisfied than their younger counterparts (Thomas, Turner, Rumsey, Dowell, & Sandy, 1997). There is some evidence that having appearance-altering surgeries before the teen years contributes to better self-esteem and less social isolation (Pertschuk & Whitaker, 1982).

Teenagers who view themselves "realistically," that is, in agreement with their peers and familiar adults, tend to be better adjusted. Generally teenagers have been found to have more negative feelings about themselves than younger children. Brantley and Clifford (1979) asked teenagers to report what they thought their parents felt and experienced when they were born. Teens with a history of cleft said that their parents experienced predominantly negative emotions and that their parents did not care to nurture them. Relative to teens with asthma, obesity, or no physical problems, adolescents with a history of cleft reported their parents had higher levels of apprehension about and felt less pride in them.

Physical appearance concerns are consistently greater in persons with a history of cleft across the life span, but in later adolescence and adulthood, women report greater feelings of self-consciousness than their male counterparts. Clifford, Crocker, and Pope (1972) found that dissatisfaction with appearance centered on the face, especially the mouth. Adults with a history of cleft lip were less satisfied with facial appearance than those with a history of cleft palate only, while people with a history of cleft palate were more displeased with their speech than those with a history of cleft lip only. More dissatisfaction with their mouth, teeth, lips, voice, and speech was expressed by both cleft groups than by the

control group of adults with no a history of cleft.

Adults with a history of cleft continue to report some levels of psychological distress. Ramstad, Ottem, and Shaw (1995a) surveyed Norwegian adults with a history of cleft and found higher levels of anxiety and depression than in unaffected controls. Their symptoms were strongly associated with more concerns about appearance, dentition, speech, and the hope of more treatment. The same researchers (1995b) also reported that adults with a history of cleft were less likely to marry than adults without a history of cleft and that when they did marry, it was often later in life. This was particularly true of the group with bilateral cleft lip and palate. Other studies in other countries have found similar results. Although education and employment per se did not differ between those with a history of cleft and the controls, people with a history of cleft appeared to make less money.

It should be noted that the rates of diagnosed psychiatric disorders for children and teens with a history of cleft appears no different than that of the population of children as a whole. In one study of the 600 most disturbed children in a large urban school district, not one had a cleft. More typical studies comparing children with a history of cleft to children with other physical problems and to children with no medical difficulties have found little difference among the groups. Research to identify a "cleft palate personality" has consistently failed to yield evidence of a consistent or specific organization or style of personality in children, adolescents, or adults with a history of cleft. The biggest risk appears to be for social competence problems, including those relating to development of friendships and participation in organizations (Richman & Eliason, 1982).

SOCIETAL ISSUES

Physical Attractiveness

One of the forces at work for a child with a cleft is society's response to facial difference. Physical attractiveness, especially facial beauty, is an area that has been well researched, with findings that are among the most reliable and robust in the psychological literature. Some characteristics that people see as attractive or unattractive are cross-cultural; for example, there is no group of people known to find highly blemished skin to be attractive. Other characteristics considered attractive vary considerably among cultures, but even then, attractiveness tends to focus on facial features and body shape. There is some evidence that mouth shape is especially important across cultures, even though the specific standard for beauty may differ. Dental differences certainly carry meaning for adults, although this is less clear in the case of children.

Within a culture, there is considerable consensus about general characteristics of attractiveness. This consensus develops early. By preschool age, children know the standards of beauty that the adults hold and share those values. In fact, until recently one of the items on a commonly used intelligence test for children required them to choose the picture of the "pretty" woman from two choices. This could serve as a developmental test only because the cultural concept of beauty normally is learned prior to age 4.

More important than the consensual nature of cultural standards of beauty are the meanings associated with being considered either attractive or unattractive. In a nutshell, beauty is equated with goodness. Attractive people are rated as smarter, more friendly, nicer, more likely to be a good friend, and kinder than those who are less attractive. Ethnologists have found that characteristics in babies, such as a round head, large eyes, and short and narrow features are rated as "cute" (witness how most people respond to pandas) and elicit caregiving behaviors from adults. Infants considered to be highly attractive tend to be rated as more likable, smarter, and less problematic. The significance of these meanings lies in their power to shape the behavior and attitudes of people, directly and indirectly. These, in turn, become part of the feedback loop that shapes how an individual behaves and views himself or herself.

Physical attractiveness is important across the life span. Cute babies are attributed characteristics that their less attractive peers are not. Preschoolers prefer attractive children as their friends and the social power of attractiveness continues to increase until the early grade school years and then tends to hold steady until adolescence. Teachers also have more favorable expectations of attractive children than unattractive children (Clifford, 1975). Teachers may respond differentially to more physically attractive children and their grades are often higher than those of less attractive peers. Being seen with attractive people increases a person's social desirability. Attractive teens are more likely to be elected to school office than other youth and, as no surprise to most people, date more frequently and have a higher number of partners. Unattractive people are more likely to be found guilty of crimes and get less help from strangers in time of need. Physical attractiveness affects the likelihood of being hired for a job, even when public contact is not a major factor. It may also influence job performance evaluations. The power of physical attractiveness appears to hold in middle and older age as well, but this is less well established. People sometimes hope that this influence only holds at first impression, but research suggests that this is not the case. Although physical attractiveness is only one of many variables contributing to the social responses to a person, it is a powerful force indeed.

Speech Quality

The quality of a person's speech is a factor rather similar to physical attractiveness. First, the quality of speech impacts the social judgments of others, which in turn helps shape behaviors and attitudes. Second, good speech appears to be associated with the assumption that the speaker has positive characteristics. While children are less likely to initiate conversations with those with impaired speech, adults associate children's speech problems with undesirable personal characteristics. Many adults with dysarthric speech have reported that, no matter what they are saying, they feel their comments are discounted or that they are assumed to be retarded or "stupid." This experience has also been noted by adults with acquired speech disorders. Although cultural differences exist in these stereotypes, listeners often believe that people with speech disorders are more likely to be emotionally disturbed (Bebout & Bradford, 1992).

It also appears that speech quality and facial appearance interact with each other in determining how a person is perceived by others. Facial attractiveness may not change ratings of speech quality, but impaired speech seems to lower ratings of physical attractiveness of the speaker. Hypernasality appears to be particularly unattractive to listeners, so that ratings of social desirability of a speaker decrease steadily as nasality increases. Clifford (1987), a well-known psychologist studying effects of cleft lip and palate, concluded that the combination of facial appearance and hypernasality contributed to "a lack of perceived competence" in individuals with a history of cleft.

Hearing Impairment

Having a hearing impairment can add to the social judgments that people make. Many children with a history of cleft have some degree of hearing impairment, which may vary with the frequency of recurrent ear infections. Negative stereotypes exist of people who have hearing impairments, with or without visible hearing aids. More importantly however, hearing is central to many aspects of social interactions among members of the general population.

Misunderstanding of overall meaning or nuance shapes the next phase of interaction. When a person is perceived as missing the intention of a communication, he or she is often viewed as annoying or frustrating. With repetition, interactions may be avoided. This is another example of the importance of the social feedback loop.

Stigma

The concept of stigma is a common thread unifying all three areas described above. *Stigma* is the discrediting and objectifying of individuals based on difference from cultural standards. In the case of persons with craniofacial anomalies, they are evaluated in a negative fashion because of their visible difference from the cultural standards of beauty, speech, hearing, and/or social interactions. Stigma diminishes a person's social acceptability, negatively impacting self-esteem. Another effect is the reduction or blocking of social and economic opportunities. The impact of stigmatization may be felt in the absence of negative intent, as when people stare out of curiosity, ignorance, or sympathy. Essentially, it is a problem of people being defined by their stigma and coming to anticipate stigmatization as well. They then may behave accordingly, as if stigmatized, regardless of the behavior or attitudes of the other people involved in interactions. People who are disfigured are particularly vulnerable to stigma. Some studies have suggested that mouth differences may be particularly open to negativity.

Behavioral Issues Related to Medical Care

As discussed earlier in this chapter, having to undergo major medical procedures is generally stressful and often difficult for family members and patients. For some, the experience is traumatizing and for others, it is an inevitable event to be faced in a matter of fact manner. Multiple surgeries may have a cumulative effect as well.

Psychological interventions can be useful for children with cleft lip and palate for a variety of concerns related to their treatment. This can be equally true for children and families who are

functioning well, as well as for those with wider psychological issues. For a small proportion of children like Brian, described in the following Case Report, multiple surgeries or medical procedures can contribute to the development of anxiety and distress. Families of children who have very visible procedures that take considerable time, such as distraction or reverse facemask use, often benefit from coaching in how to prepare peers, answer questions, and deal with the inconvenience or discomfort. Children often dread even relatively minor procedures, such as injections or having dental caries filled. Multiple studies have demonstrated that teaching children coping skills can help to reduce both the distress associated with a procedure and the time it takes to carry it out (Nocella & Kaplan, 1982; Powers, Blount, Bachanas, & Cotter, 1993). A psychologist who works with the child's medical providers can readily accompany the child to appointments to coach them in coping during the dreaded procedure.

CASE REPORT

Brian was a 9-year-old boy with a bilateral cleft lip and palate. Brian's surgical repairs had been without apparent complications and he was able to go home at the expected time on each of the several occasions. He was an honor student at a private school considered to be one of the more rigorous in the area. He had friends and had not experienced teasing since second grade. His family was close-knit and generally supportive, except for a typical sibling rivalry with a sister. Brian had interacted well with his physicians and their staff at their offices. His family was careful to adhere to recommendations and reliably attended follow-up appointments. However, after a bone graft, which he experienced as fairly painful at the donor site, he became highly anxious at the thought of the hospital. The smell of bubble gum, which had been used as a spray on the mask before surgery, brought distress, no matter what the circumstances. A few months later, he required PE tube reinsertion. Following an uneventful outpatient procedure, Brian's anxiety about the hospital almost always led to nausea and vomiting. Episodes began with him feeling scared, developing cold hands, and having a sensation of salivation, and nausea.

The usual route from Brian's house to his grandmother's passed near the children's hospital. He developed nausea as they neared the hospital and on several occasions, the driver had to pull over to the curb so that Brian could vomit. They began driving a more convoluted, lengthy route that avoided the hospital area, which eliminated his vomiting. Brian was able to voice that he appreciated avoiding the hospital, but realized it was "stupid" to react so strongly "to nothing." An interdisciplinary team clinic appointment at the hospital was marked by his vomiting twice, once about four blocks from the hospital and once in the parking lot. He could readily say that he knew there was no surgery planned for the day, but felt that reassuring himself of that fact did nothing to curb his feelings.

Brian was referred to the team psychologist to address these symptoms. His family was supportive and hopeful that intervention would lead to greater comfort for Brian and shorter and more pleasant car travel for all. He agreed to come to sessions "to get over this," even though the psychologist's office was at the hospital. The psychologist took a detailed history of the symptoms and had him monitor his thoughts and feelings throughout the week. As a result, it was evident that Brian had become classically conditioned to respond to the hospital in a way similar to children (and adults) with cancer who vomit at the sight of the hospital before they receive the chemotherapy that makes them nauseated. Therapy sessions often included his mother who enlisted the cooperation of Brian's sister and father to carry out home assignments. Brian was treated with a combination of systematic desensitization and methods to improve and broaden his coping strategies. One of the strategies was for Brian to talk about his fears, concerns, and desires for surgery and then role-play, talking to his surgeon about questions and preferences. Then his mother made an appointment for him to talk to the plastic surgeon with whom the psychologist had previously spoken and prepared. Empowering Brian to be an active participant in his care allowed Brian some sense of control. In three sessions, Brian was able to attend therapy without nausea, and in eight sessions, he was able to visit the surgical floors without anxiety. His family resumed more direct driving routes without difficulty and Brian managed his next surgery two years later without relapse.

Another area where pediatric psychologists can be of use to children with clefts is in adhering to recommendations for daily activities. For example, parents of children who suck their thumbs past early childhood can develop ways to help their children break the difficult habit through increased awareness and a reward system (Friman & Leibowitz, 1990). Parents are taught to avoid power struggles while focusing on times when the child is not sucking his or her thumb. Similarly, children whose dental hygiene is so poor that it endangers their well-being or prevents needed and even desired orthodontia can alter the children's behaviors through psychological consultation (Dahlquist, 1985; Philippot, Lenoir, D'Hoore, & Bercy, 2005). The underlying concerns expressed through poor hygiene can also be addressed when relevant. For example, looking in the mirror while brushing teeth forces the child to confront the presence of an undesirable difference in appearance, which makes some children prefer not to brush.

SUMMARY

If a child is born with a cleft lip and/or palate, it does not mean that he or she is certain to develop major psychopathology (Christensen & Mortensen, 2002). In fact, many individuals with craniofacial conditions are amazingly resilient due to a variety of factors (Strauss, 2001). However, having a facial difference complicates life and presents challenges that children without medical problems generally do not face. These challenges are not restricted to the child, but extend to the family of the child as well. In fact, early in the child's development, the majority of the psychological "fallout" of the cleft is on the family, rather than on the child. Later, the challenges to the individual seem most often to be related to school achievement (especially reading) and peer relationships. People with a history of cleft appear to be particularly at risk for diminished social interaction and sense of social competence.

Because of the prevalence of psychological problems in children with a history of cleft and their families, it is strongly recommended that craniofacial or cleft palate teams have a psychologist or similar professional as a member. Additionally, the cognitive differences that may affect learning and social interactions can often best be addressed by the team psychologist. If a psychologist cannot be included as a member of the team, the next-best option is to have a pediatric psychologist, trained in issues related to clefts, available on a referral basis. The psychologist needs to communicate with other team members and address the behaviors and attitudes of the child and family that can interfere with an optimal treatment outcome.

FOR REVIEW, DISCUSSION, AND CRITICAL THINKING

1. What are factors that contribute to the shock of having a baby with a cleft? What are some factors that help parents to adjust? What can health care professionals do to lessen the immediate shock and distress?

2. Why is cleft palate a "chronic" medical condition? How does this affect the parents? How does it affect the child?

3. What are some issues that a child with a history of cleft lip and palate may experience in school? What are some ways that parents and healthcare providers can lessen these issues? How would you suggest that the child deal with teasing?

4. What are factors that affect self-perception of individuals with a history of cleft lip and palate? How do you explain the fact that some children with significant malformations are better adjusted than other children with minor differences?

5. How does physical attractiveness affect an individual's ability to fit into society? What is a common perception of individuals with speech problems regarding intelligence? Why do you think this occurs?

6. Describe the role of the psychologist on a craniofacial team and the potential benefit of psychological services to the patient and other team members.

REFERENCES

Adachi, T., Kochi, S., & Yamaguchi, T. (2003). Characteristics of nonverbal behavior in patients with cleft lip and palate during interpersonal communication. *Cleft Palate-Craniofacial Journal, 40*(3), 310–316.

Andrews-Casal, M., Johnston, D., Fletcher, J., Mulliken, J. B., Stal, S., & Hecht, J. T. (1998). Cleft lip with or without cleft palate: Effect of family history on reproductive planning, surgical timing, and parental stress. *Cleft Palate-Craniofacial Journal, 35*(1), 52–57.

Bebout, L., & Bradford, A. (1992). Cross-cultural attitudes toward speech disorders. *Journal of Speech and Hearing Research 35*(1), 45–52.

Bradbury, E. T., & Hewison, J. (1994). Early parental adjustment to visible congenital disfigurement. *Child Care Health and Development*, 20(4), 251–266.

Brantley, H. T., & Clifford, E. (1979). Maternal and child locus of control and field dependence in cleft palate children. *Cleft Palate Journal*, 16, 183–187.

Broder, H., Richman, L. C., & Matheson, P. B. (1998). Learning disabilities, school achievement, and grade retention among children with clefts: A two-center study. *Cleft Palate-Craniofacial Journal*, 35, 127–131.

Broder, H., Smith, F. B., & Strauss, R. (2001). Developing a behavior rating scale for comparing teachers' ratings of children with and without craniofacial anomalies. *Cleft Palate-Craniofacial Journal*, 38(6), 560–565.

Broder, H., & Strauss, R. (1989). Self-concept of early primary school-age children with visible or invisible defects. *Cleft Palate Journal*, 26(2), 114–117.

Broen, P. A., Devers, M. C., Doyle, S. S., Prouty, J. M., & Moller, K. T. (1998). Acquisition of linguistic and cognitive skills by children with cleft palate. *Journal of Speech, Language, and Hearing Research*, 41(3), 676–687.

Christensen, K. & Mortensen, P. B. (2002). Facial clefting and psychiatric diseases: A follow-up of the Danish 1936–1987 facial cleft cohort. *Cleft Palate-Craniofacial Journal*, 39(4), 392–396.

Clifford, E. (1969). Paternal ratings of cleft palate infants. *Cleft Palate Journal*, 6, 235–243.

Clifford, E. (1971). Cleft palate and the person: Psychological studies of its impact. *Journal of Southern Medical Association*, 12, 1516–1520.

Clifford, E. (1987). *The cleft palate experience: New perspectives on management*. Springfield, IL: Charles C. Thomas.

Clifford, E., Crocker, E. C., & Pope, B. A. (1972). Psychological findings in the adulthood of 98 cleft palate children. *Journal of Plastic and Reconstructive Surgery*, 50, 234.

Clifford, M. M. (1975). Physical attractiveness and academic performance. *Child Study Journal*, 5, 201–209.

Coy, K., Speltz, M. L., and Jones, K. (2002). Facial appearance and attachment in infants with orofacial clefts: A replication. *Cleft Palate-Craniofacial Journal*, 39(1), 66–72.

Dahlquist, L. M. (1985). The effects of behavioral intervention on dental flossing skills in children. *Journal of Pediatric Psychology*, 10(4), 403–412.

Estes, R. E., & Morris, H. L. (1970). Relationships among intelligence, speech proficiency, and hearing sensitivity in children with cleft palates. *Cleft Palate Journal*, 7, 763–773.

Friman, P. C., & Leibowitz, J. M. (1990). An effective and acceptable treatment alternative for chronic thumb- and finger-sucking. *Journal of Pediatric Psychology*, 15(1), 57–65.

Goodstein, L. D. (1960). MMPI differences between parents of children with cleft palate and parents of physically normal children. *Journal of Speech and Hearing Research*, 3, 31–38.

Goodstein, L. D. (1961). Intellectual impairment in children with cleft palates. *Journal of Speech and Hearing Research*, 4, 287–294.

Kapp-Simon, K. (1986). Self-concept of primary school age children with cleft lip, cleft palate or both. *Cleft Palate Journal*, 23 (1), 24–27.

Koomen, H., & Hoeksma, J. (1993). Early hospitalization and disturbances of infant behavior and the mother-infant relationship. *Journal of Child Psychology and Psychiatry*, 34(6), 917–934.

Lamb, M., Wilson, F., & Leeper, H. (1973). The intellectual function of cleft palate children compared on the basis of cleft type and sex. *Cleft Palate Journal, 10*, 367.

Middleton, G. N., Lass, N. J., Starr, P., & Pannbacker, M. (1986). Survey of public awareness and knowledge of cleft palate. *Cleft Palate Journal, 23*, 58–63.

Nocella, J., & Kaplan, R. M. (1982). Training children to cope with dental treatment. *Journal of Pediatric Psychology, 7*(2), 175–178.

Nopoulos, P., Choe, I., Berg, S., Van Demark, D., Canady, J., & Richman L. (2005). Ventral frontal cortex morphology in adult males with isolated orofacial clefts: Relationship to abnormalities in social function. *Cleft Palate-Craniofacial Journal, 42*(2), 138–144.

Pertschuk, M. J., & Whitaker, L. A. (1982). Social and psychological effects of craniofacial deformity and surgical reconstruction. *Clinical Plastic Surgery, 9*(3), 297–306.

Philippot, P., Lenoir, N., D'Hoore, W., & Bercy, P. (2005). Improving patients' compliance with the treatment of periodontitis: A controlled study of behavioural intervention. *Journal of Clinical Periodontology, 32*(6), 653–658.

Pillemer, F. G., & Cook, K. V. (1989). The psychosocial adjustment of pediatric craniofacial patients after surgery. *Cleft Palate Journal, 26*(3), 201–207.

Powers, S. W., Blount, R. L., Bachanas, P. J., & Cotter, M. W. (1993). Helping preschool leukemia patients and their parents cope during injections. *Journal of Pediatric Psychology, 18*(6), 681–695.

Ramstad, T. E., Ottem, E., & Shaw, W. C. (1995a). Psychosocial adjustment in Norwegian adults who had undergone standardised treatment of complete cleft lip and palate: II. Self-reported problems and concerns with appearance. *Scandinavian Journal of Plastic and Reconstructive Surgery and Hand Surgery, 29*(4), 329–336.

Ramstad, T. E., Ottem, E., & Shaw, W. C. (1995b). Psychosocial adjustment in Norwegian adults who had undergone standardized treatment of complete cleft lip and palate: I. Education, employment and marriage. *Scandinavian Journal of Plastic and Reconstructive Surgery and Hand Surgery, 29*(3), 251–257.

Richman, L. (1978). Parents and teachers: Differing views of behavior of cleft palate children. *Cleft Palate Journal, 15*, 360–364.

Richman, L. C., & Eliason, M. (1982). Psychological characteristics of children with cleft lip and palate: Intellectual, achievement, behavioral, and personality variables. *Cleft Palate Journal, 19*, 249.

Richman, L. C., & Millard, T. (1997). Brief report: Cleft lip and palate: Longitudinal behavior and relationships of cleft conditions to behavior and achievement. *Journal of Pediatric Psychology, 22*(4), 487–494.

Richman, L. C., & Ryan, S. M. (2003). Do the reading disabilities of children with cleft fit into current models of developmental dyslexia? *Cleft Palate-Craniofacial Journal, 40*(2), 154–157.

Richman, L. C., Ryan, S., Wilgenbusch, T., & Millard, T. (2004). Overdiagnosis and medication for attention-deficit hyperactivity disorder in children with cleft: Diagnostic examination and follow-up. *Cleft Palate-Craniofacial Journal, 41*(4), 351–354.

Sank, J., Berk, N. W., Cooper, M. E., & Marazita, M. I. (2003). Perceived social support of mothers of children with clefts. *Cleft Palate-Craniofacial Journal, 40*(2), 165–171.

Slifer, K. J., Beck, M., Amari, A., Diver, T., Hilley, L., Kane, A., & McDonnell, S. (2003). Self-concept and satisfaction with physical appearance in youth with and without oral clefts. *Children's Health Care*, 32, 81–101.

Slifer, K. J., Amari, A., Diver, T., Hilley, L., Beck, M., Kane, A., & McDonnell, S. (2004). Social interaction patterns of children and adolescents with and without oral clefts during a videotaped analogue social encounter. *Cleft Palate-Craniofacial Journal*, 41(2), 175–184.

Speltz, M. G., Armsden, G. C., & Clarren, S. S. (1990). Effects of craniofacial birth defects on maternal functioning postinfancy. *Journal of Pediatric Psychology*, 15(2), 177–196.

Strauss, R. P. (2001). "Only skin deep": Health, resilience, and craniofacial care. *Cleft Palate-Craniofacial Journal*. 38(3), 226–30.

Strauss, R. P., & Fenson, C. (2005). Experiencing the "good life": Literary views of craniofacial conditions and quality of life. *Cleft Palate-Craniofacial Journal*, 42(1), 14–18.

Strauss, R. P., Sharp, M. C., Lorch, S. C., & Kachalia, B. (1995). Physicians' communication of "bad news": Parent experiences of being informed of their child's cleft lip/palate. *Pediatrics*, 96(1), 82–89.

Thomas, P. S., Turner, S. R., Rumsey, N., Dowell, T., & Sandy, J. R. (1997). Satisfaction with facial appearance among subjects affected by a cleft. *Cleft Palate-Craniofacial Journal*, 34(3), 226–231.

Tobiasen, J. M. (1988). Psychosocial outcome of craniofacial surgery in children: Discussion. *Plastic and Reconstructive Surgery*, 82, 745–746.

Tobiasen, J. M. (1989). Scaling facial impairment. *Cleft Palate Journal*, 26(3), 249–254.

Van Staden, F., & Gerhardt, C. (1995). Mothers of children with facial cleft deformities: Reactions and effects. *South American Journal of Psychology*, 25(1), 39–46.

Weigl, V., Rudolph, M., Eysholdt, U., & Rosanowski, F. (2005). Anxiety, depression, and quality of life in mothers of children with cleft lip/palate. *Folia Phoniatrica et Logopaedica*, 57(1), 20–27.

PART 3

INTERDISCIPLINARY CARE

CHAPTER

11

THE TEAM APPROACH TO ASSESSMENT AND TREATMENT

CHAPTER OUTLINE

INTRODUCTION

I ndividuals with craniofacial anomalies, including cleft lip and palate, often demonstrate multiple complex issues, including early feeding and nutritional problems, developmental delay, hearing loss, abnormal speech and/or resonance, dentofacial and orthodontic abnormalities, aesthetic issues, and possible psychosocial problems (American Cleft Palate-Craniofacial Association, 1996). It is not possible for one professional to deal with all of these areas of concern. In fact, these patients often have the need for medical, surgical, dental, speech pathology, and psychological treatment. Patients with craniofacial anomalies not only require evaluation and treatment from a variety of professionals, they also need follow-up over a long period of time (Paynter, Wilson, & Jordan, 1993). The entire habilitative process can last from infancy into adulthood. Even the most knowledgeable of families prefer a coordinated team approach of appointments and procedures (Jeffery & Boorman, 2001). Team care is therefore very important to achieve the best treatment outcome in a way that is best for the family.

The main purpose of this chapter is to impress upon the reader of the importance of the team approach in the management of patients with cleft lip/palate or craniofacial anomalies. This chapter discusses the advantages of and some of the problems with the team management. The types and characteristics of teams are described. Finally, information is given on how to find a specialty team in order to refer a child for further assessment and intervention as appropriate.

NEED FOR TEAM MANAGEMENT

There are many qualified professionals throughout the United States and the world who can care for patients with craniofacial anomalies. However, as part of the habilitation process, it is common that the treatment of one professional has an impact on the treatment of other professionals. In addition, the sequence of treatment from each discipline must be considered for a variety of reasons. Therefore, services to this population of patients must be provided in a coordinated and integrated manner over a period of years for maximum benefit to the patient. In order to accomplish this, the team approach to management is required for these patients. With the team approach, the patient is more likely to receive quality services, continuity of care, and long-term follow-up in order to achieve the best ultimate outcome. In addition, the team approach allows the care to focus on the whole child, and not just the cleft or one particular abnormality. Therefore, the multidisciplinary team approach for the management of these patients is widely accepted (David, Anderson, Schnitt, Nugent, & Sells, 2006; Schnitt, Agir, & David, 2004; Thomas, 2000).

The importance of team management for patients with cleft lip and palate was first recognized by H. K. Cooper, who founded the Lancaster Cleft Palate Clinic in the early 1930s (Krogman, 1979). Many cleft palate or craniofacial teams were formed across the country in subsequent years. In 1987, the Surgeon General of the United States recognized the need for a team approach to the management of patients with special health care needs, and articulated this need in a report (Surgeon General's Report, 1987). This report emphasized that these children require comprehensive, coordinated care provided by health care systems that are accessible and responsive to the patients and their families.

In response to this report, the Maternal and Child Health Bureau provided funding to the American Cleft Palate-Craniofacial Association (ACPA) to develop recommended practices in the care of patients with craniofacial anomalies. In order to accomplish this, a large group of various professionals from around the country was convened for a consensus conference in 1991. This meeting resulted in the publishing of a comprehensive document by the ACPA containing parameters for evaluation and treatment of patients with clefts or craniofacial anomalies (American Cleft Palate-Craniofacial Association, 1993, 2004). One of the fundamental principles contained in this document is that the management of patients with craniofacial anomalies is best provided by an interdisciplinary team of specialists, especially when these specialists see a significant number of patients each year and therefore develop expertise through experience (p. 5).

There is general consensus among professionals regarding the importance of a team approach to the care of patients with cleft lip/palate or craniofacial anomalies. This approach has the advantages of access to multiple disciplines, centralization of services, long-term treatment planning from birth to adulthood, better continuity of care, comprehensive documentation from all professionals involved in the patient's care, interdisciplinary evaluations, follow-up studies, and interdisciplinary research and quality assurance (Tindlund & Holmefjord, 1997). The team approach makes the care of patients easier for the provider and

more effective for the patient. The goal of the cleft or craniofacial team, therefore, is to "insure that care is provided in a coordinated, consistent manner with proper sequencing of evaluations and treatments within the framework of the patient's overall developmental, medical and psychological needs" (American Cleft Palate-Craniofacial Association, 1996).

CHARACTERISTICS OF TEAMS

Types of Teams

A team of professionals can be multidisciplinary or interdisciplinary, depending on the working relationship of the members and the structure of the team. A *multidisciplinary team* is a group of professionals from various disciplines who work independently in evaluating and treating patients with complex medical needs. The members of this type of team have well-defined roles and cooperate with each other, but there is little communication and interaction among the team members (Bardach et al., 1984; Strauss, 1999). The biggest problem with a multidisciplinary team is that the patient receives a series of evaluations and recommendations, but there is no integration of the information or recommendations.

On the other hand, an *interdisciplinary team* is a group of professionals from various disciplines who work together to coordinate the care of a patient. With this model, there is collaboration, interaction, communication, and cooperation among the different specialists who are involved in the patient's care. There may or may not be a joint evaluation, but there definitely is a joint plan of care. This is developed when all members of the team come together to discuss the findings, impressions, and recommendations. The final plan of care is negotiated and based on the integration of all the recommendations (Strauss, 1999). With this approach, the sequence of procedures and approximate timelines can be outlined for the patient and the family. Therefore, the interdisciplinary team model is felt to be the most effective one for management of patients with craniofacial anomalies.

A cleft palate or craniofacial team that works together for a period of time may even evolve into *transdisciplinary team*. This type of team has members that truly understand the other disciplines and how they relate to the total care of the patient. Although team members cannot perform duties across disciplines, they can have an understanding of the various disciplines in order to see the "big picture." This is certainly a benefit for the ultimate care of the patient.

Cleft palate or craniofacial teams often serve as the primary *treating team* for their patients. In larger centers, the team may also serve as a *consulting team*. In the role as a consulting team, the team members provide a second opinion as a group regarding the total care of the patient. This is forwarded to the treating professionals for consideration. The treating professionals may be in the local community or far away. Regardless, there must be excellent communication between the team and the practitioners who will be following the patient for treatment and follow-up care.

Team Membership and Structure

In order to meet the complex needs of the patients and their families, cleft palate or craniofacial teams typically include medical, surgical, dental, speech, and psychosocial professionals. Table 11–1 lists the various professionals who are often members of a cleft or craniofacial team, and it gives a description of each professional's role in the management of

---

TABLE 11–1 Professional Roles within a Cleft Palate or Craniofacial Anomaly Team

Audiologist: The audiologist is the person who is responsible for testing the child's hearing and middle ear function. Since individuals with craniofacial anomalies are at high risk for structural ear anomalies, middle ear disease, and hearing loss, the audiologist works with the otolaryngologist in monitoring the hearing and middle ear function of these individuals.

Pediatric Dentist: The role of the pediatric dentist (sometimes called pedodontist) is to be responsible for the general care of the child's teeth, and the prevention and treatment of tooth decay. The pediatric dentist ensures that the child develops habits of good oral hygiene for the promotion of healthy teeth and gums. Even the primary teeth are important to protect and preserve since they act as placeholders for the permanent teeth. The pediatric dentist may be involved with managing misaligned cleft segments prior to the lip closure. When the child is in the primary or mixed dentition stages, the pediatric dentist is often the one to improve early malocclusion, which often includes moving the maxillary segments through palatal expansion.

Geneticist: A geneticist (dysmorphologist) is responsible for assessing patients with a history of cleft, velopharyngeal dysfunction, or craniofacial anomalies for a pattern that indicates a known syndrome. Once a syndrome is identified, the geneticist counsels the family regarding the diagnosis, the recurrence risk for additional offspring of both the family and the patient, and the prognosis.

Nurse: The nurse's role on the team is to assess the child's overall physical development. The nurse can determine if the child is growing normally and is in good general health. The nurse is often the professional who assists the family in developing compensatory feeding techniques. Finally, the nurse is usually the professional who counsels the family regarding surgical procedures and answers their specific questions.

Oral Surgeon: The oral surgeon is the specialist who does bone grafts to the alveolar cleft areas when there is deficient bone in the line of the cleft. This professional also performs the orthognathic surgeries, including maxillary expansions and mandibular setbacks, to normalize the occlusion between the maxillary and mandibular arches.

Orthodontist: The orthodontist treats dental and skeletal malocclusion and promotes normal jaw relationships. The orthodontist is responsible for aligning misplaced teeth and adjacent tissues to improve the dental and facial aesthetics and to improve the function of the dentition.

(continues)

TABLE 11–1 *(continued)*

Otolaryngologist: The otolaryngologist, also known as the ear, nose, and throat specialist (ENT), is responsible for monitoring middle ear function and hearing, and treating middle ear disease, which is common in children with a history of cleft or craniofacial anomalies. The otolaryngologist also assesses the structural aspects of the oral cavity, oropharynx, nasal cavity, and upper airway—and treats anomalies, including adenotonsillar hypertrophy, pharyngeal masses, or vocal fold abnormalities. The otolaryngologist may be the surgeon involved in the nasal and oral repairs and reconstruction. The otolaryngologist also manages upper airway obstruction, which is particularly common in infants with Pierre Robin sequence.

Pediatrician: The pediatrician is responsible for assessing the patient's overall medical health, growth, and development. The pediatrician determines whether other aspects of medical care should be done prior to surgical intervention.

Plastic Surgeon: The plastic surgeon is responsible for the surgical repair of the lip, palate, and facial anomalies, and is also responsible for the surgery for correction of velopharyngeal dysfunction. This surgeon may perform cranial surgery, bone grafts, and orthognathic surgery on the jaws. The plastic surgeon is responsible for not only the repair of the defects, but also for the improvement through surgery of the patient's overall facial aesthetics, feeding function, and speech.

Prosthodontist: Prosthodontics is a branch of dentistry that deals with the restoration of natural teeth or the replacement of missing teeth. The prosthodontist can develop prosthetic devices to replace or improve the appearance of surrounding oral and facial structures. The prosthodontist can also manufacture and fit devices to assist with feeding and with velopharyngeal closure.

Psychologist: The psychologist assesses the patient's psychosocial needs, and assists the patient and family in dealing with the medical, social, and emotional challenges that occur due to the patient's anomalies. The psychologist often assists the physician in determining the preparedness of the patient for each surgical procedure.

Social Worker: The social worker helps families to deal with the many problems associated with the child's anomalies. The social worker may be the one to coordinate appointments and may also assist the families in dealing with insurance and other funding sources. The social worker may help the family to manage their stress and emotional reactions to the many problems and issues associated with the child's treatment.

Speech-Language Pathologist (SLP): The speech-language pathologist counsels the parents or guardians regarding what to expect with communication skills and how to stimulate normal development at home. The speech-language pathologist evaluates feeding and swallowing, general development, speech, language, resonance, and velopharyngeal function, and makes recommendations for treatment when problems are identified. The speech-language pathologist provides therapy for communication problems and disorders of feeding or swallowing.

Team Coordinator: The team coordinator typically represents the team in any interactions with parents, other health care professionals, and the community. This person is responsible for planning the meetings and scheduling patients for each meeting. The coordinator compiles the recommendations from each professional and puts this together in a comprehensive team report. The coordinator helps to counsel the family regarding the recommendations and ensures that there is follow-up on recommendations that are made by team members.

these patients. (Figure 11–1 shows the team members of the Craniofacial Center at Cincinnati Children's Hospital Medical Center.)

In 1996, the membership of the ACPA established basic standards for what constitutes a cleft or craniofacial team (American Cleft Palate-Craniofacial Association, 1996). Those teams that meet these standards are listed in the ACPA Membership-Team Directory, which is published annually (American Cleft Palate-Craniofacial Association, 2007), and also on the ACPA Web site (http://www.cleftline.org).

One standard requirement for meeting the ACPA standards is that each team must have a coordinator, who is usually a nurse or other health care professional. This person facilitates the scheduling of all team meetings, as well as the documentation of impressions and recommendations for each patient. The coordinator ensures that the recommendations are implemented and may also be the person who represents the team in communicating with the patient or family. Other requirements include regular team meetings and participation in

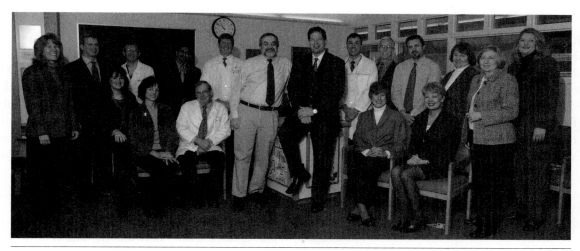

FIGURE 11–1   Team members of the Craniofacial Center at Cincinnati Children's Hospital Medical Center, 2006.

continuing education programs about clefts or craniofacial anomalies.

As part of the basic standards, ACPA determined which professionals should be members of the team in order to qualify as either a cleft palate team (CPT) or a craniofacial team (CFT) and be listed as such in the team directory. The ACPA minimum standards for team membership are as follows:

- **Cleft Palate Team (CPT):** ACPA has determined that a Cleft Palate Team (CPT) must have a surgeon, an orthodontist, a speech-language pathologist, and at least one additional specialist. Other members might include an audiologist, geneticist (dysmorphologist), nurse, oral surgeon (maxillofacial surgeon), otolaryngologist (ear, nose, and throat specialist), orthodontist, pediatrician, prosthodontist, psychologist, or social worker. ACPA also requires this type of team to evaluate at least 50 patients per year and have at least one surgeon who operates on at least 10 primary clefts per year.

- **Craniofacial Team (CFT):** A Craniofacial Team, as defined by ACPA, must consist of a craniofacial surgeon, an orthodontist, a mental health professional, and speech-language pathologist. Other members may include a neurosurgeon and ophthalmologist, in addition to those professionals included in a cleft team.

ACPA has some additional categories as follows:

- **Evaluation and Treatment Review Team (ERT):** This team provides evaluation services but not clinical care.

- **Low Population Density Team (LPD):** This team provides clinical care in rural regions where there are few services available.

- **Interim Team (I-CPT or I-CFT):** This is a team that provides clinical care and is in transition.

- **Geographical Listed Teams (GLT):** This category is used for teams that do not fall under the previous categories.

ACPA has made no specific recommendations for a team structure for children who have abnormal resonance (with or without a history of cleft palate) as the primary presenting concern. Patients with velopharyngeal dysfunction, regardless of etiology, are often managed effectively by a cleft palate or craniofacial team. However, a subset of these professionals can form a specialty team as follows:

- **Velopharyngeal Dysfunction (VPD or VPI) Team:** A team for evaluation of velopharyngeal function should include a speech-language pathologist, an otolaryngologist (or a plastic surgeon), and ideally a geneticist. The geneticist is important because many children with VPD of unknown origin have a previously unidentified syndrome, which is most commonly velocardiofacial syndrome.

In 1996, the American Cleft Palate-Craniofacial Association conducted a survey of all known cleft palate and craniofacial teams in the United States and Canada (Strauss, 1998). Of the 296 contacted, 247 (83.4%) responded by filling out a self-assessment survey. Based on the results of that survey, it was determined that 105 (42.5%) were functioning as cleft palate teams, and 102 (41.3%) were functioning as craniofacial teams. The remaining 12 teams (4.9%) were either new teams, teams with low numbers due to their geographic location, or teams that merely consult, but do not provide treatment.

In addition to the professionals on the team, the parents or family are also key players in determining the treatment plan for the patient. It is important that the professionals on the team gain the support and cooperation from the families. In fact, all decisions for treatment must be based on the patient's and family's wishes, in addition to the clinical indications (Sharp, 1995). If the family members are not active participants in the decision-making process, compliance with the team's recommendations can be affected (Nackashi & Dixon-Wood, 1989; Pannbacker & Scheuerle, 1993; Paynter, Jordan, & Finch, 1990; Paynter et al., 1993). On the other hand, appropriate family involvement can significantly improve compliance with the recommendations, which can ultimately improve the outcomes of treatment (Paynter et al., 1990; Paynter et al., 1993).

Team Leadership

The qualifications, personality, and skill of the team leader are highly important in determining the function and success of the team. There is little room for authoritarianism in clinical team leadership. Instead, the leader must be able to ensure that all team members are respected equally, and that their opinions are heard and considered for the best patient outcome. Having a dominant team member can result in decisions that are made based on that person's opinion rather than on team consensus. It is the responsibility of the team leader to be sure that that does not happen and that all members' opinions are heard and considered before decisions regarding the patient's care are made (Strauss & Broder, 1985). The most effective teams function by consensus, even though each professional may view the needs of the patient differently (Noar, 1992; Strauss, 1999).

Team Responsibilities

In order to provide a truly integrated system of patient care, the ACPA has made a number of recommendations regarding the responsibilities of the team in its Parameters document (American Cleft Palate-Craniofacial Association, 1993). For example, it is recommended that each team should have an office with a secretary or coordinator and a designated phone number.

The office should maintain all team documents and patient records. Patients should be evaluated at regular intervals, depending on the needs of the patient and the family. Although the patients may be examined individually by the professionals on the team, regularly scheduled team meetings must be held for discussion and negotiation of the plan of care. Communication of recommendations to the patient and family must be made verbally and in written form. There must be ongoing communication with the direct care providers in the patient's home community. The team should provide patients with information regarding resources for other services and financial assistance as needed. Finally, the teams should provide educational programs for families, other care providers, and the general public.

In a diverse society, team members must be sensitive to the ethnographic and cultural characteristics of the families that they serve. These factors may determine the way in which families understand and view the medical issues, and the way they follow the recommendations of the team (Louw, Shimbambu, & Roemer, 2006). To provide the most effective services, team intervention must be family-focused and culturally sensitive.

Team Quality

The quality of the services provided by a team is difficult to measure or quantify. In many cases, quality is determined solely by the perception of the "customers." Although this is an important indicator of quality, there are other more measurable ways to assure quality of services. The guidelines listed in the Parameters document (American Cleft Palate-Craniofacial Association, 1993) can help a team achieve and maintain the basic requirements for an appropriate team, as determined by professional consensus from around the country.

Another way to ensure quality is for the team to develop and participate in a performance improvement program. In a 1999 survey of cleft and craniofacial teams in the North America, 50% reported that they have a quality assurance program in place to measure treatment outcomes (Strauss, 1999). This type of a program provides a mechanism for teams to monitor, self-evaluate, and improve various aspects of their patient care. Clinical pathways and algorithms of care have also been developed by some teams (Stal, Klebuc, Taylor, Spira, & Edwards, 1998b).

The quality of the team is greatly determined by the quality of each individual member. It is important that all members of the team are licensed and certified in their individual areas of specialty. The education and experience required for specialization are determined by the various professional associations, specialty boards, and licensure boards. Each team must assure that all members possess not only the appropriate and current credentials for practice, but also the requisite experience and skill in the evaluation and treatment of patients in the specialty area of craniofacial anomalies. If the professionals are not well trained in this specialty area, their good intentions may not be enough to result in good decisions. In fact, these "experts" can actually do more harm than good due to their lack of specialty experience in the area of craniofacial anomalies (Sidman, 1995).

Another factor that affects the quality of a team is the number of patients seen per year and the number of team meetings per year. This has an impact on the experience base of the team and on the time commitment given by the team members to craniofacial anomalies. In addition, teams with a large patient base usually have more members than those with few patients and they also have more disciplines represented on the team. Therefore, it is more likely that the patient's various treatment needs will be adequately and appropriately served by the team. Of course, when the patient requires services by professionals not represented on the team, members must have the knowledge and resources to refer the patient to appropriate professionals outside of the immediate team.

The stability of the team and how long team members serve on the team can also be a factor to consider. Since the patient's treatment typically begins at birth and may continue until adulthood, the consistency and longevity of team members becomes important for the consistency and continuity of care.

It is especially important that all members of the team stay current with recent developments in their respective disciplines, particularly as it relates to cleft and craniofacial care. Active membership in the American Cleft Palate-Craniofacial Association (ACPA) and attendance at annual meetings of this association and other similar associations (local, national, and international) is the best way to be informed. In addition, it is important to be familiar with the literature regarding the current techniques used for the evaluation and treatment of craniofacial anomalies. An interest in continuous learning helps the team members to provide the best possible care for the patients.

Finally, the extent to which the team involves the parents or caregivers in the decision-making process affects the overall team quality. It has been found that when parents have a high opinion of the team and the services provided, compliance with recommendations is greatest. However, if the parents have a low opinion of the team, compliance is negatively affected (Paynter et al., 1990).

Team Process

The cleft or craniofacial team typically becomes involved in the management of the child's needs soon after birth. This begins with parent counseling and the management of feeding issues and airway problems in the neonatal period. Team care should then continue until the physical growth of the individual has been completed, which is usually between the ages of 18 and 21. Care can continue through adulthood if there are remaining medical, surgical, dental, psychological, or communication problems that can be improved or resolved by the team members.

The method of scheduling and evaluating patients as a team differs in different settings. In most cases, each professional evaluates the patient through a separate consultation or screening, but this often occurs on the same day in a clinic setting. When the evaluations are done in a clinic, there is the opportunity for several professionals to work together in evaluating the patient (Figure 11–2). The interdisciplinary team members then meet to discuss impressions and recommendations, and to negotiate a plan of treatment (Figure 11–3). The treatment priorities and appropriate sequence of treatment is then determined. The coordinator, or another designated team member, is responsible for communicating the recommendations with the family and making sure that appropriate appointments are scheduled.

Although the team coordinator may be the primary contact person for the family, each person on the team is responsible for counseling the family about the plan of treatment relative to that discipline, as well as any concerns the family might have. It has been shown that when the family members are involved and informed regarding the health care decisions for their children, this can reduce stress and improve treatment outcomes (Paynter, Edmonson, & Jordan, 1991; Walesky-Rainbow & Morris, 1978). The ultimate treatment plan is determined by the recommendations of the team members; the concerns, needs, and goals of the

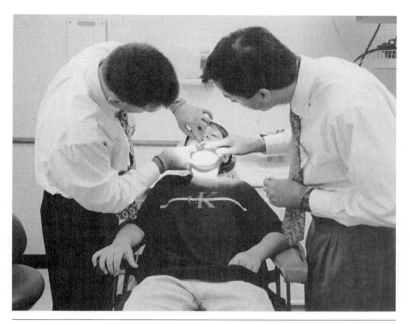

FIGURE 11–2   The team approach to assessment.

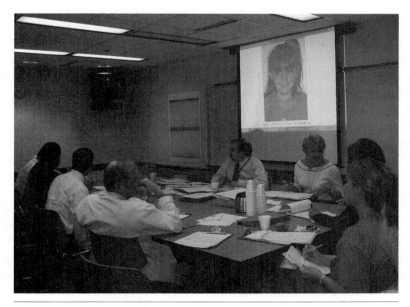

FIGURE 11–3   Face-to-face discussions in team conferences are important for coordinated patient care.

patient and the patient's family; and the limitations and restrictions of the third-party payment sources.

Advantages of and Potential Problems with the Team Approach

Advantages of the Team Approach

The team approach to management offers many advantages to the patient and the patient's family (American Cleft Palate-Craniofacial Association, 1993; Borah, Hagberg, Jakubiak, & Temple, 1993; Chen, Chen, Wang, & Noordhoff, 1988; Colburn & Cherry, 1985; Kline, 1997; Lang, Neil-Dwyer, Evans, & Honeybul, 1998; Marsh, 1982; McWilliams, Morris, & Shelton, 1990; Pinsky & Goldberg, 1977; Sharp, 1995; Stal, Chebret, & McElroy, 1998a; Strauss, 1998; Strauss, 1999; Strohecker, 1993; Will, Aduss, Kuehn, & Parsons, 1989). First of all, the team offers an evaluation of the whole child that is completed through the individual evaluations of many professionals. The team evaluation is comprehensive, yet done with fewer visits and usually at a lower cost than individual evaluations. The plan of care is devised by professionals who work together and understand each other's disciplines. There is shared decision-making among the team members and decisions are based on more information than one professional would have compiled independently (Sharp, 1995). There is usually better follow-up and monitoring of care, since this is the responsibility of the team coordinator. Teams usually consist of "experts" in the field who can provide state-of-the-art care. Teams promote better services through parent groups, special camps, and the provision of pamphlets

and other educational materials. There is usually one main contact person on the team who can assist the family in communicating problems, questions, or concerns.

There are also many advantages of the team approach for the professionals. First, the team approach saves time by expediting the collaboration process. It also increases inter-professional communication. This helps to develop good working relationships among the team members and increases the knowledge of each professional. One of the most significant advantages of the team approach is that it makes it possible to keep good serial records (Brogan, 1988). The team can also be an effective vehicle for collaboration in research and publications. Some states have developed networks of teams for the purpose of collaboration in research endeavors and continuing education (Abdoney, Habal, Scheuerle, & Rans, 1988; Will & Aduss, 1987; Will & Parsons, 1991).

Potential Problems with the Team Approach

Although the advantages of the team approach far outweigh any disadvantage, there are some common inherent problems associated with interdisciplinary teams. One factor that can affect the function of the team is the perceived or ascribed status of various team members relative to other members. This can be based on characteristics such as age, gender, discipline, experience, or accomplishments (Cohn, 1991). If team members are not considered equals in status on the team, then the individuals with the ascribed higher status will tend to exert more influence on the decisions of the group than those members of lower status (Cohn, 1991). This can have a negative impact on the quality of the group decision making. For the team to be effective, there must be an atmosphere of equality and mutual respect among all of the team members.

Problems can also occur if the individual roles are not clearly defined within the team. If the roles are not clear, there may be interdisciplinary competition or "turf issues" at times. For example, there is often an overlap of skills between the plastic surgeon, the oral surgeon, and the otolaryngologist. As a team, it is helpful to define who does what, when it's done, and under what circumstances. This avoids conflicts over such things as who does the bone graft, who does the orthognathic surgery, or who does the secondary surgery for velopharyngeal dysfunction.

A different but equally disruptive problem occurs when there are members on the team who are hypersensitive to feedback. This can be a problem, for example, when a surgical procedure was not as successful as was hoped, and needs to be revised. Team members must be able to speak honestly without concern of "hurting someone's feelings." They must also be able to express differences of opinion without hesitation.

Disagreements in the philosophy of care or in treatment protocols can have a major impact on the team's performance. Communication among members regarding procedures and protocols must take place so that there is consensus regarding the standards of care and continuum of care within the team. If necessary, an algorithm of care can be developed to help team members reach consensus on the management of various diagnoses and patient concerns.

All of the potential problems of the interdisciplinary team can and should be overcome for the team to be successful. This requires ongoing communication, honesty, and mutual respect. Ultimately, the focus of the team should be on the care and well-being of the patients, and not on individual agendas and egos of the team members.

How to Be an Effective Team Member

Effective interdisciplinary team members are usually those who are very competent and knowledgeable in their particular discipline. When working on an interdisciplinary team that requires specialty knowledge, such as a craniofacial team, each member must have specialty expertise in that area. At the same time, an effective team member must show a strong interest in the knowledge of other disciplines, and have a desire to learn from other disciplines.

All team members should show respect for others and their opinions, especially when there is disagreement. Each team member must feel free to express his or her honest opinion, without the fear of offending someone. It is important to place quality patient care and appropriate patient management first and not be willing to compromise this due to a concern about personal feelings or personal agendas. When mistakes are made, as they will be, it is important that each team member feels comfortable enough to be able to admit mistakes, without worry about undue criticism. In addition, the team members must be comfortable enough with each other to be able to admit what they don't know in order to further learning and professional competence.

It is important that team members are dependable and reliable, especially since all professionals are very busy. It is not well received when one person holds up the process or lets the other members down.

Finally, the use of humor can be very effective in developing camaraderie, and can also help to enhance respect and working

Case Report

The Value of the Team Approach

The value of a team approach to management is illustrated by the following case history: Barbara was born with a bilateral complete cleft lip and cleft palate. The lip and palate repairs were done at the appropriate time. She had had speech therapy in grade school, but she was discharged from therapy with the notation that she was "doing as well as can be expected, given her velopharyngeal mechanism." Unfortunately, she was not followed by a craniofacial team at the time, and no referral was made for further assessment and treatment.

Barbara was finally seen at the age of 16 by the craniofacial team at Cincinnati Children's Hospital Medical Center. Following the team evaluation, many treatment recommendations were made.

- The orthodontist reported that the patient had a Class III malocclusion with anterior open bite and linguaverted maxillary incisors. His recommendation was to align the maxillary arch with orthodontics.
- The speech-language pathologist reported that the speech was characterized by hypernasality and nasal air emission. Given those findings, the speech-language pathologist recommended a nasopharyngoscopy assessment and a pharyngeal flap for correction of velopharyngeal insufficiency (VPI). This was to be followed by postoperative speech therapy to correct articulation errors that were compensatory as a result of both the malocclusion and the VPI.
- The oral surgeon reported that with the discrepancy between the position of the maxillary and mandibular arches, a Le Fort I maxillary advancement was indicated to move the maxilla in appropriate position.
- The plastic surgeon noted that there was redundant vermilion in the line of the cleft and that the Cupid's bow needed revision with an Abbe flap.
- The psychologist reported that, after talking with Barbara at length, she discovered that one of the things that really bothered Barbara about herself was her flattened nose.

Given all of these concerns and recommendations, the plan of care had to be designed with the best overall results in mind. In order to achieve that, the appropriate sequencing of procedures had to be determined.

In this case, the first step was for the orthodontist to bring the teeth into alignment in preparation for the orthognathic (jaw) surgery. Bringing the teeth into proper alignment made the occlusion and profile actually worse, but this was an important first step for the best ultimate results. The next step was for the oral surgeon to perform a Le Fort I maxillary advancement. This normalized the occlusion and gave more support for the upper lip and base of the nose. Once the jaws were in alignment, the plastic surgeon did a pharyngeal flap to correct the velopharyngeal insufficiency, and then he performed the lip and nose revision. About six weeks after the surgery, Barbara began speech therapy to correct the remaining compensatory articulation errors. She was discharged from therapy with normal speech after less than two months of therapy.

With this planned sequence, Barbara had the best overall outcome for both aesthetics and speech. On the other hand, if the pharyngeal flap had been done prior to maxillary advancement, the position and effectiveness of the flap could have been compromised with the maxillary advancement. The maxillary advancement could also have had a detrimental effect on the lip and nose if those revisions had been done first. Therefore, the sequence and coordination of treatment is very important in patients who require care from multiple specialists.

relationships among the team members. Team members who use humor in their interactions with each other usually work more effectively together and this has a positive effect on the quality of services that are ultimately provided to the patients.

RESOURCES FOR SERVICES

How to Find a Cleft Palate or Craniofacial Team

Craniofacial teams are located all around the country, but particularly within teaching hospitals or pediatric hospitals. In most cases, it is not important that the team be located near the patient's home. In general, the team will need to see the patient for evaluation and consultation only once or twice a year during the active treatment process. Routine treatment, such as general dental care, orthodontics, speech therapy, and pediatric care can usually be provided by professionals in the patient's own community, as long as there is regular communication and consultation with the team members. The closest cleft palate or craniofacial team can be determined by contacting the Cleft Palate Foundation (CPF), which is associated with the American Cleft Palate-Craniofacial Association. Information regarding this organization and others is listed in the Resources section in this book.

Funding Sources

Funding for the evaluation and treatment of cleft lip, cleft palate, and other craniofacial anomalies can come from a variety of sources. Private insurance companies will usually cover most of the expenses associated with the medical care of the patient if the patient was born when the policy was in effect. Financial assistance can also be obtained through federal and state programs such as Champus, Medicaid, the patient's state's Children's Special Health Services, the Bureau of Vocational Rehabilitation, and through selected Shriners' Hospitals across the country. Some private and nonprofit organizations provide funds or special services to meet the needs of children with clefts or craniofacial anomalies. Resources for financial aid can often be obtained through a social worker or team coordinator.

Identifying sources of funding and making sure that there is adequate funding are an important components in treatment planning. Recommending many expensive procedures that are not covered by insurance and are out of the family's financial reach is truly a disservice to the patient and the family.

CHALLENGES TO THE SPECIALTY TEAM CONCEPT

With changes in health care financing, there are some additional challenges to the team approach for the management of complex patients. Most people would agree that the fee-for-service system of health care funding is ineffective in either assuring quality or controlling costs. However, the change to a managed care system has resulted in some additional concerns about the quality and costs of health care, particularly as it applies to specialty services.

Although the managed care system was designed to help to control the cost of health care, many critics would argue that this is hard to do when most of the managed care organizations exist as for-profit corporations. In fact, in many cases, the investors and the administrators of these organizations are reaping substantial profits. This may occur at the expense of the patients, who are not always receiving the services that they need. Critics of managed care would also argue that this system discourages the use of specialists in the care of complex disorders (Strauss, 1999). In fact, there are financial disincentives for primary care providers to seek specialty care for their patients. The managed care organizations seek to control costs by limiting the number and type of professionals that the patient can see and the number and type of procedures that the patient can have. This certainly has an impact on the specialty team approach.

An additional concern is that some third-party payers limit access to physicians who are outside the network. If there are no specialists within the network to cover the particular medical needs, this may seriously affect the quality of care provided to the patient. This is an even greater problem when a whole team of professionals is required for quality care.

Some patients or parents are unable to move or change jobs due to a concern about changing insurance coverage. Managed care organizations will often refuse to cover preexisting conditions when the policy is new. As a result, the care of patients with cleft palate or craniofacial anomalies may not be covered. In addition, there is an incentive for managed care organizations to seek to enroll groups of patients who are a low financial risk because they have few health problems. This may result

in excluding the individuals who really need insurance coverage for medical services.

As the health care system continues to evolve in this country, it is difficult to predict the future and what it holds for specialty team care or even general medical care. With the help of the efforts of professionals and various advocacy groups, it is hoped that the system will be refined so that the specific needs of the patient become a priority.

Summary

Over the last 50 years, the team approach to the management of individuals with craniofacial anomalies has evolved from a good idea to the accepted standard of care. Although there are some inherent difficulties that can occur when a group of professionals must work together, the advantages of this approach far outweigh the disadvantages. Without the interaction of various professionals using a team approach, the treatment of patients would become fragmented, and the outcomes would be negatively affected. Hopefully, as our health care system continues to change and develop, the team approach to cleft and craniofacial care will be supported and will thrive.

For Review, Discussion, and Critical Thinking

1. Why is team management preferable to individual management of children with craniofacial anomalies?

2. List the typical members of a cleft palate–craniofacial team and their specific roles.

3. How soon should a child been seen by a cleft team and for how long?

4. What guidelines are available for standards of team care and where can they be found?

5. Your patient is 4 years old and has a collapsed maxillary arch, anterior crossbite, and midface retrusion. He has very poor oral hygiene and large tonsils. Speech is characterized by consistent nasal emission

and compensatory productions. The child is very afraid of doctors and cries every time he comes to the hospital. Discuss the interdisciplinary management of this child. Which professionals will be involved in treatment and how can one type of treatment affect the other treatments?

6. What are the particular advantages of and potential problems with providing care through a team?

7. What could you do to be an effective team member?

References

Abdoney, M., Habal, M. B., Scheuerle, J., & Rans, N. P. (1988). Cleft palate teams and the craniofacial centers in Florida: A state network. *Florida Dental Journal*, 59(2), 25–27, 53.

American Cleft Palate-Craniofacial Association. (1993). Parameters for evaluation and treatment of patients with cleft lip/palate or other craniofacial anomalies. *Cleft Palate-Craniofacial Journal*, 30(Suppl.), 1–16.

American Cleft Palate-Craniofacial Association. (1999). *Membership-Team directory*. Chapel Hill: American Cleft Palate-Craniofacial Association.

Bardach, J., Morris, H., Olin, W., McDermott-Murray, J., Mooney, M., & Bardach, E. (1984). Late results of multidisciplinary management of unilateral cleft lip and palate. *Annals of Plastic Surgery*, 12(3), 235–242.

Borah, G. L., Hagberg, N., Jakubiak, C., & Temple, J. (1993). Reorganization of craniofacial/cleft care delivery: The Massachusetts experience. *Cleft Palate-Craniofacial Journal*, 30(3), 333–336.

Brogan, W. F. (1988). Team approach to the treatment of cleft lip and palate. *Annals of the Academy of Medicine, Singapore*, 17(3), 335–338.

Chen, Y. R., Chen, S. H., Wang, C. Y., & Noordhoff, M. S. (1988). Combined cleft and craniofacial team: Multidisciplinary approach to cleft management. *Annals of the Academy of Medicine, Singapore*, 17(3), 339–342.

Cohn, E. R. (1991). Commentary on Team Acceptance of Recommendations by Dixon-Wood et al. *Cleft Palate-Craniofacial Journal*, 28(3), 290–292.

Colburn, N., & Cherry, R. S. (1985). Community-based team approach to the management of children with cleft palate. *Child Health Care*, 13(3), 122–128.

David, D. J., Anderson, P. J., Schnitt, D. E., Nugent, M. A., & Sells, R. (2006). From birth to maturity: A group of patients who have completed their protocol management. Part II. Isolated cleft palate. *Plastic and Reconstructive Surgery*, 117(2), 515–526.

Jeffery, S. L., & Boorman, J. G. (2001). Patient satisfaction with cleft lip and palate services in a regional centre. *British Journal of Plastic Surgery*, 54(3), 189–191.

Kline, R. M., Jr. (1997). Management of craniofacial anomalies. *Journal of the South Carolina Medical Association*, 93(9), 336–341.

Krogman, W. M. (1979). The cleft palate team in action. In H. K. Cooper, R. L. Harding, W. M. Krogman, M. Mazaheri, & R. T. Millard (Eds.), *Cleft palate and cleft lip: A team approach to clinical management and rehabilitation of the patient* (pp. 144–161). Philadelphia: W. B. Saunders.

Lang, D. A., Neil-Dwyer, G., Evans, B. T., & Honeybul, S. (1998). Craniofacial access in children. *Acta Neurochirurgica, 140*(1), 33–40.

Louw, B., Shibambu, M., & Roemer, K. (2006). Facilitating cleft palate team participation of culturally diverse families in South Africa. *Cleft Palate-Craniofacial Journal, 43*(1), 47–54.

Marsh, J. L. (1982). Interdisciplinary care for craniofacial deformities. *Missouri Medicine, 79*(9), 623–628, 630.

McWilliams, B. J., Morris, H. L., & Shelton, R. L. (1990). *Cleft Palate Speech*. Toronto: B. C. Decker.

Nackashi, M., & Dixon-Wood, V. (1989). The craniofacial team: Medical supervision and coordination. In K. Bzoch (Ed.), *Communicative disorders related to cleft lip and palate* (pp. 63–73). Boston: College-Hill Press.

Noar, J. H. (1992). A questionnaire survey of attitudes and concerns of three professional groups involved in the cleft palate team. *Cleft Palate-Craniofacial Journal, 29*(1), 92–95.

Pannbacker, M., & Scheuerle, J. (1993). Parents' attitudes toward family involvement in cleft palate treatment. *Cleft Palate-Craniofacial Journal, 30*(1), 87–89.

Paynter, E. T., Edmonson, T. W., & Jordan, W. J. (1991). Accuracy of information reported by parents and children evaluated by a cleft palate team. *Cleft Palate-Craniofacial Journal, 28*(4), 329–337.

Paynter, E. T., Jordan, W. J., & Finch, D. L. (1990). Patient compliance with cleft palate team regimens. *Journal of Speech and Hearing Disorders, 55*(4), 740–750.

Paynter, E. T., Wilson, B. M., & Jordan, W. J. (1993). Improved patient compliance with cleft palate team regimes. *Cleft Palate-Craniofacial Journal, 30*(3), 292–301.

Pinsky, T. M., & Goldberg, H. J. (1977). Potential for clinical cooperation between dentistry and speech pathology. *International Dental Journal, 27*(4), 363–369.

Schnitt, D. E., Agir, H., & David, D. J. (2004). From birth to maturity: A group of patients who have completed their protocol management. Part I. Unilateral cleft lip and palate. *Plastic and Reconstructive Surgery, 113*(3), 805–817.

Sharp, H. M. (1995). Ethical decision-making in interdisciplinary team care. *Cleft Palate-Craniofacial Journal, 32*(6), 495–499.

Sidman, J. D. (1995). The team approach to cleft and craniofacial disorders—The down side [editorial]. *Cleft Palate-Craniofacial Journal, 32*(5), 362.

Stal, S., Chebret, L., & McElroy, C. (1998a). The team approach in the management of congenital and acquired deformities. *Clinics in Plastic Surgery, 25*(4), 485–491, vii.

Stal, S., Klebuc, M., Taylor, T. D., Spira, M., & Edwards, M. (1998b). Algorithms for the treatment of cleft lip and palate. *Clinics in Plastic Surgery, 25*(4), 493–507, vii.

Strauss, R. P. (1998). Cleft palate and craniofacial teams in the United States and Canada: A national survey of team organization and standards of care. The American Cleft Palate-Craniofacial Association (ACPA) Team Standards Committee. *Cleft Palate-Craniofacial Journal, 35*(6), 473–480.

Strauss, R. P. (1999). The organization and delivery of craniofacial health services: The state of the art. *Cleft Palate-Craniofacial Journal, 36*(3), 189–195.

Strauss, R. P., & Broder, H. (1985). Interdisciplinary team care of cleft lip and palate: Social and psychological aspects. *Clinics in Plastic Surgery, 12*(4), 543–551.

Strohecker, B. (1993). A team approach in the treatment of craniofacial deformities. *Plastic Surgery Nursing, 13*(1), 9–16.

Surgeon General's Report. (1987, June). *Children with special needs.* Washington, DC: Office of Maternal and Child Health, U.S. Department of Health and Human Services, Public Health Service.

Thomas, P. C. (2000). Multidisciplinary care of the child born with cleft lip and palate. *ORL-Head & Neck Nursing, 18*(4), 6–16.

Tindlund, R. S., & Holmefjord, A. (1997). Functional results with the team care of cleft lip and palate patients in Bergen, Norway. The Bergen Cleft Palate-Craniofacial Team, Norway. *Folia Phoniatrica et Logopedica, 49*(3/4), 168–176.

Walesky-Rainbow, P. A., & Morris, H. L. (1978). An assessment of informative-counseling procedures for cleft palate children. *Cleft Palate Journal, 15*(1), 20–29.

Will, L. A., & Aduss, M. K. (1987). Illinois Association of Craniofacial Teams: A new state organization. *Cleft Palate Journal, 24*(4), 339–341.

Will, L., Aduss, M. K., Kuehn, D. P., & Parsons, R. W. (1989). The team approach to treating cleft lip/palate and other craniofacial anomalies in Illinois. *Illinois Dental Journal, 58*(2), 112–115.

Will, L. A., & Parsons, R. W. (1991). Characteristics of new patients at Illinois cleft palate teams. *Cleft Palate-Craniofacial Journal, 28*(4), 378–383; Discussion 383–384.

ASSESSMENT PROCEDURES: SPEECH, RESONANCE, AND VELOPHARYNGEAL DYSFUNCTION

Note: Chapters on instrumental assessment procedures (Nasometry, Speech Aerodynamics, Videofluoroscopy, and Nasopharyngoscopy) provide general information for the graduate student, and also very specific information regarding procedures and interpretation for the practicing clinician. It is recommended that professors select certain sections of these chapters for graduate students who just need an overview of instrumental procedures.

CHAPTER

12

ASSESSMENT USING "LOW-TECH" AND "NO-TECH" PROCEDURES

INTRODUCTION

The evaluation of resonance and velopharyngeal function must begin with a speech pathology evaluation. In this evaluation, a perceptual assessment is done to determine whether resonance is normal or abnormal. Resonance can be said to be abnormal if the quality or the intelligibility of speech is affected by inappropriate transmission of acoustic energy in the vocal tract. A speech pathology evaluation is also necessary to determine if there are any other characteristics of velopharyngeal dysfunction, such as nasal air emission or compensatory articulation productions. The perceptual evaluation of speech and resonance should be done by a qualified and experienced speech-language pathologist.

Listener judgment is the most important test of velopharyngeal dysfunction as it relates to impaired communication. In fact, in a survey of speech-language pathologists in the United States and Canada, 90% of those associated with a cleft palate team reported that they rely primarily on listener judgment, oral examination, and articulation testing in the diagnosis of velopharyngeal insufficiency (Schneider & Shprintzen, 1980). If there is no abnormality, as judged by a perceptual evaluation, then it does not matter what the instrumental procedures show. It is only when the perceptual evaluation shows an abnormality that treatment is ever initiated.

The goal of the perceptual evaluation is to determine if an abnormality exists, and if so, the type, severity, and possible cause of the disorder. Based on the results of the evaluation, further assessment may be recommended using instrumental procedures to determine the specific cause of the problem. The ultimate goal of the evaluation is to determine an appropriate treatment plan.

The purpose of this chapter is to review the perceptual evaluation process for individuals who have a history of cleft lip/palate or craniofacial anomalies. This information also applies to individuals who have a resonance disorder due to other causes. This chapter provides practical suggestions for a thorough assessment of resonance and the articulation correlates to velopharyngeal dysfunction.

DIRECT VERSUS INDIRECT MEASURES FOR EVALUATION

Prior to discussing the perceptual assessment procedures, it may be helpful to describe the types of measures available for assessment of resonance and velopharyngeal function. There are two basic categories of procedures for evaluation of velopharyngeal function: those that give direct information and those that give indirect information.

Procedures that give direct information are those that allow the examiner to visualize aspects of velopharyngeal function. These direct measures include videofluoroscopy and nasopharyngoscopy procedures. Through these procedures, the examiner can view the anatomical and physiological defects that cause velopharyngeal dysfunction. Because there is a wide spectrum of anatomic and physiologic causes for velopharyngeal dysfunction, it is important to obtain this information so that the appropriate and most effective treatment can be determined. Although the structures and function of the velopharyngeal valve can be seen through these measures, the evaluation of what is seen is still subjective and open to interpretation. More information can be found in Chapter 16, "Videofluoroscopy," and Chapter 17, "Nasopharyngoscopy."

In contrast to direct measures, procedures that provide indirect information do not allow visualization of the structures. However, these indirect measures give objective data regarding the results of velopharyngeal function, such as airflow, air pressure, or acoustic output. The nasometer and pressure/flow equipment are examples of instrumentation that provide indirect, yet objective information. The advantage of objective data is that it can be compared to standardized norms for interpretation. In addition, these instruments can be used to collect objective data for pre- and posttreatment comparisons. See Chapters 14 and 15 on nasometry and aerodynamics for more information.

Although instrumental assessment is important, the most important tool that we have for making decisions regarding velopharyngeal function and the need for management is the examiner's ear (Moller, 1991; Shprintzen & Golding-Kushner, 1989). From a thorough analysis of speech, a determination can be made regarding the status of velopharyngeal function and its potential for change. In the perceptual evaluation, the ear is used to analyze the acoustic product of velopharyngeal function in order to make inferences about the adequacy of the velopharyngeal mechanism. If the human ear can be considered an instrument in the broadest sense of the word, then listener judgment should be considered an indirect measure of velopharyngeal function (Dalston, 1997). Although a perceptual assessment is an indirect approach, it has face validity in that velopharyngeal dysfunction is usually not a problem unless it affects speech.

TIMETABLE FOR ASSESSMENT

All children with a history of a cleft or craniofacial condition are at risk for communication disorders. If the child had a cleft of the primary palate, this risk is due to the possibility of dental abnormalities. If the cleft was of the secondary palate, the risk is related to the possibility of a fluctuating hearing loss that may accompany eustachian tube malfunction and velopharyngeal dysfunction. As noted in Chapter 6, there may also be other problems, such as mental retardation or neurological dysfunction, especially if the child has a craniofacial syndrome. The structural and functional problems that are typical of cleft and craniofacial conditions can cause problems in the areas of articulation, language, phonation, and resonance at different times in development. Therefore, periodic assessments are needed (Smith & Guyette 2004).

First Year

The first year of a child's life is usually a time of great joy for the parents. However, when the infant has a congenital anomaly, there is also significant anxiety over what will happen in the future and the ultimate results of treatment. Most people cope better with information rather than with uncertainty. Therefore, the parents should be counseled by various professionals, usually cleft palate team members, soon after the birth and again early in the first year. These professionals should explain the diagnosis, the effect of the anomalies on function, what might happen in the future, what will be done about it, and the ultimate prognosis.

During the first year, the primary speech pathology concerns are feeding and the prerequisites for verbal communication. The family should be assisted with feeding modifications as necessary. In addition, the infant's development should be monitored through parent report, direct observation, or the use of infant scales. If problems in development are noted, further assessment and intervention should be initiated immediately.

During the first year, the speech-language pathologist should counsel the family on methods of speech and language stimulation. It should be emphasized that under that age of 3, language development should be the primary focus. In other words, the quantity of speech is more important than the quality of speech during those early years. However, instructions for stimulating sound production after the palate repair are also important to include in this discussion. The speech-language pathologist should reinforce this discussion with a handout that summarizes the information and provides additional suggestions.

At Cincinnati Children's Hospital Medical Center, these counseling sessions are done through the Infant/Toddler Meetings, where six to eight sets of parents attend each session. At these meetings, various team members give a brief lecture and then are available for questions and discussion. A particular benefit of these group meetings is that the parents are able to meet other families who are going through a similar experience and develop a support network. Many long-term relationships have developed through some of these meetings.

Annual Screenings and Periodic Evaluations

Children with a history of cleft lip/palate or craniofacial anomalies should receive at least a screening evaluation of speech and language skills on an annual basis until the age of 4 years (American Cleft Palate-Craniofacial Association, 1993). This is often done during the annual visit to the cleft palate or craniofacial team. If problems are suspected during these assessments, the child should be scheduled for a more in-depth evaluation.

Around the age of 3, the child should receive a comprehensive evaluation of speech and language. If the child is communicating with connected speech and is able to produce a variety of sounds, this is also the appropriate time to evaluate resonance and velopharyngeal function. On the other hand, if the child's speech development and expressive language development are delayed, the assessment of resonance and velopharyngeal function should be done at a later time in order to obtain accurate results.

In addition to the annual evaluations, a perceptual assessment, along with instrumental measures, should be done prior to any surgery that is designed to improve speech, such as a pharyngeal flap, or surgery that might affect speech, such as orthognathic surgery. It is very important to document baseline information regarding speech and resonance prior to the surgical procedure. A postoperative assessment should also be done to determine the effect of surgery on speech and whether any further treatment is indicated.

THE DIAGNOSTIC INTERVIEW

Whether a comprehensive evaluation is being done or merely a screening evaluation in a cleft palate clinic, the examiner can obtain valuable information from the patient or family (Hirschberg & Van Demark, 1997). Therefore, the perceptual evaluation is usually preceded by an interview with the patient or family member as appropriate. Many clinics send the family a preevaluation questionnaire in order to obtain medical and development history, and to determine the current concerns about speech. This information helps the examiner to prepare for the evaluation and can shorten the interview process. However, even if background information was received through a questionnaire or medical record, at least a brief interview should be done prior to the formal assessment.

Examples of interview questions for pediatric patients can be found in Table 12–1.

Parents are usually very good observers of their own children, and can often effectively compare their child's communication skills with those of siblings or peers. A study by Glascoe (1991) showed that identification of the parent's concern and skillful observation of the

---

TABLE 12–1 Sample Questions for Use in a Diagnostic Interview

Current Concern

- What concerns you about your child's speech?
- When did you first become concerned?
- Who referred your child for the evaluation and what was that person's concern?

Articulation

- What types of sounds does your child use during vocal play—vowels only or some consonants?
- If consonants, what are some of the consonants that you hear?
- Are they produced individually or over and over?
- Does the child jabber or use jargon?
- Does your child leave out sounds in words?
- Do you understand your child's speech all of the time, most of the time, some of the time, or hardly at all?
- How well do strangers understand your child's speech?
- Are there any particular sounds that are difficult for your child to produce?

Resonance

- Does your child sound "nasal" to you? If yes, does it sound like your child is talking through the nose, or does it sound like your child has a cold?
- When did you first notice the problem with nasality?
- If the onset was sudden, what event preceded it?
- Does it vary with the weather, allergies, fatigue, or any other factor?
- Do you ever hear air coming through the nose during speech?

Language

- Does your child communicate with gestures, single words, short phrases, incomplete sentences, or complete sentences?
- How many words does your child usually put together in an utterance?
- Does your child leave out the little words (such as "of," "to," "the," or "is") in the sentence?
- Is your child communicating as well as other children his or her age?
- Have you ever had a concern about how well your child understands the speech of others or follows directions?

TABLE 12–1 *(continued)*

Medical History

- Was your child born with any congenital problems? If so, what were they? How and when were they treated?
- Does your child have any medical problems, medical diagnoses, or conditions?
- What surgeries has your child undergone?
- Does your child take any medications on a regular basis? If so, what are they for?
- Does your child hear normally? When was the last hearing test?
- Has your child had many ear infections? If so, how were they treated?
- Does your child have any problems with vision?
- Where is your child on the growth chart?

Developmental History

- Was your child quiet, about average, or very vocal as an infant?
- Did you have any concerns about initial speech development?
- Did your child begin to use words before or after his/her first birthday?
- When your child was learning to sit up, stand, and walk, did he or she seem normal or behind other children?
- Did your child walk before or after his/her first birthday?
- Does your child have any difficulty learning in preschool or school?

Feeding and Oral-Motor Skills

- Does your child have any difficulty chewing, sucking, or swallowing?
- Is there a history of feeding problems?
- Does your child drool or keep his or her mouth open during the day?

Airway

- Does your child snore at night?
- Does your child ever gasp for breath at night or sleep restlessly?
- Does your child like to breathe through the mouth or through the nose?
- Is your child's breathing ever noisy during the day?
- Does your child have allergies, asthma, or chronic congestion?

Treatment History

- Has your child ever had a speech evaluation or speech therapy?
- Is your child currently receiving speech therapy? If yes, what are the goals?
- Has your child's speech improved in the last six months? If so, in what way?

child is often sufficient to identify many speech and language problems. A simple rule of thumb is that if the parents are worried about their child's speech, there probably is a good reason.

Language Screening

Because children with a history of cleft or craniofacial anomalies are at risk for early language delay, it is important that these children receive regular language screenings throughout the preschool years. This can be done at the time of the yearly visits to the cleft palate team. If language problems are suspected from the screening evaluation or if the parents have concerns about language development, a comprehensive language evaluation should be done. A comprehensive evaluation should also be done if the child has additional risk factors for language disorders, such as hearing loss, developmental delay, or neurological problems. This type of evaluation cannot be done adequately in a clinic setting; therefore, a separate appointment with the speech-language pathologist is usually needed. If a language disorder is identified, intervention should be initiated as soon as possible to ensure the best outcome.

The methods for language evaluation are beyond the scope of this text. Instead, the interested reader should consult one of the many books available on this subject. However, a discussion regarding screening methods may be helpful, particularly as it applies to a clinic setting.

Language Screening through Parent Questionnaire

One way to screen the language of infants and toddlers is to seek information from the parents through a questionnaire format. The questions must be understandable enough for the parents to answer with confidence and detailed enough to be of value to the examiner. Scherer and D'Antonio (1995) investigated the efficacy of a parent questionnaire as a component of early language screening using the MacArthur Communicative Development Inventory (Fenson et al., 1989). They found that the parent questionnaire can be a valid means of screening language development as compared with other methods.

Informal Language Screening

Although formal screening tests provide structure and a set format, they are not necessary for the experienced examiner. It should be kept in mind that the purpose of a screening test is to determine whether more comprehensive testing is indicated. Most experienced examiners can make this determination through a parent interview, observations of the child, and informal testing. The behaviors of the child, as noted through observation and report, can be compared to norms to estimate the child's developmental level. An informal screening assessment can be done by most experienced examiners without the need for special materials or tests.

Informal language screening can be done by:

- Observing play behaviors, and the type and complexity of gestures (Scherer & D'Antonio, 1997).

- Asking the child to point to certain objects or follow certain commands.

- Having interesting toys available and observing spontaneous vocalizations and utterances.

- Listening to the child's spontaneous speech while he or she is talking to the parent.

- Asking questions or asking for explanations. (See Table 12–2 for examples.)

TABLE 12–2   Sample Questions and Requests for Eliciting Speech

What do you like best…
- Puppy dogs or kitty cats?
- Baby dolls or teddy bears?
- Cupcakes or cookies?
- Chocolate-chip cookies or peanut-butter cookies?
- Singing or dancing?
- Baseball or basketball?
- Playing inside or outside?

What do you want to be when you grow up? Why?

What does a fireman do? What does a policeman do? What does a teacher do?

Tell me how you make a peanut-butter-and-jelly sandwich.

Explain the game of baseball to me.

- Having the child repeat sentences, such as those listed in the articulation screening test. (See Table 12–3.) Even in repeating, the child will usually revert to his or her own form of syntax and morphology, which gives an indication of expressive language abilities.

Through these simple methods, the examiner should be able to determine the primary mode of communication (i.e. gestures, signs, single words, short utterances, short sentences, or complete sentences). If the child is communicating with sentences, the examiner should also be able to determine whether the sentences are complete or merely telegraphic; what the approximate mean length of utterance (MLU) is; and whether there are errors of syntax or morphology.

Formal Language Screening Tests

There are several formal screening tests that allow the examiner to sample the child's communication abilities using a structured format. Some examples of screening tests include the *Receptive-Expressive Emergent Language Scale (REEL)* (Bzoch & League, 1991), the *Early Language Milestone (ELM) Scale* (Coplan, 1987), and the *Rossetti Infant-Toddler Language Scale* (Rossetti, 1990). These tests are used to screen children from birth to age 3 through observation and parent report. *The Fluharty Preschool Speech and*

TABLE 12–3   Sample Sentences for Assessment of Articulation, Nasal Emission, and Resonance

Have the individual repeat the following sentences:

p	Popeye plays in the pool.
b	Buy baby a bib.
m	My mommy made lemonade.
w	Wade in the water.
y	You have a yellow yo-yo.
h	He has a big horse.
t	Take Teddy to town.
d	Do it for Daddy.
n	Nancy is not here.
k	I like cookies and cake.
g	Go get the wagon.
ng	Put the ring on her finger.
f	I have five fingers.
v	Drive a van.
l	I like yellow lollipops.
s	I see the sun in the sky.
z	Zip up your zipper.
sh	She went shopping.
ch	I ride a choo-choo train.
j	John told a joke to Jim.
r	Randy has a red fire truck.
er	The teacher and doctor are here.
th	Thank you for the toothbrush.
blends	splash, sprinkle, street

Language Screening Test (Fluharty, 1978) can be used to screen children from the ages of 2 to 6 in the areas of articulation, vocabulary, and receptive and expressive language.

SPEECH SAMPLES

When assessing articulation, resonance, and velopharyngeal function, it is important to select an appropriate speech sample to obtain the information that is needed for a definitive diagnosis. When testing a child, the speech sample must also be developmentally appropriate in the areas of speech sound production and syntax.

Formal Articulation Tests

The speech evaluation should begin with an articulation test. One purpose of the articulation test is to determine the cause of the speech problem (structure versus function). Another purpose is to provide data that the clinician can use to develop an appropriate treatment plan for therapy. The *Iowa Pressure Articulation Test*, a part of the *Templin-Darley Tests of Articulation* (Templin & Darley, 1960), and the *Bzoch Error Pattern Diagnostic Articulation Tests* (Bzoch, 1979) were specifically designed to assess the effects of VPI. However, any articulation test can be used for this purpose.

Although a formal articulation test with single articulatory targets is usually easiest for the novice clinician, normal speech does not usually consist of single words. Therefore, an informal test of articulation at the sentence level is often more appropriate.

Syllable Repetition

The examiner may want to test phonemes at the syllable level to isolate the effects of other sounds and to determine if there is phoneme-specific

nasal air emission. This is done by having the child produce consonant phonemes (particularly plosives, fricatives, and affricates) in a repetitive manner (i.e., "pa, pa, pa; pee, pee, pee; ta, ta, ta; tee, tee, tee," etc.). Each of the pressure-sensitive phonemes should be tested with both a low vowel and then again with a high vowel. This type of test allows the examiner to assess both articulation and the presence of nasal emission on each individual phoneme. It also allows the examiner to determine whether hypernasality occurs more on high vowels than on low vowels, or even whether it is vowel-specific (Andrews & Rutherford, 1972).

Sentence Repetition

The examiner should have a battery of sentences that test each consonant phoneme, such as those found in Table 12–3. It is best if these sentences contain phonemes that are similar in articulatory placement (such as "Take Teddy to town"). By asking the child to repeat these sentences, the examiner can quickly and easily test articulation, nasal emission, and resonance in a connected speech environment. This is much faster than a single-word articulation test, and is actually a more valid test of normal speech production (Hirschberg & Van Demark, 1997).

When evaluating for nasal emission and the other related characteristics (weak consonants or short utterance length), the sample should contain many pressure-sensitive consonants, particularly those that are voiceless (such as "Sissy sees the sun in the sky"). When testing for hypernasality, the sample should contain a high number of voiced, oral sounds. To separate out the effects of nasal air emission or compensatory errors, the examiner could use a sample with a large number of low-pressure consonants (such as "How are you? Where are you? Why are you here?"). Sample sentences with low-pressure

---

TABLE 12–4 Sample of Low-Pressure Sentences for Evaluation of Resonance without the Complication of Nasal Air Emission

Have the individual repeat the following sentences:

How are you?

Who are you?

Where are you?

Why are you here?

You are here.

They are here.

Where are they?

They are where you are.

TABLE 12–5 Sentences for Evaluation of Hyponasality, Denasality, or Cul-de-Sac Resonance

Have the individual repeat the following sentences:

My mama made lemonade for me.

My name is Amy Minor.

My mama takes money to the market.

Many men are at the mine.

Ned made nine points in the game.

My nanny is not mean.

Nan needs a dime to call home.

My mom's home is many miles away.

Many men are needed to move the piano.

---

sounds can be found in Table 12–4. To test for hyponasality, the examiner should use sentences with a high frequency of nasal phonemes (such as "My mama made lemonade for me"). Sample sentences loaded with nasal sounds can be found in Table 12–5.

At times, young children are very reluctant to imitate sentences or even speak in the evaluation. If this is the case, it is helpful to ask the child either/or questions as noted in Table 12–2. This will often get the child started in talking and the child is more likely to repeat after that.

Counting and Rote Speech

Connected speech can be difficult to obtain when evaluating young children. However, connected speech can often be elicited by having the child count or recite the alphabet. Counting from 60 to 70, or simply repeating "60, 60, 60, 60" can be particularly informative because these numbers contain a combination of high vowels (/i/), sibilants, plosives, and even a triple blend (/kst/). These sounds require a build-up and continuation of intraoral air pressure, which can particularly tax the velopharyngeal mechanism and may overwhelm a tenuous velopharyngeal valve. Counting from 70 to 79 can be diagnostic as this series contains a nasal phoneme followed by an alveolar plosive. If there are timing difficulties, this may become apparent in this speech sample as assimilated hypernasality. If there are concerns regarding possible hyponasality, counting from 90 to 99 allows the examiner to assess the production of the nasal /n/ in connected speech.

Spontaneous Connected Speech

Although a single word test helps the examiner to isolate the production of individual phonemes, it is important to assess articulation, and particularly resonance, in connected speech. Connected speech increases the demands on the velopharyngeal valving system to achieve and maintain closure. As a result, hypernasality and nasal emission will be more apparent in connected speech than in single words. An increase in articulation errors is also common during the production of continuous utterances.

Some children are naturally loquacious and little or no effort is needed to elicit connected speech. Other children need some prodding. The examiner should begin by asking the child questions that require only a short response. Either/or questions (e.g., "What do you like best, baseball or basketball?") can be particularly helpful in getting the child to talk. Once the child is responding, questions that require a longer response can be asked (e.g., "How do you play the game of baseball?"). If this fails, it may be best to allow the parent to try to engage the child in conversation while the examiner appears to be not listening.

WHAT TO EVALUATE

Articulation

In assessing articulation it is important to correctly identify the type of errors (i.e., compensatory, obligatory, or just abnormal placement). It is also important to assess the potential cause of the errors (abnormal structure, apraxia or oral-motor dysfunction, phonological disorder, delayed development, or normal developmental error). Finally, the examiner should determine if there is nasal air emission during the production of pressure-sensitive phonemes, or nasalization of other oral consonants. All of this information is important because it is used as a basis for determining appropriate treatment.

As noted previously, an obligatory error is one where the articulation placement (the function) is normal, but the abnormality of the structure causes distortion of speech. For example, when there is a large velopharyngeal opening, the placement of articulation may be normal, but manner of production is altered

from oral to nasal due to the lack of velopharyngeal closure. As a result, attempts to produce voiced plosives may result in the production of their nasal cognates (m/b, n/d, ng/g). Even voiceless plosives and other oral sounds can be nasalized due to the open velopharyngeal valve. Whenever there is a predominate use of nasal phonemes during connected speech, the examiner should suspect a significant velopharyngeal opening due to these obligatory errors.

Compensatory articulation errors are common in individuals with VPI; therefore, it is important to specifically look for these errors in this population. When compensatory errors occur as a result of VPI, the manner of production is usually maintained. However, the placement of production is moved posteriorly to the pharynx where there is airflow. A description of various compensatory errors is found in Chapter 7, and therefore, will not be repeated here. In addition, Trost-Cardamone (1987) has an instructional videotape in which compensatory productions are nicely demonstrated.

Some compensatory productions can be coarticulated with the normal oral sound. For example, the child may appear to be producing a normal /p/ phoneme with bilabial closure, while coarticulating the plosive portion with a glottal stop. A pharyngeal fricative can be coarticulated with closed teeth for substitution of the /s/ sound. To determine the true placement of the sound, the examiner should listen carefully and then try to imitate the sound. By imitating the production, the examiner can often determine the place of production and, therefore, identify the compensatory error. The examiner should also watch the production of each phoneme. Glottal stops, for example, will result in visible exaggerated laryngeal movements that can also be felt on the individual's neck during articulation.

Glottal stops can also be confused with a simple consonant omission. To make a distinction between a glottal stop and an omission, it should be remembered that glottal stops are produced with a quick sound and rapid voice onset time. If the phoneme is completely omitted, the voice onset is smooth with the initiation of the vowel. There is also an obvious difference between a consonant omission and glottal stop in the duration of the following vowel. If the phoneme is merely omitted, the vowel will be longer in duration than if the consonant is substituted by a glottal stop. A final clue to the production of glottal stops is the observation of increased laryngeal activity that can be seen in the throat area. Again, this can be felt if the examiner places a hand on the individual's throat as he or she is speaking.

A pharyngeal fricative can sound similar to a lateral lisp to an inexperienced listener. To make this distinction, the examiner should determine whether the air stream is in the oral or pharyngeal area. If the examiner cannot find the air stream at either side of the dental arch, then the sound is probably produced in the pharynx.

The scoring of an articulation test is traditionally done by using phonetic diacritics from the International Phonetic Alphabet (IPA) (Bronsted et al., 1994). However, this system does not include symbols for compensatory productions that are typical of individuals with velopharyngeal dysfunction. Therefore, a set of diacritic symbols for compensatory productions was proposed by Trost (1981) and Trost-Cardamone (1997). The examiner may choose to learn and use these diacritics. However, it may be easier to just use the words (i.e., glottal stop, pharyngeal fricative) rather than the symbol to describe the errors. This also enhances communication with others who are unfamiliar with these symbols.

Stimulability

An assessment of stimulability is an important component of the perceptual evaluation because some articulation errors actually cause nasal air emission and even hypernasality (Moller, 1991). In fact, it has been shown radiographically that during the production of glottal stops, there is less velopharyngeal movement than during the production of oral sounds (Henningsson & Isberg, 1991). In addition, individuals who use a posterior nasal fricative as a substitution for sibilants show a velopharyngeal opening on nasopharyngoscopy during production of these sounds.

Articulation errors that cause nasal air emission or hypernasality are the result of faulty placement and are not caused by a primary velopharyngeal valving disorder. Therefore, the child will usually be stimulable for an elimination of nasal air emission or hypernasality with a change in articulatory placement. If the child is able to produce the sound without nasal air emission or hypernasality merely by changing placement, this suggests a good prognosis for correction with speech therapy.

Nasal Air Emission

As part of the articulation assessment, the speech-language pathologist should assess for the presence of audible nasal air emission. If it is present, it is important to determine whether the nasal emission is low in intensity, which is usually the result of a larger velopharyngeal opening, or whether it is the "bubbly" nasal rustle (turbulence), which is the result of a small opening (Kummer, Briggs, & Lee, 2003; Kummer, Curtis, Wiggs, Lee, & Strife, 1992). The examiner should also note the occurrence of a nasal snort, which is produced most often with /s/ blends. A nasal grimace commonly accompanies nasal air emission and this should be reported if it is observed.

The consistency of the nasal air emission should be noted during the articulation test. If nasal air emission occurs during the production of most pressure-sensitive phonemes, then it is considered consistent. If it occurs occasionally on most pressure-sensitive phonemes, then it is inconsistent. If it occurs consistently, but only on specific phonemes, then it may be phoneme-specific nasal air emission (PSNAE), which is related to faulty articulation rather than VPI.

It is always important to assess for nasal air emission in connected speech. Many individuals are able to achieve velopharyngeal closure for short segments and therefore, nasal air emission may not be noted on even the sentence level during the examination. Because connected speech increases the demands on the velopharyngeal mechanism, nasal air emission is more likely to be noted at this level.

Weak Consonants

The adequacy of intraoral air pressure should be evaluated by listening to the force of production of the pressure-sensitive consonants. Having the individual repeat sentences loaded with these consonants is a good way to test oral pressure. If these consonants seem to be weak in intensity and pressure, it might be assumed that intraoral air pressure is compromised due to significant nasal air emission. Weak consonants are usually associated with both nasal air emission and hypernasality, and are due to a large velopharyngeal opening.

Short Utterance Length

If there is significant nasal air emission, it can also have an effect on utterance length. This can be determined by observing the phrasing of utterances in connected speech. If the individual seems to take breaths frequently during speech, this may be due to the loss of air pressure through the velopharyngeal valve and the need to replenish this air pressure more frequently. Utterance length can be tested by

asking the individual to count to 20. Most normal speakers will count at least to 15 on one breath. If more than two breaths are needed, this may indicate a significant loss of air pressure during speech due to VPI.

Oral-Motor Dysfunction

Characteristics of velopharyngeal dysfunction may occur as a result of apraxia of speech. Individuals with apraxia of speech have difficulty coordinating the movements of the various subsystems of speech, including the velopharyngeal valve. This can cause errors in the closing of the valve for oral sounds and the opening of the valve for nasal sounds. These errors tend to increase with an increase in utterance length or phonemic complexity. Therefore, the examiner should note the difference in resonance between short, simple utterances and longer, phonemically complex utterances.

Oral-motor dysfunction is common in individuals with craniofacial syndromes, and seems to be particularly prevalent in individuals with velocardiofacial syndrome (VCFS). Because patients with VCFS are at risk for both VPI and apraxia, the examiner should be careful to determine the cause of abnormal resonance in these patients.

There are several formal tests of apraxia that go from a nonspeech oral level up to the sentence level of production (Hickman, 1997; Kaufman, 1995), but this can also be tested informally. The individual can be asked to repeat individual oral movements (e.g., lateralizing the tongue) and to sequence movements (e.g., moving the tongue to the corner of the mouth and then to the upper lip). Diadochokinetic exercises can be used to assess the ability to sequence syllables. The individual can be asked to repeat two syllable combinations (e.g., "puh tuh, puh tuh") or three syllable combinations (e.g., "puh tuh kuh, puh tuh kuh, puh tuh kuh").

CASE REPORT

Velocardiofacial Syndrome and Oral-Motor Dysfunction

Katie, age 2 years 3 months, had a diagnosis of velocardiofacial syndrome. Medical history was consistent with this diagnosis and included a submucous cleft, a ventricular septal defect (VSD), and an interrupted aortic valve. Katie was very small for her age and was under the 10th percentile for both weight and height. She had a history of airway problems as an infant. Early feeding problems were also reported and Katie continued to have difficulty with certain textures.

Although the development of gross motor milestones was essentially within normal limits, speech and language development were delayed and fine motor skills were abnormal. Although she could put words together and even sing nursery rhymes, Katie's speech was mostly unintelligible. Therefore, she communicated primarily by gestures, signs, and pointing to pictures. According to the parents, Katie's understanding of language, however, seemed normal.

A speech assessment revealed a severe articulation disorder and hypernasality. Katie's phonemic repertoire was extremely limited and consisted of nasal consonants (/m/, /n/), /h/, glottal stops, and vowels. Occasionally she was able to produce a /d/ approximation. Vowels were on target most, but not all of the time. When attempting to imitate sounds or oral placement, there was evidence of significant oral-motor dysfunction. Although Katie was able to produce nasal sounds in isolation, she was unable to produce them in certain word positions or with certain vowels. She was also unable to combine them for words such as "mommy," "money," "naming," or "many." When attempting to imitate oral pressure sounds or blow, there was only nasal air emission.

Although it was felt that Katie would need surgical intervention for correction of the velopharyngeal dysfunction, given her age, her size, her history of airway obstruction, and the evidence of severe oral-motor dysfunction, it was decided to delay the surgery for a few months until she was a little bigger. In the meantime, speech therapy (with active involvement of the parents) was recommended to improve articulation placement and ability to combine different articulation positions.

Although nonsense syllables are fine to use for assessment, real words usually work better. The child can be asked to repeat certain words repetitively (e.g., "patty cake," "puppy dog," "teddy bear," "baby doll," "kitty cat," "bubble gum," "basketball," "peanut butter and jelly," etc.). If there is significant hypernasality, the use of words with nasal sounds (e.g., "money," "mommy," "many more," etc.) helps to isolate the oral-motor dysfunction from the VPI.

Resonance

Resonance should be judged as either normal, hypernasal, hyponasal, denasal, cul-de-sac, or mixed by listening to spontaneous speech. As a general rule, if nasal sounds are heard more frequently than normal or if they are substituted for oral-type sounds, the resonance is hypernasal. On the other hand, if oral-type sounds are heard as a substitution for nasal sounds, the resonance is hyponasal. If necessary, the examiner can have the individual repeat sentences loaded with oral sounds and then repeat sentences loaded with nasal sounds if the type of resonance is hard to determine in spontaneous speech. Cul-de-sac resonance sounds as if the voice is muffled and remains in the head. For comparison, a type of cul-de-sac resonance can be simulated by imitating hypernasal speech while closing the nose. Mouth breathing or a history of upper airway obstruction may suggest either hyponasality or cul-de-sac resonance.

Determining the type of resonance is very important, but determining the severity is usually irrelevant. This is because severity doesn't impact treatment protocols (Bzoch, 1979). Despite this, several authors have suggested the use of an equal-appearing interval scale, with up to seven levels, to rate the severity of deviant resonance (McWilliams, Morris, & Shelton, 1990; Subtelny, Van Hattum, & Myers, 1972). Although these rating scales have a high degree of face validity, the reliability of these scales is in question. In fact, the more levels on the scale, the less reliable the scale will be. As a compromise, the examiner may choose to use a simple 4-point scale that includes normal, and then mild, moderate, and severe as descriptors of severity.

In some cases, hypernasality is inconsistent. It may occur primarily on high vowels because the high tongue position reduces oral resonance and increase transpalatal nasal resonance. If the back of the tongue is too high during the production of high vowels, there may be vowel-specific hypernasality.

Phonation

As noted in Chapter 7, dysphonia is common in individuals with VPI or craniofacial anomalies (McWilliams, Lavorato, & Bluestone, 1973; McWilliams, Morris & Shelton, 1990). Therefore, the examiner should listen for characteristics of dysphonia, including hoarseness, breathiness, glottal fry, hard glottal attack, inappropriate pitch level, restricted pitch range, diplophonia, or inappropriate loudness (Kummer & Marsh, 1998). When present, these abnormalities can be rated on a severity scale from mild to severe (Stemple, Glaze, & Gerdeman, 1995; Wilson, 1987). The ability to

sustain phonation for 10 seconds or longer should also be observed. Dysphonic characteristics may not be noted until the end of the prolonged vowel as the child begins to run out of air. Finally, the quality of breath support and the type of breathing pattern should be noted.

SIMPLE "LOW-TECH" AND "NO-TECH" EVALUATION PROCEDURES

Experienced clinicians may be able to evaluate all of the above characteristics by merely listening to spontaneous speech or repetition of sentences. The assessment of experienced evaluators tends to be very reliable (Paal, Reulbach, et al., 2005). However, less-experienced clinicians may find it helpful to employ some supplemental tests to more clearly define the speech characteristics and the potential cause. Therefore, the following is a list of simple "low-tech" and "no-tech" evaluation procedures that may be useful.

Visual Detection

- *Mirror Test*: A mirror can be held under the nares during speech in order to evaluate nasal air emission based on condensation (Figure 12–1). The examiner should place the mirror under the child's nose during the production of pressure-sensitive sounds. If the mirror clouds up, it indicates nasal air emission. Unfortunately, this is not a very practical technique because the mirror fogs as soon as the child breathes at the end of an utterance. In addition, it shows nasal emission, but there is no way to know if it was consistent or just occurred on one phoneme.

- *Air Paddle*: The examiner can actually see nasal emission by using an "air paddle," as first described by Bzoch (1979). An air

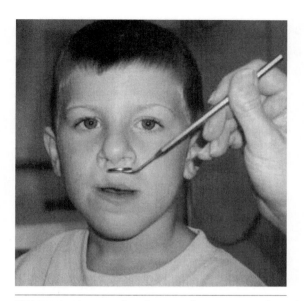

FIGURE 12–1 A dental mirror for testing nasal air emission. A dental mirror can be held under the nares during speech in order to evaluate nasal air emission. The evaluation is based on the appearance of condensation and should be done carefully to be sure the condensation is not from breathing. Also, this test does not indicate the sound during which the nasal emission occurred.

paddle can be cut from a piece of paper and placed underneath the nares during the production of repetitive syllables with pressure-sensitive consonants (i.e., "pa pa pa; ta ta ta; ka ka ka") (Figure 12–2). It is best to use voiceless consonants since these consist of more air pressure and are therefore most likely to show nasal air emission. If the paddle moves during the production of these sounds, this indicates that there is nasal air emission.

- *See Scape*: A See-Scape™ (Pro-Ed, 1986, Austin, Texas) allows the examiner to view the occurrence of nasal air emission. A nasal olive is placed in the child's nostril. The nasal olive is attached to a flexible tube that is connected to a rigid vertical tube. As the child repeats pressure-sensitive phonemes, a styrofoam

stopper rises in the vertical tube if there is nasal air emission (Figure 12–3). It is important to keep in mind that, at the end of the utterance, the child will exhale slightly through the nose. Therefore, the stopper may rise slightly at this point, but this is normal.

Tactile Detection

- *Feeling the Sides of the Nose*: Vibration from hypernasality and nasal air emission can often be felt by placing the index fingers lightly on the individual's nose, in the area of the cartilage (Figure 12–4). This feeling can be simulated by prolonging an /m/ and feeling the vibration on the nasal cartilage.

Auditory Detection

Although visual and tactile detection can be helpful, by far the best evaluation procedures are to use auditory detection since what is being evaluated is an auditory event. In addition, the auditory tests are more reliable.

- *Nose Pinch (Cul-de-Sac) Test*: The nose pinch test has been called the "Cul-de-Sac Test" by Bzoch and others (Bzoch, 1979, 1997; Haapanen, 1991). It is done by having the child produce a speech segment with the nose unoccluded, and then repeat the same speech segment with the nostrils pinched closed (Figure 12–5). To assess hypernasality with this test, the child is asked to prolong a vowel or repeat a sentence that is devoid of nasal consonants. In normal speech, there should be no perceptible difference in the quality of the production because the nasal cavity is already closed by the velopharyngeal valve. If there is a dysfunctional velopharyngeal valve, the

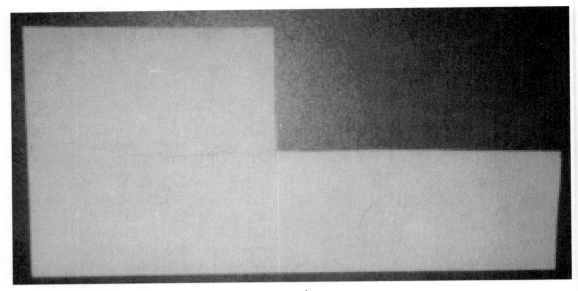

A

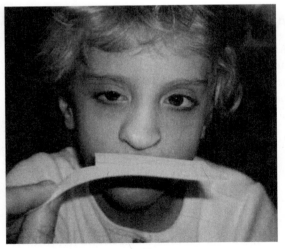

B

FIGURE 12–2 (A and B) A. An "air paddle" to be used in testing for nasal air emission. The paddle can be cut (or even torn) from a piece of paper. B. The paddle is placed underneath the nares during the production of repetitive syllables that have pressure sensitive consonants. If the paddle moves during speech, this indicates nasal air emission.

sound will resonate in the nasal cavity but be blocked by the closed nose, causing cul-de-sac resonance. If the velopharyngeal valve is functioning normally, there should be no change in resonance with the closed nose. Therefore, a difference in quality with closure of the nares indicates hypernasality. To assess for nasal air emission, the child is asked to repeat syllables or sentences loaded with pressure-sensitive consonants. If there is an increase in oral pressure with closure of the nose, this is suggestive of significant nasal air emission. Finally, to assess hyponasality, the child is asked to produce a nasal sound repetitively (such as "ma, ma, ma").

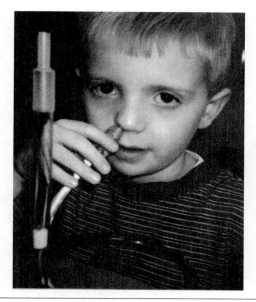

FIGURE 12–3 The use of a See-Scape™ (Super Duper, Greenville, SC) for testing nasal air emission. The patient places the nasal olive at the entrance to the nostril. If there is nasal air emission during speech production, the styrofoam stopper will rise in the tube.

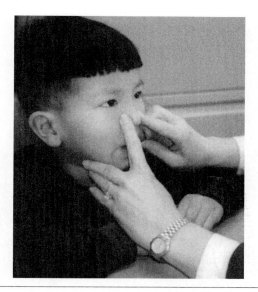

FIGURE 12–4 A tactile test of nasal air emission and hypernasality. Nasal air emission or hypernasality can sometimes be felt by placing the index fingers lightly on the individual's nose, in the area of the cartilage that is just below the bone. As the child repeats pressure-sensitive consonants or says "60, 60, 60," the examiner can feel the vibration of nasal air emission or hypernasality.

If there is little or no difference in the quality of the speech with the nose closed, this suggests significant hyponasality.

- *Stethoscope*: If a stethoscope is available, it can be especially helpful in evaluating the characteristics of velopharyngeal dysfunction. The drum of the stethoscope can be placed on either side of the nose or under the nose. If there is hypernasality or nasal emission during the production of oral sounds, this can be clearly heard through the stethoscope (Figure 12–6). The stethoscope is even more effective if the drum is removed and the tubing is placed at the entrance of one nostril. The only disadvantage of this method is that the tubing needs to be appropriately disinfected between patients.

- *Straw*: A straw is the ultimate low-cost, low-tech instrument. Yet, it is extremely

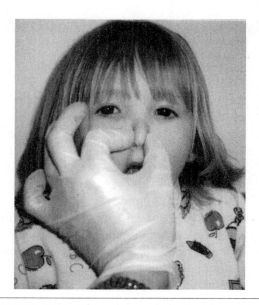

FIGURE 12–5 The nose pinch or "cul-de-sac test." The examiner asks the patient to produce a speech segment and then repeat the segment with the nostrils occluded.

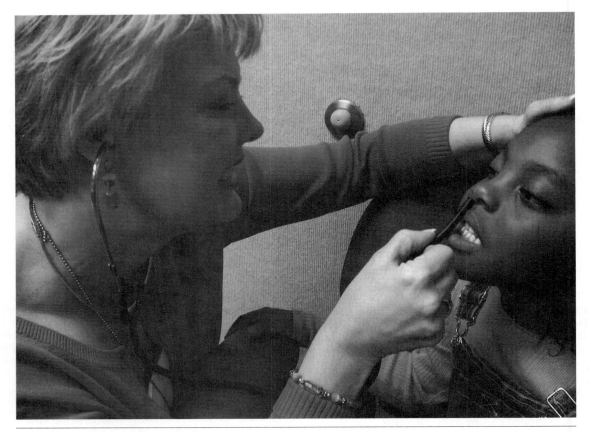

FIGURE 12–6 The use of a stethoscope. The drum is taken off the end so that the tube is placed near the opening of the nostril. This requires disinfection after each use.

helpful and reliable in detecting hyper-nasality and nasal emission. Both of these can be detected by placing the short end of the bending straw in the child's nostril and the other end near the examiner's ear (Figure 12–7). Another use of the straw is detection of a lateral lisp, which is often confused with nasal air emission. In this case, the examiner can place a straw at different positions on the side of the dental arch during the production of a prolonged sibilant. If the air stream is lateralized, it will be heard through the straw at the side of the dental arch, rather than in the front.

- *Listening Tube*: A plastic tube works just like the stethoscope or the straw in helping to detect hypernasality and nasal emission. One end of the tube is placed at the entrance to the child's nostril, and the other end is placed near the examiner's ear as the child produces oral syllables or sentences (Figure 12–8). The advantage of the tube is that you can make it any length for comfort. The disadvantage is that the examiner needs to be careful to not to forget which end went in the child's nose and which end went in his or her ear. In addition, the tube needs to be either disinfected or discarded after use.

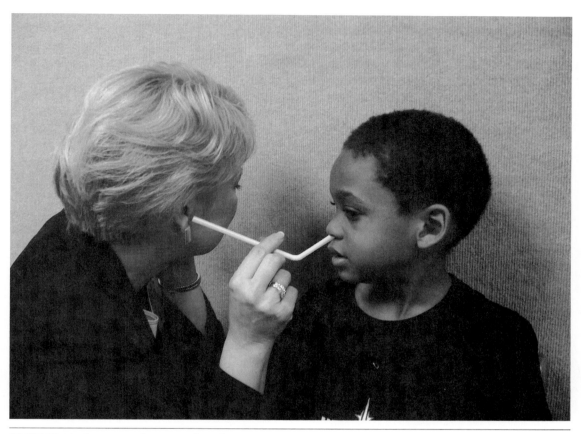

FIGURE 12–7   A straw for a test of nasal air emission and hypernasality. A straw is placed in the child's nostril as he or she produces pressure-sensitive sounds. If there is nasal air emission or hypernasality, this can be heard through the straw.

It should be noted that of all of these tests, using some kind of tube (stethoscope, listening tube, or straw) is by far the best way to evaluate hypernasality, nasal emission, and velopharyngeal function for several reasons. First, the examiner is able to hear nasal emission that is inaudible in regular speech. It also allows the examiner to hear the nasal emission in a noisy environment. Even if the velopharyngeal valve is only slightly inefficient in closing, this inefficiency can be heard as a click when using a straw or listening tube. (This suggests a risk for hypernasality with adenoid atrophy or maxillary advancement.)

The examiner can determine when the nasal emission occurs and on what sounds. The "equipment" is cheap, reliable, dependable, and readily available. Finally, this method has face validity in that it involves an auditory assessment of an auditory event.

Differential Diagnosis of Cause

Hypernasality and nasal air emission can be caused by VPI, an oronasal fistula, or by an articulation disorder. The cause of the problem is important to determine because it will have a

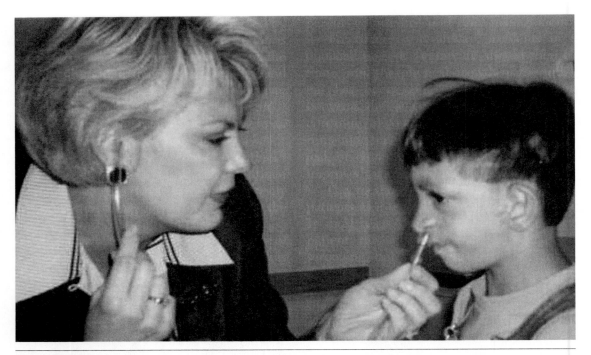

FIGURE 12–8 A "listening tube" for a test of nasal air emission and hypernasality. One end of a plastic tube is place in the child's nostril or at the entrance to the nostril, and the other end is place in the examiner's ear. As the child produces sounds or sentences, the examiner can hear occurrences of nasal air emission or hypernasality.

direct impact on the treatment recommendations (Garrett, Deal, & Prathanee, 2002).

If there is an oronasal fistula, the size is one factor that can determine the effect on speech. If the fistula is small, it may not be symptomatic at all because the airflow in the oral cavity is horizontal to the opening (refer to Figure 2–13). If the fistula is 5 mm or more in diameter, nasal air emission may be noted with the production of pressure-sensitive consonants. If the fistula is very large, there may be hypernasality as well (refer to Figure 7–3).

The position of the fistula can also determine whether there is an effect on speech. If the fistula is in the area of the incisive foramen, which is very common, there may be nasal air emission during the production of lingual-alveolar sounds due to the fact that the tongue pushes air into the opening as it elevates for production. A midpalatal fistula can result in the use of a palatal-dorsal placement for many sounds as a compensatory strategy for closing the fistula with the tongue. A posterior fistula may be less symptomatic because there are fewer posterior sounds in speech to force the air stream upward.

To determine if a fistula is symptomatic, the examiner can compare the occurrence of nasal air emission on anterior sounds versus posterior sounds. If there is no difference, then the source of the nasal air emission is probably the velopharyngeal valve. However, if there is more nasal emission on anterior sounds than on the sounds that are posterior to the fistula, this suggests the fistula as the cause.

Another way to evaluate the effect of a fistula is to temporarily close it with chewing gum or Fruit Rollups (Janet Middendorf, personal communication, May 4, 2005). The gum and tissues surrounding the fistula need to be dried with a tissue or Q tip for the substance to stick. A comparison of the speech can then be done with and without occlusion. A reduction in nasal air emission or hypernasality with fistula occlusion indicates that the fistula is symptomatic for speech. If hypernasality or nasal air emission are still noted with total occlusion of the fistula, then VPI is implicated as the cause.

One complicating factor in evaluating VPI in the presence of a fistula is the combined effect of the two. When there is a leak in the system as a result of a fistula, this can cause the velopharyngeal mechanism to function less efficiently (Moller, 1991). Therefore, unless the fistula is closed or obturated, it can be difficult to evaluate the capabilities of velopharyngeal mechanism. It often takes a multidisciplinary approach to determine the symptomatology that is directly due to the fistula, and to formulate the appropriate treatment plan (Folk, D'Antonio, & Hardesty, 1997).

When there is hypernasality or nasal emission, the examiner must also determine if the cause is structural, or due to misarticulations. For example, a nasal rustle commonly occurs due to a small velopharyngeal opening. However, it also occurs in association with the production of a posterior velar fricative. The first is a structural cause that requires surgical intervention. The second is due to mislearning and therefore requires speech therapy. Therefore, determining the cause of the nasal emission is very important. This is done by assessing consistency of occurrence and stimulability.

If the nasal emission is phoneme-specific in that it occurs only on certain sounds (particularly sibilants), this is due to misarticulation. If hypernasality is phoneme-specific in that it only occurs on high vowels (particularly /i/), this indicates faulty articulation, as well. Stimulability testing can also be very helpful in making the correct diagnosis as to cause. If nasal emission or hypernasality are eliminated with a change in articulation placement, this confirms that the cause is faulty articulation and not VPI. For specific suggestions on changing articulatory placement to eliminate nasal air emission, see Chapter 21.

CASE REPORT

Phoneme-Specific Nasal Air Emission

Jeff was a 36-year-old man with a history of "nasality," although he was not born with a cleft palate. His parents were told that he would need surgery to correct the problem, but they opted not to have that done. In his early 20s, Jeff sought another opinion and was again told that he would require surgery for correction. Due to his hesitancy to go through with the procedure, the surgery was never done. When he came to our clinic at the age of 36, Jeff reported that his speech had been a barrier in his work and social life and therefore, he was finally ready for the surgery.

Upon examination, the velum appeared to be normal. An assessment of speech revealed the substitution of a posterior nasal fricative for sibilant sounds (/s/, /z/, /sh/, /ch/, /j/), which caused nasal air emission on those sounds. All other speech sounds were produced correctly with normal air pressure and showed no evidence of nasal air

(continues)

(continued)

emission. Resonance was normal. Given these findings, it was surmised that this patient was demonstrating phoneme-specific nasal air emission rather than velopharyngeal insufficiency/incompetence (VPI).

To test stimulability, Jeff was instructed to produce an isolated /t/ sound repetitively and in a forceful manner, while feeling the air pressure during production. Then he was told to produce the /t/ sound repetitively with the teeth closed. He was able to do this easily with good oral pressure and no nasal air emission. After doing this several times, he was instructed to produce the /t/ with the teeth closed and then prolong the end, making it a /tsssss/. Again, he was able to do this easily, and the resulting /s/ sound was produced orally with no nasal air emission. The final step was to eliminate the starter /t/. This was the hardest part for Jeff, but within a few minutes, he was able to produce the /s/ and all of the other sibilants in isolation with normal oral pressure and no nasal air emission.

Rather than undergoing a surgical procedure, as had been recommended several times in the past, Jeff was enrolled in speech therapy. Within a few months, he had eliminated the use of posterior nasal fricatives and was producing sibilants normally without nasal air emission. The nasality was eliminated without the need for surgery.

This case illustrates the importance of a differential diagnosis. In Jeff's case, the nasal emission was due to misarticulation, rather than VPI. It is fortunate that he did not follow through with the recommendation for surgery, since that would not have corrected the problem. On the other hand, it is unfortunate that he was misdiagnosed previously and that the appropriate form of speech therapy was not done when he was a child.

FOLLOW-UP

Recommendations

Upon completion of the evaluation the examiner must make appropriate recommendations considering the cause of the abnormal speech characteristics. Table 12–6 has a list of possible recommendations that can be considered for each cause. Based on the particular speech characteristics, the examiner can estimate velopharyngeal gap size (see Table 7–1). If there is nasal emission and hypernasality, this suggests a large velopharyngeal opening that will require surgical intervention. On the other hand, if there is a nasal rustle that is phoneme-specific or if there are articulation errors that are not obligatory, speech therapy would be appropriate.

Depending on the evaluation results, additional assessments may be recommended from other professionals. The examiner might also recommend other diagnostic procedures, such as a sleep study, a videofluoroscopic swallow study, or an endoscopic evaluation of swallowing. Treatment recommendations might include surgical management, prosthetic management, or speech therapy. A special preschool or educational setting may be part of the overall treatment plan.

Prior to making the referrals for additional evaluations or for other forms of treatment, the speech-language pathologist should always discuss the recommendations with the primary care physician and the referring physician. This is not only common courtesy, but is consistent with the "medical model" where the primary care physician manages the child's overall plan of care.

Finally, recommendations should always be based on the cause and severity of the speech or resonance disorder, its effect on the child's quality of life, the potential for improvement, the associated risks, and the desires of the child and the family. The examiner must be careful not to impose his or her own value system and personal preferences on the child

---

TABLE 12–6 Possible Recommendations Regarding Treatment Based on Cause

Velopharyngeal Insufficiency (Structural Abnormality)

- Surgery (postoperative speech therapy as needed)
- Prosthesis—speech bulb
- Speech therapy for articulation and compensatory productions

Velopharyngeal Incompetence (Physiological Abnormality)

- Surgery (postoperative speech therapy as needed)
- Prosthesis—palatal lift
- Speech therapy (particularly if acquired) and therapy for articulation and compensatory productions

Velopharyngeal Mislearning

- Speech therapy only

Symptomatic Fistula

- Surgery
- Prosthesis—obturator
- Speech therapy for articulation and compensatory production

---

and the family. They are the ones who have to live with the consequences of the decision.

Family Counseling

Counseling the family (and child as appropriate) following the evaluation is one of the most important desired outcomes of the evaluation (Smith & Guyette, 2004). Handouts with labeled drawings are particularly useful in helping the family to understand the anatomy, the problem with speech, and any surgical procedures that are being proposed. Many centers give out their own handouts and brochures that contain specific information regarding their program and facility (see Appendix 12–1). In addition, many informational brochures are available

through the Cleft Palate Foundation (CPF) of the American Cleft Palate-Craniofacial Association. (See Appendix A and Appendix B of this book.)

Evaluation Report

Many professionals have recommended standardization of assessment protocols, and standardization of the methods of rating and recording evaluation results (Golding-Kushner et al., 1990; Hirschberg & Van Demark, 1997; Sell, Harding, & Grunwell, 1999). For clinicians who wish to store clinical information in a standardized manner, the American Cleft Palate-Craniofacial Association has a database that is available to members (American Cleft Palate-Craniofacial Association, 1504 East Franklin Street, Suite 102, Chapel Hill, NC, 27514-2820). Despite general agreement that standardization is needed, in practice, there is still great variability among centers and between providers in the way evaluation results are reported.

The speech evaluation is only as good as the information in the report, since that is what is primarily communicated to the family and other professionals. Therefore, the report must be accurate, succinct, clear, and concise. Many professionals fail to consider their "customers" when writing the report. Long reports are usually not read and are definitely not appreciated by busy professionals. The report should contain appropriate language and medical terminology, but should also be understandable to the readers. Diacritic symbols are not understood by nonprofessionals. Therefore, the letters or word descriptions should be used when communicating with others. The report should focus on the evaluation results, the examiner's impressions, and the recommendations. Most of all, it is important to be correct and confident in the stated conclusions and recommendations, as this will often result in surgical management.

Summary

A perceptual assessment of speech and resonance gives the examiner information regarding the presence of VPI and its effect on speech production. It is important to assess articulation in order to determine if there are any obligatory or compensatory errors resulting from velopharyngeal dysfunction. The examiner should determine if there is nasal emission, and if this is causing weak consonants and short utterance length. If resonance is abnormal, the examiner should determine the type of resonance, but not be particularly concerned about rating the severity. Phonation should also be assessed because dysphonia is common in individuals with VPI.

Although there are instrumental procedures to evaluate velopharyngeal function, the ear remains the best method for judging abnormal speech and resonance. To augment the perceptual assessment, the use of a tube (stethoscope, listening tube, or straw) is the most appropriate and effective method of assessing the speech correlates of velopharyngeal dysfunction.

For Review, Discussion, and Critical Thinking

1. When should the child first be seen by the speech-language pathologist? What should be the focus of concern when the child is a newborn? What should be the focus of concern when the child is a toddler? At what age can velopharyngeal function be evaluated? Why can't it be evaluated earlier?

2. What type of information is important to obtain in the diagnostic interview with the parent or guardian?

3. Discuss different types of speech stimuli that can be used in an assessment and the advantages of each type.

4. List the types of errors that should be identified in the articulation test. Why is it important to identify the type of error?

5. Why is it important to test stimulability? If the child responds well to stimulation, what might that suggest?

6. What sounds would you test for nasal emission? Why?

7. Describe methods for informally detecting nasality. What is the advantage of auditory detection over visual or tactile detection? What is the advantage of using a straw or listening tube over using a mirror for detection of nasal emission?

8. Your patient has normal resonance, but inconsistent nasal emission. He has a small fistula in the middle of the palate. What would you do to determine if the nasal emission is due to the fistula, or due to velopharyngeal insufficiency?

9. Why is a differential diagnosis of the cause of abnormal resonance or nasal emission so important? Discuss possible repercussions of making the wrong diagnosis.

References

American Cleft Palate-Craniofacial Association. (1993). Parameters for evaluation and treatment of patients with cleft lip/ palate or other craniofacial anomalies. *Cleft Palate-Craniofacial Journal, 30* (Suppl.), 1–16.

Andrews, J. R., & Rutherford, D. (1972). Contribution of nasally emitted sound to the perception of hypernasality of vowels. *Cleft Palate Journal*, 9, 147–156.

Bronsted, K., Grunwell, P., Henningsson, G., Jansonius, K. J. K., Meijer, M., Ording, U., Sell, K., Vermeij-Zieverink, E., & Wyatt, R. (1994). A phonetic framework for the cross-linguistic analysis of cleft palate speech. *Clinical Linguistics and Phonetics*, 8, 109–125.

Bzoch, K. R. (1979). Measurement and assessment of categorical aspects of cleft palate speech. In K. R. Bzoch (Ed.), *Communicative disorders related to cleft lip and palate* (Vol. 2, pp. 161–191). Boston: Little, Brown and Company.

Bzoch, K. R. (1997). Clinical assessment, evaluation and management of 11 categorical aspects of cleft palate speech. In K. R. Bzoch (Ed.), *Communicative disorders related to cleft lip and palate* (Vol. 4, pp. 261–311). Austin, TX: Pro-Ed.

Bzoch, K. R., & League, R. (1991). *Receptive-Expressive Emergent Language Test: A method for assessing the language skills of infants* (2nd ed.). Austin, TX: Pro-Ed.

Coplan, J. (1987). *Early Language Milestone (ELM) Scale*. Austin, TX: Pro-Ed.

Dalston, R. M. (1997). The use of nasometry in the assessment and remediation of velopharyngeal inadequacy. In K. R. Bzoch (Ed.), *Communicative disorders related to cleft lip and palate* (Vol. 4, pp. 331–346). Austin, TX: Pro-Ed.

Fenson, L., Dale, P. S., Reznick, J. S., Thal, D., Bates, E., Hartung, P., Pethick, S., & Reilly, J. S. (1989). *The MacArthur Communicative Development Inventory*. San Diego, CA: Development Psychology Lab, San Diego State University.

Fluharty, N. B. (1978). *Fluharty Preschool Speech and Language Test*. Boston: Teaching Resources Corporation.

Folk, S. N., D'Antonio, L. L., & Hardesty, R. A. (1997). Secondary cleft deformities. *Clinics in Plastic Surgery*, 24(3), 599–611.

Garrett, J. D., Deal, R. E., & Prathanee, B. (2002). Velopharyngeal assessment procedures for the Thai cleft palate population. *Journal of the Medical Association of Thailand*, 85(6), 682–692.

Glascoe, F. P. (1991). Can clinical judgment detect children with speech-language problems? *Pediatrics*, 87(3), 317–322.

Golding-Kushner, K. J., Argamaso, R. V., Cotton, R. T., Grames, L. M., Henningsson, G., Jones, D. L., et al. (1990). Standardization for the reporting of nasopharyngoscopy and multiview videofluoroscopy: A report from an International Working Group. *Cleft Palate Journal*, 27(4), 337–347; Discussion 347–338.

Haapanen, M. L. (1991). A simple clinical method of evaluating perceived hypernasality [Erratum appears in *Folia Phoniatrica* 1991, 43(4), 203]. *Folia Phoniatrica*, 43(3), 122–132.

Henningsson, G., & Isberg, A. (1991). A cineradiographic study of velopharyngeal movements for deviant versus nondeviant articulation. *Cleft Palate-Craniofacial Journal*, 28(1), 115–117; Discussion 117–118.

Hickman, L. A. (1997). *Apraxia profile: A descriptive assessment tool for children*. San Antonio, TX: Communication Skill Builders.

Hirschberg, J., & Van Demark, D. R. (1997). A proposal for standardization of speech and hearing evaluations to assess velopharyngeal function. *Folia Phoniatrica et Logopedica*, 49(3/4), 158–167.

Kaufman, N. R. (1995). *Kaufman Speech Praxis Test for Children (KSPT)*. Detroit, MI: Wayne State University Press.

Kummer, A. W., Briggs, M., & Lee, L. (2003). The relationship between the characteristics of speech and velopharyngeal gap size. *Cleft Palate-Craniofacial Journal, 40*(6), 590–596.

Kummer, A. W., Curtis, C., Wiggs, M., Lee, L., & Strife, J. L. (1992). Comparison of velopharyngeal gap size in patients with hypernasality, hypernasality and nasal emission, or nasal turbulence (rustle) as the primary speech characteristic. *Cleft Palate-Craniofacial Journal, 29*(2), 152–156.

Kummer, A. W., & Marsh, J. H. (1998). Pediatric voice and resonance disorders. In A. F. Johnson & B. H. Jacobson (Eds.), *Medical speech-language pathology: A practitioner's guide*. New York: Thieme.

McWilliams, B. J., Lavorato, A. S., & Bluestone, C. D. (1973). Vocal cord abnormalities in children with velopharyngeal valving problems. *Laryngoscope, 83*(11), 1745–1753.

McWilliams, B. J., Morris, H. L., & Shelton, R. L. (1990). Diagnosis of phonation and resonance. In B. J. Williams, H. L. Morris, & R. L. Shelton (Eds.), *Cleft palate speech* (pp. 311–319). Philadelphia: B. C. Decker.

Moller, K. T. (1991). An approach to the evaluation of velopharyngeal adequacy for speech. *Clinics in Communication Disorders, 1*(1), 61–65.

Paal, S., Reulbach, U., Strobel-Schwarthoff, K., Nkenke, E., & Schuster, M. (2005). Evaluation of speech disorders in children with cleft lip and palate. *Journal of Orofacial Orthopedics, 66*(4): 270–278.

Rossetti, L. (1990). *The Rossetti Infant-Toddler Language Scale*. East Moline, IL: LinguiSystems.

Scherer, N. J., & D'Antonio, L. L. (1995). Parent questionnaire for screening early language development in children with cleft palate. *Cleft Palate-Craniofacial Journal, 32*(1), 7–13.

Scherer, N. J. & D'Antonio, L. L. (1997). Language and play development in toddlers with cleft lip and/or palate. *American Journal of Speech-Language Pathology, 6* (4), 48–54.

Schneider, E., & Shprintzen, R. J. (1980). A survey of speech pathologists: Current trends in the diagnosis and management of velopharyngeal insufficiency. *Cleft Palate Journal, 17*(3), 249–253.

Sell, D., Harding, A., & Grunwell (1999). GOS.SP.ASS.'98: An assessment for speech disorders associated with cleft palate and/or velopharyngeal dysfunction (Revised). *International Journal of Language and Communication Disorders, 34*(1), 17–33.

Shprintzen, R. J., & Golding-Kushner, K. J. (1989). Evaluation of velopharyngeal insufficiency. *Otolaryngologic Clinics of North America, 22*(3), 519–536.

Smith, B., and Guyette, T. W. (2004). Evaluation of cleft palate speech. *Clinics in Plastic Surgery, 31*(2), 251–260.

Stemple, J. C., Glaze, L. E., & Gerdeman, B. K. (1995). *Clinical voice pathology: Theory and management*. San Diego, CA: Singular Publishing Group.

Subtelny, J. D., Van Hattum, R. J., & Myers, B. B. (1972). Ratings and measures of cleft palate speech. *Cleft Palate Journal, 9*(1), 18–27.

Templin, M. C., & Darley, F. (1960). *Screening and diagnostic tests of articulation*. Iowa City, IA: Bureau of Educational Research and Service Extension Division, State University of Iowa.

Trost, J. E. (1981). Articulatory additions to the classical description of the speech of persons with cleft palate. *Cleft Palate Journal, 18*(3), 193–203.

Trost-Cardamone, J. E. (1987). *Cleft palate misarticulations: A teaching tape* [Video-tape]. Northridge, CA: California State University, Northridge, Instructional Media Center.

Trost-Cardamone, J. E. (1997). Diagnosis of specific cleft palate speech error patterns for planning therapy of physical management needs. In K. R. Bzoch (Ed.), *Communicative disorders related to cleft lip and palate* (Vol. 4, pp. 313–330). Austin, TX: Pro-Ed.

Wilson, D. K. (1987). *Voice problems of children* (Vol. 3). Baltimore, MD: Williams & Wilkins.

Appendix 12–1

The Effects of Cleft Lip/Palate on Communication Development: Information for Parents

By Ann W. Kummer, Ph.D.

A history of cleft lip or palate can affect the child's ability to develop verbal communication skills. The following aspects of verbal communication may be defective:

- **Articulation (Speech)**—the physical production of sounds to form spoken words

- **Language**—the message conveyed back and forth in talking. This includes the ability to understand the speech of others (receptive language) and the ability to express thoughts through words and sentences (expressive language)

- **Voice**—the sound that results from the vibration of the vocal cords (phonation)

- **Resonance**—the vibration of voiced sound in the oral cavity (mouth) and nasal cavity (nose)

There are three main causes of communication disorders in children with a history of cleft lip and palate. These are as follows:

1. Dental Abnormalities

If the cleft extended into the gum ridge, dental development may be affected, causing the following:

- Missing teeth in the area of the cleft

- Extra (supernumerary) teeth

- Malocclusion (poor closure of the top and bottom jaws)

Dental abnormalities may cause speech errors as follows:

- A lisp-type of distortion on sibilant sounds (/s/, /z/, /sh/, /ch/, /j/)

- Difficulty producing lip sounds (/p/, /b/, /m/)

- Difficulty producing teeth-to-lip sounds (/f/, /v/)

- Difficulty producing tongue-tip sounds (/t/, /d/, /n/, /l/)

These distortions can usually be corrected with a combination of dental and orthodontic treatment, and speech therapy.

2. HEARING LOSS

The eustachian tube connects the middle ear and the back of the throat. It opens with swallowing. This allows fluids to drain out of the middle ear and equalizes air pressure in the ear with the environment. Children with a history of cleft palate often have chronic ear infections (otitis media) because the muscle in the soft palate that is responsible for opening the eustachian tube does not function well. As a result, negative pressure and fluids build up in the middle ear, causing ear infections and a conductive hearing loss. A conductive hearing loss can affect the child's ability to develop language and even speech skills.

To avoid middle ear problems, pressure-equalizing (PE) tubes are often inserted in the eardrum at an early age. This helps to prevent fluids from building up in the ear that cause infection and hearing loss.

3. VELOPHARYNGEAL DYSFUNCTION (VPD)

(Also Known as Velopharyngeal Insufficiency or Incompetence—VPI)
In order to close off the nose from the mouth during speech, several structures come together to achieve "velopharyngeal closure." These include the following:

- Velum (soft palate)
- Lateral pharyngeal walls—side walls of the throat

- Posterior pharyngeal wall—the back wall of the throat

When the velopharyngeal valve closes, the speaker is able to build up air pressure and sound in the mouth to produce various consonant sounds and vowel sounds. Velopharyngeal closure also occurs during other activities, such as swallowing, gagging, vomiting, sucking, blowing, and whistling.

After a cleft palate repair, the velum (soft palate) may still be too short or may not move well enough to reach the posterior pharyngeal wall (back wall of the throat). This results in velopharyngeal dysfunction (VPD) which causes problems with speech.

Effects of Velopharyngeal Dysfunction on Speech

Velopharyngeal dysfunction can cause the following speech characteristics:

- Hypernasality (too much sound in the nose during speech)
- Nasal air emission during consonant production
- Weak or omitted consonants due to inadequate air pressure in the mouth
- Compensatory articulation productions (speech sounds produced in a different way)

Treatment of Velopharyngeal Dysfunction (VPD)

Treatment of VPD usually includes surgical intervention and speech therapy. Prosthetic devices can also be used on a temporary or permanent basis in some cases.

SUMMARY

Communication disorders due to cleft lip or palate can be successfully treated with early and appropriate treatment. Prior to age 3, language development should be the primary focus. After age 3, speech, voice, and resonance should be evaluated and treated if necessary. If therapy or surgery is indicated, it is usually done in the preschool years so that speech is normal, or close to normal, by the time the child begins school. The team approach to management is particularly important for the best overall outcome since the coordination of multiple professionals is required to meet a variety of needs.

CHAPTER

13

OROFACIAL EXAMINATION

INTRODUCTION

An orofacial examination (sometimes called an oral-peripheral examination or perioral examination) involves assessment of oral structures and other facial structures that may be relevant for speech. An intraoral examination (sometimes called an oral mechanism examination) is part of a complete orofacial examination.

A complete orofacial examination should always be done as part of a speech or resonance evaluation, especially if they child has a history of cleft or a craniofacial anomaly. However, many speech-language pathologists are unsure of how to perform this type of exam or what to look for in the exam. By performing regular orofacial examinations, speech-language pathologists will increase their familiarity with normal oral structures and be able to recognize abnormalities more easily (Thomas & Bender, 1993).

Knowledge of the oral structures and their potential effect on speech production and resonance is extremely important in order to make appropriate recommendations for treatment. If there are structural factors that cause or contribute to the deviant speech or resonance, these structural problems should be corrected if possible prior to starting speech therapy. In some cases, correcting the structure can result in a correction of the speech without the need for further intervention. In other cases, the compensatory productions need to be corrected with therapy after the structure is normalized.

In performing an intraoral assessment, the examiner should be *aware,* however, that a judgment regarding velopharyngeal function cannot be made based on an intraoral examination (Smith & Guyette, 2004). Velopharyngeal closure occurs behind the velum, usually on the plane of the hard palate. Therefore, it is well above the level that is viewed through the oral cavity. In addition, the examiner cannot see the point of maximum lateral pharyngeal wall movement from an intraoral perspective. In fact, at the oral level, the lateral pharyngeal walls may actually appear to bow outward during phonation. Finally, velopharyngeal function cannot be judged during a sustained vowel, such as "ah." Instead, the function of the velopharyngeal mechanism must be evaluated based on the movement and closure during connected speech.

Despite these limitations, the examiner can evaluate all of the oral structures that can affect speech and resonance production, including the status of labial competence, dental occlusion, the hard palate, the oral surface of the velum, the uvula, the tonsils, and the tongue. Therefore, an intraoral assessment can result in valuable information that can impact the examiner's overall impressions and recommendations from the assessment.

This chapter will discuss methodology for a comprehensive examination of relevant structures and function for the production of normal speech and resonance. In addition, appropriate procedures for infection control will be discussed.

General Methodology

Tools for an Orofacial Examination

An intraoral examination can often be done effectively without the need for any instruments. However, there are some instruments that are very helpful and should be available for oral examinations. The tools for an intraoral examination include the following:

- **Gloves:** for protection of the patient and the examiner.

- **Flashlight:** for illumination of the oral cavity.

- **Tongue blades:** to assist in holding the tongue down (when necessary) in order to observe the velum and uvula and to put between the buccal sulcus to observe dentition. Flavored tongue blades are now available and seem to be better received by young patients.

- **Dental mirror:** to use like a tongue blade in depressing the tongue. Also for looking up into the pharynx, or for inspecting the palate for a fistula.

- **Alcohol swabs or towelettes:** for cleaning contaminated instruments or equipment.

Visual Inspection of the Oral Cavity

If done correctly, a physical examination of morphology and function of the oral cavity can reveal important information. An adequate examination therefore involves more than a quick look in the mouth. It involves careful inspection of the structures that relate to speech production and a view of these structures during function.

When conducting an intraoral examination, most health care professionals ask the patient to say "ah" in order to inspect the structure. This vowel works well for evaluation of the hard palate and the anterior oral structures, but is less appropriate for evaluating the structure of the velum and the uvula. Although the "ah" vowel is considered a low vowel, it is primarily the jaw and tip of the tongue that are in a low position. The back of the tongue can be high and retracted so that it obstructs the view of the posterior section of the oral cavity and pharynx. Furthermore, this vowel makes it impossible to bring the tongue forward and out of the way for an adequate view. Because of these problems, a tongue blade is usually required to depress the back of the tongue so that it is low enough for the examiner to view the tip of the uvula.

If the vowel "aah" is used for the examination instead, the patient can be instructed to stick the tongue out and down as far as it will go (Figure 13–1). A young child can be instructed to point his tongue to his shoes or to try to touch his chin with his tongue. Although this does not allow the examiner to see "typical" velar movement, it does provide the examiner with a better view of the velum, uvula, and pharynx as the base of the tongue moves down and forward. This can be especially important when evaluating for a submucous cleft, because the examiner can see down to the posterior border of the velum and can better evaluate the integrity of the muscles of the velum. In addition to providing a better view, this technique allows the examiner to see the structures without the use of a tongue blade in most cases. Many patients, including adults, have a strong aversion to the use of tongue blades for fear of gagging, and therefore, this technique is appreciated.

If a tongue blade is needed, however, the blade should be placed approximately three-quarters of the way back. If the blade is placed

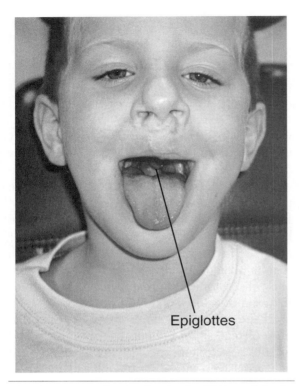

Epiglottes

FIGURE 13–1 The vowel "aah" should be used for the examination of the oral cavity. The patient should be instructed to stick the tongue out and down as far as it will go. A young child can be asked to point it to his shoes. Although this does not allow the examiner to see "typical" velar movement, it does provide the examiner with a better view of the velum, uvula, and pharynx as the base of the tongue moves down and forward. Note the epiglottis at the base of the tongue.

too far forward, which is a common mistake, it causes the posterior part of the tongue to mound up so as to obscure, rather than expose, the pharynx. If the tongue blade is placed behind the *circumvallate papilla*, a line of prominent taste buds that form an inverted "V" on the posterior tongue, it often elicits a gag reflex. The gag can give the examiner a good view, but it is a quick view and this technique is not appreciated by the patient. The correct technique for using a tongue blade is to press the tongue downward firmly, while scooping it

forward at the same time. The tongue is a strong, muscular organ, so firm pressure is often required to push against resistance.

As the individual phonates in producing a single vowel, there may be vigorous movement of the velum, or very little movement, even in normal speakers. To stimulate movement in order to see the pharynx and the tip of the uvula, the child can be asked to produce the vowel repetitively or to pant like a puppy dog (Beste, 1999). If this does not seem to stimulate movement, then the examiner can ask the child to do a big yawn with the tongue protruded. This will help to elevate the velum to its fullest extent.

Positioning of the patient is another consideration when performing an intraoral examination. The patient's head should be tilted slightly backward so that the examiner can look directly to the back of the pharynx. The examiner's eye level should be at the level of the patient's oral cavity. If the patient is an infant or is very young, it is sometimes helpful to have the parent or caregiver hold the child in a supine position with the head slightly lower than the rest of the body. This gives the examiner a good view from above. In addition, it will usually promote an open mouth posture, but the tongue may fall back into the pharynx, requiring the use of a tongue blade. In rare occasions when an examination is needed and the patient refuses to open his or her mouth, the examiner should place the tongue blade between the upper and lower incisors and apply steady pressure. The muscles closing the mouth are powerful, but fatigue rapidly, so that constant, firm pressure will allow insertion of the tongue blade within a few seconds. When the blade reaches the posterior tongue, the gag reflex will cause the mouth to open fully. Alternatively, closing the nares will force the mouth to open for breathing.

If the patient can cooperate adequately, the examiner should be able to evaluate the oropharynx, velar morphology and mobility, and the tonsils. In some cases, the tip of the epiglottis can even be seen.

IMPORTANT OBSERVATIONS

When conducting an orofacial or intraoral examination, it is important to keep in mind that there are normal variations in structure. Therefore, the examiner may observe characteristics that are unusual, but not necessarily abnormal. In addition, there may be abnormalities that have no relevance to speech or resonance. While the examiner should focus on assessing for abnormalities that can contribute to a speech or resonance disorder, other abnormalities should also be noted. This is particularly important if they require additional referral and follow-up (i.e., dental caries) or they provide evidence for the diagnosis of a syndrome (i.e., hypertelorism). Although the speech-language pathologist is not qualified to make a diagnosis of a syndrome based on observations of abnormalities, the speech-language pathologist can and should discuss the observations with the primary care physician and referring physician. A genetics evaluation may be suggested if that has not been done.

An orofacial examination begins with observation of the external anatomy, particularly the anatomy of the face. The facial structures should be observed initially at rest. The examiner should then watch the facial gestures, the tongue, and the teeth during articulation. In addition to observing the mouth, the examiner should inspect the eyes, ears, nose, and facial profile for evidence of abnormality or dysmorphology.

Eyes

The spacing between the eyes can be abnormal in certain craniofacial syndromes. Normally, the eyes should be about one eye's width apart. An individual with a craniofacial syndrome may demonstrate excessive spacing between the eyes, called *hypertelorism*, or too little spacing between the eyes, which is called *hypotelorism* (Figure 13–2). The opening between the eyelids, called *palpebral fissures*, should also be observed. Narrow palpebral fissures are a phenotypic feature in congenital conditions, such as velocardiofacial syndrome (Figure 13–3). Finally, the presence of *epicanthal folds* might be noted. These are excess folds of tissue that extend from the upper eyelid to the lower part of the orbit at the inner *canthus* or corner of the eye. This is often seen in Down syndrome and other syndromes,

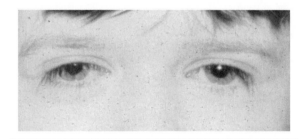

FIGURE 13–2 Hypertelorism (wide spaced eyes) which is common with several syndromes.

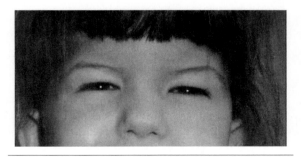

FIGURE 13–3 Narrow palpebral fissures (eye openings) in a child with velocardiofacial syndrome.

although epicanthal folds are normal in the Asian population.

Ears

The shape and location of the ears should be observed. Many craniofacial syndromes include malformed ears, such as a simplified helix, or *microtia* (Figure 13–4 and refer to Figure 8–1B), which is hypoplasia or absence of the pinna or auricle of the ear. This is often accompanied by *aural atresia*, which is the congenital absence of the external auditory canal. Aural atresia usually results in a conductive hearing loss, and of course, this can have an impact on the quality of speech and possibly resonance when it's bilateral. Ears that are low set, or below the level of the eyes, may also be suggestive of a syndrome.

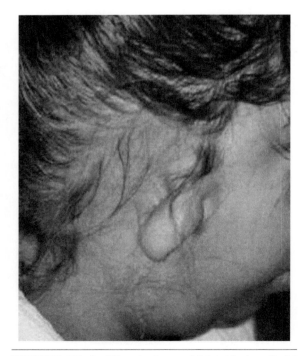

FIGURE 13–4 Microtia in a child with hemifacial microsomia.

Nose and Airway

The *nasal bridge*, or *nasion*, is the bony structure that is located between the eyes and corresponds to the nasofrontal suture. This structure should be examined because a flat nasal bridge can affect the nasal airway, causing upper airway obstruction and hyponasality. A bulbous nasal tip is often associated with syndromes. On the other hand, a flattened nasal tip may be noted if the columella is short due to a history of cleft lip. The nares should be inspected for evidence of stenosis that could affect nasal breathing and cause hyponasality.

Upper airway obstruction is common in individuals with a history of cleft palate or craniofacial anomalies. When there was a unilateral cleft lip and palate, septal deviations often occur. Upper airway obstruction can cause a chronic open mouth posture and anterior tongue position, which can ultimately result in an anterior open bite. The mandible may be positioned down and forward in order to open the airway further. Additional characteristics of upper airway obstruction include suborbital coloring, which makes the patient appear to be tired; pinched nostrils; and a face that appears elongated and narrow due to the position of the mandible. These characteristics have been referred to as the *"adenoid facies,"* because they are commonly seen in individuals with upper airway obstruction due to adenoid enlargement. Other signs of upper airway obstruction include strident breathing, snoring at night, sleep apnea, and of course, hyponasality.

To test the nasal airway, the examiner can ask the patient to close the lips and breathe nasally for a several minutes. The examiner should observe whether there is any difficulty with nasal breathing. Prior to opening the mouth, the patient should then inspire deeply through the nose, and then exhale through the nose. Again, the examiner should observe any difficulty. The patency of each nostril can be assessed by having the child close one nostril and then forcibly inspire through the other nostril. If there is obstruction, this will be difficult to do and will result in a high pitched sound, with the highest sound in the most obstructed nostril. Another test is to ask the patient to prolong an /m/ with the lips closed to see if there is blockage. If there is significant blockage, the patient will be unable to do this easily.

Facial Bones and Profile

The bony structures of the face are important to assess, particularly as they relate to each other. Flattened *zygomas* (cheekbones), are often seen in individuals with a history of cleft lip and palate or other craniofacial syndromes. The facial profile can give an indication of the dysmorphology of the other facial bones. This can be evaluated by having the patient turn so that the examiner is viewing the side of the person's face. For a normal profile, imaginary points on the forehead, bridge of the nose, base of the nose, and chin button should all line up in a vertical plane. If these points do not line up, the examiner should determine whether this is due to protrusion or retrusion of particular facial bones, particularly the maxilla or mandible. Discrepancy in the relationship between the maxilla and mandible can be particularly problematic for speech. Since the tongue always resides within the arch of the mandible, the position of the maxilla in relationship to the mandible can affect the amount of space available for the tongue tip to articulate (Figure 13–5).

Lips

The lips should be assessed for the ability to achieve bilabial closure at rest and during

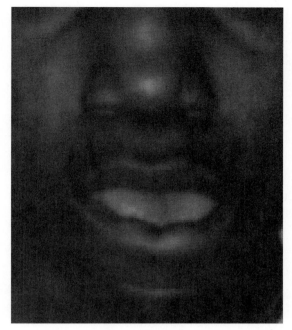

A

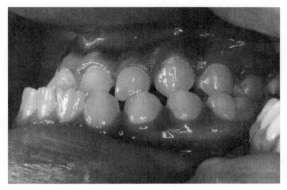

B

FIGURE 13–5 (A and B) Prognathic mandible and Class III malocclusion. This results in an anterior tongue position relative to the position of the maxilla.

speech. If the upper lip is short relative to the length of the maxilla, bilabial closure may be difficult to achieve and maintain (Figure 13–6). The lip may even be relatively short due to a protruding premaxilla (Figure 13–7). As a result, during the production of bilabial

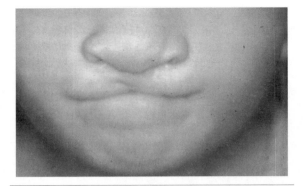

FIGURE 13–6 Short upper lip making bilabial competence an effort.

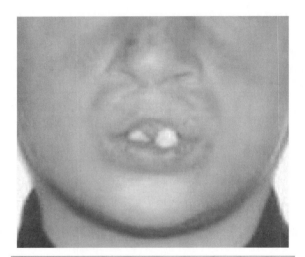

FIGURE 13–7 Protruding premaxilla which affects bilabial competence at rest and during speech.

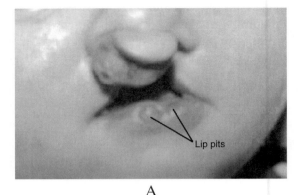

A

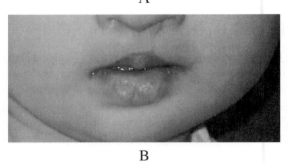

B

FIGURE 13–8 (A and B) Bilateral lip pits which indicate Van der Woude syndrome. This is an important finding because this syndrome is autosomal dominant.

sounds, the individual may substitute labiodental sounds. When there is a history of cleft lip, there may be excess scarring, the Cupid's bow may be asymmetrical or flat, or the vermilion may extend into the philtral suture lines. The examiner should always look for *lip pits*, which are small depressions in the bottom lip (Figure 13–8 A and B). This finding is indicative of Van der Woude syndrome, which also includes cleft palate. This syndrome has a 50%

recurrence risk for future pregnancies and therefore, the finding of lip pits is significant.

If the lips are apart and the upper lip is not short, the problem may be related to a skeletal discrepancy and resultant malocclusion. The open mouth posture may also be due to poor facial tone or oral-motor dysfunction. There may be drooling associated with the lack of adequate tone or motor skills. A chronic open mouth posture can actually increase the production of saliva, which further exacerbates the drooling.

There may be reduced mobility of the lips due to scarring. To assess labial movement, the patient can be asked to sustain exaggerated /i/ and /u/ sounds. The examiner should observe the symmetry and range of lip and facial movements. Observing the patient produce quick repetitions of the /p/ or /b/ sounds will allow the examiner to assess the ability to make rapid movements with the lips (Mason & Simon, 1977).

Additional External Anatomy

Additional external anomalies should be noted, since they may be relevant to a syndrome. Some anomalies may not be readily seen, but may be recorded in the medical history or reported by the parents. When velocardiofacial syndrome is suspected, an examination of the fingers may reveal the characteristic long and slender digits (Figure 13–9). The child's size and stature may also be important to note, since short stature is another phenotypic feature of this syndrome.

Hard Palate

To examine the hard palate, it is best to have the patient put the head back as far as possible

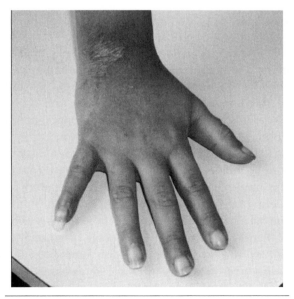

FIGURE 13–9 Long and tapered fingers which are often found with velocardiofacial syndrome.

so that the entire hard palate and velum can be visualized. For very young children, it is often helpful to have the child lay on the parent's lap with the head back over the parent's knees.

Once the palate can be seen, the mucosa of the hard palate should be observed. It should be uniform in color. The incisive papilla and rugae in the anterior portion of the hard palate can be noted. At the junction of the hard and soft palate, bilateral midline depressions may be observed. These are the *foveae palati*, which are openings to minor salivary glands (Jones, 1989).

As part of the examination, the position of the alveolar ridge, as it relates to the position of the tongue tip, should be determined. If the alveolar ridge is not just above the tongue tip, as commonly occurs when there is significant maxillary retrusion or protrusion, difficulty with the production of lingual-alveolar sounds might be expected. The palatal vault should also be evaluated, especially in relationship to the size of the tongue. If the palatal vault is low and flat, this can reduce the space available for the lingual articulation. This can also be a problem if the maxillary arch is narrow relative to the tongue size. To compensate for intraoral crowding, the mandible will often lower and the tongue may be forced down and forward.

If the patient has a history of cleft palate, the examiner should rule out the presence of an oronasal (palatal) fistula in the line of the cleft (Figure 13–10). A tongue flap, which is used to close a large fistula may be noted (Figure 13–11). If the fistula is small, it may be difficult to see due to the angle of an intraoral view. Therefore, a dental mirror can be especially helpful in visualizing the surface of the palate (Figure 13–12). The size of a fistula is often difficult to estimate because it may appear narrow on the oral surface but open considerably on the nasal surface. With gloved fingers, the examiner can sometimes feel the

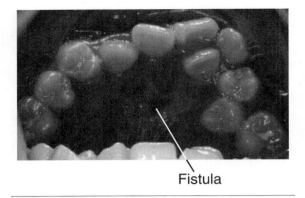

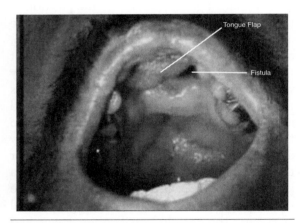

FIGURE 13–10 A small oronasal fistula in the area of the incisive foramen.

FIGURE 13–11 Tongue flap which was done to correct a large oronasal fistula. There is still a remaining opening on the patient's left.

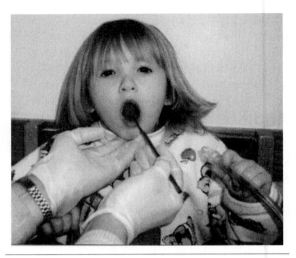

FIGURE 13–12 A dental mirror can be especially helpful in visualizing the palate in order to see a palatal fistula.

extent of a large palatal fistula. Occasionally, there is a furrow or a small depression in the palate. This may appear to be a fistula, but it may actually be a blind pouch that does not go through to the nasal cavity. If a palatal fistula is noted anywhere in the palate, its size and location are important to note because these are the primary determinants of whether the fistula will be symptomatic for nasal regurgitation or for speech.

If the patient or parent report that the coloring of food is sometimes seen in the nostril area, this is an indication of a patent fistula, most likely a nasolabial fistula. (Chocolate milk, chocolate pudding, and spaghetti seem to be primary offenders!) It should be noted that regurgitation of food does not usually occur with velopharyngeal insufficiency/incompetence. A nasolabial fistula is in the alveolar bone, just under the upper lip and in the line of the cleft. It is often left there purposely by the surgeon until the bone graft is done around age 6 or 7. To inspect for a nasolabial fistula, the examiner should use a tongue blade or dental mirror to gently raise the upper lip. The fistula can be palpated by feeling the anterior gum ridge under the buccal sulcus with a gloved finger. This type of fistula does not affect speech because it is out of the way of articulation and does not cause a reduction in intraoral air pressure.

If a submucous cleft is suspected, palatal palpation can be done to determine if there is a

CASE REPORT

Oronasal Fistula

Gerald presented as a new patient at the age of 11. He had a history of bilateral complete cleft lip and palate, which were repaired in another state. He had also had a pharyngeal flap for correction of velopharyngeal insufficiency at the age of 4. Gerald received speech therapy for several years in school. The mother reported that her primary concern was Gerald's nasality.

Upon examination, Gerald's speech was found to be minimally intelligible. His articulation pattern consisted of backing of anterior phonemes. Many compensatory productions were used. Resonance was hyponasal and mouth breathing was noted, suggesting upper airway obstruction. An obstructing pharyngeal flap was suspected.

The surprise came with the intraoral inspection, however. When examining the hard palate, a very large palatal fistula was observed. However, this was packed with food. Gerald was taken to the otolaryngologist, who spent some time cleaning out the fistula and the nasal cavity.

Once the fistula was cleaned out and opened, the speech was reevaluated and found to be hypernasal with nasal air emission. The pattern of backing of phonemes was obviously developed as a means to compensate for the position of the open fistula. Nasopharyngoscopy showed both lateral ports around the flap to be stenosed, which was the cause of the hyponasality and upper airway obstruction when the fistula was impacted. With this information in mind, a fistula repair and lateral port revisions were recommended.

This case study illustrates the importance of an intraoral examination. At times, observations made in the intraoral examination relate directly to the cause of the speech or resonance disorder.

notch in the border of the hard palate. Palpation might also be done to further explore a fistula in order to determine whether it is patent. If the examiner is inexperienced or not well trained in this area, palatal palpation can be difficult not only for the examiner, but even more so for the patient. The key to successful palpation is to be gentle and slow in feeling the palatal structures. Surprises in the area of the gag reflex are not well received by the child! However, carefully feeling the roof of the mouth with a gloved finger does not cause pain or even discomfort. If there is an open cleft or a fistula, it should be remembered that this is a variation in the structure and not a wound.

In preschool and school aged children, it is best to use the fifth (or little) finger for palpation (Figure 13–13). This finger is long enough to reach the back of the palate of children in this age group. In addition, this finger is narrow enough to feel a small notch in the palatal bone. For teenagers and adults, the fifth finger is usually not long enough to reach to the back of the hard palate. Therefore, the index finger must be used.

To begin the examination, it is important to wash hands thoroughly and then to don gloves. For a young child, the examiner should begin by merely rubbing or stimulating the outside gums above the maxillary teeth. This helps the patient to become more comfortable and accepting of the examiner's finger in the mouth. The examiner should then stimulate the alveolar ridge behind the teeth by moving

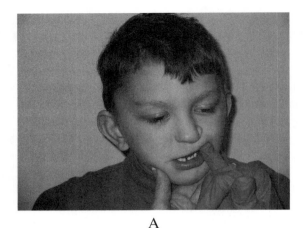

A

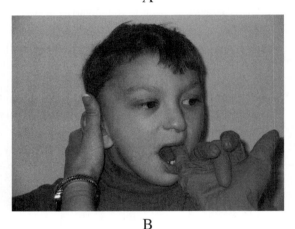

B

FIGURE 13–13 (A and B) A. Method for palpating the hard palate. Using the little finger for children, the examiner can start by putting the finger under the lips and palpating the gum ridge. B. The finger is then moved between the cheek and gum, around the molars, and then along the back end of the hard palate, until it is in midline.

the finger from the front of the ridge to the back in the area of the molars. Once the patient is comfortable with that amount of stimulation, the examiner should glide the finger directly behind the last molar, and then slowly move the finger horizontally along the back edge of the hard palate until it reaches the midline. This is the point where

the notch should be felt if it exists. To feel for the notch, the examiner should try to gently probe the midpoint of the posterior border of the hard palate. With the little finger, the examiner is more likely to feel a small or narrow defect than if the larger index finger is used.

Occasionally, an intraoral examination will reveal a palatal torus. A *torus* is a slow-growing nodular protuberance of bone that can occur in either the hard palate or mandible. There is evidence that both types of tori (plural form of torus) are hereditary. They occur almost twice more often in females than in males (Yeatts & Burns, 1991). A *palatal torus*, also called a *torus palatinus* is a bony protuberance in the midline of the hard palate (Figure 13–14). This type of torus is frequently symmetric, occurring in the midline of the hard palate, and has either a flat, spindled, nodular, or lobular configuration. It is of little clinical significance and is rarely a source of discomfort, unless the mucosal surface becomes ulcerated. A palatal torus usually does not interfere with speech or any other function, unless it is very large.

Velum and Uvula

In an intraoral examination, the clinician should determine velar integrity. As noted previously, a normal velum may have a white line down the middle, called the *median palatine raphe*. This is the area where the levator veli palatini muscles interdigitate in the midline. If there is a repaired cleft palate, it is important to rule out whether there is a fistula in the velum in addition to the hard palate. The position of the fistula relative to the velar dimple is important to determine. (The *velar dimple* is the point on the oral side of the velum that corresponds to the place where it bends during velopharyngeal closure. It is

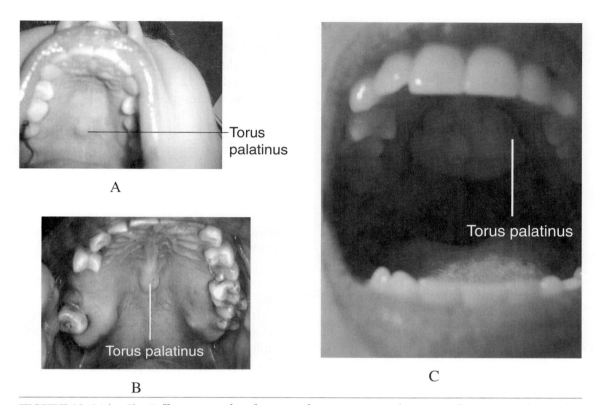

FIGURE 13–14 (A–C)   Different examples of a torus palatinus. Figure C shows a very large torus palatinus that grew to this size following the use of osteoporosis medication. It was interfering with speech and therefore, surgically removed.

formed by the contraction of the levator muscles.) If the fistula is anterior to the velar dimple, it is likely to be symptomatic because this location is near the area of maximum air pressure as it enters the oral cavity. On the other hand, a fistula that is posterior to the area of the velar dimple will not affect resonance because it is below the area of velopharyngeal closure and in the area of velar redundancy (the area of velar contact against the posterior pharyngeal wall).

If there is no history of cleft palate, the examiner should always look for characteristics of a submucous cleft. The most common sign of a submucous cleft is a bifid uvula with two separate tags, or a hypoplastic uvula that is short and stubby (Figure 13–15). In some cases, the uvula may appear to be intact due to the fact that the saliva helps to "glue" the tags of a bifid uvula together. If the examiner suspects that the uvula is bifid but is unsure, this can often be determined by taking a tongue blade gently behind the uvula and then flipping it forward (Mason & Simon, 1977). If there are two tags, they will separate with this maneuver. This must be done very carefully

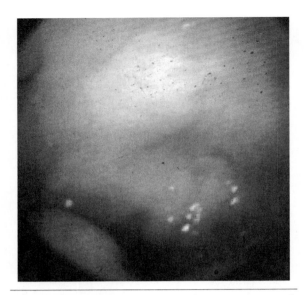

FIGURE 13–15 Hypoplastic uvula in a patient with submucous cleft.

and only with a very cooperative individual. It should be remembered, however, that a bifid uvula is a relatively common finding in the general population and can occur without a velar abnormality or hypernasal speech (Bagatin, 1985; Meskin, Gorlin, & Isaacson, 1964; Saad, 1980; Shapiro, Meskin, Cervenka, & Pruzansky, 1971; Wharton & Mowrer, 1992). It is important to counsel these individuals that they are at increased risk for hypernasality following an adenoidectomy.

Additional signs of a submucous cleft include a zona pellucida, which is a bluish-appearing area in the middle of the velum. This appearance is due to the fact that the velum is thin and somewhat transparent as a result of the lack of muscle in this area. A thin velum is important to note because it can be the cause of nasal resonance due to transmission of sound energy through it.

If there is a submucous cleft that extends through the velum, the velum may appear to "tent up" in an inverted V-shape during phonation (Figure 13–16). This is due to the fact that the levator veli palatini muscles have a forward attachment and are inserted on the edge of the posterior hard palate, rather than in the midline of the velum. This inverted V defect may extend all the way into the bony hard palate and be noted without phonation. By palpating the posterior nasal spine, the examiner may feel a notch in the bony structure that would suggest a submucous cleft that extends into the hard palate.

Even when there is no apparent evidence of a submucous cleft through an intraoral examination, it cannot be ruled out. There may be an occult submucous cleft in the muscles or mucosa on the nasal side of the velum. This can only be detected though nasopharyngoscopy or during a surgical procedure.

After examining the basic morphology of the velum, both velar length and mobility should be observed during phonation. The "effective length" of the velum is determined by the position of the velar dimple during velopharyngeal closure (Mason & Grandstaff, 1971). The *velar dimple* is the area where the levator veli palatini muscle interdigitates in the velum. When it contracts, it pulls the velum up and back during phonation and forms the dimple. Of note is the fact that when two lateral dimples are observed during phonation, this suggests diastasis of the levator veli palatini muscles, which is consistent with a submucous cleft (Boorman & Sommerland, 1985).

During sustained phonation, the velar dimple should appear to be back approximately 80% of the length of the velum (Mason & Grandstaff, 1971; Mason & Simon, 1977). The section of the velum that is anterior to the dimple is the effective length because it spans the length of the pharynx to obturate the nasopharyngeal port during speech. The section of the velum that is posterior to the velar

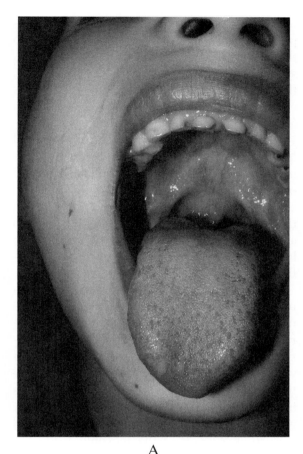

A

B

FIGURE 13–16 (A and B) During phonation, the velum appears to "tent up" in an inverted V-shape, suggesting a submucous cleft.

dimple serves to maintain firm closure across a vertical surface. If the velar dimple is closer to the hard palate rather than to the uvula, this suggests that the place of velar bend may not be back far enough for the velum to reach the posterior pharyngeal wall. The effective length is therefore short, which can cause velopharyngeal insufficiency. On the other hand, the velar dimple may be very close to the uvula, causing the uvula to flip back during phonation. This suggests that there is little vertical surface of the velum to maintain firm contact against the pharyngeal wall. This too can cause velopharyngeal insufficiency.

During phonation, the velum should raise symmetrically in a superior and posterior direction. Asymmetrical velar movement may suggest velopharyngeal incompetence due to unilateral paralysis or *paresis* (weakness) of the velum. During phonation, the velum will pull up on the unaffected side and droop on the affected side. With asymmetrical velar movement, the uvula will point to the unaffected, functional side. The examiner should particularly rule out unilateral velar paralysis or paresis in individuals with hemifacial microsomia. This finding is very important to note prior to planning surgical intervention since this will cause a lateral, rather than central, velopharyngeal gap.

When poor velar movement is noted during phonation, this may suggest velopharyngeal incompetence. Eliciting the gag reflex may confirm the presence of neuromotor function and also show the maximum excursion of the velum and pharyngeal walls. However, this does not correlate well with movement potential for speech.

In individuals with a history of cleft palate, poor velar movement can be due to abnormal function of the levator veli palatini, despite the palate repair. It may also be caused neuromotor dysfunction related to dysarthria, apraxia, or velar paralysis or paresis. Enlarged adenoids can even interfere with the upward movement of the velum during speech. On the other hand, poor velar movement may be an insignificant finding, If the individual has a sagittal form of closure, velar movement is less important. In addition, there may be an anterior inclination of the pharyngeal wall above the oral level of view, making extensive velar movement unnecessary.

Regardless of the appearance of the velum or its mobility, the examiner should remember that one can only guess at the implication for velopharyngeal function. This is because the oral view is below the level of velopharyngeal closure, and it is impossible to know the curve of the posterior pharyngeal wall or the basic closure pattern from an intraoral perspective alone.

Epiglottis

The epiglottis can often be viewed during an intraoral assessment of a young child as he or she protrudes the tongue to say "aah" (refer to Figure 13–1). The epiglottis is located just below the base of the tongue and is relatively high in the hypopharynx in young children. As the tongue goes forward, the epiglottis is pulled upward toward the oropharyngeal isthmus. The epiglottis is not usually seen in adults, since the larynx descends in the neck with age, minimizing its ability to be viewed during oral examinations.

Posterior and Lateral Pharyngeal Walls

The depth of the posterior pharyngeal wall can sometimes be judged relative to the possible length of the velum during phonation. In cases of severe velopharyngeal insufficiency, the examiner can almost look up into the nasopharynx, especially with a dental mirror, due to the severe discrepancy between velar length and pharyngeal depth. However, in most cases, the examiner can only guess how the pharynx curves as it courses superiorly and then anteriorly to form the nasal cavity. The pharynx may appear to be very deep on the oral level, but may curve sufficiently during the incline so that velopharyngeal closure can be obtained. In addition, the velum may be closing against the adenoid pad rather than the posterior pharyngeal wall. The best way to assess the depth of the pharynx is through lateral radiography, preferably lateral videofluoroscopy.

Lateral and posterior pharyngeal wall movement can be observed during phonation. There may be very vigorous movement of the pharyngeal walls, which may indicate good pharyngeal movement higher up in the area of velopharyngeal closure. This can also substantiate that the nervous supply to the pharynx is intact. However, there is no way to know whether there is complete velopharyngeal closure as a result of the movement. On the other hand, poor movement of the pharyngeal walls is not necessarily an indication of a problem. In fact, at the oral level, the lateral pharyngeal walls may actually bow outward during phonation, while bowing inward at a higher plane to assist with closure.

At times, a Passavant's ridge can be observed to bulge forward from the posterior pharyngeal wall during phonation. This ridge appears with muscular contraction of the entire velopharyngeal sphincter. An up-and-down movement of the posterior pharyngeal wall can often be observed with the Passavant's ridge (Finkelstein, Hauben, Talmi, Nachmani, & Zohar, 1992). They termed this the "shutter sign" and noted that it occurs when the individual phonates or during the gag reflex.

Unfortunately, if a Passavant's ridge can be observed from an intraoral view, it is not positioned high enough to assist with velopharyngeal closure. Therefore, in this case, it is no more than an interesting observation. The inferior border of the adenoid pad can occasionally, although infrequently, be observed on the posterior pharyngeal wall. It appears as lobulated tissue just behind and under the point of velar contact.

Tonsils

As noted previously, the tonsils are located between the anterior and posterior faucial pillars. They tend to be largest in preschool or school-age children. They usually begin to gradually atrophy as the child gets older and may suddenly shrink around puberty. Tonsils are virtually nonexistent in most adults.

With the oral examination, the presence of tonsils should be noted. If they are present, their relative size can be judged on a 4-point scale. If the tonsils are absent, the rating would be 0. Tonsils that are small and fit within the confines of the faucial pillars are considered to be grade 1 in size. If the tonsils extend to the edge of the pillars, they are rated as grade 2. If they are beyond the pillars, they are rated as grade 3, and if they are very large and meet in midline, they would be judged as a grade 4 in size (refer to Figure 8–10). The tonsils are generally not a problem for speech unless they extend beyond the faucial pillars or are so large that they interfere with the transmission of sound into the oral cavity.

The two tonsils are not always symmetrical in size. In fact, one may be significantly larger than the other. When this is the case, the size of each should be judged. In addition, if one tonsil is very large, the examiner should note whether it is affecting velar movement. A very

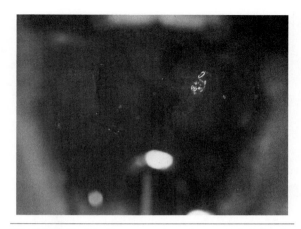

FIGURE 13–17 Large tonsil on the patient's left side. Note the deviation of the uvula. This suggests that the tonsil is intruding into the oropharynx.

large tonsil can pull the velum upward on that side or even intrude into the pharynx and interfere with velopharyngeal closure. When the velum is stretched upward by the tonsil, the uvula will point to the side of the large tonsil (Figure 13–17). Markedly asymmetric tonsils may be a sign of malignancy and therefore, require further evaluation.

Dentition and Occlusion

Dental occlusion should always be assessed as part of an intraoral examination since occlusion can have a significant effect on articulation. Malocclusion is a common contributor to speech problems in patients with a history of cleft palate. Anterior and lateral crossbites, missing teeth, and supernumerary teeth are often seen in this population.

To examine the dentition, the examiner should first assess the skeletal relationships between the maxillary and the mandibular arches during biting. The best way to examine the relationships of the two arches is to have the patient bite down on the "back teeth." The

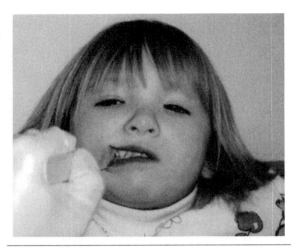

FIGURE 13–18 By inserting a tongue blade between the lateral teeth and the cheeks, the examiner can pull the cheeks away from the teeth to view the occlusal relationships.

examiner should make sure that the bite is with the molars, and not with the incisors. Then by inserting a tongue blade between the lateral teeth and the cheeks, the examiner can pull the cheeks away from the teeth to view the occlusal relationships (Figure 13–18).

The position of the molar teeth is important to observe since once they erupt, they become the key to alignment for the rest of the dentition (Mason & Simon, 1977). In normal occlusion, the mandibular molar should line up to be one-half of a tooth in front of the maxillary molar. If one or more molars have not yet erupted or have been extracted, the examiner can look at the relationships between the canine teeth in the same way. A normal occlusal relationship is termed a Class I occlusion according to Angle's classification (Bloomer, 1971). If the mandible is behind where it should be in relationship to the maxillary arch, this is considered a Class II occlusal relationship. On the other hand, if the mandible is forward in relationship to the maxilla, this is considered a Class II malocclusion.

In addition to assessing the anterior-posterior skeletal relationships, the examiner should determine if there is any evidence of dental malocclusion (see Chapter 9). In the cleft population, crossbite, where the maxillary teeth are inside the mandibular teeth, is very common. There can be an anterior crossbite, involving the maxillary incisors, or a lateral crossbite, due to a narrow maxillary arch relative to the mandibular arch. The examiner should rule out a deep bite, where there is excessive vertical overlap, since this can cause crowding in the oral cavity and restrict tongue movement. The examiner should also note an overjet where the incisors are labioverted, or an underjet where the incisors are linguaverted.

If the individual had a bilateral cleft of the lip and alveolus, the position of the premaxilla should be assessed. In many cases, the premaxilla is positioned in a way that affects speech. It may be in an anterior position so that it makes bilabial closure very difficult if not impossible, or it may be retruded so that the teeth are linguaverted. In this case, labiodental sounds could be affected. An open bite, where the maxillary teeth do occlude or overlap the mandibular teeth, should be noted since this can affect the position of the tongue at rest and during speech. The effect of these dental conditions on tongue position and movement during speech is very important to determine since this will have an impact on the recommendations for speech therapy versus physical management.

The examiner should note the presence of supernumerary teeth, especially if the tooth is in a place where it might interfere with tongue movement, and whether there are any missing teeth in the line of the cleft or elsewhere. The status of oral hygiene should also be determined. When the examiner observes poor oral hygiene or obvious caries, a referral for dental care must be included in the overall recommendations following the assessment.

Tongue

Both the structure and the function of the tongue should be assessed. The size of the tongue should be evaluated in relationship to the mandibular arch, the palatal arch, and the overall oral cavity space. It should be remembered that the infant's tongue is considerably larger relative to the oral cavity space than the tongue of an older child or adult. In addition, the tongue reaches maturation at around the age of eight, while the mandible continues to grow for several more years (Mason & Simon, 1977). Therefore, at various points during development, the tongue may appear to be relatively large. However, if the tongue is significantly larger than the oral cavity space so that it doesn't fit with attempts to close the teeth, this might indicate a macroglossia (Figure 13–19). A large tongue relative to the mandibular space can affect the dentition, so this should also be evaluated. The tongue should be further evaluated for multiple lobes if there is a history of a syndrome (Figure 13–20). If the patient has

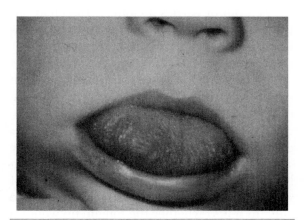

FIGURE 13–19 Macroglossia in a patient with Beckwith-Wiedemann syndrome.

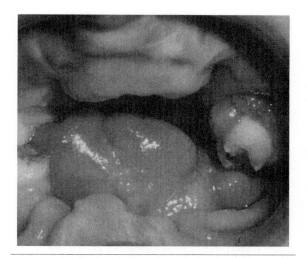

FIGURE 13–20 Lobulated tongue in a patient with orofaciodigital (OFD) syndrome.

had a tongue flap for closure of an oronasal fistula, the scarring and effect on function should be noted. Usually, even with extensive scarring, there is little effect on articulation.

The lingual frenulum under the tongue should be inspected for the location of its attachment. If there is ankyloglossia, the tongue tip will course inward during protrusion so that it resembles the top of a heart (Figure 13–21). When ankyloglossia is noted, the examiner should determine if this affects tongue tip elevation for production of /l/, or tongue tip protrusion for production of /th/. It can also affect the production of the Spanish /r/ sound. However, an effect on speech is not common. In fact, the /l/ sound can be produced with the tongue tip down and the dorsum up, and the /th/ sound can be produced with the tongue tip against the back of the incisors. In fact, although there is a common assumption that ankyloglossia affects speech production, there is no evidence in the literature to support this contention. Instead, it is more likely that it will affect early feeding by causing difficulty latching on to the nipple, and later feeding by

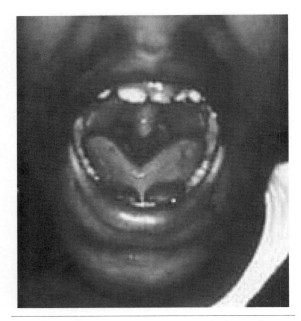

FIGURE 13–21 Ankyloglossia. Note the heart shape at the tip of the tongue.

restricting the ability to move a bolus around in the mouth (Kummer, 2005). The potential effect on "French kissing" should also be mentioned.

Oral-Motor Function

In examining the function of the tongue, the examiner can request the child to protrude, elevate, depress, and lateralize the tongue tip. The examiner can also evaluate the function of the lips by having the patient purse or smack the lips. However, what is most important is to evaluate the individual's ability to sequence motor movements for speech. This can be done through the use of diadochokinetic exercises, which require the person to produce a sequence of syllables rapidly. The syllables "puh," "tuh," and "kuh" have been used for years to assess motor movements for speech. The examiner can use one syllable and have

the patient produce it over and over (i.e., puh, puh, puh, puh, etc.) or the syllables can be combined (i.e., puhtuhkuh, puhtuhkuh, puhtuhkuh, etc.). Using meaningless syllables can be difficult for young children, however. Therefore, having the child repeat common multisyllabic words over and over (i.e., patty cake, kitty cat, puppy dog, teddy bear, basketball, or baseball bat) may be more effective.

In diadochokinetic testing, it is more important to look at the accuracy of production than the number of repetitions. If consonants are omitted, substituted, or reversed with an increase in utterance length or phonemic complexity, the possibility of verbal apraxia should be considered.

During the examination, the examiner should also look for more subtle signs of oral-motor dysfunction, such as those that might indicate dysarthria. Some of the signs include a chronic open mouth posture in the absence of upper airway obstruction. Usually when there is an open mouth posture, the tongue is also in an anterior position in the mouth. With the open mouth and anterior tongue position, drooling is a common observation. This can be subtle, with just a little moisture on the chin, or it can be copious so that the child wears a bib or carries a cloth. If the child has feeding difficulties by history or by observation, this could also be an indication of oral-motor dysfunction.

If the individual demonstrates an open mouth posture and anterior tongue position, the possibility of a tongue thrust should be ruled out, especially if there is also an anterior open bite. This can be determined by gently stimulating the tip of the tongue with a tongue blade, and then having the child take a drink of water. After the swallow, the examiner asks the child to report whether the tongue tip went up (against the alveolar ridge), forward (against or between the incisors), or down (against the mandibular incisors). If the child consistently reports that the tongue goes forward or down with the swallow, a tongue thrust should be suspected (Neiva & Wertzner, 1996). If the child is unable to report the direction of the tongue movement, this can be observed by asking the child to swallow with the lips open. At times, it is necessary to use a tongue blade to hold the lips apart. If there is an anterior open bite, observing the tongue movement during swallowing is usually easy.

Putting It All Together

Once the oral and peripheral examination is complete, the examiner must put the information together for a diagnostic profile. In particular, it is important to determine if there are physical factors that could potentially be interfering with articulation and resonance.

If multiple anomalies are noted in addition to a speech or resonance disorder, the examiner should consider the possibility of a syndrome if one has not already been diagnosed. Because speech, resonance, and learning problems are some of the primary characteristics of velocardiofacial syndrome, it is very common for the speech-language pathologist to be the first to identify individuals with this syndrome (Carneol, Marks, & Weik, 1999).

INFECTION CONTROL DURING THE EXAMINATION

A discussion of the intraoral examination would not be complete without a section on infection control. Knowledge of infection control is important to protect the health care provider and prevent the spread of infection to those individuals who are being served. Speech-language pathologists should practice good infection control procedures because they are in close physical contact with the individuals in their care, and they are often working around and even in the mouth. Unfortunately, most speech-language pathologists have had little training on appropriate infection control procedures unless they have obtained it from on-the-job experience (Bankaitis, Kemp, Krival, & Bandaranayake, 2006; Mosheim, 2005).

There are four communicable diseases that make up the biggest concern in the health care environment, and can also cause concern in other settings, including schools. These include the human immunodeficiency virus (HIV), hepatitis B virus (HBV), cytomegalovirus I (CMV), staphylococcus bacteria, and tuberculosis (TB). Professionals must also be concerned about the transmission of minor diseases, such as a cold or influenza. Pediatric settings are a particular concern since children generally have poor personal hygiene habits, and yet are very susceptible to infection (Krewedl, 1991).

In 1988, the Centers for Disease Control and Prevention (CDC) in Atlanta published guidelines for infection control (Centers for Disease Control and Prevention, 1988). These were first called *Universal Blood and Body Fluid Precautions* and are now called *Standard Precautions*. The basic premise of Standard Precautions is that ANY body fluid may contain contagious microorganisms. The American Speech-Language-Association Hearing Association (ASHA) adopted these guidelines and recommended them to its membership in 1990 (ASHA, 1990). Standard precautions contain recommended procedures that are designed to protect the patient, the professional, and all others in a health care environment from the spread of infection These procedures are based on the assumption that every patient and health care provider is a potential carrier of an infectious disease (Centers for Disease Control and Prevention, 1987, 1988).

Handwashing

The role of the human hands in the transmission of infection was recognized even before the establishment of microbiology as a science (Kerr, 1998). For many years, handwashing has been considered the single most important means of preventing the spread of infection in a health care setting (Centers for Disease Control and Prevention, 1986; Gallagher, 1999; Ginsberg & Clarke, 1972; Horton, 1995; Kiernan, 1999). Handwashing reduces the number of potential pathogens on the hands and interrupts the opportunity of transferring organisms to patients. If all health care providers used the proper technique for handwashing and this became a habit, infection rates in health care facilities would drop dramatically (Brown & Persivale, 1995). The Centers for Disease Control (1986) have issued guidelines on appropriate handwashing in a hospital environment. Unfortunately, it is widely acknowledged that health care workers are not always compliant in washing their hands as often as they should (Pittit, Mourouga, & Perneger, 1999). This is one reason why *nosocomial infections* (those infections that are acquired while in the hospital) continue to be a principal cause of morbidity and even mortality in health care settings.

It is best if hands are washed in front of the parents and child. This models appropriate hygienic behavior (Bellet, 1996). Hands should be washed before and after every patient contact and especially before and after an intraoral examination. In addition, hands should be washed after contact with potentially contaminated surfaces, after accidental contact with body fluids, and any time the hands are soiled. The use of examination gloves does not eliminate the need for handwashing (Bowman & Nicholas, 1990; Hopkins, 1989; Ripper,

1988; Shogren, 1988). It is important to wash hands before putting on gloves since there can be a perforation in the glove that is not readily visible. It is also necessary to wash hands after glove removal, since the warm, moist environment in the glove is conducive to rapid bacterial multiplication (Mayone-Ziomek, 1998).

Routine handwashing is accomplished by wetting hands with water and applying an antibacterial soap. The hands should be washed using friction for a minimum of 10–15 seconds, and then rinsed thoroughly with water to remove any residual soap. The hands should be dried thoroughly with fresh paper towels. The towels should be used to turn off manual faucets in order to avoid recontamination.

If soap and water are not immediately available or if hands are not visibly dirty or contaminated, antimicrobial handwipes or gels can be used for antisepsis. Antimicrobial handwashing products (e.g., 2% chlorhexidine gluconate, triclosan) should be used before contacts with newborns, immunocompromised patients, patients on high-risk units, and prior to an invasive procedure.

Gloves

With the universal precautions approach to infection control, the examiner should assume that all human secretions, including saliva, could potentially be infectious or contain bloodborne pathogens. Therefore, the examiner must wear personal protective equipment (PPE) when performing any task that has the risk of contact with the patient's secretions. Protection must be worn when the professional is engaged in any type of evaluation or treatment that requires physical contact with the mouth or nose of patient.

The best form of protection for the examiner is a pair of gloves. Until recently, latex gloves were used in most health care settings. However, latex allergies have become very common. To minimize the sensitization of health care workers and exposure to latex-sensitive patients, most institutions have now eliminated the use of latex gloves. Gloves should always be worn during an intraoral examination and also while performing a nasopharyngoscopy exam. They should fit tightly because loosely fitted gloves interfere with the manipulation of objects. Gloves should be changed immediately if holes, rips, or tears are visible and as needed during the patient's care. Because all gloves are designed for single-patient use, they are discarded in the waste can after each patient. When removing gloves, they should be pulled off so that they are inside out, and then immediately discarded (Figure 13–22). This prevents physical contact with the contaminated surface of the gloves.

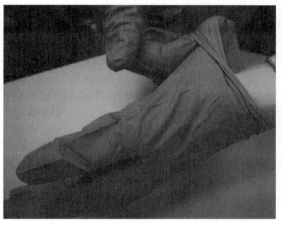

A

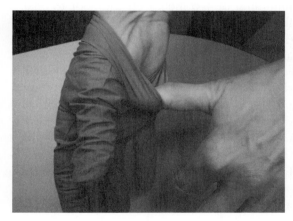

C

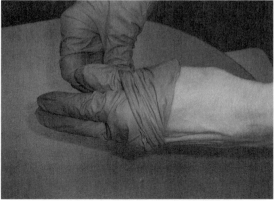

B

FIGURE 13–22 (A–C) Proper way to remove gloves. A. Grab the glove at the wrist. B. Pull the glove off so that it is inside out. C. Put thumb under the wrist of the second glove and pull it off inside out.

Patient Equipment and Supplies

Tongue blades, dental mirrors, and other tools for an intraoral assessment should not be placed directly on a desk or table after use. Instead, these tools should be placed on a clean paper towel or tissue until they can be cleaned. Patient equipment and supplies should be stored in a clean and safe manner that protects the items from exposure or contamination to body fluids, known soiled items, dust, particulate matter, and even moisture. Supplies should always be stored a minimum of 4–6 inches off the floor to enable floor cleaning and to protect from accidental damage due to rolling carts, being stepped on, and contamination with floor cleaning solutions.

Disposable items, such as tongue blades, should be used for intraoral examinations or manipulation whenever possible. It is easier to dispose of an item and use a new one for the next person than to have to wash and disinfect the item between uses. Items that are manufactured to be disposable can usually not be adequately washed or disinfected. Therefore, all disposable items are for single-patient use and should be discarded immediately after use. It is important to discard these items appropriately and not leave contaminated items sitting on a desk or table.

A dental mirror, which is not disposable, should be thoroughly cleaned after use with hot soapy water or placed in a dishwasher. Disinfection can then be done by wiping the dental mirror with alcohol. Both ethyl alcohol and isopropyl alcohol have a broad spectrum of antimicrobial activity that counteracts vegetative bacteria, fungi, and viruses (including HIV) (Widmer & Frei, 1999). In addition, alcohol has many qualities that make it suitable for low-level and intermediate-level disinfection, including the fact that it is fast acting (15–30 seconds), and it readily evaporates. Sterilization, as opposed to disinfection, is required to destroy bacterial spores. However, the dental mirror is contaminated with saliva only and intact mucous membranes are resistant to bacterial spores. Therefore, sterilization is not necessary for a dental mirror being used as described. (Note that sterilization is required for other dental instruments that have the potential for exposure to blood.)

Surface Disinfection

All therapy or patient care rooms should be equipped with spray disinfectant products and disinfectant towelettes (Bankaitis, Kemp, Krival, & Bandaranayake, 2006). Flat surfaces, such as tables and armchairs, can be contaminated with saliva or mucous during a session. Therefore, they should be cleaned and disinfected with a disinfection agent between patients.

SUMMARY

The structure and function of the oral articulators and the oral cavity have a direct impact on the quality and intelligibility of speech. In addition, the function of the velopharyngeal valve is critical for normal speech and resonance. Therefore, when speech or resonance problems are noted, a thorough intraoral examination must be done. The examiner must rule out structural abnormalities that may require surgical or orthodontic treatment prior to the initiation of speech therapy. In addition, a keen eye and a thorough examination can help to detect previously undiagnosed conditions.

For Review, Discussion, and Critical Thinking

1. Describe the best method for viewing all oral structures with the least amount of stress or discomfort for the patient.

2. What is the purpose of palatal palpation? Describe how this is done and what should be felt.

3. What would you look for when observing eyes, ears, nose, lips, and facial bones? Why are these observations an important part of a speech pathology examination?

4. What observations of the velopharyngeal mechanism can be made through an intraoral examination? Why can't you view velopharyngeal function by looking in the mouth?

5. Describe a method for evaluating dental occlusion. Why is it important to assess occlusion? What are the implications for treatment recommendations?

6. Describe methods of infection control when performing an intraoral examination.

References

American Speech-Language-Hearing Association, (1990). AIDS/HIV: Implications for speech-language pathologists and audiologists. *ASHA*, 46–48.

Bagatin, M. (1985). Submucous cleft palate. *Journal of Maxillofacial Surgery*, 13(1), 37–38.

Bankaitis, A. U., Kemp, R. J., Krival, K., & Bandaranayake, D. (2006) *Infection control for speech-language pathology*. St. Louis, MO: Auban.

Bellet, P. S. (1996). Physical examination. In R. C. Baker (Ed.), *Pediatric primary care*. Philadelphia: Lippincott Williams & Wilkins.

Beste, D. J. (1999). Special considerations in the assessment of the pediatric otolaryngology patient. In R. T. Cotton & C. M. Myer, III (Eds.), *Practical pediatric otolaryngology*. Philadelphia: Lippincott-Raven.

Bloomer, H. (1971). Speech defects associated with dental malocclusions and related abnormalities. In L. Travis (Ed.), *Handbook of speech pathology and audiology*. New York: Appleton.

Boorman, J. G., & Sommerland, B. C. (1985). Levator veli palati and palatal dimples: Their anatomy, relationship, and clinical significance. *British Journal of Plastic Surgery*, 38, 326–332.

Bowman, A. M., & Nicholas, T. J. (1990). Improving compliance with universal blood and body fluid precautions in a rural medical center. *Journal of Nursing Quality Assurance*, 5(1), 73–81.

Brown, J. W., & Persivale, E. J. (1995). Managing the front line of infection control: Handwashing. *Director*, 3(1), 36–37.

Carneol, S. O., Marks, S. M., & Weik, L. (1999). The speech-language pathologist: Key role in the diagnosis for velocardiofacial syndrome. *American Journal of Speech-Language Pathology*, 8(1), 23–32.

Centers for Disease Control and Prevention. (1986). Guidelines for handwashing and hospital environmental control. *Infection Control*, 7(4), 231–235.

Centers for Disease Control and Prevention. (1987). Recommendations for prevention of HIV transmission in health-care settings.

Morbidity and Mortality Weekly Review, 36 (Suppl. 25).

Centers for Disease Control. (1988). Perspectives in disease prevention and health promotion. *Morbidity and Mortality Weekly Review*, 37, 377–388.

Federal Register. (1991). *Occupational exposure to bloodborne pathogens: Final rule.* Occupational and Safety Health Administration, 29 CFR Part 1910.1030.

Finkelstein, Y., Hauben, D. J., Talmi, Y. P., Nachmani, A., & Zohar, Y. (1992). Occult and overt submucous cleft palate: From peroral examination to nasendoscopy and back again. *International Journal of Pediatric Otorhinolaryngology*, 23(1), 25–34.

Gallagher (1999). This is the way we wash our hands. *Nursing Times*, 95(10), 62–65.

Ginsberg, F., & Clarke, B. (1972). Handwashing is simple, effective infection control, so why won't people wash their hands? *Modern Hospital*, 119(4), 132.

Hopkins, C. C. (1989). AIDS. Implementation of universal blood and body fluid precautions. *Infectious Disease Clinics of North America*, 3(4), 747–762.

Horton, R. (1995). Handwashing: The fundamental infection control principle. *British Journal of Nursing*, 4(16), 926, 928, 930–933.

Jones, J. A. (1989, October 30). Integrating the oral examination into clinical practice. *Hospital Practice*, pp. 23–30.

Kerr, J. (1998). Handwashing. *Nursing Standards*, 12(51), 35–39; Quiz 41–42.

Kiernan, M. (1999). Handwashing in infection control. *Community Nurse, 5*(7), 19–20.

Krewedl, A. (1991, August 23). Infection control in pediatric settings. *Advance*, pp. 26–27.

Kummer, A. W. (2005, December 27). To clip or not to clip? That's the question. *The ASHA Leader*, 10(17), 6–7, 30.

Mason, R. M., & Grandstaff, H. L. (1971). Evaluating the velopharyngeal mechanism in hypernasal speakers. *Language, Speech, and Hearing Services in the Schools*, 2(4), 53–61.

Mason, R. M., & Simon, C. (1977). An orofacial examination checklist. *Language, Speech, and Hearing Services in the Schools*, 8(3), 155–163.

Mayone-Ziomek, J. M. (1998). Handwashing in health care. *Dermatological Nursing, 10* (3), 183–188.

Meskin, L., Gorlin, R., & Isaacson, R. (1964). Abnormal morphology of the soft palate: The prevalence of a cleft uvula. *Cleft Palate Journal*, 3, 342–346.

Mosheim, J. (2005, October 24). Infection control: Protocols protect the clinician and patient. *Advance for Speech-Language Pathologists & Audiologists*, pp. 7–9.

Neiva, F. C., & Wertzner, H. F. (1996). A protocol for oral myofunctional assessment: For application with children. *International Journal of Orofacial Myology*, 22, 8–19.

Pittit, D., Mourouga, P., & Perneger, T. V. (1999). Compliance with handwashing in a teaching hospital. Infection control program. *Annals of Internal Medicine*, 130(2), 126–130.

Ripper, M. (1988). Universal blood and body fluid precautions. *Journal of Advances in Medical Surgical Nursing*, 1(1), 21–25.

Saad, E. F. (1980). The underdeveloped palate in ear, nose and throat practice. *Laryngoscope*, 90(8, Pt. 1), 1371–1377.

Shapiro, B. L., Meskin, L. H., Cervenka, J., & Pruzansky, S. (1971). Cleft uvula: A microform of facial clefts and its genetic basis. *Birth Defects Original Article Series*, 7(7), 80–82.

Shogren, E. (1988). An ounce of prevention is worth a pound of cure: Using universal blood and body fluid precautions in your work setting. *MNA Accent*, 60(2), 35–36.

Smith, B., & Guyette, T. W. (2004). Evaluation of cleft palate speech. *Clinics in Plastic Surgery*, 31(2), 251–260.

Thomas, J. E., & Bender, B. S. (1993). What to look for after you say "Open wide." *Postgraduate Medicine*, 93(7), 109–110.

Wharton, P., & Mowrer, D. E. (1992). Prevalence of cleft uvula among school children in kindergarten through grade five. *Cleft Palate-Craniofacial Journal*, 29(1), 10–12; Discussion 13–14.

Widmer, A. F., & Frei, R. (1999). Decontamination, disinfection, and sterilization. In P. R. Murray, E. J. Baron, M. A. Pfaller, F. C. Tenover, & R. H. Yolken, (Eds.), *Manual of clinical microbiology* (pp. 138–164). Washington, DC: ASM Press.

Yeatts, D., & Burns, J. C. (1991). Common oral mucosal lesions in adults. *American Family Physician*, 44(6), 2043–2050.

CHAPTER

14

NASOMETRY

CHAPTER OUTLINE

INTRODUCTION

Nasometry is a method of measuring the acoustic correlates of resonance and velopharyngeal function through a computer-based instrument. Nasometry testing gives the examiner a *nasalance score*, which is the percentage of nasal acoustic energy of the total (nasal plus oral) energy. Because nasometry does not include visualization of the velopharyngeal structures, it is considered an *indirect measure*. The advantage of the nasometry is that it provides objective data that can be compared to standardized norms for interpretation. Nasometry is useful in the evaluation of resonance since it supplements what is heard through the perceptual evaluation and what is seen through direct instrumental measures. It can also be a valuable treatment tool because it provides visual feedback for the patient. Finally, it can be used effectively for pre- and posttreatment comparisons.

The purpose of this chapter is to describe nasometry and its use in the evaluation and treatment of individuals with resonance disorders.

NASOMETRY AND ITS CLINICAL USES

Development of Nasometry

The first instrument to measure nasal and oral acoustic energy was developed by Samuel Fletcher in 1970. This instrument was called TONAR, which is an acronym for The Oral-Nasal Acoustic Ratio (Fletcher & Bishop, 1970). The TONAR was later updated, revised, and then renamed the TONAR II (Fletcher, 1976a; Fletcher, 1976b). Although the TONAR instruments provided objective data regarding the acoustic product of speech, the data acquisition was somewhat unreliable (Dalston, 1997).

Samuel Fletcher, along with colleagues Larry Adams and Martin McCutcheon at the University of Alabama, Birmingham, developed the Nasometer based on his early work; it was then introduced by Kay Elemetrics Corp. in 1987 (Fletcher, 1970; Fletcher, Adams, & McCutcheon, 1989). In 2002, a second version of the Nasometer was released as Nasometer II,

Model 6400 (KayPENTAX, Lincoln Park, NJ). This is the model that is used today. Although the Nasometer II is fundamentally the same as the original version, it captures data through analog and digital circuitry, rather than just analog circuitry. Additionally, Nasometer II captures the speech signal which can be played back.

Two other instruments have been developed to measure nasalance: the NasalView (Tiger Electronics, Seattle, WA) and the OroNasal System (Glottal Enterprises Inc., Syracuse, NY). Both instruments measure acoustic energy from the oral cavity and the nasal cavity in a similar manner as the Nasometer. However, these instruments are not widely used and there is no normative data. In addition, it has been shown that there are significant differences in the nasalance scores of these instruments and therefore, they are not interchangeable with the Nasometer or with each other (Bressmann, 2005; Lewis & Watterson, 2003). Given these findings and the fact that the Nasometer is more widely used, the remainder of this chapter will focus on nasometry using Nasometer II, Model 6400.

What Is a Nasometer?

A *Nasometer* (KayPENTAX, Lincoln Park, NJ) is a computer-assisted instrument that measures the relative amount of nasal acoustic energy in an individual's speech. The Nasometer provides an easy, noninvasive method for obtaining objective data regarding resonance. As such, it can be a valuable tool in both the evaluation of resonance disorders and in treatment of functional resonance problems.

The Nasometer provides a visual representation of resonance in real time, and also gives descriptive data of the relative amount of nasal resonance in speech for a data set or passage. This is done by measuring the acoustic energy in both the nasal (N) cavity and the oral (O) cavity during speech, and calculating a ratio of nasal over total (nasal plus oral) acoustic energy. This ratio is converted to a percentage value and is called the *nasalance score*. The nasalance score can be depicted, therefore, as follows:

$$\text{Nasalance} = N \div (N + O) \times 100.$$

When an individual's score is compared to normative data, a judgment can be made regarding the normalcy of resonance. High scores, in comparison to normative data, suggest hypernasality; low scores, in comparison, suggest hyponasality.

In addition to the objective data, the Nasometer II provides a visual display of the data on the computer screen in the form of a nasogram. The *nasogram* is a contour display that shows the individual data points in sequence as they were collected in real time during the production of a passage. The nasogram is recorded and can be saved for later review along with the auditory playback feature. The contour display can be changed to a bar graph, which is helpful in

therapy. For young children, there are also games and animated graphics to help keep the child engaged.

Purpose and Clinical Uses

Since its introduction, the Nasometer has been a useful tool in the evaluation of resonance and velopharyngeal function (Dalston, 1991b; Dalston, 1991c; Dalston, 1997; Hardin, et al., 1992; Karnell, 1995). It has even been used to evaluate resonance of children with hearing impairment (Tatchell, Stewart, & Lapine, 1991). Nasometry is used to assess upper airway obstruction and hyponasality through their acoustic correlates during speech (Dalston et al., 1991a; Dalston, et al., 1991b; Hardin, Van Demark, Morris, & Payne, 1992; Hong, Kwon, & Jung, 1997; Nieminen, Lopponen, Vayrynen, Tervonen, & Tolonen, 2000; Parker, Clarke, Dawes, & Maw, 1990) and has been suggested as a means of selecting at-risk individuals for adenoidectomy (Gonzalez-Landa, Santos Terron, Miro Viar, & Sanchez-Ruiz, 1990; Kummer, Myer, Smith, & Shott, 1993; Parker, Maw, & Szallasi, 1989; Williams, Eccles, & Hutchings, 1990; Williams, Preece, Rhys, & Eccles, 1992).

Very often, nasometry is used to measure changes in resonance following surgical procedures (David, Blalock, & Argenta, 1999; Dejonckere & van Wijngaarden, 2001; Gonzalez Landa, Sanchez-Ruiz, Perez Gonzalez, Santos Terron, & Miro Viar, 2000; Gray, Pinborough-Zimmerman, & Catten, 1999; Haapanen, 1992; Haapanen, Kalland, Heliovaara, Hukki, & Ranta, 1997; Soneghet et al., 2002; Van Lierde, De Bodt, Baetens, Schrauwen, & Van Cauwenberge, 2003; Van Lierde, Monstrey, Bonte, Van Cauwenberge, & Vinck, 2004; Whitehill, 2001).

It is also used to show the effects of various forms of therapy, including CPAP (Sweeney, Sell, & O'Regan, 2004) and prosthetic management (Rieger, Wolfaardt, Seikaly, & Jha, 2002).

Equipment

Hardware and Software

The basic Nasometer II equipment is illustrated in Figure 14–1. The Nasometer requires the use of a host PC computer. Laptops are not recommended due to their variability in the sound card performance and specifications. The system components include a Nasometer II external module, a headset with a sound separator plate, two directional microphones, cables, software, and a Santa Cruz sound card.

The equipment connection and software installation instructions can be found in the *Nasometer II, Model 6400 Installation, Operations and Maintenance Manual* (KayPENTAX, 2003).

Calibration

Prior to its first use, and at periodic intervals, the Nasometer should be calibrated according to the manufacturer's instructions. This is necessary to be sure that the data collection

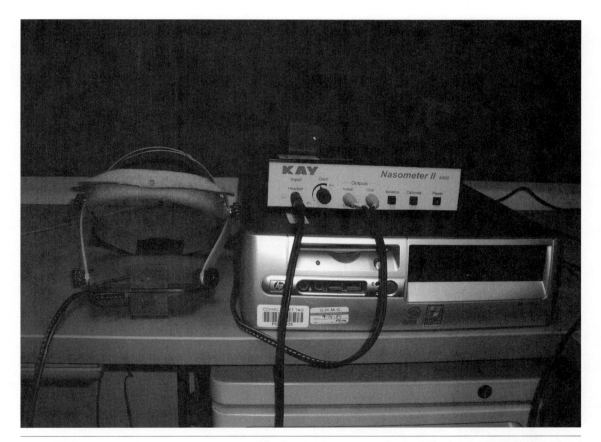

FIGURE 14–1 Basic Nasometer equipment. The Nasometer requires the use of either an IBM-compatible or Apple computer, a Nasometer box, which is connected by a cable to an interface printed circuit board in the computer, and a headset that is worn by the individual during data collection. Nasometer software is installed on the computer's hard drive.

and analyses are accurate. The Nasometer comes with a calibration stand that holds the headset during the calibration process. The headset is placed in the calibration stand located on the top of the Nasometer II external hardware module. The provided calibration slot ensures that both microphones are equidistant from the calibration speaker (approximately 6 inches) (Figure 14–2). When a tone from the external module is presented to the microphones, both the nasal and oral microphones should register the tone equally. If the two microphones are not balanced so that the tone registers above or below the 50% mark, calibration adjustments are made in the Nasometer II software to balance any detected sensitivity differences between the two microphones. Calibration is not required often, but it should be done periodically to insure a proper balance for accurate data collection.

NASOMETRIC PROCEDURES

For comprehensive information about nasometric procedures, the reader should consult the Nasometer II Manual. Although extensive

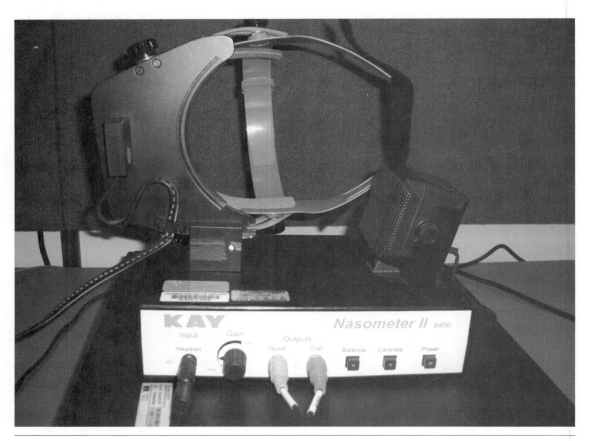

FIGURE 14–2 Calibration. During calibration, the headset should be placed so that both microphones are equidistant from the Nasometer box and about 12 inches in front of the calibration speaker.

instruction regarding nasometry procedures is beyond the scope of this text, some basic information is important to cover.

Placing the Headset

The Nasometer headset (Figure 14–3) is designed to be worn by the individual during data collection. Prior to placing the headset on the individual's head, the examiner should wipe the sound separator plate and plastic guard with an alcohol towelette or a germicidal wipe to prevent the spread of infection. The headset is then plugged into the external module.

The headset is placed on the individual and secured using the top adjustment band and the Velcro strip in the back. When the headset is in place, the sound separator plate should be between the upper lip and the nose. The microphones should be directly in front of the mouth and the nose and the plate should be perpendicular to the face (or in a horizontal position). An angle in excess of 15 degrees in either direction can affect the integrity of the data (KayPENTAX, 2003). Once the plate is in proper position, the top and then the bottom adjustment knobs are tightened to keep the plate in place and add further stability. The plastic tubing along the plate promotes a tight seal

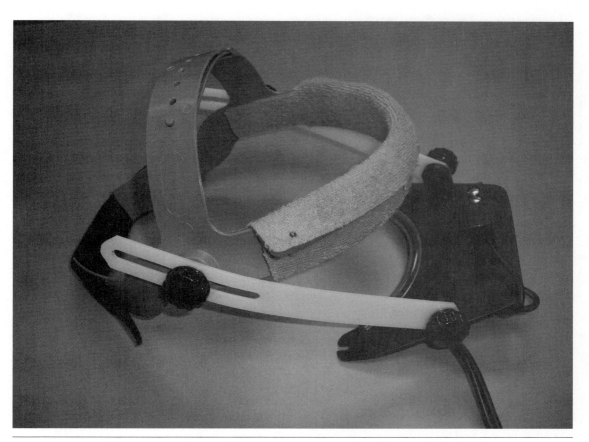

FIGURE 14–3 The Nasometer headset that is worn by the patient during data collection.

while softening the force against the face. The proper placement of the headset is seen in Figure 14–4.

Positioning the headset on small children can be a challenge. If possible, parents should be sent both information describing the exam and even a picture prior to the appointment so they can help to prepare the child. At Cincinnati Children's Hospital Medical Center, we send the child a coloring book prior to the evaluation. In the book, one page explains the nasometry procedure (Figure 14–5). This helps to reduce any fear that the child may have about wearing the headset.

During the exam, the child can be told that he will be able to play a computer game and wear a "superhero" mask. He will talk to the computer, but since computers don't have ears, he will have to talk into the microphones (computer ears). When the computer can hear him talk, it will make lots of blue "mountains." It helps to have the child feel the plate and the plastic tubing that will come in contact with the face. The examiner can explain that this part of the headset will "hug" around the face so that it will stay on by itself. To further reduce fears of putting the headset on the face, it is often helpful to have the headset hug the child's leg,

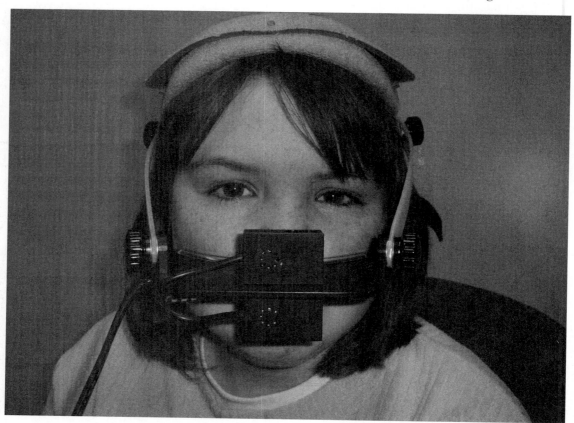

A

FIGURE 14–4 (A and B) Placement of the headset on the patient. The headset is positioned so that the sound separator plate is perpendicular to the face or in a horizontal position. The microphones should be directly in front of the mouth and the nose. (*continues*)

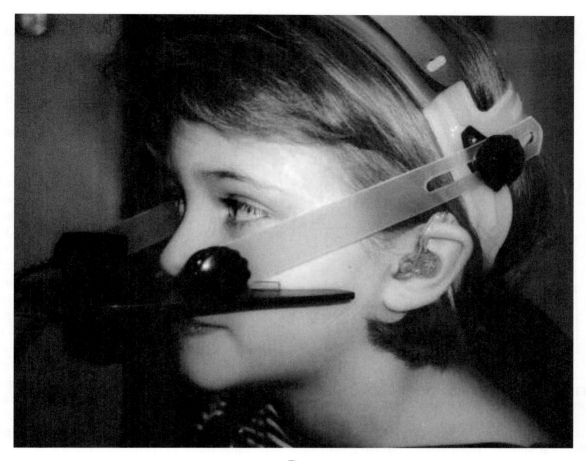

B

FIGURE 14–4 **(A and B)**   *(continued)*

arm, forehead, and chin first. Once the headset is on, the examiner should praise the child and comment on how great he or she looks.

Despite the examiner's best efforts, there are times when the child will refuse to put the headset on. When this occurs, the parent can hold the sound separator plate at the appropriate position on the child's face while the child repeats a few syllables or short utterances from the SNAP Test-R (Kummer, 2005). Even a brief speech sample will result in the collection of data that can be useful.

Data Collection and Standardized Passages

Once the headset is in place, the individual is asked to read or repeat standardized speech passages (Figure 14–6). To start data collection, the examiner presses the F12 button and to stop data collection, the examiner presses the space bar. The microphones pick up acoustic energy from the oral cavity and the nasal cavity simultaneously. The sound separator plate provides sufficient sound separation between

Do you like computer games?

We hope so because the speech pathologist has one for you to play. With this game, you get to wear a super hero mask that fits around your face.

When you talk into microphones on the mask, you will see funny blue lines on the computer screen.

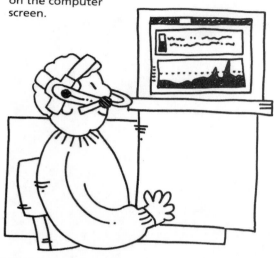

FIGURE 14–5 Page out of a coloring book used to prepare the patient for the examination.

the oral and the nasal signals (about 25 dB of separation), but there is some spillover.

In order to compare the individual's performance with normative data, a standardized speech segment must be used. There are several standardized passages that can be selected. These can be displayed on the screen (Figure 14–7).

The first nasometric norms were established for the following three passages; the Zoo Passage (Fletcher, 1972), the Rainbow Passage (Fairbanks, 1960), and Nasal Sentences (Fletcher, 1978). These passages and their norms (mean scores and standard deviations) for Nasometer II can be found in Appendix 14–1.

The Zoo Passage consists of sentences that are devoid of nasal phonemes. Therefore, this passage allows the examiner to determine if velopharyngeal closure can be achieved and maintained throughout connected speech. Of course without nasal consonants, this passage does not test the effects of the timing of closure with the transitions between nasal and oral phonemes. If there are problems with velopharyngeal timing or movement, this is more likely to be demonstrated with the Rainbow Passage. In this passage, 11.5% of the consonants are nasal consonants, which is representative of the percentage of nasal consonants in normal Standard American English. If hyponasality is suspected, the Nasal Sentences passage is used since it is heavily loaded with nasal consonants. In fact, 35% of the phonemes in this passage are nasal consonants, which is more than three times as many nasal sounds as would normally occur in standard American English. This passage allows the examiner to test the individual's ability to open the velopharyngeal port for normal nasal resonance. In addition to giving information regarding resonance, this score also has implications for the presence of nasal obstruction.

Although the original passages are still commonly used, particularly with adults, they have certain disadvantages. They are hard to use with individuals who cannot read, have a limited attention span, or may be noncompliant. The Zoo and Rainbow Passages are long and awkward and some of the sentences are semantically and syntactically complex. Some of the words are difficult to pronounce, especially for children who have incomplete phonological acquisition. This increases the possibility of production errors. When the passage is produced with articulation substitutions or deletions, the nasalance score associated with it loses some validity. A pause with the use of "um" is particularly problematic. The phonetic heterogeneity of these passages also limits their use in many ways. This makes

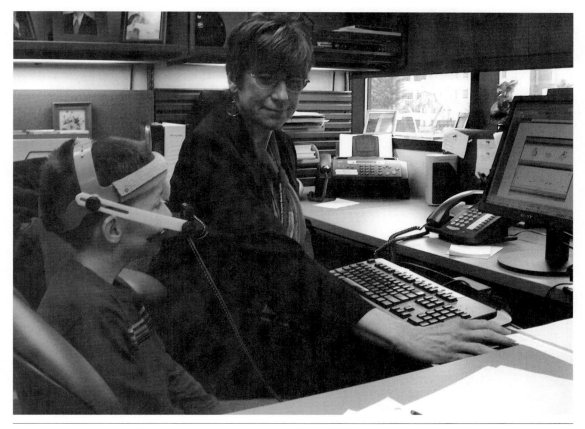

FIGURE 14–6 Nasometer procedure for data collection. The individual is asked to read or repeat certain speech passages for data collection.

it impossible to isolate the effects of phoneme-specific nasal emission or hypernasality since the nasalance score is computed based on the average score for a variety of phonemes. In addition, there is no way to isolate the effects of a fistula versus velopharyngeal dysfunction on the nasalance score.

In an effort to determine the best and most efficient way to collect nasometric data while avoiding the pitfalls of the original passages, some investigators have found that reliable measures of nasalance can be obtained using much shorter stimuli (Kummer, 2005; MacKay & Kummer, 1994; Watterson, Lewis,

& Foley-Homan, 1999; Wozny, Kuehn, Oishi, & Arthur, 1994). In addition, it has been reported that the clinically relevant information provided in the Rainbow Passage can be obtained using the other speech samples (Dalston & Seaver, 1992). Therefore, it can be eliminated from the test battery in most cases.

Given the limitations of the first three standardized passages, the *Simplified Nasometric Assessment Procedures (SNAP Test)* (Kummer, 2005; MacKay & Kummer, 1994) was developed in a pediatric setting for the purpose of providing more appropriate

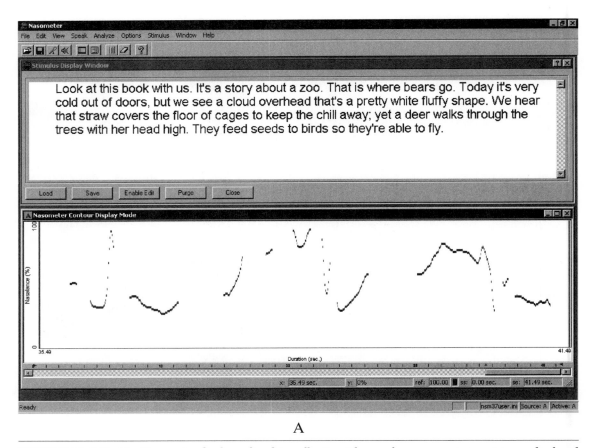

Look at this book with us. It's a story about a zoo. That is where bears go. Today it's very cold out of doors, but we see a cloud overhead that's a pretty white fluffy shape. We hear that straw covers the floor of cages to keep the chill away; yet a deer walks through the trees with her head high. They feed seeds to birds so they're able to fly.

A

FIGURE 14–7 (A–C) Nasometer displays after data collection. The nasalance percentage points are displayed on the computer screen in real time as the individual is speaking. For normal speech and the production of only oral sounds, the data points are usually between the 10 to 20 percentage points above the baseline. A. A contour display of results. (*continues*)

standardized passages for children. It was also designed to enhance the diagnostic value of nasometry by allowing the examiner to test nasalance using specific phonemes, and thus avoid the problem of phonetic heterogeneity. Normative data was first obtained using the Nasometer I Model 6200. With the introduction of Nasometer II, another normative study was conducted and the test form was revised. The SNAP Test-R (2005) with normative data for Nasometer II can be found in Appendix 14–2.

The SNAP Test-R consists of a battery of passages divided into three subtests: *Subtest I:*

Syllable Repetition/Prolonged Sounds Subtest; *Subtest II: Picture-Cued Subtest*; and *Subtest III: Paragraph Subtest.* Any or all of these subtests can be used by the examiner, but are usually selected based on the age of the child, the anticipated level of cooperation, the child's level of literacy, and the specific characteristics or etiologies that need to be evaluated.

Subtest I, the *Syllable Repetition/Prolonged Sounds Subtest,* includes 14 consonant-vowel (CV) syllables of pressure-sensitive consonants (plosives, fricatives, or affricates) combined with

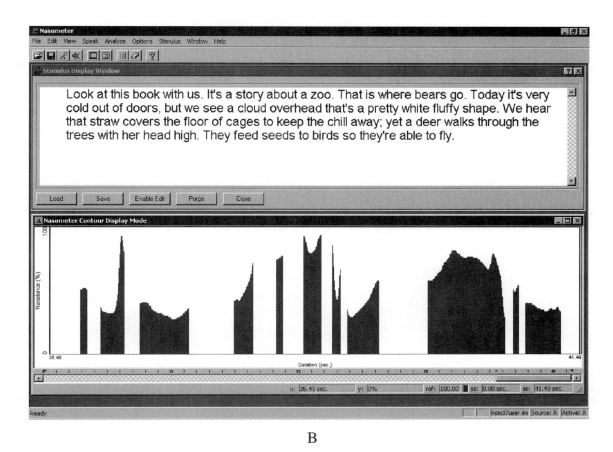

B

FIGURE 14–7 (A–C) (*continued*)   B. A filled contour display of the same data. (*continues*)

either the low vowel /a/ or the high vowel /i/ (pronounced "eee"). (Note: The high vowel is written phonetically as /i/ on the test form.) In addition, it includes syllables with nasal sounds (/m/ and /n/), two prolonged vowels and two prolonged consonants. Subtest I provides phonetic specificity for in-depth analysis. To administer this subtest with the syllables, the individual is asked to repeat the syllables at a "normal" speed until the screen is full of relatively even peaks and the first couple of syllables have disappeared off the screen. Approximately six to eight syllables should be produced during the two-second period. The prolonged sounds should be produced until the screen is full.

Subtest I is particularly appropriate for individuals who have a short attention span, poor cooperation, or a limited phonemic repertoire. If the child cannot produce velar sounds (/k/, /g/), for instance, then the velar passage would not be used. In addition, this subtest has excellent diagnostic value because it allows the examiner to isolate out the effects of misarticulation by evaluating nasalance on specific phonemes or phoneme groups. For example, by comparing the relative nasalance

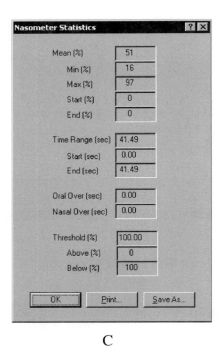

Nasometer Statistics

Mean (%)	51
Min (%)	16
Max (%)	97
Start (%)	0
End (%)	0
Time Range (sec)	41.49
Start (sec)	0.00
End (sec)	41.49
Oral Over (sec)	0.00
Nasal Over (sec)	0.00
Threshold (%)	100.00
Above (%)	0
Below (%)	100

OK   Print...   Save As...

C

FIGURE 14–7 (A–C) (*continued*) C. Summary statistics of these results. The statistic that is listed as the "mean" is actually the mean of all of the percentage points for the entire passage.

on sibilant phonemes (particularly /s/) versus plosives sounds, the examiner can make a judgment as to whether nasal emission is phoneme-specific or is more generalized due to velopharyngeal dysfunction. By comparing the relative nasalance on high vowels versus low vowels, the examiner may determine that there is nasality on high vowels and not on low vowels, suggesting a high tongue position or thin velum as possible causes. Finally, if the individual has an anterior fistula and its effects on speech and resonance are unknown, the examiner can compare the nasalance score on anterior sounds (ta, ta, ta or sa, sa, sa) with those obtained on the posterior sounds (ka, ka, ka). Higher nasalance scores on anterior versus posterior sounds suggest that the fistula is symptomatic for speech.

Finally, the nasal phonemes can be used effectively to evaluate individuals who have evidence of hyponasality due to upper airway obstruction. These syllable strings can be particularly useful in testing individuals following placement of a pharyngeal flap, which has the potential to cause these problems. Low scores on the nasal syllables can be an indication of both hyponasality and upper airway obstruction that should be medically evaluated and treated.

Subtest II, the *Picture-Cued Subtest,* contains passages that are essentially phonetically homogeneous. For each passage, a carrier phrase is used with pictures to form complete sentences. These pictures can be displayed on the screen (Figure 14–8). Each passage has three pictures for eliciting three sentences. Each sentence is said twice, making six sentences per passage. In this subtest, there is a passage that focuses on each of the following: bilabial plosives, lingual-alveolar plosives, velar plosives, sibilant fricatives, and nasals. To administer this subtest, the examiner can model the three sentences of the passage for the child and then ask the child to say the sentences with the pictures used as cues. The child should repeat the set of three sentences so that there are a total of six sentences produced for the passage. The examiner may use the images displayed on the computer screen or may make use of printed copies of the pictures. The sentences could also be printed if the patient is a reader.

Subtest II allows the examiner to elicit a form of connected speech, yet it is standardized and normed, and very simple to use, even with young children. The pictures are easy to identify and the same carrier phrase is used for each set in order to reduce the chance of production errors and increase validity. Because each set is phonologically homogeneous, this further aids the examiner in the diagnostic process.

Subtest III, the *Paragraph Subtest,* consists of two short, simple, easy-to-read passages

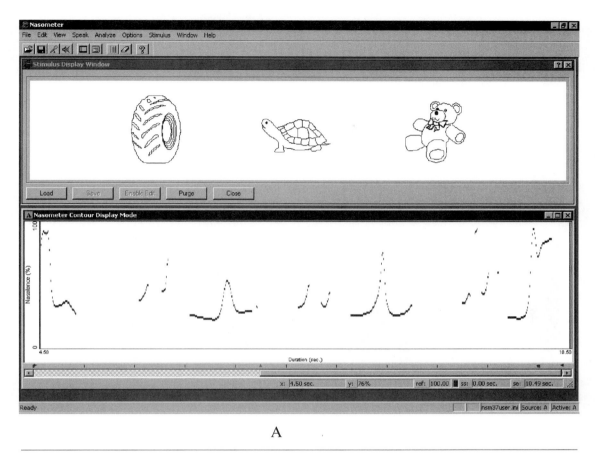

A

FIGURE 14–8 (A and B) Nasometer data from the Picture-Cued Subtest of the SNAP Test. The pictures are displayed on the screen. A. Contour display. (*continues*)

(Figure 14–9). These passages can either be read or repeated after the examiner. The first passage contains primarily plosive phonemes while the second passage contains a high incidence of sibilant (fricative and affricate) phonemes. The examiner can select either or both passages, depending on the articulation ability of the individual and the diagnostic goals of the examiner. These passages are more heterogeneous phonetically than the other two subtests, but are still more homogeneous than the "phonetically-balanced" passages that are often used in clinical nasometry.

Normative Studies of Passages

Normative data for Nasometer I has been gathered from thousands of normal English-speaking speakers using standardized passages (i.e., Zoo, Rainbow, Nasal Sentences, and passages from the SNAP Test-R). Similar passages with normative data have also been developed in many other English dialects, such as Australian English (van Doorn & Purcell, 1998), and other languages including Cantonese (Whitehill, 2001), Finnish (Haapanen, 1991), Flemish (Van Lierde, Wuyts, De Bodt, & Van Cauwenberge,

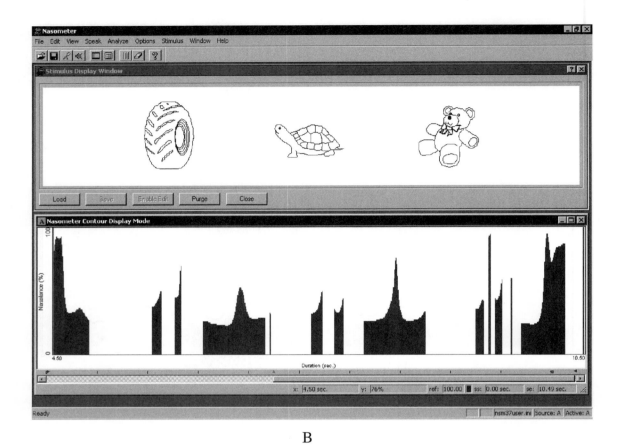

B

FIGURE 14–8 (A and B) (*continued*)   B. Filled contour display.

2001; Van Lierde, Wuyts, De Bodt, & Van Cauwenberge, 2003), German (Muller, Beleites, Hloucal, & Kuhn, 2000), Hungarian (Hirschberg et al., 2005), Irish (Sweeney et al., 2004), Japanese (Tachimura, Mori, Hirata, & Wada, 2000), Marathi (Nandurkar, 2002), Spanish (Anderson, 1996; Nett & Ochoa, 2004; Nichols, 1999), and Thai (Prathanee, Thanaviratananich, Pongjunyakul, & Rengpatanakij, 2003).

Some studies suggest that nasalance scores can vary with language (Anderson, 1996; Leeper et al., 1992; Nichols, 1999; Santos-Terron, Gonzalez-Landa, & Sanchez-Ruiz, 1990; van Doorn & Purcell, 1998). These studies should

be interpreted with caution however because when different passages are used, as is necessary with a different language, there is a difference in the phonemic composition. Passages with more high vowels and voiced consonants will have higher nasalance scores normally in comparison to passages with more low vowels or more voiceless consonants. Therefore, comparison of scores between languages is difficult.

Some normative studies have suggested that nasalance scores vary with dialect when the same passage is used (Leeper, Rochet, & MacKay, 1992; Seaver, Dalston, Leeper, & Adams, 1991), and even with racial group or

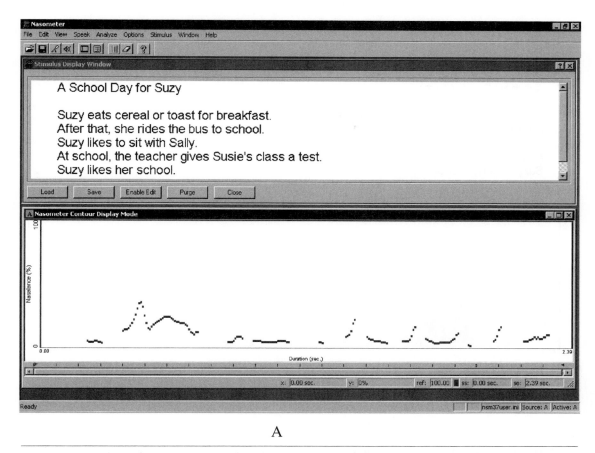

A

FIGURE 14–9 (A and B) Nasometer data from the Paragraph Subtest of the SNAP Test. A. Contour display. (*continues*)

culture (Mayo, Floyd, Warren, Dalston, & Mayo, 1996). Since consonants are produced essentially the same, regardless of dialect, these differences must be in the production of the vowels. Nasalized vowels are presumably the cause of a "nasal twang" in some dialects. It might be assumed that dialects, accents, or even languages that use more high vowels or a higher tongue position might be expected to have higher nasalance scores as compared to those with a greater incidence of low vowels or a lower tongue position (Lewis & Watterson, 2003). There may also be a differ-

ence in dialects between the timing of closure when transitions are made between nasal consonants and vowels (Mayo et al., 1996). No difference has been found with gender (Litzaw & Dalston, 1992).

Since the introduction of the Nasometer II, normative studies were repeated. These studies found slight differences in the mean scores between the two versions (Kummer, 2005; Watterson, Lewis, & Foley-Homan, 1999), but these differences are slight and usually not clinically significant. The new norms should be used with Nasometer II however.

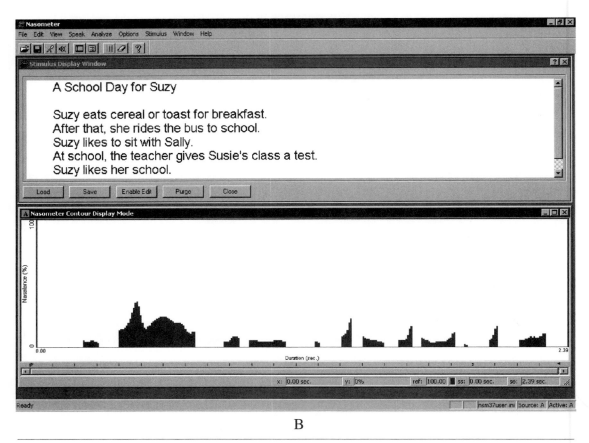

B

FIGURE 14–9 (A and B) (*continued*)   B. Filled contour display.

NASOMETRIC RESULTS

Display of the Speech Signal

As the individual is speaking, the speech signal enters the microphones and the program computes the nasalance score which, as noted previously, is the percentage of nasal acoustic energy of the total energy. This percentage is displayed on the bottom of the screen in real time. The default is the Contour Display mode (Nasogram) (Figures 14–7A, 14–8A, and 14–9A), where the percentage nasalance is displayed on the vertical (*x*) axis and time is

on the horizontal (*y*) axis. The contour can be filled in as an option as well (Figures 14–7B, 17–8B, and 14–9B). The Bar Display mode also shows nasalance on the horizontal axis but only one frame of data shows at a time and it is displayed in real time (Figure 14–10).

Result Statistics

Once the passage has been read or repeated, the examiner can obtain descriptive statistics for that segment of speech. This is done by clicking on **Analyze** from the menu and then on **Compute Result Statistics,** which will bring

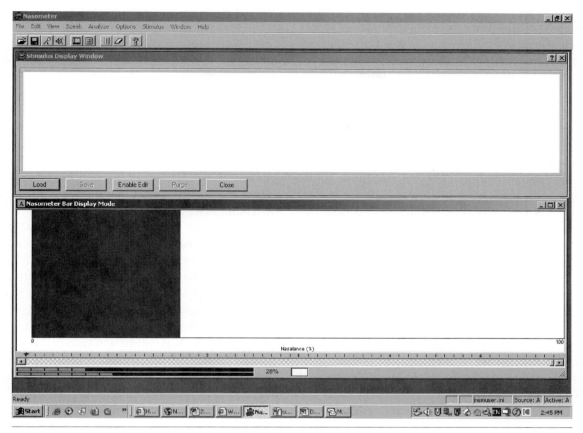

FIGURE 14–10   Horizontal bar graph shows nasalance results in real time. It can be used to provide feedback in therapy.

up a statistics box (Figure 14–7C). Among others, the statistics box contains the following:

- Mean (%)—the mean nasalance percentage points for the entire passage

- Min (%)—the lowest nasalance value in the data, excluding zero values

- Max (%)—the highest nasalance value in the data

- Threshold (%)—An assigned target nasalance value that is indicated by the placement of the reference cursor

- Above (%)—the percentage of the nasalance trace that is greater than the ratio

value set by the location of the reference cursor

- Below (%)—the percentage of the nasalance trace that is less than the ratio value set by the location of the reference cursor

For evaluation, the most important statistic is the mean nasalance score. It is this score that is compared to normative data to determine if there is a problem, and if so, the approximate degree of severity. The minimum and maximum percent nasalance scores give the range of nasalance and can help the examiner to judge the variability of resonance. The slope can be used to estimate the rate of velopharyngeal closure. For treatment, the threshold can be useful in setting a target for the individual to achieve.

Because there is variability in the scores of normal speakers and the scores do not always match perceptual impressions, Bressman and colleagues (Bressmann et al., 2000) suggested adding two new measures to the nasometric evaluations: the *nasalance distance*, which they define as the range between maximum and minimum nasalance; and the *nasalance ratio*, which is the minimum nasalance divided by maximum nasalance. These numbers give an indication of the variability of nasalance within a passage.

Prior versions of the Nasometer included the standard deviation of the passage in the statistics. In a study to evaluate the value of the standard deviation scores, it was found that the standard deviation score could not distinguish speakers beyond a gross normal and abnormal resonance diagnostic category (Vallino-Napoli & Montgomery, 1997). Although the standard deviation score might give some indication of the amount of variability of resonance during production of the passage, it was concluded that the standard deviation value serves little overall clinical utility. Instead, the mean nasalance score continues to be the best measure of nasalance.

Sensitivity and Specificity of the Nasalance Score

There have been several studies to evaluate the sensitivity and specificity of the nasalance score as it is correlated to another measure that serves as the guide. The *sensitivity* refers to the extent to which the score is able to correctly identify individuals with abnormal resonance. The *specificity* refers to the extent to which the score correctly excludes individuals with normal speech from the abnormal group.

Dalston and colleagues (Dalston et al., 1991c) conducted a study to determine the extent to which nasometric results using Nasometer I corresponded with aerodynamic estimates of velopharyngeal orifice area. Using an oral speech passage and a cutoff nasalance score of 32, the sensitivity of the Nasometer scores in correctly identifying the presence or absence of velopharyngeal areas in excess of 0.10 cm^2 was 0.78 and 0.79, respectively. As a second part of the study, the nasalance results were compared to clinical judgments of hypernasality. Again, using the score of 32 as the threshold of abnormality, the sensitivity and specificity of nasometry in correctly identifying subjects with more than mild hypernasality in their speech was 0.89 while the specificity was 0.95. Hardin and others (Hardin et al., 1992) conducted a similar study, but used a cutoff score of 26. In this study a sensitivity coefficient of 0.87 and a specificity coefficient of 0.93 were obtained. Ninety-one percent of the nasometry-based classifications accurately reflected listener judgments of hypernasality. Watterson, McFarlane, and Wright (1993) also found a significant correlation between nasalance and judgments of hypernasality on an oral speech passage. These results suggest that the Nasometer is an appropriate instrument that can be of value in assessing individuals suspected of having velopharyngeal impairment.

Dalston and associates (Dalston et al., 1991b) conducted a complementary study to determine the extent to which nasometric scores corresponded with clinical judgments of hyponasality and aerodynamic measurements of nasal cross-sectional area. Among the 38 adult subjects with moderate to severe nasal airway impairment as identified with aerodynamic studies, the sensitivity of the nasalance scores in correctly identifying these individuals was 0.38, whereas the specificity was 0.92. Among a group of 76 individuals, the sensitivity and specificity of nasometry in correctly identifying the presence or absence of hyponasality, as determined by perceptual assessment, was 0.48 and 0.79 respectively. However, when individuals with audible nasal emission were eliminated from analysis, the sensitivity rose to 1.0 and the specificity rose to 0.85. This study suggests that the sensitivity of nasometry in the identification of hyponasality with nasal air emission is not as strong as the sensitivity for identification of hypernasality.

Karnell (1995) suggested that one reason for a lack of agreement between perceptual measures and the nasalance results is that nasometry does not permit discrimination between nasal acoustic energy due to hypernasality and nasal acoustic energy due to turbulent nasal airflow. Hypernasal resonance occurs on vowels and nasal air emission occurs during the production of consonants. However, the presence of either can give the impression of "hypernasality," as judged by the listener. To test resonance, without the effect of nasal air emission, he used a "low-pressure" speech sample that contained only consonants that do not require intraoral air pressure. The nasalance results from this sample were compared to the results of the "high pressure" sentences from the Zoo Passage. He found that the scores for some individuals were significantly different in the two passages. From this study, he suggested that those individuals with hypernasal resonance will obtain elevated nasalance scores on the low-pressure and high-pressure speech samples, since the resonance occurs primarily on the vowels. In contrast, those individuals with normal resonance but with nasal air emission, especially the turbulent nasal rustle, will have low scores or normal scores on the low-pressure sample, but will have higher nasalance scores on the speech sample with high-pressure consonants. This observation seems true in our clinical experience and is another reason to consider the nasalance score based on what is heard perceptually.

INTERPRETATION OF NASOMETRIC RESULTS

Expected Nasalance Results

In isolating the degree of nasalance by phoneme, the nasalance score does not seem to vary between the low-pressure and high-pressure sounds (Watterson, Lewis, & Deutsch, 1998). Nasalance does vary, however, depending on whether the sound is voiced or voiceless. For voiceless oral consonants, the nasalance score is actually 0. This can be noted by the fact that when the individual with normal speech sustains an /s/ or /sh/, there is no tracing on the screen. Although there is no nasal resonance (or nasalance) on voiceless consonants, there is variable nasalance on voiced sounds. This can be seen on the screen when prolonging a voiced consonant, such as /z/.

In addition to voiced consonants, all vowels have some nasal resonance, as can be seen on the screen when prolonging a vowel. The degree of nasalance varies, depending on the type of vowel produced (Lewis & Watterson, 2003). There is more nasalance on high vowels than on low vowels, as can be noted on the SNAP Test-R (Kummer, 2005). In fact, the nasalance for /i/ (eee) is usually at least 10 percentage points higher than that for the low vowel /ah/.

One might question how it is possible to have nasal resonance, as represented by nasalance, on oral consonants when the velopharyngeal valve is completely closed. There are actually two reasons for nasalance on voiced oral consonants. One is that the sound separator plate cannot totally block reception of the signal from one side of the plate to the other side. Therefore, there is always some spillover between the microphones during the production of voiced phonemes, particularly vowels (KayPENTAX, 2003). The other reason is due to transpalatal transmission of sound during production of voiced phonemes, particularly vowels (Gildersleeve-Neumann & Dalston, 2001). This can be proved by prolonging an oral vowel and watching the nasalance tracing; then repeating the same vowel with the nose occluded. The nasalance score will drop as much as 20 percentage points. It can be assumed that the hard palate is like a brick wall and allows little sound to go through it. On the other hand, the soft palate is more like a curtain—allowing some sound to pass through into the nasal cavity.

The reason that high vowels have more nasal resonance than low vowels is due to the fact that the high tongue position results in a smaller oral cavity size and increased impedance of the sound as it passes through the oral passage. At the same time, there is increased bombardment of sound against the velum, so more sound goes through the soft tissues (S.G. Fletcher, personal communication, May 12, 1999). In contrast, when the tongue is low in the oral cavity for the production of low vowels, there is considerably less impedance of the sound and the size of the oral cavity is larger so that oral resonance is more pronounced.

In evaluating nasal resonance, a prolonged nasal sound often results in scores that are in the 90s. However, when nasal consonants are combined with oral consonants in connected speech, the resulting nasalance score is between 50% to 70%.

Interpretation of the Nasalance Score

When various phonemes are combined together for connected speech, the resultant average nasalance score for speakers with normal resonance will depend on the passage and its phonemic content of voiced versus voiceless consonants and high versus low vowels. Therefore, it is difficult to compare norms for different passages.

When one of the standardized passages is used, the nasalance score of the individual can be compared to normative data for that particular passage in order to determine if the score is close to normal or obviously abnormal. Unfortunately, this is still difficult because there is no single score that serves as an absolute or definitive cutoff point between normal and abnormal resonance. Since nasalance and resonance are on a continuum, there is a borderline area between clearly normal and clearly abnormal.

For Nasometer I, Vallino-Napoli and Montgomery (1997) suggested that a mean nasalance score in the high 20s could be used to differentiate speakers with borderline velopharyngeal function from those who are normal speakers. Also for Nasometry I, Dalston, Warren, and Dalston (1991c) used the score of 32 as the threshold of normal, but later, Dalston, Neiman, and Gonzalez-Landa (1993) used the score of 28 as the threshold between normal and abnormal. Suggested thresholds are given for the various passages of the SNAP-R which was normed on Nasometer II. In looking at all the norms for a passage devoid of nasal phonemes, it can be said that a score under about 20% does not have hypernasality, scores between 20% to 30% are in the borderline range, and scores over 30% can be considered clearly abnormal.

Given the large borderline range and the variability of scores based on phonemic content of the passage, the results of nasometric testing must always be interpreted by the speech pathologist in the context of the perceptual and intraoral assessment. This is important because many factors can affect the nasalance score. For example, an individual's nasalance score can be in the normal range, even in the presence of audible nasal air emission, if there is normal resonance. On the other hand, the nasalance score may be about two standard deviations above the normative mean, yet that person may still have very acceptable speech.

If there is obstruction in the vocal tract causing cul-de-sac resonance, the obstruction may impede the transmission of resonance in both the oral and the nasal cavities, resulting in an essentially normal nasalance score because the nasalance score is a ratio of the two. When there is a combination of hyponasality and hypernasality, both aspects are combined for the average nasalance score (Dalston et al., 1991a). When there is nasal turbulence (or a nasal rustle), this may result in a high nasalance score due to the degree of nasal distortion, even though it may be due to a small velopharyngeal opening. On the other hand, a large velopharyngeal opening may give a moderate nasalance score due to the lack of intensity of both oral and nasal acoustic energy.

A breathy vocal quality or low volume can even influence the nasalance score to some degree.

Articulation errors can also affect the nasalance score. If pharyngeal fricatives or posterior nasal fricatives are substituted for sibilant phonemes, the nasal emission associated with these articulation productions will produce an elevated nasalance score, particularly on passages that contain a large number of sibilants. The same is true if nasal sounds are substituted for oral sounds (for example, the substitution of /ng/ for /l/). Although these errors are due to faulty articulation placement rather than true velopharyngeal dysfunction, this can not always be distinguished by the Nasometer if heterogeneous passages are used. Since there are so many factors that can affect the nasalance score, nasometry should always serve as a supplement to clinical judgment, but not as a substitute for it.

With prior information from the perceptual and oral examination, the examiner can interpret the nasalance scores with more confidence. In addition, certain patterns of scores can be diagnostic, as can be seen through the following case studies:

CASE REPORTS

Case #1

Oral Passages	Nasalance Score
Bilabial Plosives	11
Lingual-Alveolar Plosives	11
Velar Plosives	13
Sibilant Fricatives	46

Diagnosis: Since all passages are normal with the exception of the sibilants, phoneme-specific nasal emission on sibilants should be suspected.

(continues)

(Continued)

Case #2

Oral Passages	Nasalance Score
Bilabial Plosives	15
Lingual-Alveolar Plosives	48
Velar Plosives	13
Sibilant Fricatives	43

Diagnosis: Velar phonemes are normal but anterior phonemes show high nasalance scores. This may indicate normal velopharyngeal function, but also a symptomatic fistula that is above the tongue tip.

Case #3

Oral + /a/ Syllables	Nasalance Score
pa, pa, pa…	5
ta, ta, ta…	8
ka, ka, ka…	8
sa, sa, sa…	7
a, a, a…	7

Oral + /i/ (eee) Syllables	Nasalance Score
pi, pi, pi…	38
ti, ti, ti…	37
ki, ki, ki…	37
si, si, si…	39
i, i, i…	37

Diagnosis: Since low-vowel syllables are normal and high-vowel syllables are abnormally high, phoneme-specific hypernasality on high vowels should be suspected due to an abnormally high tongue position. Another possibility is a thin velum.

Interpretation of the Nasogram

The configuration of the nasogram can be useful when the results of the entire passage are displayed on the screen. Some general guidelines in interpretation are as follows:

During production of an oral passage:

- Normal oral resonance is typically around 15–20 percentage points.

- The expected difference between vowels /a/ and /i/ (eee) is about 10 points when combined with oral consonants and about 20 points with nasal consonants.

- The higher the contour is on the screen, the more hypernasality to expect.

- If most of the data points appear normal (and the nasalance score is normal) but there are occasional high peaks, this suggests normal resonance but inconsistent nasal emission.

- A gradual rise in the curve throughout the passage suggests muscle fatigue, which could indicate neuromotor problems.

- There should be no data points during production of a prolonged /s/ or /sh/. If there is a break in velopharyngeal closure, this will be seen on the screen.

- If either /s/ or /sh/ are high and others are normal, consider phoneme-specific nasal emission due to a pharyngeal fricative or posterior nasal fricative.

- If lingual-alveolars and bilabials are significantly higher than velars, this could be due to the effect of a fistula.

- If vowels are high, but prolonged /s/ is zero, this could be due to a thin velum, high tongue position, or vowel-specific nasality.

During production of a nasal passage:

- If the data points are low and remain toward the bottom of the screen, this indicates hyponasality and can also suggest upper airway obstruction.

The nasogram can be particularly helpful in counseling individuals and their families. With the visual display, it is easier for the examiner to explain both what is happening during speech as well as the relative severity of the problem.

USE IN TREATMENT

In addition to its utility as diagnostic tool, nasometry is very useful in treatment. It can provide the individual with valuable real-time visual feedback and tangible goals during the treatment process. It can be particularly helpful in eliminating nasal emission or hypernasality that is functional or phoneme-specific. In some cases, it can even help to eliminate a nasal rustle (turbulence) if it is due to a very small, inconsistent velopharyngeal opening, particularly after surgical repair. As a form of biofeedback, it can be used to modify resonance in certain cases of velopharyngeal incompetence (Heppt, Westrich, Strate & Mohring, 1991). The games that are provided as part of the software help to motivate young patients (Figure 14–11).

When using nasometry in therapy, the speech pathologist can access different display formats, including the filled contour display, bar display, or inverted contour display, depending on the therapy task (Figure 14–12). The green reference cursor line can be placed on the nasogram according to the needs of the patient and the therapy goals. The patient works with a goal of keeping the nasalance trace below the reference line level during speech. After the speech task has been completed, the clinician can open the statistics box to obtain the percentage above and below the threshold. This can serve as a basis for charting progress.

To address specific errors, such as a nasal rustle on a pressure-sensitive phoneme, it is often helpful to contrast minimal paired words with and without the /s/ phoneme. Instruct the child that the /s/ phonemes should not be visible. Therefore, words such as "mile" and "smile" should look similar, as noted in Figure 14–13.

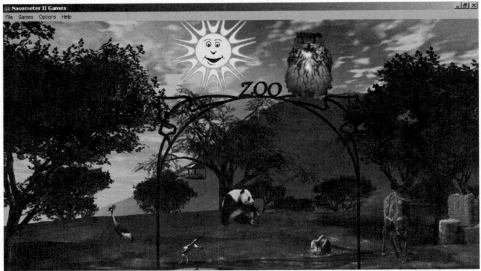

Look at this book with us. It's a story about a zoo. That is where bears go. Today it's very cold out of doors, but we see a cloud overhead that's a pretty white fluffy shape. We hear that straw covers the floor of cages to keep the chill away; yet a deer walks through the trees with her head high. They feed seeds to birds so they're able to fly.

A

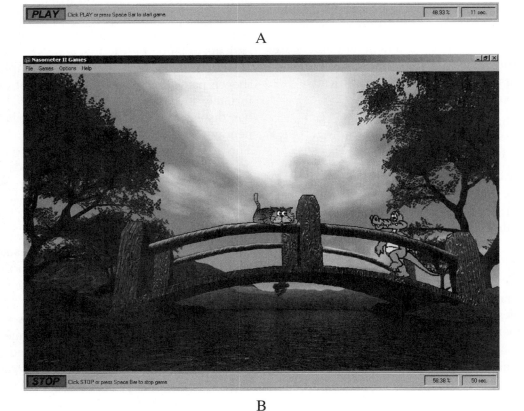

B

FIGURE 14–11 (A and B) Nasometer games. All games provide biofeedback, with the ability to set a nasalance threshold. When achieving the desired threshold, the child is rewarded with an emerging picture.

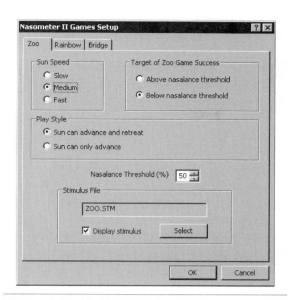

When there is a nasal rustle, an obvious difference can be noted in the tracings, as can be seen in Figure 14–14.

In therapy, the child is instructed to eliminate the tracings that are the result of the /s/ phoneme. One great advantage of the Nasometer is that the tracing with the audio can be replayed for the child again and again. This allows the child to see and hear the nasal rustle.

Although the Nasometer is a great tool for providing biofeedback in therapy, it should be noted that biofeedback is only effective if the individual's velopharyngeal mechanism is anatomically and physiologically capable of achieving normal velopharyngeal closure. For more

FIGURE 14–12 You can change the options on the Nasometer games to meet the needs of each therapy session.

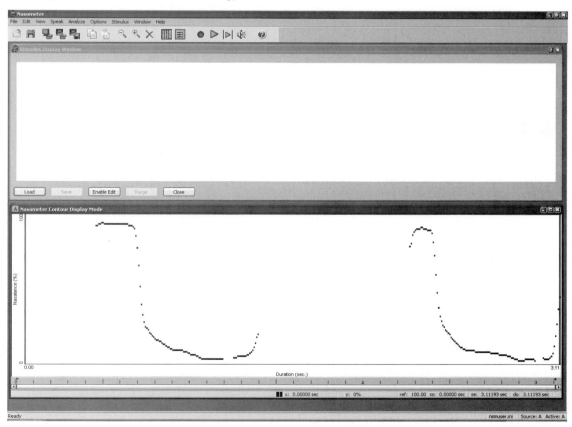

FIGURE 14–13 Normal speech production of the word "mile" and then "smile." Note that the two tracings are very similar in appearance due to the fact that there is no nasalance on the /s/ sound. (Courtesy of Janet Middendorf, M.A.)

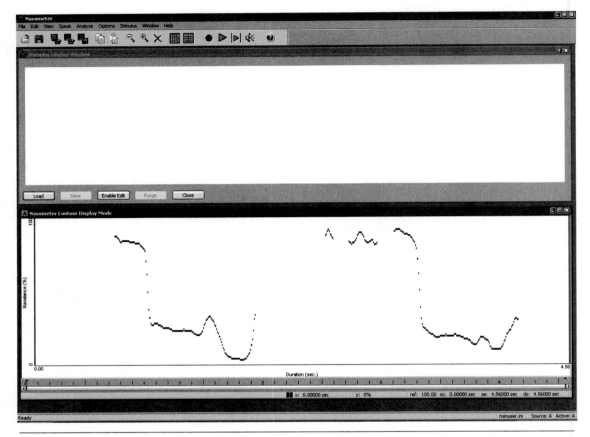

FIGURE 14–14 Production of the word "mile" and then "smile" with a nasal rustle on /s/. Note that in this case, the tracings are different. There is a high squiggly line at the beginning of the word "smile" due to the nasal rustle on /s/. (Courtesy of Janet Middendorf, M.A.)

information regarding the use of nasometry in treatment, please refer to Chapter 21.

SUMMARY

Nasometric testing is an easy, noninvasive procedure used to obtain objective data regarding the results of velopharyngeal function. The nasalance score can be compared to normative data in order to gauge the type and degree of abnormality. Nasometry is an excellent means of substantiating the subjective findings of the speech pathologist. In addition, the Nasometer provides a visual display that is helpful in counseling individuals and families. Finally, nasometry is an excellent means for providing visual biofeedback regarding the results of velopharyngeal function during speech and therefore, it can be very useful during treatment.

Although nasometry can be a very valuable part of an evaluation of resonance and velopharyngeal function, it should not be viewed as an independent diagnostic measure. Since the nasalance score can be affected by articulation errors, production errors, mixed nasality, and other factors, the objective measurements provided by nasometry should be interpreted based on an accompanying perceptual evaluation by a qualified speech pathologist. In addition, just like with aerodynamic instrumentation, nasometry can give objective scores, but cannot show the cause of velopharyngeal dysfunction, or the location and size of the defect in the same manner that the direct measures can do. Therefore, the results of the nasometry testing must be integrated into a test battery for a complete evaluation of velopharyngeal function.

FOR REVIEW, DISCUSSION, AND CRITICAL THINKING

1. What is the Nasometer and what are the equipment components?

2. What does the nasalance score measure? How is it calculated?

3. What are the standardized tests for use with nasometry? What type of passage should be used for testing hyponasality? What type of passage would be appropriate for testing hypernasality?

4. If the child has only plosives in his phonemic repertoire, what passages could be used?

5. Why is the nasalance score not 0 with normal speech and with normal velopharyngeal closure?

6. If the child has a high nasalance score on the sibilants passage, but other scores are normal, what might you conclude? What would you recommend?

7. If a child with a history of cleft palate has a high nasalance score on plosives and lingual-alveolars, but a normal score on velars, what might you suspect to be the cause? What would you do next? What would you recommend?

8. Why is the nasalance score 0 during prolongation of the /s/ sound?

9. Which passage would have the highest nasalance score in normal speech: "pee, pee, pee" or "pa, pa, pa"? Why?

REFERENCES

Anderson, R. T. (1996). Nasometric values for normal Spanish-speaking females: A preliminary report. *Cleft Palate-Craniofacial Journal*, 33(4), 333–336.

Bressmann, T. (2005). Comparison of nasalance scores obtained with the Nasometer, the NasalView, and the OroNasal System. *Cleft Palate-Craniofacial Journal*, 42(4), 423–433.

Bressmann, T., Sader, R., Whitehill, T. L., Awan, S. N., Zeilhofer, H. F., & Horch, H. H. (2000). Nasalance distance and ratio: Two new measures. *Cleft Palate-Craniofacial Journal*, 37(3), 248–256.

Dalston, R. M. (1997). The use of nasometry in the assessment and remediation of velopharyngeal inadequacy. In K. R. Bzoch (Ed.), *Communicative disorders related to cleft lip and palate* (Vol. 4, pp. 331–346). Austin: Pro-Ed.

Dalston, R. M., Neiman, G. S., & Gonzalez-Landa, G. (1993). Nasometric sensitivity and specificity: A cross-dialect and cross-culture study. *Cleft Palate-Craniofacial Journal*, 30(3), 285–291.

Dalston, R. M., & Seaver, E. J. (1992). Relative values of various standardized passages in the nasometric assessment of patients with velopharyngeal impairment. *Cleft Palate-Craniofacial Journal, 29*(1), 17–21.

Dalston, R. M., Warren, D. W., & Dalston, E. T. (1991a). The identification of nasal obstruction through clinical judgments of hyponasality and nasometric assessment of speech acoustics. *American Journal of Orthodontics and Dentofacial Orthopedics, 100*(1), 59–65.

Dalston, R. M., Warren, D. W., & Dalston, E. T. (1991b). A preliminary investigation concerning the use of nasometry in identifying patients with hyponasality and/or nasal airway impairment. *Journal of Speech and Hearing Research, 34*(1), 11–18.

Dalston, R. M., Warren, D. W., & Dalston, E. T. (1991c). Use of nasometry as a diagnostic tool for identifying patients with velopharyngeal impairment [published Erratum appears in *Cleft Palate-Craniofacial Journal,* 1991, *28*(4), 446]. *Cleft Palate-Craniofacial Journal, 28*(2), 184–188; Discussion 188–189.

David, L. R., Blalock, D., & Argenta, L. C. (1999). Uvular transposition: A new method of cleft palate repair. *Plastic and Reconstructive Surgery, 104*(4), 897–904.

Dejonckere, P. H., & van Wijngaarden, H. A. (2001). Retropharyngeal autologous fat transplantation for congenital short palate: A nasometric assessment of functional results. *Annals of Otology, Rhinology, & Laryngology, 110*(2), 168–172.

Fairbanks, D. (1960). *Voice and articulation drill book* (pp. 127). New York: Harper and Row.

Fletcher, S. G. (1970). Theory and instrumentation for quantitative measurement of nasality. *Cleft Palate Journal, 7,* 601–609.

Fletcher, S. G. (1972). Contingencies for bio-electronic modification of nasality. *Journal of Speech and Hearing Disorders, 37,* 329–346.

Fletcher, S. G. (1976a). "Nasalance" vs. listener judgments of nasality. *Cleft Palate Journal, 13,* 31–44.

Fletcher, S. G. (1976b). Theory and use of Tonar II: A status report. *Biocommunications Research Reports, 1,* 1–38.

Fletcher, S. G. (1978). *Diagnosing speech disorders from cleft palate.* New York: Grune & Statton, Inc.

Fletcher, S. G., Adams L., & McCutcheon. (1989). Cleft palate speech assessment through oral-nasal acoustic measures. In K. R. Bzoch (Ed.), *Communicative disorders related to cleft lip and palate* (pp. 246–257). Boston: College Hill Press.

Fletcher, S. G., & Bishop, M. E. (1970). Measurement of nasality with tonar. *Cleft Palate Journal, 7,* 610–621.

Gildersleeve-Neumann, C. E., & Dalston, R. M. (2001). Nasalance scores in noncleft individuals: Why not zero? *Cleft Palate-Craniofacial Journal, 38*(2), 106–111.

Gonzalez Landa, G., Sanchez-Ruiz, I., Perez Gonzalez, V., Santos Terron, M. J., & Miro Viar, J. L. (2000). [Clinical and nasometric study of velopharyngeal function in two-stage palatoplasty]. *Acta Otorrinolaringologica Espanola, 51*(7), 581–586.

Gonzalez-Landa, G., Santos Terron, M. J., Miro Viar, J. L., & Sanchez-Ruiz, I. (1990). [Post-adenoidectomy velopharyngeal insufficiency in children with velopalatine clefts]. *Acta Otorrinolaringology Espanola, 41*(3), 159–161.

Gray, S. D., Pinborough-Zimmerman, J., & Catten, M. (1999). Posterior wall augmentation for treatment of velopharyngeal insufficiency. *Otolaryngology–Head & Neck Surgery, 121*(1), 107–112.

Haapanen, M. L. (1991). Nasalance scores in normal Finnish speech. *Folia Phoniatrica, 43*(4), 197–203.

Haapanen, M. L. (1992). Nasalance scores in patients with a modified Honig velopharyngeal flap before and after operation. *Scandinavian Journal of Plastic and Reconstructive Surgery and Hand Surgery, 26*(3), 301–305.

Haapanen, M. L., Kalland, M., Heliovaara, A., Hukki, J., & Ranta, R. (1997). Velopharyngeal function in cleft patients undergoing maxillary advancement. *Folia Phoniatrica et Logopedica, 49*(1), 42–47.

Hardin, M. A., Van Demark, D. R., Morris, H. L., & Payne, M. M. (1992). Correspondence between nasalance scores and listener judgments of hypernasality and hyponasality. *Cleft Palate-Craniofacial Journal, 29*(4), 346–351.

Heppt, W., Westrich, M., Strate, B., & Mohring, L. (1991). [Nasalance: A new concept for objective analysis of nasality]. *Laryngorhinootologie, 70*(4), 208–213.

Hirschberg, J., Bok, S., Juhasz, M., Trenovszki, Z., Votisky, P., & Hirschberg, A. (2005). Adaptation of nasometry to Hungarian language and experiences with its clinical application. *International Journal of Pediatric Otorhinolaryngology, 70*(5), 785–98.

Hong, K. H., Kwon, S. H., & Jung, S. S. (1997). The assessment of nasality with a nasometer and sound spectrography in patients with nasal polyposis. *Otolaryngology–Head & Neck Surgery, 117*(4), 343–348.

KayPENTAX (2003). *Installation, operations, and maintenance manual: Nasometer II, Model 6400*, Lincoln Park, NJ: KayPENTAX.

Karnell, M. P. (1995). Nasometric discrimination of hypernasality and turbulent nasal airflow. *Cleft Palate-Craniofacial Journal, 32*(2), 145–148.

Kummer, A. W. (2005). The MacKay-Kummer SNAP Test-R: Simplified nasometric assessment procedures. KayPENTAX. Retrieved 3/3/07, from http://www.kayelemetrics.com/snaptestr.htm

Kummer, A. W., Myer, C. M. I., Smith, M. E., & Shott, S. R. (1993). Changes in nasal resonance secondary to adenotonsillectomy. *American Journal of Otolaryngology, 14*(4), 285–290.

Leeper, H. A., Rochet, A. P., & MacKay, I. R. A. (1992). Characteristics of nasalance in Canadian speakers of English and French. *Proceedings of the International Conference on Spoken and Language Processes, 5*, 49–52.

Lewis, K. E., & Watterson, T. (2003). Comparison of nasalance scores obtained from the Nasometer and the NasalView. *Cleft Palate-Craniofacial Journal, 40*(1), 40–45.

Litzaw, L. L., & Dalston, R. M. (1992). The effect of gender upon nasalance scores among normal adult speakers. *Journal of Communication Disorders, 25*(1), 55–64.

MacKay, I. R. A., & Kummer, A. W. (1994). Simplified nasometric assessment procedures. In Kay Elemetrics Corp. (Ed.), *Instruction manual: Nasometer Model 6200–3* (pp. 123–142). Lincoln Park, NJ: Kay Elemetrics Corp.

Mayo, R., Floyd, L. A., Warren, D. W., Dalston, R. M., & Mayo, C. M. (1996). Nasalance and nasal area values: Crossracial study. *Cleft Palate—Craniofacial Journal, 33*(2), 143–149.

Muller, R., Beleites, T., Hloucal, U., & Kuhn, M. (2000). Objektive Messung der normalen Nasalanz im sachsischen Sprachraum. *HNO, 48*(12), 937–942.

Nandurkar, A. (2002). Nasalance measures in Marathi consonant-vowel-consonant syllables with pressure consonants produced by children with and without cleft lip and palate. *Cleft Palate-Craniofacial Journal, 39*(1), 59–65.

Nett, K., & Ochoa, J. (2004). *Preliminary nasometric values for bilingual Spanish/English children with normal resonance.* Presentation at the American Speech-Language-Hearing Association, Philadelphia, November 19, 2004.

Nichols, A. C. (1999). Nasalance statistics for two Mexican populations. *Cleft Palate-Craniofacial Journal, 36*(1), 57–63.

Nieminen, P., Lopponen, H., Vayrynen, M., Tervonen, A., & Tolonen, U. (2000). Nasalance scores in snoring children with obstructive symptoms. *International Journal of Pediatric Otorhinolaryngology, 52* (1), 53–60.

Parker, A. J., Clarke, P. M., Dawes, P. J., & Maw, A. R. (1990). A comparison of active anterior rhinomanometry and nasometry in the objective assessment of nasal obstruction. *Rhinology, 28*(1), 47–53.

Parker, A. J., Maw, A. R., & Szallasi, F. (1989). An objective method of assessing nasality: A possible aid in the selection of patients for adenoidectomy. *Clinical Otolaryngology, 14*(2), 161–166.

Prathanee, B., Thanaviratananich, S., Pongjunyakul, A., & Rengpatanakij, K. (2003). Nasalance scores for speech in normal Thai children. *Scandinavian Journal of Plastic and Reconstructive Surgery and Hand Surgery, 37*(6), 351–355.

Rieger, J., Wolfaardt, J., Seikaly, H., & Jha, N. (2002). Speech outcomes in patients rehabilitated with maxillary obturator prostheses after maxillectomy: A prospective study. *International Journal of Prosthodontics, 15*(2), 139–144.

Santos-Terron, M. J., Gonzalez-Landa, G., & Sanchez-Ruiz, I. (1990). Nasometric patterns in the speech of normal child speakers of Castilian Spanish. *Revista Espanola de Foniatrica, 4*, 71–75.

Seaver, E. J., Dalston, R. M., Leeper, H. A., & Adams, L. E. (1991). A study of nasometric values for normal nasal resonance. *Journal of Speech and Hearing Research, 34*(4), 715–721.

Soneghet, R., Santos, R. P., Behlau, M., Habermann, W., Friedrich, G., & Stammberger, H. (2002). Nasalance changes after functional endoscopic sinus surgery. *Journal of Voice, 16*(3), 392–397.

Sweeney, T., Sell, D., & O'Regan, M. (2004). Nasalance scores for normal-speaking Irish children. *Cleft Palate-Craniofacial Journal, 41*(2), 168–174.

Tatchell, J. A., Stewart, M., & Lapine, P. R. (1991). Nasalance measurements in hearing-impaired children. *Journal of Communication Disorders, 24*(4), 275–285.

Tachimura, T., Mori, C., Hirata, S. I., & Wada, T. (2000). Nasalance score variation in normal adult Japanese speakers of midwest Japanese dialect. *Cleft Palate-Craniofacial Journal, 37*(5), 463–467.

Vallino-Napoli, L. D., & Montgomery, A. A. (1997). Examination of the standard deviation of mean nasalance scores in subjects with cleft palate: Implications for clinical use. *Cleft Palate-Craniofacial Journal, 34*(6), 512–519.

Van Doorn, J., & Purcell, A. (1998). Nasalance levels in the speech of normal Australian children. *Cleft Palate-Craniofacial Journal, 35*(4), 287–292.

Van Lierde, K. M., De Bodt, M., Baetens, I., Schrauwen, V., & Van Cauwenberge, P. (2003). Outcome of treatment regarding articulation, resonance, and voice in Flemish adults with unilateral and bilateral cleft palate. *Folia Phoniatrica et Logopedica, 55*(2), 80–90.

Van Lierde, K. M., Monstrey, S., Bonte, K., Van Cauwenberge, P., & Vinck, B. (2004).

The long-term speech outcome in Flemish young adults after two different types of palatoplasty. *International Journal of Pediatric Otorhinolaryngology*, 68(7), 865–875.

Van Lierde, K. M., Wuyts, F. L., De Bodt, M., & Van Cauwenberge, P. (2001). Nasometric values for normal nasal resonance in the speech of young Flemish adults. *Cleft Palate-Craniofacial Journal*, 38(2), 112–118.

Van Lierde, K. M., Wuyts, F. L., De Bodt, M., & Van Cauwenberge, P. (2003). Age-related patterns of nasal resonance in normal Flemish children and young adults. *Scandinavian Journal of Plastic and Reconstructive Surgery and Hand Surgery*, 37(6), 344–350.

Watterson, T., Lewis, K. E., & Deutsch, C. (1998). Nasalance and nasality in low-pressure and high-pressure speech. *Cleft Palate-Craniofacial Journal*, 35(4), 293–298.

Watterson, T., Lewis, K. E., & Foley-Homan, N. (1999). Effect of stimulus length on nasalance scores. *Cleft Palate-Craniofacial Journal*, 36(3), 243–247.

Watterson, T., McFarlane, S. C., & Wright, D. S. (1993). The relationship between nasalance and nasality in children with cleft palate. *Journal of Communication Disorders*, 26(1), 13–28.

Whitehill, T. L. (2001). Nasalance measures in Cantonese-speaking women. *Cleft Palate-Craniofacial Journal*, 38(2), 119–125.

Williams, R. G., Eccles, R., & Hutchings, H. (1990). The relationship between nasalance and nasal resistance to airflow. *Acta Otolaryngology (Stockholm)*, 110(5/6), 443–449.

Williams, R. G., Preece, M., Rhys, R., & Eccles, R. (1992). The effect of adenoid and tonsil surgery on nasalance. *Clinical Otolaryngology & Allied Sciences*, 17(2), 136–140.

Wozny, C. G., Kuehn, D. P., Oishi, J. T., & Arthur, J. L. (1994, November). *Effect of passage length on nasalance values in normal adults*. Paper presented at the American Speech-Language-Hearing Association, New Orleans, LA.

APPENDIX 14–1

STANDARD NASOMETRIC PASSAGES SUPPLIED BY KAYPENTAX

ZOO PASSAGE*

Look at the book with us. It's a story about a zoo. That is where bears go. Today it's very cold out of doors, but we see a cloud overhead that's a pretty, white, fluffy shape. We hear that straw covers the floor of cages to keep the chill away; yet a deer walks through the trees with her head high. They feed seeds to birds so they're able to fly.

*The Zoo Passage excludes nasal consonants.

RAINBOW PASSAGE*

When the sunlight strikes raindrops in the air, they act like a prism and form a rainbow. The rainbow is a division of white light into many beautiful colors. These take the shape of a long round arch, with its path high above, and its two ends apparently beyond the horizon.

There is, according to legend, a boiling pot of gold at one end. People look, but no one ever finds it. When a man looks for something beyond his reach, his friends say he is looking for the pot of gold at the end of the rainbow.

*In the Rainbow passage, 11.5% of the consonants are nasal consonants.

NASAL SENTENCES*

Mama made some lemon jam.

Ten men came in when Jane rang.

Dan's gang changed my mind.

Ben can't plan on a lengthy rain.

Amanda came from Bounding, Maine.

*The Nasal Sentences Passage is loaded with nasal phonemes so that 35% of the total phonemes in these sentences are nasal consonants. This is more than three times as many as would be expected in standard American English sentences.

Normative data for standardized passages collected on 40 adult subjects using Nasometer II (KayPENTAX, 2003):

Test Passage	Mean Nasalance	*SD* of Mean
Zoo Passage	11.25	5.63
Rainbow Passage	31.47	6.65
Nasal Sentences	59.55	7.96

APPENDIX 14–2

SCORE SHEET FOR THE SNAP TEST-REVISED

THE MACKAY-KUMMER SNAP TEST-R
SIMPLIFIED NASOMETRIC ASSESSMENT PROCEDURES
REVISED 2005

Name:	Date:
Age:	Examiner:

Subtest I: Syllable Repetition/Prolonged Sounds Subtest

Instructions: Repeat or prolong until the screen is full.

Oral + /a/ Syllables	Norms	*SD*	Score (Threshold: ≥15)
pa, pa, pa…	6	3	
ta, ta, ta…	7	4	
ka, ka, ka…	7	4	
sa, sa, sa…	7	5	
ʃa, ʃa, ʃa…	7	4	

Oral + /i/ (eee) Syllables	Norms	*SD*	Score (Threshold: ≥35)
pi, pi, pi…	17	7	
ti, ti, ti…	17	7	
ki, ki, ki…	18	8	
si, si, si…	17	8	
ʃi, ʃi, ʃi… (sh)	16	8	

Nasal + /a/ Syllables	Norms	*SD*	Score (Threshold: ≤40)
ma, ma, ma…	53	13	
na, na, na…	53	11	

Nasal + /i/ (eee) Syllables	Norms	*SD*	Score (Threshold: ≤60)
mi, mi, mi…	72	13	
ni, ni, ni…	74	11	

Prolonged Sounds	Norms	*SD*	Score (Threshold: +/–2 *SDs*)
Prolonged /a/	6	3	
Prolonged /i/ (eee)	19	9	
Prolonged /s/	0	0	
Prolonged /m/	93	3	

SNAP Test-Revised, page 2.
Name: _____

Subtest II: Picture Cued Subtest

Instructions: Produce a sentence with the carrier phrase and picture. Do each twice.

Oral Passages	Norms	SD	Score (Threshold: ≥22)
Bilabial Plosives	11	5	
Lingual-Alveolar Plosives	11	5	
Velar Plosives	13	6	
Sibilant Fricatives	12	5	
Nasal Passage	**Norms**	**SD**	**Score (Threshold: ≤45)**
Nasals	54	9	

Subtest III: Paragraph Subtest

Instructions: Read or repeat each passage.

Passages (Reading)	Norms	SD	Score (Threshold: ≥25)
Bilabial Plosives (w/nasals)	16	5	
Passages (Reading)	**Norms**	**SD**	**Score (Threshold: ≥20)**
Sibilant Fricatives (w/o nasals)	10	4	

Notes:

_____

_____

_____

Important: The threshold value for each test is an approximation of the beginning of a borderline range of abnormal resonance. These values were estimated based on standard deviations (about two higher for orals, about one lower for nasals) and clinical experience. It should be noted that a small number of normal speakers will score outside two standard deviations of the mean for both orals and nasals. Therefore, the suggested threshold values should be used as general guidelines and not as absolute markers between normal and abnormal resonance. The scores on nasometry should always be used as a means to support clinical judgment, but never to replace it.

Pick up the . . .

 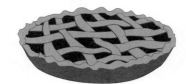 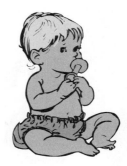

Take a . . .

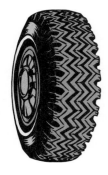 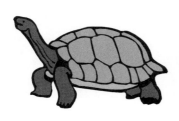 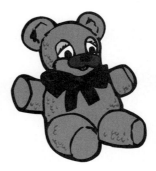

Go get a . . .

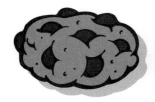 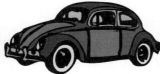 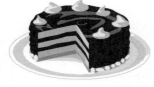

Suzy sees the . . .

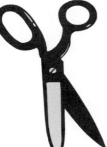 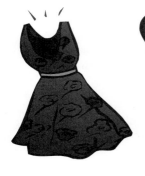 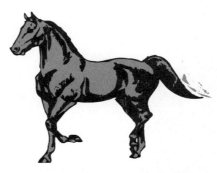

Mama made some . . .

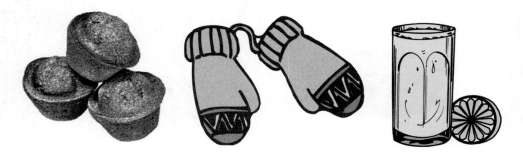

CHAPTER

15

SPEECH AERODYNAMICS

DAVID J. ZAJAC, PH.D.

CHAPTER OUTLINE

INTRODUCTION

Aerodynamics is the branch of physics that deals with the mechanical properties of air and other gases in motion. Because speech production requires a buildup and release of air pressure at the various valving points in the vocal tract, aerodynamic principles can be used to study the speech process.

The purpose of this chapter is to first discuss the aerodynamics of normal speech production. This chapter will then review the principles and procedures of the pressure-flow technique. The use and value of the pressure-flow technique in evaluating the nasal airway and velopharyngeal function will then be described.

WHY AERODYNAMIC ASSESSMENT?

Aerodynamic processes are indeed responsible for all acoustic aspects of speech production. Beginning with inspiration, air enters the lungs due to the expansion of the thoracic cavity and the generation of negative air pressure relative to the atmosphere. During expiration, positive subglottal pressure (P_S) is generated due to passive relaxation of the thorax and, if needed, active contraction of the muscles of respiration. Positive P_S is responsible for the rapid displacement of the vocal folds that results in the quasiperiodic release of air for all voiced speech sounds. The articulators of the upper vocal tract further modify airflow for sound production. During production of the stop-plosive /p/, for example, the lips momentarily impede airflow resulting in a buildup and release of pressure. The acoustic bursts resulting from the release of the articulators provide important intensity and frequency cues to the place of articulation of stop consonants. In addition, the articulators create relatively prolonged noise by constricting the size of the upper vocal tract. During production of the fricative /s/, for example, the tongue approximates the alveolar ridge,

resulting in a reduction of cross-sectional area and the generation of turbulent airflow.

Adequate production of speech requires an effective velopharyngeal (VP) mechanism. During production of oral pressure consonants, the VP mechanism must separate the oral and nasal cavities. Conversely, during production of nasal consonants, the VP mechanism must allow some degree of oral-nasal coupling. As indicated by Sussman (1992) and others, the following perceptual speech symptoms commonly occur in individuals with cleft palate due to VP dysfunction: (1) weak pressure consonants, (2) nasal air emission, (3) hypernasality, (4) hyponasality, and (5) compensatory articulation (pp. 211–212). Although the first two symptoms have clear aerodynamic foundations, their perceptual characteristics are not well defined. Both occur during oral consonant production due to the physical coupling of the oral and nasal cavities. Sussman (1992) described weak pressure consonants as sounds that "appear muffled and lack clarity." As indicated by Peterson-Falzone, Hardin-Jones, and Karnell (2001), nasal air emission may or may not be audible depending on the status of the nasal passages. Even when audible, nasal air emission may be masked by or attributed to acoustic deviations resulting from faulty oral articulation, especially those related to sibilant production. Clearly, aerodynamics should be considered an essential assessment method to determine the extent of "weak pressure consonants" and "nasal air emission." Although hypernasality and hyponasality are complex acoustic-perceptual phenomena associated with vowels and nasal consonants, respectively, they too may have identifiable aerodynamic substrates.

Because of the aforementioned factors, we believe that aerodynamic techniques should form an important part of the diagnostic procedures for individuals when VP inadequacy is suspected. Indeed, as noted by Peterson-Falzone et al. (2001), a comprehensive evaluation of VP function must include both perceptual and instrumental techniques. As described below, when aerodynamic techniques are appropriately employed, they provide objective documentation of intraoral air-pressure levels, rates of nasal air emission, and estimates of VP orifice size during consonant production. In addition, aerodynamic methods can be used to provide information on (a) the timing aspects of VP function during certain phonetic contexts and (b) the patency of the nasal airways during breathing. Such information can provide a firm basis for diagnostic decisions and/or postmanagement evaluation of individuals with cleft palate and/or VP dysfunction.

The following sections describe (a) basic principles of the pressure-flow technique, (b) instrumentation and calibration of equipment, (c) aerodynamic assessment of nasal respiration, and (d) aerodynamic assessment and characteristics of speech production in cleft palate. The first two sections lay the groundwork and theory of aerodynamic assessment techniques. The third section is included because, as indicated, the nasal airway is an important component relative to the perceptual aspects of speech production. The final section provides a detailed examination of aerodynamic characteristics of normal and cleft palate speech.

BASIC PRINCIPLES OF THE PRESSURE-FLOW TECHNIQUE

Warren and DuBois (1964) were the first to describe the use of aerodynamic principles to study the dynamics of the velopharyngeal (VP) mechanism during speech. Their procedure has often been referred to as the pressure-flow technique. By placing small-bore catheters in the oral cavity and in the nostril, respectively, along with the insertion of a flow tube into the remaining nostril, estimation can be made of the cross-sectional area of the VP port. The technique, therefore, provides an indirect method of determining the presence and extent of VP inadequacy.

Derivation of the "Orifice Equation"

As described by Warren and DuBois (1964), the cross-sectional area of a constriction or an orifice can be calculated if the differential pressure across the orifice and rate of airflow are measured simultaneously. In an ideal situation (see Figure 15–1), the static pressures (i.e., pressures associated with the moving airstream) are determined before the orifice (Point A) and at a point near the constriction (Point B). The difference between these pressures is the dynamic pressure loss. Assuming that airflow is steady or nonturbulent, the area of the orifice can be calculated using the dynamic pressure loss and a modification of Bernoulli's equation as follows:

$$A = \hat{V}/[2(p_1 - p_2)/D]^{1/2}$$

Pressure ports

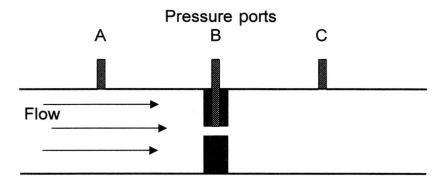

FIGURE 15–1 The area of a constriction can be calculated if the rate of airflow and the pressure loss across the constriction are measured. Either the dynamic pressure loss (from A to B) or the stagnation pressure loss (from A to C) are measured.

where A is orifice area in cm^2, $\hat{V}$ is airflow in ml/s, p_1 is static pressure in dynes/cm^2 before the orifice, p_2 is static pressure in dynes/cm^2 at the orifice, and D is the density of air (.001 gm/cm^3). As indicated by Warren and DuBois (1964), however, ideal or "theoretical" conditions do not exist in the human anatomy. In addition, because of practical limitations involving the placement of pressure probes, the static pressure at the constriction cannot be measured. The pressure-flow technique, therefore, uses a stagnation pressure (i.e., pressure associated with a low-velocity or nonmoving airstream) detected at Point C in Figure 15–1 to determine the pressure loss. As noted by Yates, McWilliams, and Vallino (1990), "the pressure loss created by the orifice is nearly equal to the dynamic pressure at the orifice" if the flow velocities before and after the orifice are small. Because these conditions are assumed in the human anatomy, and indirectly confirmed by Zajac and Yates (1991), the substitution of a stagnation pressure for a dynamic pressure is used in the pressure-flow technique.

As further noted by Warren and DuBois (1964), the substitution of a pressure measured downstream of the orifice is valid "if the kinetic energy of the gas passing through the orifice is lost due to turbulence on the nasal side of the orifice." Because the "theoretical" equation does not take turbulence into account, the calculated area will differ from the actual area. To overcome this problem, Warren and DuBois (1964) introduced a "correction factor k." This was a dimensionless coefficient, 0.65, derived from model tests of the upper vocal tract. Using short tubes that varied in area from 2.4 to 120.4 mm^2, they determined that an average value of 0.65 would suffice for the range of areas typically encountered in speakers with inadequate VP structures.[1]

Based on their model tests, Warren and DuBois (1964) modified the "theoretical" equation as follows:

$$A = \hat{V}/k[2(p_1 - p_2)/D]^{1/2}$$

where k is 0.65. Although Warren and DuBois (1964) referred to this as a "working equation," it has subsequently become known as the "orifice equation."

Application of the Pressure-Flow Technique

Air pressures during consonant production can be associated with a moving airstream (e.g., the fricative /s/) or a nonmoving air volume (e.g., the stop-plosive /p/). To detect these air pressures, small-bore catheters must be positioned behind the articulators of interest. To detect static pressures associated with fricative sounds, care must be taken to ensure that the opening of the catheter is positioned perpendicular to the direction of airflow. To detect stagnation pressures associated with stop consonants, the orientation of the catheter within the vocal tract is inconsequential—as long as it is behind the articulator of interest—due to equal pressure being exerted in all directions (Baken & Orlikoff, 2000). Practical placement of the catheters, therefore, is an important issue that will be addressed below.

Warren and DuBois (1964) originally used a balloon-tipped catheter placed in the posterior oropharynx (see Figure 15–2A and B). The catheter was passed through a nostril and secured by a cork at a level just below the resting velum. The catheter was then connected to a calibrated differential air pressure transducer referenced to atmosphere. A larger plastic tube was fitted to the speaker's other nostril and connected to a calibrated flowmeter. Because the balloon-tipped catheter was positioned behind the tongue, stagnation pressures associated with the place of articulation of all stop sounds (i.e., bilabial, alveolar, and velar) could easily be detected. These pressures reflected the driving pressure before the VP orifice, corresponding to Point A in Figure 15–1. Warren and DuBois (1964) noted that the use of a thin-walled balloon reduced pressure measurements by approximately 3% as compared with an open-tip catheter. The balloon

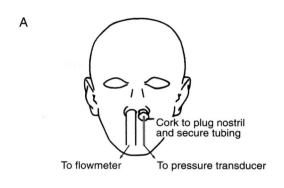

A

Cork to plug nostril and secure tubing

To flowmeter   To pressure transducer

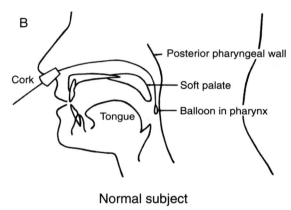

B

Posterior pharyngeal wall

Cork

Soft palate

Balloon in pharynx

Tongue

Normal subject

FIGURE 15–2 (A and B) The pressure-flow method as originally described by Warren and Dubois (1964). A. Front view. B. Side View. A balloon-tipped catheter was placed in the oropharnyx.

was used, however, to eliminate the possibility of saliva occluding the catheter. An additional advantage of using a transnasal placement of a catheter is that it does not interfere with tongue movements during articulation.

A disadvantage of the pressure-flow technique as illustrated in Figure 15–2 is that the differential pressure recorded during speech also includes a nasal pressure component when the VP portal is open. To overcome this problem, Warren and DuBois (1964) first instructed the speaker to breathe lightly through the nose with the lips closed. The differential pressure and nasal airflow values obtained during breathing were then plotted as x and y coordinates. As noted by Warren and DuBois (1964), although the differential pressure in theory also contains a VP orifice component during breathing, at low rates of nasal airflow typical of speech, this component is too small to be recorded. During speech, the measured flow rate for a specific segment is used to determine the nasal pressure component from the breathing plot. This pressure is then subtracted from the differential pressure obtained during speech.

In a subsequent report by Warren (1964), the pressure-flow technique was modified to permit direct estimation of the differential pressure across the VP orifice during speech production. As illustrated in Figure 15–3, a catheter was placed in the oral cavity to detect oral-pharyngeal pressure below the VP orifice and another catheter was placed in one of the nostrils. The latter catheter was held by a cork stopper that also served to occlude the nostril and create a stagnation pressure downstream (i.e., above) of the VP orifice. The oral and nasal catheters were connected to a calibrated differential pressure transducer. The remaining nostril was used to detect nasal airflow as described above.

A final modification of the pressure-flow technique was described by Warren, Dalston, Trier, and Holder (1985). Instead of recording differential oral-nasal pressure by means of a single transducer, they recorded oral and nasal

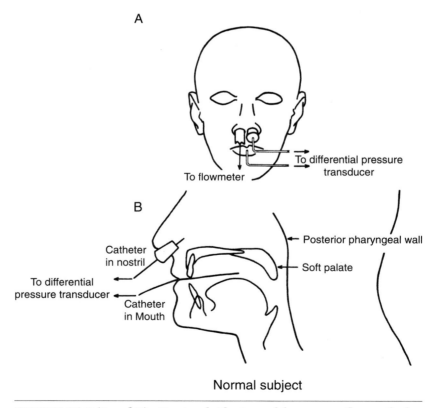

A

To flowmeter

To differential pressure transducer

B

Catheter in nostril

To differential pressure transducer

Catheter in Mouth

Posterior pharyngeal wall

Soft palate

Normal subject

FIGURE 15–3 (A and B) Front and side views of the pressure-flow method as modified by Warren (1964). Open-end catheters were placed in the nostril and the oropharnyx.

pressures separately by using two pressure transducers—each referenced to atmosphere. The differential pressure needed for the orifice equation was then calculated from the oral and nasal pressure values. An advantage of this modification was that true oral air pressure was obtained that could be compared to normative data. An estimate of subglottal pressure, therefore, could also be inferred from the oral pressure value during production of voiceless stop consonants.

INSTRUMENTATION AND CALIBRATION

Equipment

Contemporary measurement of air pressure and flow during speech production requires the use of appropriate transducers. Transducers convert the detected air pressure or flow into electrical signals for further processing. Transducers vary in construction, design, and performance characteristics. Figure 15–4 illustrates two types of differential air pressure transducers useful for speech work. A variable capacitance transducer (Figure 15–4A) consists of a diaphragm and an insulated electrode that forms a variable capacitor. As pressure is applied to the high (center) port relative to the low (or atmospheric) port, capacitance increases in proportion. Two of the transducers shown in Figure 15–4A have a pressure range of 0–15 inches of water (approximately 0–38 cm H_2O), useful for recording most pressures associated with speech activities. The upper limit of these transducers, for example, is approximately twice as high as pressures associated with even loud speech. The other two transducers shown have a pressure range of 0–0.5 inches of water, useful for recording the typically low airflow rates associated with

speech. Solid state transducers are illustrated in Figure 15–4B. Again, two of the transducers have relatively high ranges required for speech pressures while two have lower ranges appropriate for recording speech airflow. Both types of transducers have good response times (especially the solid state) and exhibit little drift (especially the variable capacitance).

The recording of speech airflow also requires the use of a heated pneumotachograph. This instrument, illustrated in Figure 15–5, provides a resistance by channeling airflow through a bundle of small diameter tubes housed within a larger conduit. The two pressure taps are connected to the ports of a differential pressure transducer. As indicated above, because the pressure drops associated with rates of airflow during speech are relatively low, a pressure transducer with a range of 0–0.5 or 0–1.0 inches of water is appropriate. The rate of airflow through the pneumotachograph is determined by measuring the differential pressure drop. Higher rates of airflow will produce a proportionally higher pressure drop for the given resistance. Pneumotachographs are available in different sizes for different applications. As indicated by Baken and Orlikoff (2000), the Fleisch #1 pneumotachograph (Figure 15–5) is appropriate for many speech applications. It has a maximum useful flow rate of 1.0 L/s, a resistance of 1.5 cm H_2O/L/s, and a dead space of 15 ml.

Calibration

Calibration of pressure-flow instrumentation is required to ensure that the output of the transducers is consistent with a known input. Calibration of pressure transducers is typically done using a U-tube water manometer. This device consists of a U-shaped glass tube partially filled with water. A scale—usually in

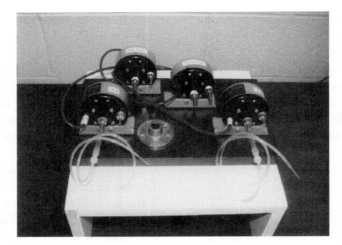

A

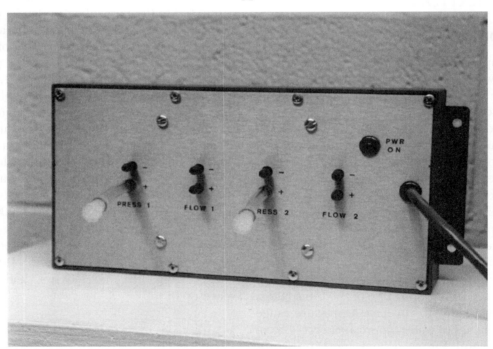

B

FIGURE 15–4 (A and B) A. Four variable-capacitance differential pressure transducers. The two in the foreground are used to measure air pressures. The two in the background are used to measure airflows. B. Four solid-state differential pressure transducers. Two are used to measured air pressures and two are used to measure airflows.

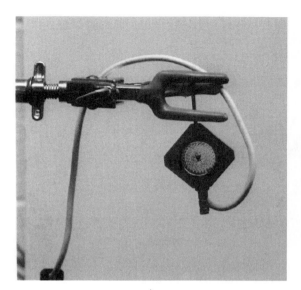

A

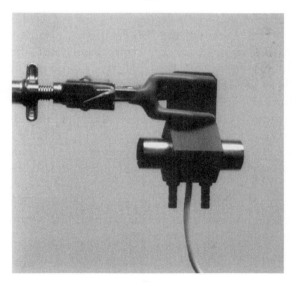

B

FIGURE 15–5 (A and B) A. Front view of a bidirectional pneumotachograph showing resistive channels. B. Side view of pneumotachograph showing static pressure ports.

centimeters of water (cm H_2O)—is positioned so that zero aligns with the meniscus of the water column. When a pressure is applied to one leg of the manometer, it depresses the

column of water in that leg while simultaneously elevating the column of water in the other leg. The amount of applied pressure is determined by summing the magnitude of displacement in both legs of the manometer. If the first column was depressed by 3 cm, for example, and the second column was elevated by 3 cm, then a total pressure of 6 cm H_2O was applied. A well-type manometer (Figure 15–6) is similar to a U-tube but provides for the direct reading of applied pressures. This type of manometer has a calibrated reservoir (the left leg in Figure 15–6) filled with water or oil. Zero on a centimeter scale is aligned with the meniscus of the reservoir. When pressure is applied to the reservoir, it causes the fluid to rise in a connected column. The height of the column of fluid indicates the applied pressure.

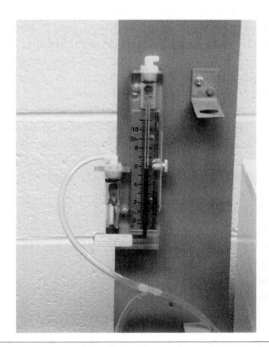

FIGURE 15–6 Well-type manometer. Applied pressure to the reservoir (left side) displaces the column of fluid on the right.

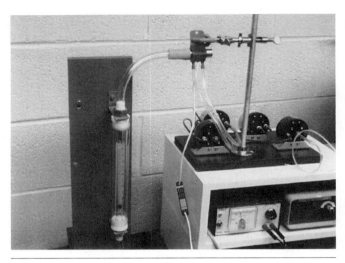

FIGURE 15–7 Calibration of pneumotachograph. A compressed air supply (not shown) delivers a known flow rate to a rotameter (left side in figure) that is coupled to a pneumotachograph and differential pressure transducer.

Calibration of the pneumotachograph is typically accomplished by using a compressed air supply and rotameter to provide a known rate of airflow as illustrated in Figure 15–7. A float or ball in the rotameter rises in proportion to the applied rate of airflow. A Gilmont rotameter is shown in Figure 15–7. This rotameter is calibrated in arbitrary units from 0 to 100. The units must be converted to ml/s (or L/s) by means of a calibration curve provided by the manufacturer. Other types of rotameters are available that are calibrated in units such as ml/s. A large volume syringe (e.g., 1–3 liters) may also be used to apply a known quantity of air across the pneumotachograph for calibration purposes. The advantage of this approach is that it eliminates the need for a compressed air supply that may not be available in all test settings.

Calibration of computer-based aerodynamic systems also involves the use of software programs that will determine and store calibration (or scale) factors for the various pressure transducers. The numerical scale factors indicate the relationship between the electrical voltage output of the transducer and the known input (i.e., the applied air pressure or flow). Currently, there are several manufacturers of speech aerodynamic equipment. They typically provide the basic components, including calibration devices and software programs, for complete assessment of patients. If clinicians are not familiar with calibration procedures, it is suggested that they seek assistance from someone with the requisite background (e.g., electrical technician, mechanical engineer) to setup and calibrate instrumentation.

ASSESSMENT OF THE NASAL AIRWAY

Nasal Airway Obstruction

Aerodynamic instrumentation can be used to evaluate nasal respiration and to quantify upper airway obstruction. Because nasal respiration involves resistance to airflow by both the nasal cavity and the velopharynx, obstruction may occur at either or both of these sites. Nasal airway obstruction is common in individuals with a history of cleft lip/palate or other craniofacial anomalies. This can be caused by maxillary retrusion, cranial base anomalies, a narrow hypopharynx, or enlarged adenoids, all of which restrict the nasopharyngeal airway. Other conditions, such as a septal deviation, choanal atresia, or a stenotic naris, restrict the size and patency of the nasal cavity. Even acute conditions, such as congestion or mucosal hypertrophy, can reduce nasal airway size. Any condition that obstructs and therefore attenuates the airflow through the nasopharynx or nasal cavity is a cause of nasal airway obstruction.

Individuals with cleft lip/palate are also susceptible to nasal airway obstruction as a consequence of the surgical procedures used to repair their defects. Indeed, work by Warren and colleagues indicated that children with repaired unilateral cleft lip and palate have significantly reduced nasal airway size as compared to noncleft children (Warren, Hairfield,

Dalston, Sidman, & Pillsbury, 1988). Individuals with a cleft of the soft palate who undergo secondary surgical procedures for residual velopharyngeal (VP) inadequacy are also at risk for posterior nasal airway obstruction. Such obstruction may not only result in hyponasal resonance, it may also interfere with health and daily living activities if severe enough to cause obstructive sleep apnea. Therefore, the evaluation of nasal resistance during respiration is of significance to both the speech-language pathologist and otolaryngologist.

Nasal Resistance and Rhinomanometry

Traditionally, measurements of nasal airway resistance have been obtained by using the techniques of anterior and posterior rhinomanometry. These techniques involve "the measurement of the pressure encountered by air passing through the nasal cavity" (Clement, 1984). During posterior rhinomanometry (Figure 15–8), the differential pressure between the oropharynx and

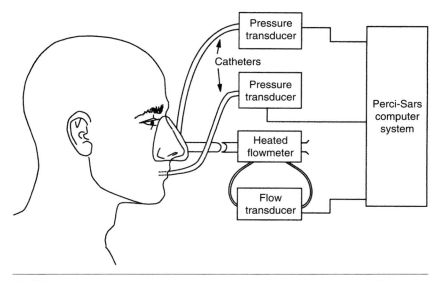

FIGURE 15–8 Posterior rhinomanometry. Both nostrils are evaluated simultaneously.

the external nostrils along with the simultaneous rate of nasal airflow are determined. The resulting nasal airway resistance measure, therefore, includes components of both the velopharynx and the nasal cavities. As previously indicated, however, the relaxed velum typically produces a negligible pressure drop during quiet breathing. During anterior rhinomanometry (Figure 15–9), the differential pressure is obtained between the exit of the nose and the atmosphere. This is achieved by occluding one of the nostrils with a cork/catheter assembly. As previously described, this condition creates a stagnation pressure downstream of the velopharynx. This pressure serves as the upstream (or driving) pressure to atmosphere. Because of the need to occlude a nostril, anterior rhinomanometry measures the resistance of only the unoccluded nostril. To

obtain resistance of the other nostril, the cork/catheter assembly and the nasal flow tube are reversed and the measurement is repeated. During either anterior or posterior rhinomanometry, it is important that the individual maintains lip closure while breathing in order to obtain valid results.

Once differential air pressure and nasal airflow measures are obtained by either anterior or posterior rhinomanometry, nasal resistance (R_n) may be calculated as:

$$R_n = P/\hat{V}_n,$$

where P is differential pressure in cm H_2O and $\hat{V}_n$ is nasal airflow in L/s. Nasal resistance, therefore, is expressed in units of cm H_2O/L/s. As noted by Clement (1984), although this formula is universally accepted for the calculation of nasal resistance, it is valid only when turbulent flow conditions are not present during nasal respiration. Depending on the degree of respiratory effort (i.e., the driving pressure provided by the lungs), airflow through the nasal cavity may be laminar or turbulent. Laminar flow is steady and smooth due to the lack of significant resistance. With the convolutions and irregularities in the passages of the nasal cavities, this causes turbulent flow. When airflow is laminar in nature, the relationship between pressure and flow is linear and the above equation for nasal resistance is valid. When airflow becomes turbulent, however, the pressure-flow relationship is quadratic and the resistance equation must be modified accordingly. To overcome this problem, many clinicians will measure nasal resistance at relatively low rates of airflow to avoid turbulent conditions and to ensure that comparisons among individuals are valid (Allison & Leeper, 1990; Berkinshaw, Spalding, & Vig, 1987; Warren, Duany, & Fischer, 1969). Berkinshaw et al. (1987), for example, suggested that a flow rate of 0.250 L/s be used because it is laminar in

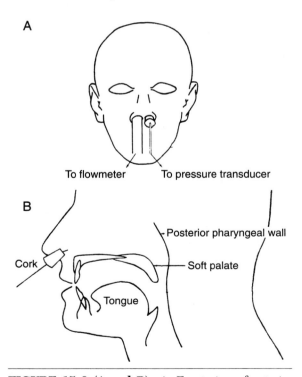

FIGURE 15–9 (A and B)   A. Front view of anterior rhinomanometry. Each nostril is evaluated separately. B. Side view.

nature and can easily be achieved by individuals even with nasal obstruction.

Estimation of Nasal Cross-Sectional Area

Warren (1984) demonstrated that the "orifice equation" could also be applied to pressure-flow measurements obtained during rhinomanometry to estimate nasal cross-sectional area. The use of an area measure effectively circumvents the problem of calculating nasal resistance when airflow is turbulent. This approach, therefore, permits the calculation of nasal area at any point and at any flow rate in the breathing cycle. The approach assumes that the calculated area reflects the smallest cross-sectional area of the nasal cavity. The anatomical location of this area—called the "nasal valve"—is approximately 1 cm posterior to the entrance of the nose (Bridger, 1970). The boundaries of the nasal valve are the septal wall medially, the alar cartilage laterally, and the anterior portion of the inferior turbinate. Collectively, these structures form the smallest constriction of the normal nasal passage. Warren and colleagues reported a nonlinear relationship between nasal cross-sectional area and nasal airflow in adults with varying degrees of nasal obstruction (Warren, Hairfield, Seaton, & Hinton, 1987). Specifically, they showed that the rate of nasal airflow was controlled by nasal cross-sectional area when the nasal airway size was less than 0.40 cm^2.

Subsequent studies by Warren and colleagues have indicated that the size of the nasal airway is age dependent (Warren et al., 1988; Warren, Hairfield, & Dalston, 1990). As with facial growth, nasal airway size appears to continue to increase up until about the age of 16–18. Warren et al. (1990), for example, used the pressure-flow technique to evaluate children between the ages of 6 and 15 years. They found that nasal airway size increased approximately 0.032 cm^2 each year, and mean nasal cross-sectional area increased from 0.21 cm^2 at age 6 to 0.46 cm^2 at age 14. The percentage of nasal breathing also increased with age in these children. Age, therefore, should always be considered when assessing the status of the nasal airway in children and adolescents.

Clinical Procedures: Posterior Rhinomanometry

The specific procedures of posterior rhinomanometry (Figure 15–8) are summarized as follows:

1. Nasal resistance and area are measured for both nostrils during inhalation and exhalation of quiet respiration.

2. A heated pneumotachograph is connected to a nasal mask, which is fitted snugly over the patient's nose. The rate of nasal airflow is measured in L/s and recorded by a computer.

3. A catheter connected to a pressure transducer is placed in the patient's mouth. This catheter detects oropharyngeal air pressure. Pressure is measured in cm H_2O and recorded by the computer.

4. A second catheter connected to a pressure transducer is inserted through the wall of the nasal mask. This catheter detects mask pressure—or the pressure external to the nostrils.

5. During the examination, the patient breathes quietly through the nose while maintaining lip closure. Simultaneous recordings are made of the rate of nasal airflow, oropharyngeal pressure, and mask pressure.

The pressure-flow breathing records from an adult without nasal obstruction are illustrated in Figure 15–10. The figure shows oropharyngeal

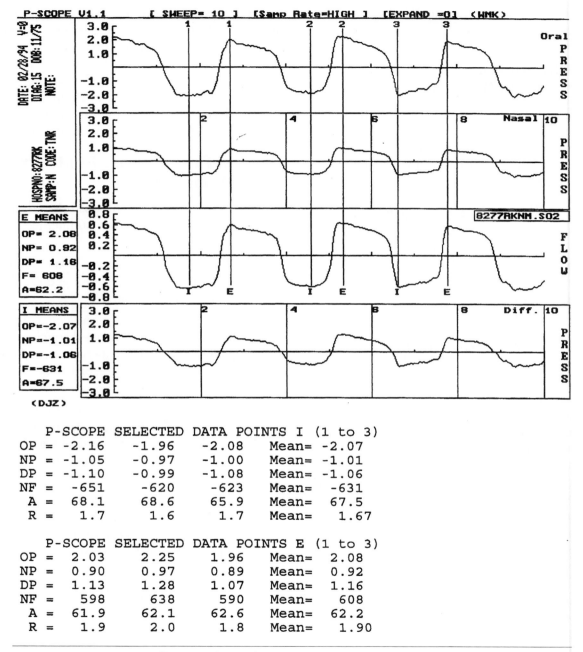

FIGURE 15–10 Pressure-flow recordings of breathing from an adult without nasal obstruction during posterior rhinomanometry. Calculated nasal area (a) is expressed in mm^2; calculated nasal resistance (R) is expressed in cm H$_2$O/L/s.

pressure, nasal (i.e., mask) pressure, nasal airflow, and calculated differential pressure from top to bottom, respectively. The three cursors labeled "I" indicate peak flow points during inspiration where measurements of nasal resistance and area were calculated. The three cursors labeled "E" show corresponding measurements made during expiration. All measurements and means are printed at the bottom of the figure. In addition, the rectangular boxes labeled "E Means" and "I Means" on the left of the figure provide a summary of the mean measurements for each parameter except nasal resistance. The mean nasal areas of the individual were 62.2 and 67.5 mm^2 during expiration and inspiration, respectively. As indicated by Warren (1984), a mean nasal area of approximately 60 mm^2 is typical of adults without nasal impairment.

Clinical Procedures: Anterior Rhinomanometry

The specific procedures of anterior rhinomanometry (Figure 15–9) are summarized as follows:

1. Nasal resistance and area are measured for each nostril separately during both inhalation and exhalation of quiet respiration.

2. A nasal flow tube connected to a heated pneumotachograph is placed snugly in one nostril of the patient. The rate of nasal airflow is measured in L/s and recorded by a computer.

3. A cork/catheter assembly connected to a pressure transducer is placed in the patient's other nostril. This catheter detects nasal cavity air pressure. Pressure is measured in cm H_2O and recorded by the computer.

4. During the examination, the patient breathes quietly through the nose while maintaining lip closure. Simultaneous recordings are made of the rate of nasal airflow and nasal cavity pressures. The nasal flow tube and cork/catheter assembly are then reversed and the procedures repeated. As noted by Riski (1988), care must be taken when using anterior rhinomanometry to ensure that an airtight seal is obtained with the nasal flow tube and that the cork/catheter assembly does not deform the nasal valve area of the unoccluded nostril.

Using the above procedures, left and right nasal areas during inspiration for the individual illustrated in Figure 15–10 were 43.8 and 17.9 mm^2, respectively. Because the individual did not have posterior nasal airway obstruction, the summation of the left and right nasal areas (61.7 mm^2) approximates the total nasal area (67.5 mm^2) obtained by posterior rhinomanometry. It must be noted, however, that if an individual has significant posterior nasal obstruction, then the two techniques will not correspond. The use of both anterior and posterior rhinomanometry, therefore, has the potential to identify the site of nasal obstruction in patients with clefts of either the primary and/or secondary palates. Although it is beyond the intended scope of this chapter, some clinicians have discussed the use of rhinomanometric techniques to partition the VP and nasal components of measured nasal resistance. The interested reader is referred to Smith, Fiala, and Guyette (1989).

SPEECH AERODYNAMICS AND VELOPHARYNGEAL FUNCTION

The pressure-flow technique is ideally suited to determine the magnitude of intraoral air pressure levels and the rates of nasal air emission during consonant production. It is important to realize, however, that intraoral air pressures vary with the type of consonant and phonetic context. Voiceless sounds are known to have greater intraoral pressure than voiced sounds due to the open glottis. In addition, intraoral air pressures tend to remain relatively constant at approximately 3.0 cm H_2O or higher, even in individuals with gross velopharyngeal (VP) dysfunction (Dalston, Warren, Morr, & Smith, 1988). This can be partly explained by the effects of increased nasal airway resistance, which is common in patients with a history of clefting as indicated above. Individuals with inadequate VP closure may also compensate for their oral pressure loss by increasing respiratory effort (Warren, Dalston, Morr, & Hairfield, 1989). Intraoral air pressures, therefore, may be affected by both increased nasal resistance and respiratory effort. Similarly, the rate of nasal airflow may be affected by increased nasal resistance. Measures of oral air pressure and/or nasal airflow, therefore, should be used with caution as indicators of VP function. The pressure-flow technique, however, circumvents these limitations by providing estimates of the size of the VP orifice that are, in theory, unaffected by changes in either respiratory effort and/or nasal resistance.

Clinical Procedures

The pressure-flow technique is noninvasive and involves minimal risk to the patient.[2] It requires, however, a certain level of cooperation in that the patient must place a flow tube in the nose and pressure catheters in the mouth and nostril. Figure 15–11 illustrates application of the pressure-flow technique with a school-age child. The specific

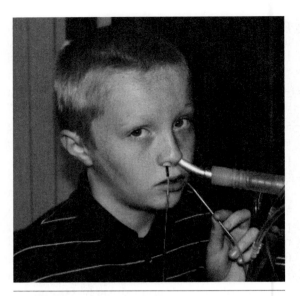

FIGURE 15–11 The pressure-flow technique to estimate velopharyngeal orifice areas during speech production.

procedures for estimating VP orifice size are as follows:

1. A plastic tube is inserted into the patient's more patent nostril. If anterior rhinomanometry has previously been performed, then the nostril with the larger area is selected. Otherwise, indirect estimation of the more patent nostril can be made using a mirror or detail reflector during quiet breathing with the mouth closed. The flow tube is connected to a heated pneumotachograph. The rate of nasal airflow is measured in L/s and recorded by a computer.

2. A cork/catheter assembly connected to a pressure transducer is placed in the patient's other nostril. This catheter detects a stagnation pressure downstream of the VP orifice. Pressure is measured in cm H_2O and recorded by the computer.

3. A catheter connected to a pressure transducer is placed in the patient's mouth. This catheter detects oral air pressure. Pressure is measured in cm H_2O and recorded by the computer.

As previously indicated, placement of the pressure catheter must be behind the articulator of interest in order to record a valid pressure. In addition, if the sound is associated with a moving airstream (e.g., /s/), then the open end of the catheter must be positioned perpendicular to the direction of airflow. Because of these requirements, clinicians most often evaluate VP function during production of the bilabial stop consonants. To evaluate the alveolar /s/ sound, the oral catheter should be occluded at the distal end, side holes placed in the catheter wall, and the catheter inserted to an area behind the alveolar ridge. Inserting the catheter from the side of the mouth during /s/ production will often reduce interference with articulation. To detect stagnation pressures associated with velar stops, a buccogingival catheter placement may be used. This approach, described below, permits valid detection of pressures associated with all oral consonants.

During the examination, simultaneous recordings are made of oral air pressure, nasal air pressure, and the rate of nasal airflow as the patient produces a series of speech samples designed to evaluate the VP mechanism. The speech samples typically employed by this author include the syllables /pi/, /pa/, /mi/, and /si/, the word "hamper," and the sentence "Peep into the hamper." The oral syllables are used because the VP mechanism must maintain closure during their repetition. The word "hamper" is tested because it contains the /mp/ sequence, which requires the speaker to rapidly adjust the VP mechanism from an open to closed configuration. Dynamic aspects of VP function, therefore, are assessed. The sentence is included to embed the word "hamper" in an utterance and thus approximate the conditions associated with continuous speech. The fricative /s/ is tested because this sound is most often associated with isolated nasal air emission seen in speakers with marginal VP function. In addition, the /s/ is also most often associated with phoneme-specific nasal air emission (PSNAE). This latter phenomenon is described below.

The following sections present actual pressure-flow recordings of speakers with adequate VP function and with varying degrees of VP inadequacy. The pressure-flow data were collected using the PERCI P-SCOPE system (MicroTronics, Inc., Chapel Hill, NC). In the recordings, oral pressure, nasal pressure, and nasal airflow are illustrated from top to bottom, respectively. In some recordings, calculated differential oral-nasal pressure is displayed. The pressures are shown in units of cm H_2O; airflow is expressed in L/s. Estimated VP areas are expressed in mm^2. Measurements were made at peak oral pressures for all oral consonants and at peak nasal flow for all nasal consonants. The locations of measurements are indicated by numbered cursors in the recordings. As indicated by Warren (1997), estimated VP areas are most accurate when the measurements are taken at the point of peak flow, where the rate of flow change is zero. Peak pressures were used for oral consonants because (a) there is typically no nasal airflow for speakers with adequate VP function, and (b) peak nasal airflow typically coincides with peak pressure for speakers with inadequate VP function. If the latter situation does not occur, however, then measurements should be made at the flow peak.

Speech Aerodynamics of Adequate Velopharyngeal Function

Figures 15–12 to 15–14 illustrate the pressure-flow recordings from an adult male speaker with adequate VP function saying the syllable /pi/, the word "hamper," and the sentence "Put the baby in the buggy," respectively. In Figure 15–12, the syllable is repeated eight times on a single breath with relatively equal stress placed on each syllable. The magnitude and shape of the oral air-pressure pulses are strikingly consistent across the repeated productions. Typically, if equal stress is not maintained throughout an utterance, the first pulse may have greater magnitude than the following pulses due to higher relaxation pressure available at the beginning of a breath group. The rise in slope of the first pressure pulse may also be steeper due to the lack of voicing from a preceding vowel. As indicated above,

voicing tends to reduce the magnitude of air pressure available to the oral cavity.

Figure 15–12 also illustrates that nasal air pressure and nasal airflow are present and in synchrony during respiration before and after the utterance. This confirms the patency of both nostrils required for valid estimation of VP orifice areas. Normal onset and offset nasal air emissions (NE) are evident at the beginning and end of the utterance. Onset NE reflects the transition of the VP mechanism from an open configuration during breathing to a closed configuration during speech. Offset NE reflects the converse transition from speech to breathing. Close examination of the nasal airflow signal reveals that the speaker exhibited approximately 40–50 ml/s of airflow during the beginning of the second pressure pulse. This type of inconsistent nasal airflow may have occurred due to several reasons. First, even in the presence of airtight VP

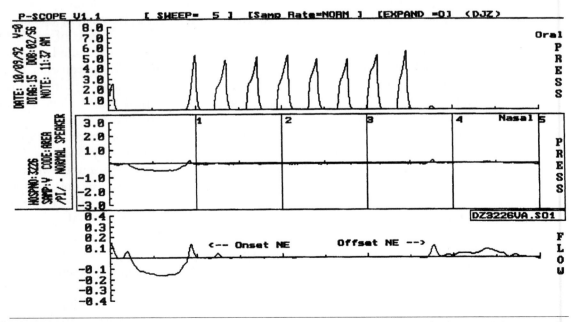

FIGURE 15–12 Pressure-flow recordings from an adult male with adequate velopharyngeal function. The syllable /pi/ was repeated eight times. Onset and offset nasal emission (NE) are evident at the beginning and end of the utterance.

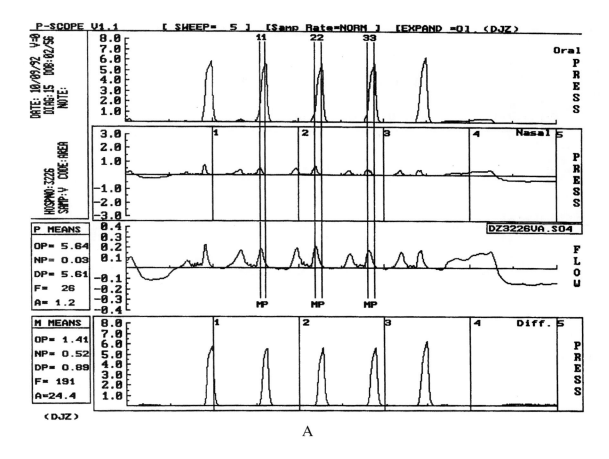

A

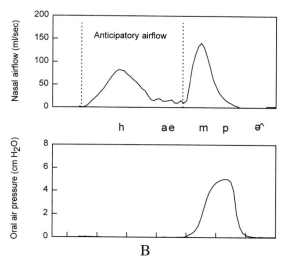

B

FIGURE 15–13 (A and B) A. Pressure-flow recordings from an adult male with adequate velopharyngeal function. The word "hamper" was repeated five times. B. Pressure-flow recordings of a single production of "hamper" with phonetic notation.

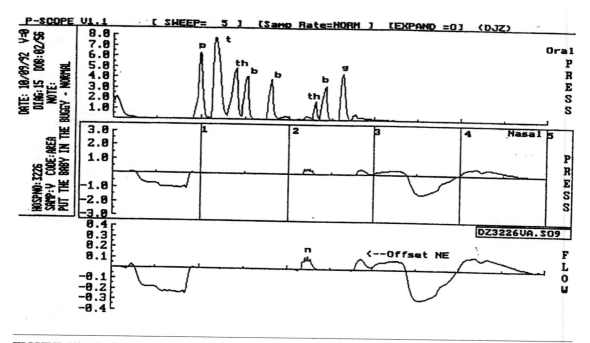

FIGURE 15–14   Pressure-flow recordings from an adult male with adequate velopharyngeal function. The sentence, "Put the baby in the buggy," was produced.

closure, muscular contractions of the velum may displace the nasal volume of air (Lubker & Moll, 1965). As noted by Thompson and Hixon (1979) and Hoit, Watson, Hixon, McMahon, and Johnson (1994), however, this phenomenon is typically characterized by both positive and negative flows with rates less than ±10 ml/s. Second, the nasal airflow may have occurred due to inadvertent movement of the flow tube. Artifact airflow resulting from compression of the flow tube, however, would also be bidirectional and relatively small in magnitude. Third, the VP mechanism of the speaker may have actually opened momentarily. As reported by Bell-Berti and Krakow (1990), velar height is reduced for vowels as compared with pressure consonants. Indeed, as noted by Moll (1962), VP closure may not be complete for all vowels, especially low vowels. Although the speaker produced the high vowel /i/, VP closure may

still have been incomplete, giving rise to nasal emission when oral pressure increased to a level that was sufficient to overcome the resistance of the nasal cavity. This last explanation may be most likely because the nasal airflow occurred following the initial vowel and did not reoccur during any of the subsequent syllables. One may speculate, therefore, that the speaker was able to implement an online adjustment that was facilitated by auditory feedback, aerodynamic feedback, or some combination of both.

It should also be noted that there may be a gender bias for inconsistent nasal emission. McKerns and Bzoch (1970) reported that males achieved VP closure with relatively less velar contact against the posterior pharyngeal wall than females. Zajac and Mayo (1996) also reported that males exhibited higher oral air pressures than females during production of "hamper." These findings suggest that subtle gender differences may exist relative to both respiratory and VP function. Such differences may cause males to be more prone to inconsistent nasal airflow than females. Although McWilliams, Morris, and Shelton (1990) also acknowledged the various reports on gender differences and VP function, they further questioned the clinical significance of the differences.

Figure 15–13A illustrates the same speaker saying the word "hamper" five times. Nasal air pressure and airflow are evident throughout the nasalized segments of each word. P-SCOPE software was used to measure oral air pressure, nasal air pressure, nasal airflow, and to calculate VP orifice areas of the /m/ and /p/ segments. The three vertical cursors labeled "M" indicate peak nasal flow where measurements were made for the /m/ segments. The three vertical cursors labeled "P" indicate peak oral pressure where measurements were made for the /p/ segments. As expected, peak nasal airflow associated with /m/ occurred before peak oral pressure for /p/. In addition, anticipatory nasal airflow occurred during the phonetic segments preceding peak nasal flow for /m/. Figure 15–13B illustrates a single production of "hamper" with accompanying notation to indicate the phonetic segments. As illustrated, nasal airflow was higher during the voiceless /h/ than during the vowel immediately preceding the nasal consonant. This was expected due to increased resistance provided by the vocal folds during voicing. Nasal airflow reached its peak during the /m/ segment when lip closure occurred. Although not shown in the illustration, the simultaneous acquisition of the speech audio signal facilitated the identification of phonetic segments. This capability is available in a newer version of the software (PERCI-SARS, MicroTronics, Inc., Chapel Hill, NC).

As indicated in the measurements of Figure 15–13A, mean oral pressure of the speaker during /p/ averaged approximately 5–6 cm H_2O. This value is typical of noncleft adult speakers saying "hamper" (Zajac & Mayo, 1996). Children typically average higher oral pressures (7–8 cm H_2O) than adults, depending on their specific age (Zajac, 2000). The reason for higher pressures is most likely due to the tendency of children to speak louder than adults. In addition, children have smaller surface areas of the vocal tract than adults. As explained by Müller and Brown (1981), a smaller surface area means that higher pressures must be generated to overcome the increased mechanical impedance to airflow. Nasal airflow of the speaker during the /p/ segments in Figure 15–13 averaged 26 ml/s and the estimated VP area was 1.2 mm^2. Although these values are typical of both children and adults (Zajac, in press), children tend to exhibit even lower rates of nasal airflow and smaller VP areas. This may be due to the fact that children typically possess greater amounts of adenoid tissue than adults. Nasal airflow of the speaker during the /m/ segments averaged 191 ml/s and the estimated VP area was 24.4 mm^2. Again, these are typical values for adult speakers. During /m/ production, children tend to show relatively reduced rates of nasal airflow and smaller VP areas. This is not surprising given that children tend to have larger adenoid tissue mass and smaller nasal cross-sectional areas than adults.

Finally, Figure 15–14 shows an example of continuous speech. The sentence "Put the baby in the buggy" was produced by the previous speaker. To record the oral pressures associated with the various consonants, a polyethylene catheter was heated and then molded so that its distal end approximated a 90° angle. The catheter was placed along the buccogingival sulcus with its angled end around the last mandibular molar, approximating the midline of the posterior oropharynx behind the tongue. This placement and orientation of the catheter permitted the valid recording of pressures associated with all consonants regardless of place of articulation. As illustrated in Figure 15–14, the voiceless consonants were associated with higher oral pressures than voiced consonants. This effect was most evident during production of /p/ and /b/, sounds that differ only in voicing. Consistent with adequate VP function, Figure 15–14 also reveals the absence of nasal air pressure and flow during the utterance except for the nasal segment.

Speech Aerodynamics of Inadequate Velopharyngeal Function

Figure 15–15 illustrates the pressure-flow recordings from a 12-year-old boy with a repaired bilateral cleft lip and palate while he repeated the syllable /pi/. Perceptually, the boy's speech was characterized by consistent but mild hypernasality, suggesting marginal VP function. Oral air pressures were somewhat reduced and variable during the utterance, ranging from approximately 2.5 to 5.5 cm H_2O. Consistent nasal emission of air occurred during the /p/ and vowel segments, averaging approximately 75 and 40 ml/s, respectively. In Figure 15–15, nasal emission during /p/ segments is reflected by the flow peaks and numbered vertical cursors. Nasal emission during vowels is reflected by the variable flow occurring between the flow peaks.

It must be noted that nasal airflow during vowel segments may not be readily detected by the pressure-flow method. This occurs because oral resistance to airflow is generally less than nasal resistance. Most of the airflow, therefore, will be shunted through the oral

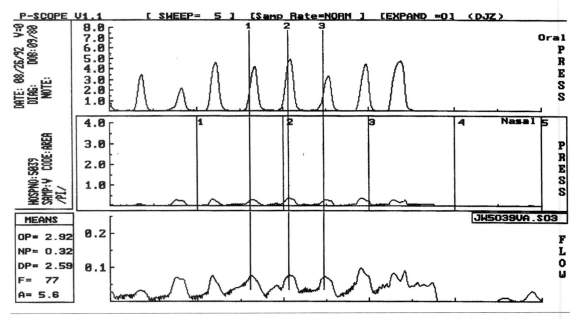

FIGURE 15–15 Pressure-flow recordings from a 12-year-old boy with repaired cleft lip and palate. The syllable /pi/ was repeated eight times. Estimates of velopharyngeal area were calculated at peak nasal airflow associated with the/p/ segments.

cavity even in the presence of a VP gap. The appearance of consistent nasal airflow during vowels in the speaker suggests the use of increased respiratory effort and/or altered lingual articulation as compensatory behaviors. Because of the consistent nasal air loss during /p/ production, however, the oral pressure measures may not be good indicators of overall respiratory effort.

The estimated size of this boy's VP gap was approximately 6 mm^2 during production of the /p/ segments. Based on this VP area, the boy's VP function would be categorized as "borderline adequate" according to criteria proposed by Warren et al. (1989). They suggested that VP areas under 5.0 mm^2 reflected adequate VP function, 5.0–9.9 mm^2 was borderline adequate, 10.0–19.9 mm^2 was borderline inadequate, and greater than 20 mm^2 was inadequate. It must be emphasized that these categories refer to the "respiratory requirements" of speech production, not perceptual aspects. The boy, whose recordings are illustrated in Figure 15–15, was capable of generating borderline-adequate oral air pressures for speech while clearly sounding hypernasal. This is an important distinction that clinicians must bear in mind when interpreting the VP area categories suggested by Warren et al. (1989). Overall, the pressure-flow records of the boy clearly indicate the marginal nature of his VP function. Borrowing a diagnostic term from Morris (1984), the boy, whose recordings are illustrated in Figure 15–15, may be considered to exhibit VP function that is "almost but not quite" adequate.

Figure 15–16 illustrates another example of a speaker with marginal VP function. The pressure-flow records are from a 7-year-old girl with a repaired bilateral cleft lip and palate while repeating the syllable /pi/. Perceptually, she exhibited inconsistent hypernasality and moderate hoarseness. The girl repeated the syllable eight times. Because the P-SCOPE

software was set to trigger automatically on a positive oral air-pressure value, only partial pressure-flow data were recorded for the first syllable. The seven numbered cursors in the figure, therefore, indicate pressure-flow measurements that were made for the last seven syllables. These measurements are listed at the bottom of the figure. Initially, the girl exhibited relatively low rates of nasal airflow during both consonant and vowel segments of the syllables. Estimated VP orifice areas during /p/ production were also well under 5 mm^2 for the second (cursor #1) and third (cursor #2) syllables. During production of the fifth syllable (cursor #4), however, VP orifice size increased dramatically to almost 40 mm^2, causing a drop in oral pressure to 1.42 cm H$_2$O. Beginning with the next syllable (cursor #5), the girl appeared to use a compensatory strategy as evidenced by a rise in oral pressure with concomitant decreases in both nasal airflow and estimated orifice size. By production of the seventh syllable (cursor #6), she had achieved essentially airtight VP closure. It should be noted that the duration of her oral air-pressure pulses increased during this process. Warren et al. (1989) have suggested that increased respiratory effort is a compensatory strategy employed by speakers with inadequate VP function. The increased duration of the oral air-pressure pulses suggests that some type of respiratory strategy occurred. Such a strategy, however, may also result in laryngeal hyperfunction and perceived dysphonia. Indeed, as previously noted, the girl exhibited vocal hoarseness. Again, using the diagnostic terms of Morris (1984), the VP function of this speaker may be categorized as "sometimes but not always" adequate.

The pressure-flow characteristics of a speaker with gross VP inadequacy are presented in Figures 15–17 and 15–18. The speaker was an almost 5-year-old girl with an

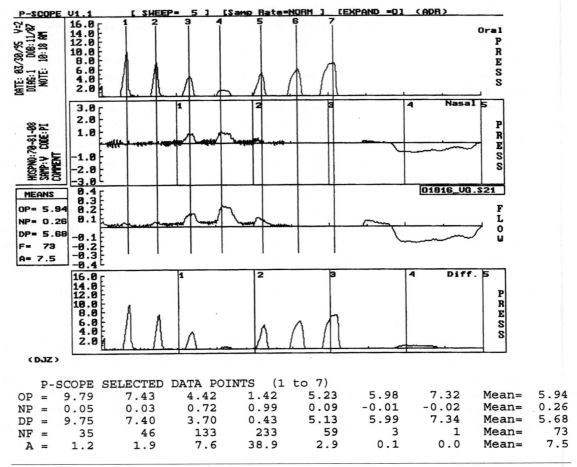

FIGURE 15–16 Pressure-flow recordings from a 7-year-old girl with repaired cleft lip and palate. The syllable / pi/ was repeated eight times.

unrepaired submucous cleft palate and hypernasal speech. Videofluoroscopy confirmed VP inadequacy. In Figure 15–17, she repeated the syllable /pa/ four times. Because of the extent of her VP inadequacy, nasal air pressures (2.86 cm H_2O) were slightly but consistently higher on average than oral air pressures (2.84 cm H_2O). This finding—relatively rare except in cases of severe inadequacy—invalidates the estimated VP orifice area shown in the figure. Nasal airflow during /p/ production was 181 ml/s on average. It should also be noted,

however, that relatively little nasal airflow was evident during vowel productions, as seen by the essentially baseline levels between the flow peaks.

In Figure 15–18, the same speaker repeated the word "hamper" five times. Because P-SCOPE software was set to an automatic trigger mode, pressure-flow data associated with the initial syllable in the first "hamper" were not recorded. The most striking feature of Figure 15–18 is the complete overlap of oral pressure, nasal pressure, and nasal airflow

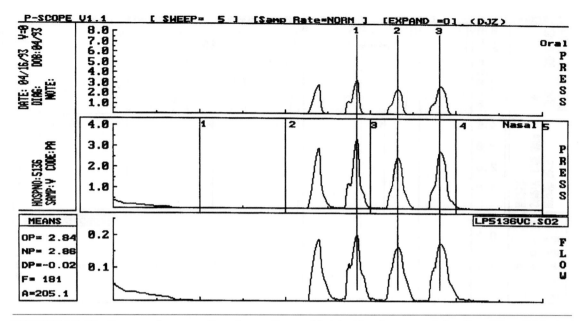

FIGURE 15–17 Pressure-flow recordings from a 5-year-old girl with submucous cleft palate. The syllable /pa/ was repeated four times.

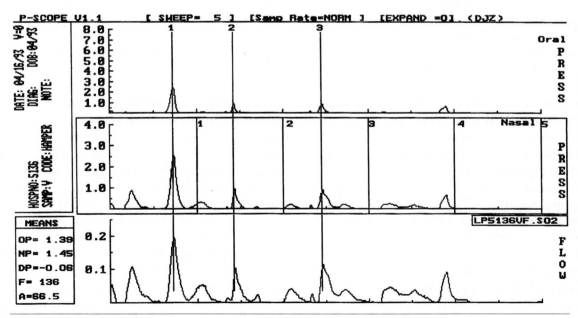

FIGURE 15–18 Pressure-flow recordings from a 5-year-old girl with submucous cleft palate. The word "hamper" was repeated five times.

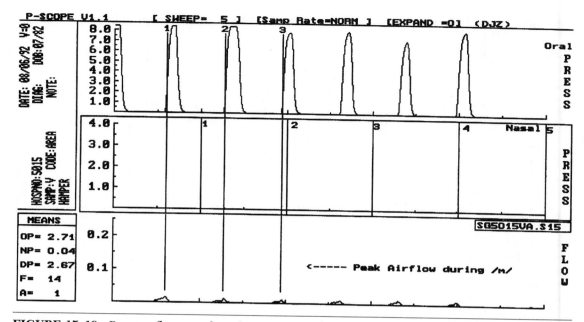

FIGURE 15–19 Pressure-flow recordings from a 10-year-old girl with a repaired cleft palate and a superior-based pharyngeal flap. The word "hamper" was repeated seven times.

during the /mp/ segments as indicated by the numbered vertical cursors. In essence, oral-nasal coupling was so complete that the speaker was unable to aerodynamically distinguish the /m/ from the /p/ segments in the words. Warren et al. (1989) showed that this overlap of pressure and airflow is a distinctive feature of inadequate VP function when orifice areas exceed 20 mm^2. Zajac and Mayo (1996) provided normative pressure-flow and timing data for the /mp/ segment in adult speakers. They reported a mean temporal separation of the nasal airflow and oral pressure pulse of approximately 70–75 ms. Finally, also demonstrated in Figure 15–18 is the speaker's inability to generate adequate oral air pressures. This is especially apparent after the initial productions of "hamper" when oral pressures dropped from approximately 2.5 cm H$_2$O (cursor #1) to 1.0 cm H$_2$O (cursor #2).

The pressure-flow recordings of "hamper" from a 10-year-old girl with a repaired cleft

palate and a superior-based pharyngeal flap are illustrated in Figure 15–19. Perceptually, the girl's speech was characterized by hyponasality, suggesting an obstructive pharyngeal flap. The aerodynamic correlate is clearly seen as a severe reduction in nasal airflow associated with the /m/ segments. In addition, expected anticipatory nasal airflow was entirely absent. Because rhinomanometric testing indicated normal nasal airway size prior to the secondary palatal surgery, these findings confirmed the suggestion of an obstructive pharyngeal flap.

Finally, Figure 15–20 illustrates the pressure-flow recordings of a 6-year-old boy without a history of cleft palate who exhibited a pattern of phoneme-specific nasal air emission (PSNE). Although the boy exhibited adequate VP function, his findings are presented because they have differential diagnostic value. The boy's speech was characterized by audible nasal air emission associated with all sibilant speech sounds. Trost (1981) has described this type of

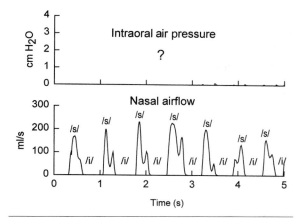

FIGURE 15–20 Pressure-flow recordings from a 6-year-old boy who exhibited a pattern of phoneme-specific nasal air emission. The syllable /si/ was repeated seven times. Oral air pressures were not detected due to deviant articulation.

articulation as a "posterior nasal fricative." All stop-plosive sounds and the /f/ and /v/ fricative sounds, however, were produced orally, indicating a learned articulatory pattern for the posterior nasal fricatives. The pressure-flow recordings in Figure 15–20 illustrate production of the target syllable /si/. Nasal airflow was evident during all expected /s/ segments (nasal pressure is not shown in the figure). More interesting, however, was the virtual lack of oral air pressures. As previously noted, oral air pressure is typically maintained at some minimal level even in the presence of severe VP inadequacy. The boy, however, had learned a pattern of phoneme-specific nasal emission that included the simultaneous articulation of a middorsum palatal stop during the posterior nasal fricative. This pattern of oral stopping was confirmed by subsequent perceptual and acoustic analyses of the separate oral and nasal audio signals obtained from the microphones of a Nasometer. In essence, the oral air pressure recordings were nearly atmospheric because the oral catheter was positioned at the alveolar ridge in anticipation of /s/. This anterior placement of

the catheter did not detect the pressure buildup at the palatal location of stop articulation.

Modifications for Young Children

The standard approach to pressure-flow testing (Figure 15–11) requires some degree of cooperation from the child and patency of both nostrils. If either or both of these conditions are lacking, the clinician may still gain valuable aerodynamic information by modifying the approach. One modification involves the acquisition of only differential oral-nasal air pressure data. As illustrated in Figure 15–21, the nasal pressure catheter is inserted into the nose while the clinician holds the oral pressure catheter behinds the lips of the child. Because nasal

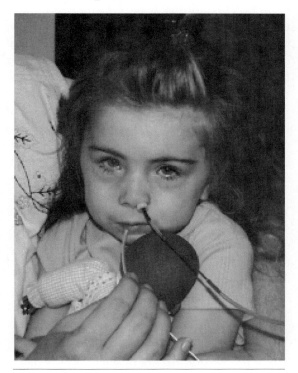

FIGURE 15–21 Determination of differential oral-nasal pressure of a young child.

airflow is not obtained, VP orifice area cannot be calculated. Adequacy of VP closure, however, can be inferred from differential pressure. According to Warren, Putnam Rochet, and Hinton (1997), VP closure is adequate if differential pressure is greater than 3.0 cm H_2O during production of /p/ in the word "hamper." VP closure is borderline if differential pressure is between 1.0 and 2.9 cm H_2O; closure is inadequate if differential pressure is below 1.0 cm H_2O. Similar to VP orifice area, differential oral-nasal pressure is relatively unaffected by changes in respiratory effort. Thus, this approach will yield valid results even with young children who typically tend to speak louder than older children and adults.

A second modification of the pressure-flow technique involves the use of a mask to obtain both nasal airflow and nasal air pressure during speech. This approach is often necessary if a child (a) is hesitant to insert tubes/catheters in the nose, and/or (b) has a unilateral nasal obstruction. The equipment configuration for this approach is the same as for posterior rhinomanometry (refer to Figure 15–8). Although an estimate of VP orifice area can be obtained, it requires a differential pressure correction. A correction is needed because the differential pressure recorded during speech also includes a nasal pressure component, similar to the original method described by Warren and DuBois (1964). The differential pressure correction, however, can be readily obtained by simply having the child breathe through the nasal mask with the lips closed around the oral pressure catheter.

Precautions and Limitations of the Pressure-Flow Technique

There are several factors of which the clinician must be aware during the acquisition and interpretation of pressure-flow measures. First, as previously indicated, to obtain accurate measures, the equipment must be properly calibrated. During the examination of patients, all tubing, masks, corks, and catheters must be intact, snugly fitted to the patient, and securely connected to other instrumental components. As Warren (1997) noted, tubing must be free of kinks and nasal masks must not be so tight that they distort the nasal valve. To estimate VP orifice size, both nostrils of the patient must be patent if the standard pressure-flow configuration (Figure 15–11) is used. Another concern is that the accuracy of VP orifice size estimations decreases significantly with openings that are 0.8 cm^2 or above (Warren, 1997). This occurs due to the limits of the pressure transducers in detecting small pressure changes. As indicated, however, most perceptual characteristics of VP inadequacy are clearly evident when orifice size exceeds 20 mm^2 (0.2 cm^2).

There is also debate in the literature about the appropriate value of the correction factor k to be used in the orifice equation. As noted by Müller and Brown (1981) and Yates et al. (1990), 0.65 may not be the most appropriate value for the geometry of the human VP orifice. Because of this uncertainty, it should be emphasized that VP area estimates are only relative measures. That is, as long as speakers exhibit similar VP orifice geometries, a relative comparison among individuals is possible using any value of k. Indeed, some researchers have omitted the k value entirely (e.g., Hixon, 1966).

Last, it must be reemphasized that, although aerodynamic procedures have the advantage of providing objective data relative to velopharyngeal closure, they do not provide direct information about perceptual aspects of speech production. As indicated throughout the previous examples, evaluation of voice quality, resonance, and articulation must be done using perceptual and/or other appropriate instrumental techniques.

SUMMARY

Since the original report by Warren and DuBois (1964), aerodynamic measures have been used by many researchers and clinicians to study the function of the velopharyngeal mechanism. The pressure-flow technique can give the examiner objective information regarding velopharyngeal function and respiratory parameters. Because of this, it should be considered an invaluable tool in the assessment of patients with cleft palate and/or suspected velopharyngeal dysfunction.

FOR REVIEW, DISCUSSION, AND CRITICAL THINKING

1. What is meant by speech aerodynamics? Why is it relevant to evaluate this in an individual with questionable velopharyngeal closure?

2. What is the pressure-flow technique? What does it measure? What information can be obtained from a pressure-flow evaluation?

3. Describe the equipment necessary for a pressure-flow examination. Where are the catheters and flow tube placed?

4. What does the orifice equation measure when there is velopharyngeal insufficiency? What does it measure when assessing upper airway obstruction?

5. Which consonant would be expected to have a higher degree of intraoral pressure, a /p/ or a /b/? Why?

6. What types of speech utterances are typically used in a pressure-flow evaluation? Why do you think that short speech segments are used instead of longer segments?

7. What is the diagnostic significance of nasal airflow measures? What is the diagnostic significance of orifice size estimates? What does a VP orifice size of 40 mm^2 suggest?

8. What are the advantages of the pressure-flow technique? What are the disadvantages?

REFERENCES

Allison, D. L., & Leeper, H. A. (1990). A comparison of noninvasive procedures to assess nasal airway resistance. *Cleft Palate Journal, 27*, 40–44.

Baken, R. J., & Orlikoff, R. F. (2000). *Clinical measurement of speech and voice* (2nd ed.). San Diego, CA: Singular.

Bell-Berti, F., & Krakow, R. A. (1990). Anticipatory velar lowering: A coproduction account. *Haskins Laboratories Status Report on Speech Research, SR-103/104,* 21–38.

Berkinshaw, E. R., Spalding, P. M., & Vig, P. S. (1987). The effect of methodology on the determination of nasal resistance. *American Journal of Orthodontic Dentofacial Orthopedics, 92,* 196–198.

Bridger, G. P. (1970). Physiology of the nasal valve. *Archives of Otolaryngology—Head & Neck Surgery, 92,* 543–553.

Clement, P. A. R. (1984). Committee report on standardization of rhinomanometry. *Rhinology, 22,* 151–155.

Dalston, R. M., Warren, D. W., Morr, K. E., & Smith, L. R. (1988). Intraoral pressure and its relationship to velopharyngeal inadequacy. *Cleft Palate Journal, 25,* 210–219.

Hixon, T. J. (1966). Turbulent noise sources for speech. *Folia Phoniatrica, 18,* 168–182.

Hoit, J. D., Watson, P. J., Hixon, K. E., McMahon, P., & Johnson, C. L. (1994). Age and velopharyngeal function. *Journal of Speech and Hearing Research, 37,* 295–302.

Lubker, J., & Moll, K. (1965). Simultaneous oral-nasal airflow measurements and cinefluorographic observations during speech production. *Cleft Palate Journal, 2,* 257–272.

McKerns, D., & Bzoch, K. R. (1970). Variations in velopharyngeal valving: The factor of sex. *Cleft Palate Journal, 7,* 652–662.

McWilliams, B. J., Morris, H. L., & Shelton, R. L. (1990). *Cleft palate speech* (2nd ed.). Philadelphia, PA: B. C. Decker.

Moll, K. L. (1962). Velopharyngeal closure on vowels. *Journal of Speech and Hearing Research, 17,* 30–77.

Morris, H. L. (1984). Marginal velopharyngeal incompetence. In H. Winitz (Ed.), *Treating articulation disorders: For clinicians by clinicians.* Baltimore, MD: University Park Press.

Müller, E. M., & Brown, W. S. (1981). Variations in the supraglottal air pressure waveform and their articulatory interpretation. In N. Lass (Ed.), *Speech and language: Advances in basic research and practice* (Vol. 4, pp. 317–389). New York: Academic Press.

Peterson-Falzone, S., Hardin-Jones, M., & Karnell, M. (2001). *Cleft Palate Speech* (3rd ed.). St Louis: MO: Mosby, Inc.

Riski, J. E. (1988). Nasal airway interference: Consideration for evaluation. *International Journal of Orofacial Myology, 14,* 11–21.

Smith, B. E., Fiala, K. J., & Guyette, T. W. (1989). Partitioning model nasal airway resistance into its nasal cavity and velopharyngeal orifice areas during steady flow conditions and during aerodynamic simulation of voiceless stop consonants. *Cleft Palate Journal, 21,* 18–21.

Sussman, J. E. (1992). Perceptual evaluation of speech production. In L. Brodsky, L. Holt, & D. H. Ritter-Schmidt (Eds.), *Craniofacial anomalies: An interdisciplinary approach.* St. Louis, MO: Mosby Yearbook.

Thompson, A. E., & Hixon, T. J. (1979). Nasal air flow during normal speech production. *Cleft Palate Journal, 16,* 412–420.

Trost, J. E. (1981). Articulatory additions to the classical description of the speech of persons with cleft palate. *Cleft Palate Journal, 18,* 193–203.

Warren, D. W. (1984). A quantitative technique for assessing nasal airway impairment. *American Journal of Orthodontics, 86,* 306–314.

Warren, D. W. (1997). Aerodynamic assessments and procedures to determine extent of velopharyngeal inadequacy. In K. R. Bzoch (Ed.), *Communicative disorders related to cleft lip and palate* (4th ed.). Austin TX: Pro-Ed.

Warren, D. W., Dalston, R. M., Morr, K., & Hairfield, W. (1989). The speech regulating system: Temporal and aerodynamic responses to velopharyngeal inadequacy. *Journal of Speech and Hearing Research, 32,* 566–575.

Warren D. W., Dalston, R. M., Trier, W. C., & Holder, M. B. (1985). A pressure-flow technique for quantifying temporal patterns of palatopharyngeal closure. *Cleft Palate Journal, 22,* 11–19.

Warren, D. W., Duany, L. F., & Fischer, N. D. (1969). Nasal pathway resistance in normal and cleft lip and palate subjects. *Cleft Palate Journal, 6,* 134–140.

Warren, D. W., & DuBois, A. (1964). A pressure-flow technique for measuring velopharyngeal orifice area during continuous speech. *Cleft Palate Journal, 1,* 52–71.

Warren, D. W., Hairfield, W. M., & Dalston, E. T. (1990). Effect of age on nasal cross-sectional area and respiratory mode in children. *Laryngoscope, 100,* 89–93.

Warren, D. W., Hairfield, W. M., Dalston, E. T., Sidman, J. D., & Pillsbury, H. C. (1988). Effects of cleft lip and palate on the nasal airway in children. *Archives of Otolaryngology—Head & Neck Surgery, 114,* 987–992.

Warren, D. W., Hairfield, W. M., Seaton, D. L., & Hinton, V. A. (1987). The relationship between nasal airway cross-sectional area and nasal resistance. *American Journal of Orthodontic Dentofacial Orthopedics, 92,* 390–395.

Warren, D. W., Putnam Rochet, A., & Hinton V. (1997). Aerodynamics. In M. McNeil (Ed.), *Clinical management of sensorimotor speech disorders.* New York: Thieme Medical Publisher.

Yates, C. C., McWilliams, B. J., & Vallino, L. D. (1990). The pressure-flow method: Some fundamental concepts. *Cleft Palate Journal, 27,* 193–198.

Zajac, D. J. (2000). Pressure-flow characteristics of /m/ and /p/ production in speakers without cleft palate: Developmental findings. *The Cleft Palate-Craniofacial Journal, 37*(5), 468–477.

Zajac, D. J., & Mayo, R. (1996). Aerodynamic and temporal aspects of velopharyngeal function in normal speakers. *Journal of Speech and Hearing Research, 39,* 1199–1207.

Zajac, D. J., & Yates, C. C. (1991). Accuracy of the pressure-flow method in estimating induced velopharyngeal orifice area: Effects of the flow coefficient. *Journal of Speech and Hearing Research, 34,* 1073–1078.

ENDNOTES

1. Although Yates et al. (1990) inferred that Warren and DuBois (1964) used "rectangular, thin plate orifices," Warren has clarified that the original model actually used short tubes to derive the k coefficient (personal communication, March 27, 2000).

2. There is always the inherent risk that patients, especially children, may accidentally harm themselves around pressure-flow (or any laboratory) equipment. Standard safety precautions, therefore, should be followed. Care should also be taken to ensure that flow tubing and/or corks do not have sharp edges that may irritate or cut the nasal skin and/or mucosa.

CHAPTER

16

VIDEOFLUOROSCOPY AND OTHER FORMS OF RADIOGRAPHY

CHAPTER OUTLINE

INTRODUCTION

Velopharyngeal dysfunction can be accurately diagnosed with a perceptual speech examination by an experienced speech pathologist. However, a wide spectrum of anatomical and physiological abnormalities can cause velopharyngeal dysfunction. Before one can determine the appropriate form of intervention, it is important to specifically define the cause of the problem and the size and location of the defect (Van Demark et al., 1985).

Videofluoroscopy is a radiographic procedure that can be used to diagnose the cause of velopharyngeal dysfunction. This technique allows visualization of all aspects of the velopharyngeal portal during speech, through the use of several standard views (Skolnick, 1970; Skolnick & Cohn, 1989; Skolnick & McCall, 1971). Because there is visualization of velopharyngeal function during speech through this procedure, it is considered a direct measure. Videofluoroscopy can help the examiner to assess both the anatomical and physiological abnormalities that are causing velopharyngeal dysfunction so that the optimal surgical or prosthetic treatment for the patient can be determined.

Videofluoroscopy was the first effective means of evaluating the entire velopharyngeal mechanism directly. It has been used for over 35 years. With the advent of nasopharyngoscopy, however, opinions vary regarding whether videofluoroscopy is the best method for evaluating velopharyngeal function (Henningsson & Isberg, 1991; Rowe & D'Antonio, 2005; Seagle, Mazaheri, Dixon-Wood, & Williams, 2002). Some centers use both videofluoroscopy and nasopharyngoscopy, while other centers no longer use videofluoroscopy, or use it only in selected cases. In February 2006, an online survey of members of the American Cleft Palate-Craniofacial Association was done through the listserv. Out of 123 respondents, 21% reported that they always use videofluoroscopy for patients with a history of cleft and 50% said they always use nasopharyngoscopy. For patients with no history of cleft, 25% said they always use videofluoroscopy and 62% said they always use nasopharyngoscopy. When asked which procedure gives the most information, 22% choose videofluoroscopy and 78% choose nasopharyngoscopy.

Although videofluoroscopy is not used as extensively as it once was, it is still used by many centers, at least occasionally. Therefore, the professionals who treat patients with velopharyngeal dysfunction need to be knowledgeable of its uses, advantages, and disadvantages.

The purpose of the chapter is to explain how radiographic images are used in the evaluation of velopharyngeal function. The specific procedures for a videofluoroscopic speech study are reviewed. Most importantly, the interpretation of the images is discussed as they relate to the diagnosis and treatment of velopharyngeal dysfunction.

RADIOGRAPHY/IMAGING

Radiography refers to the use of the roentgen ray (X-ray) to image internal body parts. As the ray goes through the body, it creates an image on the other side. The image then shows structures as light images and air space as a dark image. Due to the fact that the beam goes entirely through a structure, it will project the summation of all of the parts of that structure through which the beam passes. In other words, it will show matter whether the matter is consistent throughout or only occurs in a small portion of the line of the beam.

Conventional radiography depends on natural attenuation of the different tissues. *Attenuation* is the combined absorption and scattering of radiation proton particles by the tissues. The greater the attenuation, as in bone, the fewer radiation particles that reach the image, resulting in less exposure and hence, an image that is near the white end of the spectrum. The less attenuation (as in air) that there is, the greater the radiation particles that reach the film will be. This results in more exposure, so the image is near the black end of the spectrum.

Traditionally, radiographic images were recorded on film or videotape. Most systems now use high-resolution digital imaging. The many advantages of digital radiographs include the fact that they can be viewed on a computer, are of greater resolution, and can be stored electronically with the written report.

Most radiographic images are planar, or two-dimensional in nature. To image a volume structure adequately, it must be examined in three mutually perpendicular planes to fully appreciate that structure (Skolnick & Cohn, 1989; Skolnick, McCall, & Barnes, 1973). Of course, the velopharyngeal port is a structure of both dimension and volume.

Lateral Cephalometric Images and Cineradiography

Lateral cephalometric X-rays are still radiographic images of the midsagittal plane of the head. They are typically taken in a dental professional's office using a standard head holder. Through a process called *laminography*, which involves careful measurement of the distances and angles between particular landmarks on the image, orthodontists and oral surgeons are able to use lateral cephalometric images to study and measure the craniofacial bones and parameters of growth.

The lateral "ceph" shows the hard palate, the velum, and the posterior pharyngeal wall. In the 1950s, lateral cephalometric X-rays were used extensively in cleft palate research (Lubker & Morris, 1968; Yules & Chase, 1968; Yules, Northway, & Chase, 1968). In fact, the role of adenoid tissue in velopharyngeal closure was better understood with the use of this procedure (Subtelny & Koepp-Baker, 1956). The lateral "ceph" remains an excellent means for evaluating the status of the cervical spine, the cranial base angle, and the morphologic features of the facial skeleton by comparing findings to normative data. Cervical spine and cranial base anomalies can affect the position of the pharyngeal wall for velopharyngeal closure and therefore, if these conditions are suspected, this is a good diagnostic procedure.

However, cephalometric images are no longer used for routine assessment of velopharyngeal function for several reasons. First of all, a lateral ceph is a still image and, therefore, the movement of the velopharyngeal structures during speech cannot be evaluated with this procedure. The image must be taken with the production of a single continuant, such as /s/, which is not a good representation of true speech.

Another problem is that a lateral ceph shows only the midsagittal section of the velopharyngeal portal. Views to visualize the lateral pharyngeal walls are not possible using cephalometric images because the structures cannot be seen well with this type of radiograph. Since the velopharyngeal mechanism is a three-dimensional dynamic structure, it is therefore impossible to adequately evaluate it through the use of a lateral cephalometric X-ray alone. In fact, it has been estimated that, when judgments are based on a lateral X-ray alone, the examiner is likely to misdiagnose the presence or absence of velopharyngeal insufficiency on the order of 30% of the time, as compared with the use of a multiview technique (Williams & Eisenbach, 1981).

The use of *cineradiography* as a method for evaluating velopharyngeal function was first introduced in the early 1950s. Often referred to as a *cine study*, this technique involved taking a series of 16 to 24 frames of radiographs per second, which were recorded on motion picture film. However, there was no way to simultaneously record sound, and thus the speech, with this procedure so correlating movement patterns with speech phonemes was not possible (Shprintzen, 1995). A significant methodological advancement was made when multiview *videofluoroscopy* was first introduced.

Magnetic Resonance Imaging (MRI)

Magnetic resonance imaging (MRI) is a non-invasive method of using a magnetic field and radio waves to produce detailed images of the inside of the human body. MRI provides a very clear view of internal body structures with a remarkable level of detail. MRI has been used successfully for the evaluation of obstructive sleep apnea in pediatric patients (Abbott, Donnelly, Dardzinski, Poe, Chini, & Amin, 2004; Donnelly, 2004, 2005; Shott, 2004). MRI is an effective method of imaging and measuring the anatomy of the levator veli palatini muscle and related structures (Ettema, Kuehn, Perlman, & Alperin, 2002; Kuehn, Ettema, Goldwasser, & Barkmeier, 2004) or for diagnosing an occult submucous cleft palate (Kuehn, Ettema, Goldwasser, Barkmeier, & Wachtel, 2001). Some authors have suggested the use of MRI as a means for evaluating velopharyngeal function (Akguner, 1999; Beer et al., 2004; Kane, Butman, Mullick, Skopec, & Choyke, 2002; McGowan, Hatabu, Yousem, Randall, & Kressel, 1992; Ozgur, Tuncbilek, & Cila, 2000; Witt, Marsh, McFarland, & Riski, 2000; Yamawaki, Nishimura, Suzuki, Sawada, & Yamawaki, 1997). With improving cine MRI techniques, that motion can now be depicted and this is being used to evaluate pharyngeal motion in obstructive sleep apnea (Donnelly, 2005; Donnelly, Shott, LaRose, Chini, & Amin, 2004; Shott & Donnelly, 2004).

MRI can provide high-resolution images of the soft tissues of the velopharyngeal sphincter in all planes (Ozgur et al., 2000). Although the individual images are very clear, a primary disadvantage of MRI in evaluating velopharyngeal function is the static nature of the imaging. Movement of the structures during speech cannot be appreciated. Noise, the potential for claustrophobia during the exam, and expense are other disadvantages. Because of these disadvantages, MRI is not a standard procedure for evaluating velopharyngeal function at this time.

Videofluoroscopy

Multiview *videofluoroscopy* was first introduced by Skolnick in 1969 (Skolnick, 1969, 1970; Skolnick & McCall, 1971). Videofluoroscopy is a technique for visualizing the structures and function of the velopharyngeal mechanism. For an excellent resource on the use of videofluoroscopy in the evaluation of velopharyngeal function, please refer to the book by Skolnick and Cohn (1989).

Using multiview videofluoroscopy, the examiner can confirm the presence of a velopharyngeal opening and estimate the size of that opening. The cause of velopharyngeal dysfunction can be differentiated between a short velum or poor velar movement. Videofluoroscopy is not as helpful in assessing the extent and symmetry of lateral pharyngeal wall motion. In comparison with nasopharyngoscopy, videofluoroscopy is superior in showing the upward movement of the velum during speech. It also provides a view of the entire length of the pharyngeal wall during closure.

Videofluoroscopy is a procedure that can help to determine surgical and prosthetic options for the treatment of velopharyngeal dysfunction. It can also be helpful in assessing the placement of a prosthetic device, particularly a palatal lift. Finally, it can be used to evaluate the effects of surgical procedures, such as adenoidectomy, maxillary advancement, retropharyngeal implant, and to a limited extent, a pharyngeal flap (Shprintzen, 1995).

VIDEOFLUOROSCOPY PROCEDURE

Preparation of the Patient

Because most patients who require an evaluation of velopharyngeal function are children, special consideration must be taken in preparing the patient and the parent for the study and making them comfortable during the procedure. Many centers help to orient the family to the videofluoroscopy procedure by sending information in the mail at the time that the appointment is scheduled. Information in the form of a story book or coloring book is particularly well received by children. The speech pathologist can also help to prepare the patient and parent by describing the procedure so that they will know what to expect on the day of the appointment. Having the child practice repeating the standard phrases and sentences while simulating the various positions for the views can also give the child an idea of what to expect.

During the examination, it is important for the X-ray technologist to speak calmly to the child and reassure the child about the procedure. Telling the child what will happen before it happens is always a good idea. The parents can always help by supporting the child and possibly by offering a reward for cooperation during the study.

Purpose of Multiple Views

The velopharyngeal port is a three-dimensional structure that operates as a sphincter, with movement from all sides of the port. Therefore, it is important to view all aspects of this sphincter in order to determine the point of deficiency (Shprintzen, 1995; Shprintzen, Rakof, Skolnick, & Lavorato, 1977; Skolnick, 1975; Skolnick, McCall, & Barnes, 1973). With fluoroscopic imaging however, only two-dimensional views can be obtained. In order to view all aspects of the velopharyngeal sphincter with fluoroscopy, it is necessary to obtain multiple views. The use of three mutually perpendicular planes is usually recommended for fully evaluating the port (Skolnick & Cohn, 1989; Skolnick & McCall, 1971). These include the lateral view, the frontal view (also known as the *anterior-posterior* or *AP view*), and the *base view*. The name of the view (e.g., lateral view) denotes the direction in which the radiation beam passes through the body. In addition to the standard views, there are some supplemental views (Towne's view and oblique view) that can also be used for certain diagnostic circumstances. When multiple views are used, the examiner can evaluate the motion of all structures of the velopharyngeal valve.

Lateral View

For the *lateral view*, the beam enters the side of the head. As such, it shows the velum and posterior pharyngeal wall in a midsagittal plane. For this view, the patient is ideally placed in an upright position. The fluoroscopic table is vertically positioned and the patient stands or sits between the table and the fluoroscopic screen (Figure 16–1). The head

remains in a neutral position with the patient looking straight ahead. For a young child who has difficulty holding still, the child can lie on the table on his or her side (Figure 16–2). A special pillow is used to support and stabilize the head. The disadvantage of this position is the potential effect of gravity on velar movement, although this effect may be negligible. In order to be sure that the head is not rotated or tilted during the study, the examiner should always be sure that the rami of both sides of the mandible are superimposed on the view. This is very important because, if a true lateral view is not obtained, it may appear that there is closure when there is not, due to the position of the head.

Frontal View

The frontal view, also called the anterior-posterior or simply the AP view, allows the examiner to visualize the lateral pharyngeal

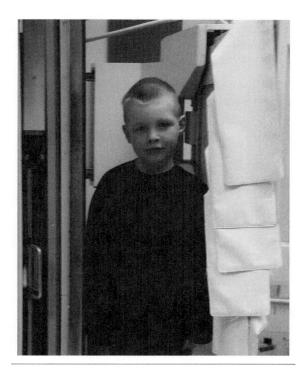

FIGURE 16–1 Patient position for the lateral view. The fluoroscopic table is vertically positioned and the patient stands or sits between the table and the fluoroscopic screen. The head remains in a neutral position with the patient looking straight ahead.

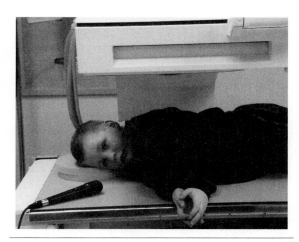

FIGURE 16–2 Alternate patient position for the lateral view. This is used if the patient needs more head support. For a young child who has difficulty holding still, the child can lie on the table on his or her side. A special pillow is used to support and stabilize the head. The disadvantage of this position is the potential effect of gravity on velar movement, although this effect may be negligible.

walls at rest and during speech. The X-ray beam is directed through the nose so that it is tangential to the plane of the velar eminence, which is usually appreciated as an arc between the lateral pharyngeal walls.

For the frontal view, the patient is positioned to face forward so that the beam is directed straight through the front of the nose. The patient can be upright, or placed in a supine position (Figure 16–3). It is very important that the head is centered for the frontal projection and is not rotated. This can be determined by observing the nasal septum and making sure that it appears to be in midline. The septum should be equidistant from the lateral margins of the maxillary cavity, and the incisor teeth should appear to be on either side of the nasal septum, allowing for deviations in structures. During nasal breathing, the lateral pharyngeal walls can be seen to bow outward on either side of the nasal septum. With speech, the lateral pharyngeal walls can be observed to bow inward where they appear to meet the area of the nasal septum.

Base View

The base view, also called an *enface view*, allows the examiner to see the entire velopharyngeal sphincter as if looking up through the port. With this orientation, the relative contributions of the velum, the lateral pharyngeal walls, and posterior pharyngeal wall to closure can be determined.

For the base view, the patient is placed on the X-ray table in a prone position. The patient is then asked to assume a "sphinx position" by pulling the head up and placing the upper body weight on the arms and elbows (Figure 16–4). The head and the back are then hyperextended so that the X-ray beam can be

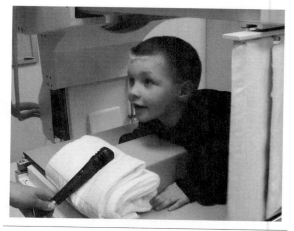

FIGURE 16–4 Patient position for the base view. The patient is placed on the X-ray table in a prone position and then asked to assume a "sphinx position" by pulling the head up and placing the upper body weight on the arms and elbows. The head and the back are then hyperextended so that the X-ray beam can be directed vertically through the base of the chin and then up through the velopharyngeal port. The correct positioning is important since the beam must be directly at right angles to the plane of closure.

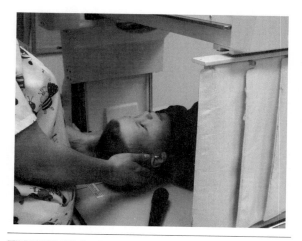

FIGURE 16–3 Patient position for the frontal or AP (anterior-posterior) view. The patient is placed in a supine position and the head is centered. This can be determined by observing the nasal septum through the fluoroscope and making sure that it appears to be in midline.

directed vertically through the base of the chin and then up through the velopharyngeal port. The correct positioning of the base view is actually very difficult, because the beam must be directly at right angles to the plane of closure. Otherwise, the port will not be visualized or the dimensions of the port will be severely distorted. The presence of large adenoids can also affect the interpretation of this view (Witt et al., 2000).

Towne's View

The *Towne's view* has been described as an alternative to the base view because it also provides an *en face* orientation (Stringer & Witzel, 1986, 1989). However, instead of looking up into the port, as is done with the base view, this view allows the examiner to look down into the port from above. The Towne's view is similar in orientation to the view that is seen through a nasopharyngoscope.

For the Towne's view, the patient is seated upright with the chin tucked and the head hyperflexed. The beam goes through the top of the head and intersects the plane of the portal in a perpendicular manner. When the adenoids are large, the Towne's view may provide a better view of the velopharyngeal portal than the base view (La Rossa, Brown, Cohen, & Spackman, 1980; Stringer & Witzel, 1986, 1989).

Oblique View

The *oblique view* might be chosen if a satisfactory base view cannot be obtained due to large adenoids or the inability to hyperextend the neck (Skolnick & Cohn, 1989). As with the base view, this view also helps the examiner to relate the movements of structures seen on the lateral view to those on the frontal view. It can also be helpful in visualizing asymmetrical movement of the lateral pharyngeal walls, which is actually quite common. It has been estimated that about 15% of patients with velopharyngeal dysfunction have asymmetrical lateral wall movement (Argamaso, Levandowski, Golding-Kushner, & Shprintzen, 1994; D'Antonio, Muntz, Marsh, Marty-Grames, & Backensto-Marsh, 1988).

The oblique view is performed by having the patient sit facing forward. With the fluoroscopy on, the patient slowly rotates the head and body as a single unit so that it moves 45% to one side, back to the midline, and then 45% to the other side. Because it is important to compare the movements on both sides with each other, a repetitive speech sample (i.e., pa, pa, pa, pa, pa) must be used.

Use of Contrast Material

The radiopaque contrast substance most commonly used to view the nasopharyngeal structures is a suspension of barium sulfate. This can be purchased as a premixed liquid or as a powder that is mixed with water. Skolnick and Cohn (1989) recommend using a consistency of heavy cream. Flavoring is often added to the mixture as well.

Barium is needed for the frontal and base views in order to view the structures adequately. It is not usually used for the lateral view, however, because the velum and posterior pharyngeal wall are actually better visualized without contrast. This is due to the fact that there is a column of air in the pharynx or space between these structures. The air is less absorbent of X-ray photons than the soft tissues of the velum and posterior pharyngeal wall. As a result, the air appears black, which provides contrast against the soft tissue density of the velum and posterior pharyngeal wall. Another reason that barium is usually not used for the lateral view is that it can mix with mucus and cause the velum to appear longer than it actually is and can also obscure the point of closure.

When the barium is added, however, it is sometimes helpful to repeat the lateral view. With the barium, a Passavant's ridge may become more obvious (Cohn, Rood, McWilliams, Skolnick, & Abdelmalek, 1984). Barium can also be helpful in illustrating the patency of an oronasal fistula on the lateral view. If the fistula is patent, the barium can often be seen as it drips from the nasal cavity through the fistula to the oral cavity (Skolnick, Glaser, & McWilliams, 1980). Having the patient swallow barium may show regurgitation up into the fistula. Finally, barium on the lateral view can sometimes outline a defect in the nasal surface of the velum as a result of a submucous cleft. Since barium can produce artifacts or occasionally obscure structures on the lateral view, it is recommend that lateral videofluoroscopy always be performed without barium first and then again with barium only if specific information is needed.

Prior to instilling the barium into the nasopharynx, the patient is asked to blow his or her nose to discharge any secretions that could interfere with the exam. One way to instill the barium into the nasal passages is through a soft rubber catheter that is inserted in a nostril and then pushed through the nose to the nasopharynx. A spray of Pontocaine in the nose a few minutes prior to inserting the catheter can help to numb the nasal cavity for more comfortable insertion. In addition, a small amount of viscous lidocaine (Xylocaine) can be applied to the tip of the catheter to help ease it through the nasal meatus. These steps are not required, however, as there is very little discomfort with the catheter insertion. A syringe is then used to place the barium through the catheter (Figure 16–5).

Another method is to simply drip the barium through the nares using a large nose dropper or

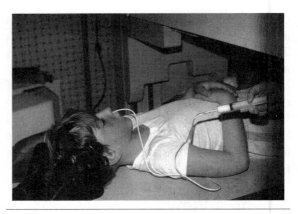

FIGURE 16–5   A method for instilling barium into the nasopharynx is through the use of a large syringe and catheter. The barium is squeezed through the catheter to the nasopharynx.

pipette. The head is hyperextended or the patient is placed in a supine position so that gravity helps to move the barium back to the nasopharynx. The patient is asked to sniff the barium and the head of the patient is rotated to be sure that the soft palate and pharyngeal walls become adequately coated with the contrast material. This is important because, without an adequate and even coating of barium over all the structures, the view may be useless to the examiner. The drip method is usually less frightening to young children, but it can delay the procedure and may not result in adequate coverage of the tissues. Regardless of the method used, approximately 1 to 3 ml of barium is needed in each nostril for adequate coverage.

When barium is introduced in the nasopharynx through the nose, it causes the eyes to water and gives the sensation that is felt when water goes into the nose. A burning sensation in the nasopharynx can last for an hour or more following its introduction. Although the barium can cause some discomfort and minor irritation, most children tolerate the procedure fairly well, especially if they are prepared for what to expect. However, if the child cries during this procedure, the secretions can wash the barium down. When that occurs, more barium needs to be passed into the nasopharynx for the study.

With all views, barium can also be helpful in the identification of small gaps that cannot otherwise be seen due to the resolution. Fortunately, air pressure going through a small opening often causes bubbling of the barium. The observation of bubbling always indicates a small gap. However, the absence of reflux and bubbling is not similarly diagnostic. When there is a larger velopharyngeal gap, there is less concentrated air pressure going through the opening and therefore, bubbling is less likely to occur.

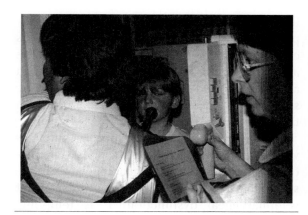

FIGURE 16–6 The X-ray technician asks the patient to repeat syllables and standard sentences. A microphone is placed near the patient's head so that it can record the speech simultaneously with the visual images.

Speech Sample

During the projection for each view, the patient should first be asked to swallow. With the act of swallowing, the velopharyngeal structures come together forcefully and are easy to identify. This helps the X-ray technologist to be sure that the orientation is correct, and it can also be useful when the study is interpreted because it orients the evaluators to the location of the structures. The technologist then asks the patient to repeat syllables or standard sentences. A microphone is placed near the patient's head so that it can record the speech simultaneously with the visual images (Figure 16–6).

The speech pathologist does not need to be present during the examination in most cases. However, it is very important that the speech sample is selected by a speech pathologist. The speech sample should include a variety of pressure-sensitive phonemes in connected speech at the sentence level. Because the /s/ sound is most often affected by velopharyngeal dysfunction, the sample should include at least one sentence with a frequent occurrence of

this sound. A sentence such as "Sissy sees the sun in the sky" can be particularly useful because it not only contains many /s/ sounds, but it also contains an /s/ blend, which further challenges velopharyngeal closure. In addition, it has some nasal sounds in the middle of the sentence, so the velum has to go up, come down, and then go up again to reach its target. It is also helpful to have the patient repeat syllables with pressure-sensitive phonemes (i.e., pa, pa, pa; pee, pee, pee; ta, ta, ta; tee, tee, tee; ka, ka, ka; kee, kee, kee; sa, sa, sa; see, see, see; etc.). Repeating "60, 60, 60" or counting from 60 to 70 are especially good speech segments to use because they require the production of fricatives and plosives, with a blend and high vowel. This type of phonemic combination is especially taxing on the velopharyngeal mechanism and therefore, it is most likely to show a problem if there is one.

There is sometimes a need to augment the standard sentences that are determined for use with each patient during a videofluoroscopic examination. For example, a longer connected speech sample might be needed when there is inconsistent velopharyngeal function or velopharyngeal dysfunction with fatigue. In this case, rote speech, such as counting or the alphabet, can be used. The speech sample can also be designed to test the patient's specific speech errors based on the observations from the speech assessment.

The composition of the speech sample is very important because, if it does not adequately tax the velopharyngeal mechanism, the study may not identify mild or inconsistent velopharyngeal dysfunction. It is tempting, therefore, to test all speech phonemes for a comprehensive speech examination. However, it is more important to keep the sample as short as possible to minimize the amount of radiation exposure to the patient (Isberg, Julin, Kraepelien, & Henrikson, 1989). If the sentences that are chosen contain many pressure-sensitive phonemes, no more than 20 seconds of speech is needed to obtain an adequate speech sample.

INTERPRETATION

Who Performs and Interprets the Study?

With good angles and good barium contrast, a videofluoroscopic speech study can be performed perfectly by the X-ray technologist. However, the study is only as good as the interpretation. Experience, skill, and careful analysis are required for interpretation of the study.

Although the radiologist or X-ray technologist actually performs the study, both the radiologist and the speech pathologist need to work together to interpret the study. The radiologist has a thorough understanding of the anatomy, physiology, and imaging of the velopharyngeal structures. The speech pathologist also understands the anatomy and physiology, but particularly understands the physiology of normal and abnormal speech. The speech pathologist has a unique perspective regarding the correlation between velopharyngeal function and the acoustic product of speech. With both perspectives, the interpretation of the study is more complete and accurate.

Interpretation of the Lateral View

On the lateral view, the examiner should observe the length, thickness, and contour of the velum, both at rest and during phonation. During phonation, the velum should elevate to the approximate level of the hard palate. There should be a bend in the velum at a point that is about two-thirds of the distance from the hard palate to the tip of the uvula. This bend, or "knee action," is at the point of insertion of the levator veli palatini muscles and occurs as the levator sling contracts to pull the velum up and back. When the velum makes contact with the posterior pharyngeal wall, the extent of contact between the velar eminence (the high point on the top of the "knee") down through the vertical part of the velum should be noted. The extent of the contact area gives an indication of the firmness of closure. If the contact area is small, it might be assumed that the closure is tenuous.

On the posterior pharyngeal wall, the presence and approximate size of an adenoid pad should be noted. The adenoid pad usually appears as a smooth, convex structure that is either on the same plane as the hard palate or slightly higher. If there is no adenoid mass, the depth and contour of the pharyngeal wall should be assessed. The examiner should note the relative depth of the pharynx during nasal breathing and then observe the anterior motion of the posterior pharyngeal wall, if this occurs, with speech. When a Passavant's ridge is present, it can be viewed during speech as a shelf-like projection on the posterior pharyngeal wall. Tonsillar tissue can be seen somewhat on this view. It appears as an oval mass that is superimposed over the area of the posterior tongue.

Tongue movement during articulation should always be assessed from this view. In some cases, the posterior portion of the tongue can be observed to assist in elevating the velum during speech. If this is occurring, then the apparent movement of the velum and the resultant closure is actually very deceiving. In addition, the movement of the tongue tip, dorsum, the posterior tongue, and even the larynx should be observed to determine if there are compensatory productions, such as glottal stops, pharyngeal plosives, pharyngeal fricatives, or middorsum palatal stops. Abnormal tongue movement, including backing of articulation or the use of the dorsum for articulation, should also be noted.

Evidence of abnormality may include a short velum relative to the posterior pharyngeal wall, a thin velum, or poor knee action of the velum during speech. Figure 16–7 shows a lateral view of a patient with a short velum relative to the posterior pharyngeal wall, resulting in velopharyngeal insufficiency. Figure 16–8 shows a velum with poor movement and little knee action, resulting in velopharyngeal incompetence. The extent of the velopharyngeal opening as a result of these abnormalities should be noted.

On the lateral view, the examiner may also note evidence of a patent oronasal fistula if barium is used. Other abnormalities may include a localized indentation on the posterior pharyngeal wall following the removal of the adenoids. The appearance of hypertrophic tonsils or adenoids that intrude into the airway would also indicate a problem.

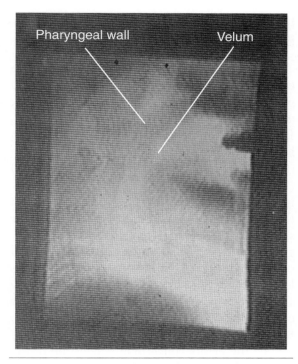

FIGURE 16–7 Lateral view showing a short velum relative to the posterior pharyngeal wall, which results in velopharyngeal insufficiency.

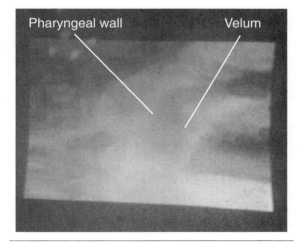

FIGURE 16–8 Lateral view showing a velum of normal length, but poor movement during speech, which results in velopharyngeal incompetence.

Interpretation of the Frontal View

The purpose of the *frontal view* is to assess the extent of lateral pharyngeal wall motion, the symmetry of movement between the two sides, and the approximate level of maximum motion. In most normal speakers, the point of maximum lateral pharyngeal wall motion is just below the plane of the velar eminence (see Figure 1–15A) (Skolnick & Cohn, 1989). Interpreting this view is a challenge because of the superimposition of the vomer and facial structures. The examiner should also remember that, because this view goes from the front to the back, the lateral wall on the right side of the screen is on the patient's left side and vice versa. The side of deficiency should be reported based on the patient's right or left, rather than on the examiner's orientation. Standard markers can be used on the image to reduce the errors concerning which side of the body is imaged.

The observation of poor lateral wall movement may suggest a problem with velopharyngeal closure. On the other hand, the patient may merely have a coronal pattern of closure, which requires only minimal lateral wall movement. Figure 16–9 shows the frontal view of a patient. The barium-coated lateral pharyngeal walls are on either side of the septum. When there is a small velopharyngeal opening, bubbling of barium is often noted on this view. The examiner should note if the point of bubbling is in the midline or skewed to one side.

In some cases, the lateral pharyngeal walls will appear asymmetrical in their position at rest and during speech. Before making this judgment, however, it is important to be sure that the orientation of the view is appropriate and that the head was not turned slightly to give a false impression. Asymmetry in lateral wall movement can cause a velopharyngeal opening

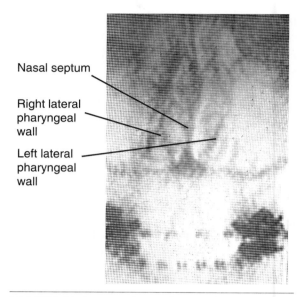

Nasal septum

Right lateral pharyngeal wall

Left lateral pharyngeal wall

FIGURE 16–9 Frontal view showing the nasal septum in midline. The lateral pharyngeal walls are well coated with barium and bow outward during nasal breathing as noted in the frame.

on the side with the least amount of movement. Another abnormality may be found when there is asymmetry in the vertical dimension. In this case, the level of maximum lateral wall movement is higher on one side than on the other. All of these observations are important to document because they have implications for appropriate surgical management.

Interpretation of the Base View

If the head is positioned properly for the base view so that the beam goes directly through the velopharyngeal port, the margins of the port appear as an oval or round structure during nasal breathing. The lateral and posterior pharyngeal walls can be seen easily with this view if there is an adequate coating of barium. The velum, which appears at the top of the oval, is harder to visualize because it does not pick up as much barium. During speech, the structures can be observed to narrow and then close the lumen as a sphincter. Depending on the basic pattern of closure, a black horizontal line (with a coronal pattern), a vertical line (with a sagittal pattern), or a circle (with a circular pattern) will remain in the middle of the closure area. Figure 16–10 shows the nasopharyngeal port through the base view. Figure 16–10A shows the port entirely open. The port begins to close in Figure 16–10B and is entirely closed in Figure 16–10C, leaving a small circle. On this view, the examiner should be careful not to confuse movement of the

tongue and vocal folds with velopharyngeal movement. In addition, the large foramen magnum can be seen on this view and this should not be mistaken for the velopharyngeal port.

When there is velopharyngeal dysfunction, the pharyngeal lumen does not appear to totally close. In fact, an opening during speech is a clear indication of velopharyngeal dysfunction. The examiner should also observe the symmetry of both sides of the port and note asymmetrical movement during speech. As with the frontal view, the left lateral wall will

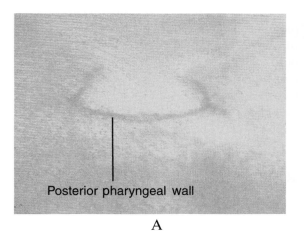

Posterior pharyngeal wall

A

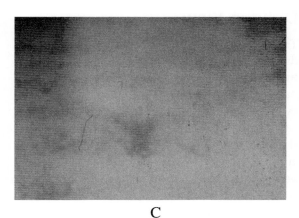

C

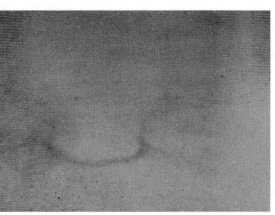

B

FIGURE 16–10 (A–C) Base view with the posterior pharyngeal wall at the bottom of the screen. A. The entire port is open for nasal breathing. B. The port is partly closed. C. The port is totally closed. This represents a circular pattern of closure.

be on the right side of the screen and vice versa. With a small velopharyngeal gap, bubbling of barium can often be seen on this view.

Interpretation of the Towne's View

Because the Towne's view is similar to the base view (only looking from above), the same observations and cautions apply. Again, the examiner should note that the patient's left lateral wall is seen on the right side of the screen and vice versa.

Interpretation of the Oblique View

The oblique view can be difficult to interpret due to the superimposition of multiple structures over the area of interest. A coating of barium can make interpretation easier, however, and a swallow prior to the speech sample can help to orient the examiner to the structures of concern. As in the frontal, base, and Towne's view, the patient's right side will be seen on the left side of the screen and vice versa.

On the oblique view, the examiner should observe each lateral wall individually. The lateral wall should be viewed at rest and then during speech to determine if it closes against the velum. A notation should be made if there is an apparent gap between the lateral wall and velum on that side. Of course, bubbling of the barium should be noted, because it indicates a small velopharyngeal opening.

Overall Results

Based on the information obtained from all views, the examiner must assimilate the information and make a determination of the extent of closure, the approximate gap size, the gap location, and the basic pattern of closure. This information is used to determine the appropriate type of treatment. If surgical intervention is planned, this information is especially important because it allows the surgeon to design the correction based on the abnormality.

Interpretation of the various views typically involves subjective analyses only. Direct measurement is difficult to do since the image on the screen is not life-sized and depends on a variety of factors. However, measurements are sometimes needed for research purposes. This can be done by putting a ruler or something of a known dimension in each view. For the view that is of interest, the examiner can then take a stop-frame at rest, and once again at the patient's best attempt at closure. The structures can then be traced off of the monitor onto a sheet of acetate paper. From this hard copy, quantifiable measurements can be made, using as a reference the object with a known dimension (Williams, Henningsson, & Pegoraro-Krook, 1997).

REPORTING THE RESULTS

Some centers report the results of videofluoroscopy with a narrative report, using a few short paragraphs. Other centers use a scale to rate various parameters of structure and function as noted on each view. The first published rating scale was developed by McWilliams-Neely and Bradley (1964). Since that time, others have made additions and modifications to this basic scale. In 1990, a group of clinicians was assembled by the American Cleft Palate-Craniofacial Association to develop a standardized method for interpreting and reporting the results from videofluoroscopy and nasopharyngoscopy (Golding-Kushner et al., 1990). A procedure was developed that attempts to quantify the movement of the velopharyngeal structures relative to each structure's resting position and the resting position of the opposing structure. This is done as a ratio rather than as an absolute measurement. For example, the resting position of the velum is at the 0.0 point and the point of closure against the pharyngeal wall is 1.0. If the velum raises and closes 50% of the opening, then velar displacement is at a rating of 0.5 along the trajectory toward the posterior pharyngeal wall. This estimation is done for each lateral wall and for the posterior pharyngeal wall as well. Although this system may be used by some, it is somewhat complicated and the inter- and even intrajudge reliability has been an issue. Therefore, it is not used by all centers.

Whether a specific rating scale is used or a narrative report is done, it is important to be consistent in the observations that are made and in the way that they are reported. This is particularly important if preoperative and postoperative studies are done for comparison.

ADVANTAGES AND LIMITATIONS OF VIDEOFLUOROSCOPY

Videofluoroscopy has the particular advantage of providing a view of the relationship between the velum and posterior pharyngeal wall through the lateral view. With this view, it is easy to determine if there is velopharyngeal insufficiency due to a short velum or velopharyngeal incompetence due to poor velar movement. In comparison with nasopharyngoscopy, videofluoroscopy is superior in showing the length of the velum and its upward movement during speech. It also provides a view of the entire length of the posterior pharyngeal wall during closure. As such, it is better than nasopharyngoscopy for looking at the pharynx below the velum during speech (Witt et al.,

2000). The fact that the study is recorded (on video or digital images) allows the study to be viewed by multiple team members after completion of the study.

A primary disadvantage of videofluoroscopy is the radiation exposure, even with the new systems that require lower doses. As with any X-ray procedure, there is always a concern about the amount of radiation exposure associated with the test. However, the aim of pediatric radiology is to keep the radiation dose to the minimum needed to obtain the required diagnostic information. Skolnick and Cohn (1989) estimated that for one minute of videofluoroscopy in the lateral view, the radiation exposure is between 0.025 rad and 0.5 rad. For the frontal and base views, which require a higher radiation level for adequate resolution, the exposure was estimated to be from 0.125 rad to 1.00 rad (Skolnick & Cohn, 1989). By way of comparison, a single lateral cephalometric X-ray is about 0.25 rad and a single CT slice is between 1 and 4 rads. In addition, digital radiographic techniques have significantly reduced the radiation dose (Vetter & Strecker, 2001). Therefore, although X-ray procedures are not innocuous and can potentially result in somatic and genetic damage, the dosage for videofluoroscopy is extremely low in comparison with many other types of X-ray procedures. In addition, the benefits gained from this procedure, despite the radiation exposure, must always be weighed against the consequences of deciding on a course of treatment without adequate information.

Another disadvantage of videofluoroscopy is that the overall resolution of a radiographic procedure is not as good as a direct view. In fact, the ability to visualize structures, such as the velum and posterior pharyngeal wall, depends on these structures being surrounded by air (Skolnick & Cohn, 1989). However, as the velopharyngeal port narrows for closure, the amount of air between the velum and pharyngeal wall is markedly reduced and finally disappears during contact. Therefore, the ability to distinguish the margins of each structure becomes more difficult, if not impossible. As a result, a small gap may not be seen at all. The only clue to its presence may be occasional bubbling of the barium. Gaps as a result of irregular adenoids cannot be seen. In addition, the X-ray beam goes through all of the structures in the plane, as noted previously, so the image represents a sum of all the parts. Therefore, if the velum touches the posterior pharyngeal wall at any point in the coronal plane, it will look as if there is complete closure, even if the velum does not contact the pharyngeal wall at all points. In addition, if the beam is not perfectly perpendicular to the opening, the gap may not be visualized.

Videofluoroscopy is not a good procedure for evaluating the placement and the results of secondary procedures, either. It is very difficult to see a pharyngeal flap or sphincteroplasty with this procedure unless there is a very good coating of barium (Figure 16–11 A–C). In fact, the presence of either could actually be missed altogether.

Although videofluoroscopy is considered less invasive than nasopharyngoscopy by some professionals, the introduction of barium into the nasopharynx can be very unpleasant. It can cause watering of the eyes and a burning sensation that can persist for an hour or more. The large equipment can also be frightening to young children.

The final disadvantage is that, although videofluoroscopy shows all of the velopharyngeal structures and their function through the use of multiple views, the examiner has to essentially extrapolate information from each view in order to imagine the three-dimensional structure and its function. Videofluoroscopy does not provide a clear view of all the structures as they function in the multidimen-

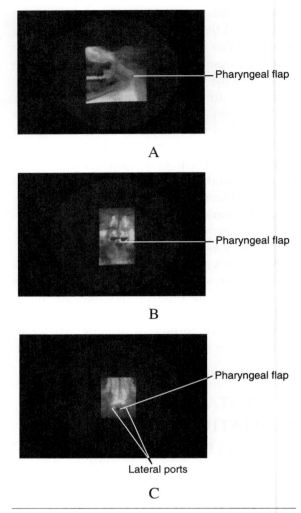

FIGURE 16–11 (A–C) Videofluoroscopy of a pharyngeal flap. A. Lateral view that shows the pharyngeal flap as a faint shadow that is low near the base of the tongue. B. Frontal or AP (anterior-posterior) view that shows the flap in midline and the lateral ports coated with barium. C. Flap noted in midline and lateral ports on each side.

sional pharynx. Because of the limitations of videofluoroscopy and the relative advantages of nasopharyngoscopy, this X-ray procedure seems to be used less frequently as a primary means of evaluating velopharyngeal function.

SUMMARY

Videofluoroscopy provides a method for directly evaluating the structures and function of the velopharyngeal valve. It allows the examiner to identify the anatomical and physiological abnormalities that cause velopharyngeal dysfunction. It also gives the examiner information regarding the size and location of the velopharyngeal opening. This information is required before an appropriate plan of intervention can be determined for each patient.

FOR REVIEW, DISCUSSION, AND CRITICAL THINKING

1. Why are lateral cephalometric X-rays no longer used for evaluation of velopharyngeal function?

2. What are the advantages and drawbacks of using magnetic resonance imaging (MRI) studies for evaluation of velopharyngeal function?

3. What are the typical views used with videofluoroscopy? For each view, describe the structures that can be evaluated. Why are multiple views necessary?

4. In evaluating an X-ray, what color are the structures and what color is the air? What causes this difference?

5. What radiopaque contrast material is commonly used during a videofluoroscopic evaluation? Which views require this substance in order to view the structures adequately? How is this substance instilled into the nasopharynx?

6. Describe what the examiner should look for when interpreting each of the views.

7. What are the advantages of videofluoroscopy? What are some of the limitations?

REFERENCES

Abbott, M. B., Donnelly, L. F., Dardzinski, B. J., Poe, S. A., Chini, B. A., & Amin, R. S. (2004). Obstructive sleep apnea: MR imaging volume segmentation analysis. *Radiology, 232*(3), 889–895.

Akguner, M., (1999). Velopharyngeal anthropometric analysis with MRI in normal subjects. *Annals of Plastic Surgery, 43*(2), 142–147.

Argamaso, R. V., Levandowski, G. J., Golding-Kushner, K. J., & Shprintzen, R. J. (1994). Treatment of asymmetric velopharyngeal insufficiency with skewed pharyngeal flap. *Cleft Palate-Craniofacial Journal, 31*(4), 287–294.

Beer, A. J., Hellerhoff, P., Zimmermann, A., Mady, K., Sader, R., Rummeny, E. J., et al. (2004). Dynamic near-real-time magnetic resonance imaging for analyzing the velopharyngeal closure in comparison with videofluoroscopy. *Journal of Magnetic Resonance Imaging, 20*(5), 791–797.

Cohn, E. R., Rood, S. R., McWilliams, B. J., Skolnick, M. L., & Abdelmalek, L. R. (1984). Barium sulphate coating of the nasopharynx in lateral view videofluoroscopy. *Cleft Palate Journal, 21*(1), 7–17.

D'Antonio, L. L., Muntz, H. R., Marsh, J. L., Marty-Grames, L., & Backensto-Marsh, R.

(1988). Practical application of flexible fiberoptic nasopharyngoscopy for evaluating velopharyngeal function. *Plastic and Reconstructive Surgery*, 82(4), 611–618.

Donnelly, L. F. (2005). Obstructive sleep apnea in pediatric patients: Evaluation with cine MR sleep studies. *Radiology*, 236(3), 768–778.

Donnelly, L. F., Shott, S. R., LaRose, C. R., Chini, B. A., & Amin, R. S. (2004). Causes of persistent obstructive sleep apnea despite previous tonsillectomy and adenoidectomy in children with Down syndrome as depicted on static and dynamic cine MRI. *American Journal of Roentgenology*, 183(1), 175–181.

Ettema, S. L., Kuehn, D. P., Perlman, A. L., & Alperin, N. (2002). Magnetic resonance imaging of the levator veli palatini muscle during speech. *Cleft Palate-Craniofacial Journal*, 39(2), 130–144.

Golding-Kushner, K. J., Argamaso, R. V., Cotton, R. T., Grames, L. M., Henningsson, G., Jones, D. L., Karnell, M. P., Klaiman, P. G., Lewin, M. L., Marsh, J. L., et al. (1990). Standardization for the reporting of nasopharyngoscopy and multiview videofluoroscopy: A report from an International Working Group. *Cleft Palate Journal*, 27(4), 337–347; Discussion 347–348.

Henningsson, G., & Isberg, A. (1991). Comparison between multiview videofluoroscopy and nasendoscopy of velopharyngeal movements. *Cleft Palate-Craniofacial Journal*, 28(4), 413–417; Discussion 417–418.

Isberg, A., Julin, P., Kraepelien, T., & Henrikson, C. O. (1989). Absorbed doses and energy imparted from radiographic examination of velopharyngeal function during speech. *Cleft Palate Journal*, 26(2), 105–109.

Kane, A. A., Butman, J. A., Mullick, R., Skopec, M., & Choyke, P. (2002). A new method for the study of velopharyngeal function using gated magnetic resonance imaging. *Plastic and Reconstructive Surgery*, 109(2), 472–481.

Kuehn, D. P., Ettema, S. L., Goldwasser, M. S., & Barkmeier, J. C. (2004). Magnetic resonance imaging of the levator veli palatini muscle before and after primary palatoplasty. *Cleft Palate-Craniofacial Journal*, 41(6), 584–592.

Kuehn, D. P., Ettema, S. L., Goldwasser, M. S., Barkmeier, J. C., & Wachtel, J. M. (2001). Magnetic resonance imaging in the evaluation of occult submucous cleft palate. *Cleft Palate-Craniofacial Journal*, 38(5), 421–431.

La Rossa, D., Brown, A., Cohen, M., & Spackman, T. (1980). Video-radiography of the velopharyngeal portal using the Towne's view. *Journal of Maxillofacial Surgery*, 8(3), 203–205.

Lubker, J. F., & Morris, H. L. (1968). Predicting cinefluorographic measures of velopharyngeal opening from lateral still X-ray films. *Journal of Speech and Hearing Research*, 11(4), 747–753.

McGowan, J. C., III, Hatabu, H., Yousem, D. M., Randall, P., & Kressel, H. Y. (1992). Evaluation of soft palate function with MRI: Application to the cleft palate patient. *Journal of Computer Assisted Tomography*, 16(6), 877–882.

McWilliams-Neely, B. J., & Bradley, D. P. (1964). A rating scale for evaluation of videotape recorded X-ray studies. *Cleft Palate Journal*, 1, 88–94.

Ozgur, F., Tuncbilek, G., & Cila, A. (2000). Evaluation of velopharyngeal insufficiency with magnetic resonance imaging and nasoendoscopy. *Annals of Plastic Surgery*, 44(1), 8–13.

Rowe, M. R., & D'Antonio, L. L. (2005). Velopharyngeal dysfunction: Evolving developments in evaluation. *Current Opinion in Otolaryngology & Head & Neck Surgery, 13*(6), 366–370.

Seagle, M. B., Mazaheri, M. K., Dixon-Wood, V. L., & Williams, W. N. (2002). Evaluation and treatment of velopharyngeal insufficiency: The University of Florida experience. *Annals of Plastic Surgery, 48*(5), 464–470.

Shott, S. R., & Donnelly, L. F. (2004). Cine magnetic resonance imaging: Evaluation of persistent airway obstruction after tonsil and adenoidectomy in children with Down syndrome. *Laryngoscope, 114*(10), 1724–1729.

Shprintzen, R. J. (1995). Instrumental assessment of velopharyngeal valving. In R. J. Shprintzen & J. Bardach (Eds.), *Cleft palate speech management: A multidisciplinary approach* (Vol. 4, pp. 221–256). St. Louis, MO: Mosby.

Shprintzen, R. J., Rakof, S. J., Skolnick, M. L., & Lavorato, A. S. (1977). Incongruous movements of the velum and lateral pharyngeal walls. *Cleft Palate Journal, 14*(2), 148–157.

Skolnick, M. L. (1969). Video velopharyngography in patients with nasal speech, with emphasis on lateral pharyngeal motion in velopharyngeal closure. *Radiology, 93*(4), 747–755.

Skolnick, M. L. (1970). Videofluoroscopic examination of the velopharyngeal portal during phonation in lateral and base projections—A new technique for studying the mechanics of closure. *Cleft Palate Journal, 7*, 803–816.

Skolnick, M. L. (1975). Velopharyngeal function in cleft palate. *Clinics in Plastic Surgery, 2*(2), 285–297.

Skolnick, M. L., & Cohn, E. R. (1989). *Videofluoroscopic studies of speech in patients with cleft palate*. New York: Springer-Verlag.

Skolnick, M. L., Glaser, E. R., & McWilliams, B. J. (1980). The use and limitations of the barium pharyngogram in the detection of velopharyngeal insufficiency. *Radiology, 135*(2), 301–304.

Skolnick, M. L., & McCall, G. N. (1971). Radiological evaluation of velopharyngeal closure. *Journal of the American Medical Association, 218*(1), 96.

Skolnick, M. L., McCall, G. N., & Barnes, M. (1973). The sphincteric mechanism of velopharyngeal closure. *Cleft Palate Journal, 10*, 286–305.

Stringer, D. A., & Witzel, M. A. (1986). Velopharyngeal insufficiency on videofluoroscopy: Comparison of projections. *American Journal of Roentgenology, 146*(1), 15–19.

Stringer, D. A., & Witzel, M. A. (1989). Comparison of multiview videofluoroscopy and nasopharyngoscopy in the assessment of velopharyngeal insufficiency. *Cleft Palate Journal, 26*(2), 88–92.

Van Demark, D., Bzoch, K., Daly, D., Fletcher, S., McWilliams, B. J., Pannbacker, M., & Weinberg, B. (1985). Methods of assessing speech in relation to velopharyngeal function. *Cleft Palate Journal, 22*(4), 281–285.

Vetter, S., & Strecker, E. P. (2001). Clinical aspects of quality criteria in digital radiography. *Radiation Protection Dosimetry, 94*(1/2), 33–36.

Williams, W. N., & Eisenbach, C. R. D. (1981). Assessing VP function: The lateral still technique vs. cinefluorography. *Cleft Palate Journal, 18*(1), 45–50.

Williams, W. N., Henningsson, G., & Pegoraro-Krook, M. I. (1997). Radiographic assessment of velopharyngeal function for speech. In K. R. Bzoch (Ed.), *Communicative disorders related to cleft lip and palate* (Vol. 4). Austin, TX: Pro-Ed.

Witt, P. D., Marsh, J. L., McFarland, E. G., & Riski, J. E. (2000). The evolution of velopharyngeal imaging. *Annals of Plastic Surgery, 45*(6), 665–673.

Yamawaki, Y., Nishimura, Y., Suzuki, Y., Sawada, M., & Yamawaki, S. (1997). Rapid magnetic resonance imaging for assessment of velopharyngeal muscle movement on phonation. *American Journal of Otolaryngology, 18*(3), 210–213.

Yules, R. B., & Chase, R. A. (1968). Quantitative cine evaluation of palate and pharyngeal wall mobility in normal palates, in cleft palates, and in velopharyngeal incompetency. *Plastic and Reconstructive Surgery, 41*(2), 124–134.

Yules, R. B., Northway, W. H., Jr., & Chase, R. A. (1968). Quantitative cine radiographic evaluation of velopharyngeal incompetence. *Plastic and Reconstructive Surgery, 42*(1), 58–64.

CHAPTER

17

NASOPHARYNGOSCOPY

INTRODUCTION

Once hypernasality or nasal air emission is identified through a perceptual speech evaluation, further assessment of velopharyngeal function is indicated. Although velopharyngeal dysfunction can be identified from the speech evaluation based on the characteristics of the speech, it is important to determine the cause, the specific size, and the location of the velopharyngeal opening. This information is needed so that the appropriate form of intervention can be determined.

Nasopharyngoscopy is a minimally invasive endoscopic procedure that allows visual observation and analysis of the velopharyngeal mechanism during speech (D'Antonio, Achauer, & Vander Kam, 1993; D'Antonio, Chait, Lotz, & Netsell, 1986; D'Antonio, Muntz, Marsh, Marty-Grames, & Backensto-Marsh, 1988; David, White, Sprod, & Bagnall, 1982; McWilliams et al., 1981; Ramamurthy, Wyatt, Whitby, Martin, & Davenport, 1997). Because the structures of velopharyngeal function can be viewed through nasopharyngoscopy, this procedure is considered a direct measure. Nasopharyngoscopy can help the examiner to assess both the anatomic and physiologic abnormalities that are causing velopharyngeal dysfunction so that the appropriate form of treatment for the individual can be identified. As such, nasopharyngoscopy can be a very powerful tool in the evaluation of velopharyngeal function and in determining the cause of velopharyngeal dysfunction when it occurs. The same endoscopic technique can also be used to evaluate swallowing, upper airway obstruction, and the structure and function of the larynx and vocal folds.

Nasopharyngoscopy has become more widely used in the last decade so that many centers now use it primarily, or even exclusively, over videofluoroscopy. A survey of members of the American Cleft Palate-Craniofacial Association was done through a listserv in 2006. In that survey, most respondents reported that they prefer nasopharyngoscopy over videofluoroscopy, especially for evaluation of velopharyngeal function in patients with no history of cleft. When asked which procedure gives the most information, 22% choose videofluoroscopy and 78% choose nasopharyngoscopy.

The purpose of the chapter is to explain how nasopharyngoscopy is used in the evaluation of velopharyngeal function. The specific procedures for assessment are reviewed, including the procedure for preparing the individual and then inserting the endoscope. The interpretation of the observations is discussed as it relates to the diagnosis of velopharyngeal dysfunction and the recommendations for treatment.

ENDOSCOPY

By definition, *endoscopy* is a procedure that allows the visualization of the interior of a canal or hollow organ by means of a special instrument called an *endoscope*. Physicians have used endoscopy for years to view anatomic structures and physiological function to make medical or surgical decisions regarding treatment. Speech pathologists are now using a form of endoscopy to assess the structures and function of the vocal tract. This particular procedure is called *naso-pharyngoscopy* or *nasendoscopy*. With this procedure, the examiner is able to observe both the anatomical and physiological correlates of articulation, phonation, resonance, and swallowing to make a determination about the cause of abnormalities. The cause of deviant speech or resonance characteristics must be known before the speech pathologist can recommend or initiate any form of treatment.

Early Endoscopic Procedures

In 1966, Taub (1966) described the use of a panendoscope for the assessment of velopharyngeal function. The *panendoscope* consisted of an optical tube that could be placed in the mouth and then turned upward for visualization of the velopharyngeal sphincter. Of course, placement of the tube in the mouth interfered with the normal production of speech, and therefore, it had an effect on velopharyngeal function as well. Unfortunately, the optical tube was too big for nasal insertion. Another problem with this procedure was that the light bulb generated a dangerous amount of heat and there was also an electrical hazard for the individual. Therefore, this procedure did not gain wide acceptance.

In 1969, Pigott, Bensen, and White (1969) described the use of a rigid endoscope that was slender enough to be inserted through the nose, but large enough to allow observation of velopharyngeal portal at rest and during speech. This endoscope provided a view of the port from above at a fixed angle. One advantage of the rigid endoscope was that it provided a wide-angle view of 70°, which can include most of the port in one view (Pigott & Makepeace, 1982). However, despite the large cone of view, only one view of the port is possible with this scope. The rigid scope cannot be maneuvered for additional assess-

ment of the lateral edges of the port or to see farther down into the pharynx or vocal tract. In addition, because the scope is very straight and the diameter of the nasal cavity is not, the rigid scope can be very difficult to insert. This can be a particular problem if the individual has a septal deviation or stenosis of the naris. The pressure of the scope on the nasal septum and turbinates can also cause significant pain for the individual. Therefore, nasopharyngoscopy with a rigid scope is not an easy procedure to administer as an examiner, and it is not well tolerated by the individual.

Flexible Fiberoptic Nasopharyngoscopy

In the mid 1970s and the 1980s, the use of a flexible fiberoptic nasopharyngoscope (FFN) began to appear in the literature. The flexible scope is smaller than the rigid scope and, as a result, has a more restricted cone of view. However, its smaller circumference makes it much easier to insert and therefore, it is easier for individuals to tolerate. This is particularly advantageous when evaluating young children.

In 1975, a side-viewing flexible endoscope was described by Miyazaki, Matsuya, and Yamaoka (1975). With this design, the scope remained in a horizontal position and the opening at the side of the scope gave the examiner the same view as with the rigid scope. However, due to the side opening, the scope could not be manipulated easily to provide a view of both the horizontal and vertical aspects of the port.

In the late 1970s and the 1980s, the end-viewing flexible endoscope was described by several authors (Croft, Shprintzen, Daniller, & Lewin, 1978; Croft, Shprintzen, & Rakoff, 1981; Shprintzen, 1979; Shprintzen et al., 1979). The tip of this scope is flexible and with the use of a lever, the examiner can turn the tip down like a periscope to view the velopharyngeal port from various angles. It can even be moved farther down the pharynx for a view of the larynx and the vocal folds. This type of endoscope is used today.

Over the past 25 years, flexible nasopharyngoscopy has become a standard of care for the evaluation of velopharyngeal dysfunction in many craniofacial centers. In 1993, D'Antonio and colleagues (D'Antonio, Achauer, & Vander Kam, 1993) conducted a national survey of craniofacial teams concerning the use of nasopharyngoscopy in the evaluation of velopharyngeal dysfunction. At that time, 90% of the responding teams indicated that nasendoscopy was available and that it was indicated for difficult diagnostic problems at the very least. Forty-one percent of teams responded that endoscopic studies were appropriate for all individuals who require secondary palatal management.

Equipment

Nasopharyngoscopy equipment includes a durable and flexible fiber optic endoscope (Figure 17–1). Endoscopes can be purchased from several manufacturers (Machida, Olympus, Pentx, and Storz). The newer endoscopes have an increased number of fiber optical elements, which significantly enhances the resolution. Anatomical features, including small capillaries, can be observed in finer detail and with more clarity than previously possible. The diameter of the scope can vary from between about 2 mm to about 4 mm. The 3.5-mm scope is commonly used since this size is easily tolerated by most individuals, including children, and it provides a wide scope of vision. However, for very young children and infants (when the procedure is done to evaluate swallowing), a smaller scope may be easier to use and better tolerated. Ideally, a variety of endoscopes should be available in a pediatric

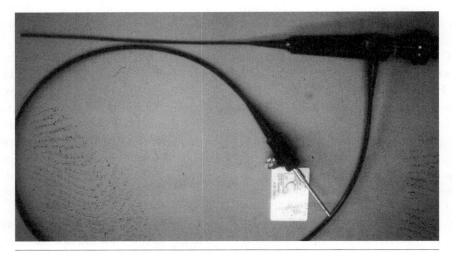

FIGURE 17–1 A flexible fiberoptic nasopharyngoscope. This instrument includes the long tubular endoscope. The body of the instrument, which is held in the examiner's hand, consists of an eyepiece and a control apparatus with a lever or wheel. The control apparatus allows the examiner to move the tip of the scope up and down like a periscope.

practice to ensure the ability to accommodate all children appropriately.

Looking at the insertion end of the scope, one can see the small lens in the middle for obtaining the image and a light source that encircles the lens. The scope is covered by a black vinyl covering with a slightly tapered tip for easy insertion. The end of the scope is very flexible and can be bent or turned easily without distorting the image.

The body of the instrument, which is held in the examiner's hand, consists of an eyepiece and a control apparatus with a lever (Figure 17–2). The control apparatus (lever or wheel) allows the examiner to move the tip of the scope up and down like a periscope. The scope has a cable that is plugged into a high-intensity halogen light source with adjustable brightness.

A light source is necessary for visualization of the structures. A special cold light source is used so that the light can travel through the scope without burning the individual as it reaches the pharyngeal area.

The endoscope and cold-light source are the bare necessities for this examination. With this equipment alone, the examiner can perform a nasopharyngoscopy procedure at bedside or almost anywhere. However, for standard evaluations in a clinic, the addition of video recording equipment is strongly recommended, and may even be required in some cases for appropriate documentation and billing.

For enhanced viewing, a high resolution miniature chip camera can be coupled to the eyepiece of the endoscope with an adapter (Figure 17–3). This type of camera is very small and lightweight. As such, it is hardly noticed by the examiner, yet it results in excellent optic quality.

The newest generation of endoscopes has a digital camera chip incorporated directly into the endoscope, therefore called a "chip in the tip" scope. It is located at the viewing end of the scope, which maximizes clarity and the field of view (Figure 17–4). These scopes provide very

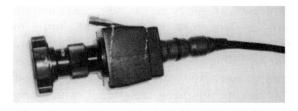

FIGURE 17–3 A very small, lightweight chip camera that can be attached directly to the eyepiece of a nasopharyngoscope.

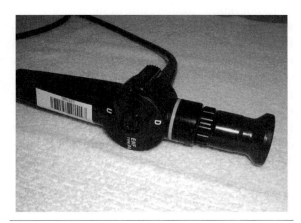

FIGURE 17–2 Eyepiece and control lever for moving the tip of the scope up and down.

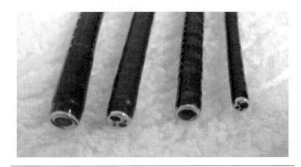

FIGURE 17–4 Nasopharyngoscopes of various sizes. The first scope on the left has a "chip in the tip" camera.

high image quality that approaches that which is obtained with rigid optical instruments.

A high resolution monitor can then be used for viewing rather than the small single-person eyepiece. This provides the examiner a better view, and also allows others (including the parents and the patient) to see the exam in real time as it is done. For some patients, nasopharyngoscopy with monitor viewing can also provide biofeedback and help the individual learn to modify speech for better velopharyngeal function.

For recording, a microphone is attached to the individual so that the speech recording is of good quality. The exam can then be recorded on videotape; in newer equipment, it can be recorded digitally. Recording is very useful because the study can always be viewed again for further analysis. One advantage of digital recording is that it can be viewed frame by frame. When the study is recorded, other professionals can view it later, including the surgeon, who may not be present during the examination. If surgical procedures are done, the recording allows for pre- and postoperative comparisons. The study can be reviewed with the parents, and even the patient, which helps the family understand the problem and proposed treatment. A high quality color printer can also be useful for a hard copy of still pictures and key examination findings. Figure 17–5 shows a complete system with monitor, video recording equipment, a cold-light source, and even stroboscopy.

Clinical Uses for Nasopharyngoscopy

Flexible fiberoptic nasopharyngoscopy is now commonly used in clinical settings for the evaluation of velopharyngeal dysfunction. Nasopharyngoscopy provides a view during speech of the nasal surface of the velum and all of the structures of the velopharyngeal valve.

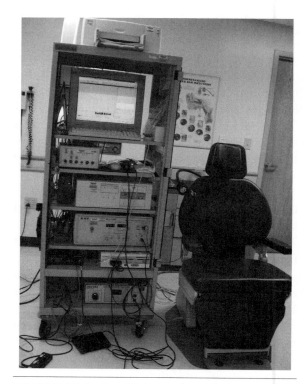

FIGURE 17–5 In addition to the endoscope, camera, and cold light source, a complete system for nasopharyngoscopy should include a computer, monitor, keyboard, speakers, video recording equipment, and a printer.

Nasopharyngoscopy results are complementary to radiographic studies, but in most cases, they are superior to those obtained through videofluoroscopy. This is due to the excellent clarity of the nasopharyngoscopy view and the maneuverability of the scope. Unlike videofluoroscopy, nasopharyngoscopy allows the examiner to see the configuration of the adenoid tissue and observe any fissures in the adenoid pad that affect the firmness of closure. Defects in the nasal surface of the velum, or the presence of an oronasal fistula, can be identified. The examiner can look directly into the port and can observe the movement of the velopharyngeal structures. Even very small gaps are easily visualized with this technique.

The observations made through nasopharyngoscopy provide a clear rationale for the design and placement of pharyngoplasty surgery (Osberg & Witzel, 1981). In fact, by determining the location of the opening, the size of the opening, and the extent of lateral pharyngeal wall motion preoperatively, the appropriate type of surgical intervention can be determined (Shprintzen et al., 1979). Nasopharyngoscopy is also an excellent technique for evaluating the effects of a secondary surgery (i.e., pharyngeal flap, sphincteroplasty, or retropharyngeal implant) because the structures and results of surgery can easily be seen.

In addition to viewing the velopharyngeal structures, flexible endoscopy allows the examiner to view the larynx and vocal folds (Karnell, 1994; Karnell & Langmore, 1998). Because laryngeal abnormalities are often found in individuals with craniofacial anomalies and there is a high incidence of vocal nodules in individuals with velopharyngeal dysfunction, this should be done routinely with each exam.

Because of the view of the pharynx and the larynx provided by nasopharyngoscopy, it is often used in the evaluation of swallowing disorders, and is sometimes referred to as the *fiberoptic endoscopic evaluation of swallowing* (FEES) procedure (Aviv et al., 1998; Bastian, 1991, 1993, 1998; Kidder, Langmore, & Martin, 1994; Langmore, Schatz, & Olsen, 1988).

Nasopharyngoscopy procedures are used not only for diagnosis, but also during the treatment process. For example, nasopharyngoscopy can be used to help to design speech prosthetic devices (D'Antonio et al., 1988; Hung & Cheng, 1989; Karnell, Rosenstein, & Fine, 1987). It can also be useful in therapy for providing biofeedback for the individual. This can help the individual to determine what is necessary for achieving velopharyngeal closure (Shelton, Beaumont, Trier, & Furr, 1978; Witzel, Tobe, & Salyer, 1988; Ysunza, Pamplona, Femat, Mayer, &

Garcia-Velasco, 1997). These uses will be discussed further in Chapter 19, which discusses prosthetic management, and Chapter 21, which discusses speech therapy.

NASOPHARYNGOSCOPY PREPARATION

Information before the Exam Day

The success of the nasopharyngoscopy procedure depends greatly on the individual's cooperation. The individual must be able to talk during the exam without crying. With proper preparation, children down to the age of 3 will generally cooperate sufficiently to obtain a useful nasopharyngoscopy examination.

In a pediatric setting, preparing the child for what to expect can make the difference between a successful examination and one that is a waste of time, money, and everyone's patience. Our center sends a coloring storybook about the procedure to the child a few weeks before the examination (see Appendix 17–1). This can help the child and the parents understand what to expect and allows the parents the opportunity to assist in preparing the child. Giving information ahead of time can also greatly reduce preparation time on the day of the exam. Cooperation tends to improve with age so that obtaining a good examination with adults is usually not a problem. However, even adults can be nervous and apprehensive about the exam. Therefore, giving them information on what to expect before the day of the exam can also be very helpful.

Perceptual Evaluation

Prior to the endoscopy evaluation, the speech pathologist should complete a perceptual evaluation. This evaluation is important so that information regarding the speech character-istics can be obtained without the discomfort of the scope in place. If there is no evidence of abnormal resonance or airway obstruction as judged through the perceptual evaluation, then the nasopharyngoscopy procedure is not done. The information derived from the perceptual evaluation helps the examiner to determine the appropriate speech stimuli for an effective nasopharyngoscopy evaluation. For example, if the individual demonstrates nasal emission on sibilants only, the examiner would want to test these sounds in particular and determine if, through instruction and biofeedback, closure can be obtained by altering the manner of production. On the other hand, if an element of hyponasality or cul-de-sac resonance is noted during the perceptual evaluation, then the examiner would want to actively look for a source of obstruction.

When working with a child, every effort should be made to help the child to feel relaxed, comfortable, and reassured throughout the evaluation. The perceptual evaluation gives the child an opportunity to do something that is painless, nonthreatening, and even fun. There-fore, it is an excellent time for the speech pathologist to develop a rapport with the in-dividual and to help the child to become comfortable in the surroundings prior to the endoscopy (D'Antonio et al., 1986; Lotz, D'Antonio, Chait, & Netsell, 1993).

Infection Control

Before even administering the topical anesthetic, the examiner should follow the Standard Precautions for the prevention of the spread of disease (ASHA, 1990; Centers for Disease Control and Prevention, 1987, 1988; *Federal Register*, 1991). This is not only for the protection of the individual, but it is also for the protection of the examiner. Considering these guidelines,

thorough hand washing should be done as the first step. The examiner should then wear gloves and keep the gloves on for the entire examination. The disinfected endoscope should always be placed on a clean surface when not in use.

Nasal Anesthesia and Decongestion

Before administering the topical anesthetic, the individual should be asked to blow his or her nose to discharge excess secretions that could interfere with the topical anesthetic or obscure the view through the nasopharyngoscope. Once the secretions have been eliminated as much as possible, the topical anesthetic is usually intro-duced into the nose. Most clinicians use some form of numbing solution prior to a nasophar-yngoscopy procedure. However, it can be done without topical anesthesia, especially with adults (Frosh, Jayaraj, Porter, & Almeyda, 1998). It is also helpful to open up the nasal passages as much as possible prior to the examination and this can be done with a topical decongestant.

Topical anesthetics and decongestants are medications that must be ordered by the physi-cian, but can be administered by the nurse, speech pathologist, or even by the parent. Because they require a physician's prescription, the speech pathologist must work in close collaboration with the physician prior to admin-istering these anesthetics. In addition, the speech pathologist should refer to the Code of Ethics of the American Speech-Language-Hearing Asso-ciation (ASHA, 1992a) and the ASHA guidelines on the administration of topical anesthetics (ASHA, 1992b) prior to beginning this practice.

Several methods for numbing the nasal cavity have been reported in the literature. Shprintzen and Golding-Kushner (1989) described a procedure where cotton packing is soaked in tetracaine (Pontocaine) and then inserted in the nose and left for approximately five minutes. Although this method is effective in numbing the nose, we have found that the process of packing the nose is often more traumatic for children than passing the scope. Other centers use a lidocaine (Xylocaine) gel, which is passed into the middle meatus with a long cotton swab. This can also be met with resistance from young children.

At Cincinnati Children's Hospital Medical Center, we recommend using a spray bottle to administer both the topical anesthesia and a decongestant at the same time (Figure 17–6). Children tolerate the introduction of numbing medicine best if a spray bottle is used. This is usually administered by the examiner, but it can also be administered by the parent or even by

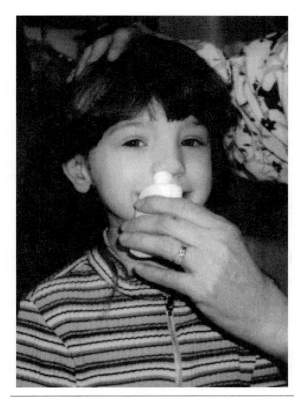

FIGURE 17–6 The use of a spray bottle to administer both the topical anesthesia and a decongestant prior to the nasopharyngoscopy procedure.

the child. It is helpful to have the child close the opposite nostril when one is sprayed and then sniff hard with the sprayed nostril to insure that the solution is distributed to the back of the nose. Three sprays are administered on each side so that there is adequate coating of the turbinates and the nasal septum. A wait of only 5 to 10 minutes is needed before the anesthetic takes effect. Because the spray coats the structures well and goes all the way to the back of the nose, anesthetic packing is usually not needed (Lotz et al., 1993).

The composition of the numbing spray and decongestant may vary. Some authors recommend the use of cophenylcaine (Douglas, 2006; Lennox, Hern, Birchall, & Lund, 1996; Smith & Rockley, 2002), whereas others dispute its benefits (Cain, Murray, & McClymont, 2002; Georgalas, Sandhu, Frosh, & Xenellis, 2005). A nasal decongestant, such as xylometazoline, is recommended by some (Sadek et al., 2001). Our center uses a one-to-one mixture of oxymetazoline (Afrin) and 2% tetracaine (Pontocaine), which also has a vasoconstrictor action. The pharmacy dispenses this mixture in individual spray bottles that are disposed of after use. Although several topical anesthetics can be used, tetracaine is preferable because it acts quickly, has infrequent side effects, and does not have a noxious odor. Fortunately, tetracaine affects the sensation, but it does not affect velopharyngeal movement, so it has no negative effect on the study. Although limited dosing information is available, 0.3 mg/kg tetracaine has not produced any complications in our population. This mixture is very effective in achieving the desired numbing effects, while opening up the nasal passages for the scope.

The numbing spray should always be administered with the patient sitting upright. If the medication is administered with the child in a reclining position, the spray may enter the hypopharynx and numb the airway, leading to aspiration and coughing episodes. The problem will spontaneously resolve after about 20 minutes, but should be avoided by keeping the patient upright during administration of the spray (J. Paul Willging, personal communication, May 12, 2006).

For additional numbing, the sides of the end of the scope can be coated with viscous lidocaine (2%), or special "slime," as we describe it for children. (It is important to slime just the sides, and not the viewing end of the scope.) This gel also acts as a lubricant to smooth the way for the scope to slide easily through the nose (Pothier, Awad, Whitehouse, & Porter, 2005). Using this technique, the examiner can ensure that the child has received adequate topical anesthesia to complete the procedure in relative comfort.

Explaining the Procedure

Prior to starting the nasopharyngoscopy procedure, the examiner should carefully explain what will be done and what to expect so that there are no surprises. If the patient is a child, it is important to talk on his or her level and to keep the atmosphere as light as possible. For example, the child can be asked if he ever picks his nose and if so, if it hurts. The size of his or her "nose-picking finger" can then be compared to the size of the end of the scope, which of course is much smaller. The child should be allowed to feel the end of the scope and even feel the sensation of the scope going up his or her sleeve.

When explaining what to expect, it is important to be honest about what might be felt. For example, the explanation might be as follows:

You will feel the scope in your nose, but because we put the medicine in there, it shouldn't hurt. Instead, you will feel a little pressure and it may feel a little uncomfortable at first. When the tube is almost where it needs to be, there is a tight spot and as the tube goes through it, it might make you want to sneeze. (In fact, many children do sneeze

at this point, so it's helpful to stand clear!) It is very important to hold still though because if you move your head too much, it might make the tube bang around inside of your nose and that might hurt a little. Once the tube is in place, you will need to repeat some silly sentences and we will watch what happens on the monitor. When you finish saying all the sentences, we can take the tube out of your nose and you are done.

Promising a reward at the end of the procedure can also provide some motivation for cooperation.

At times, children will delay the procedure out of fear. If the child has further questions on what to expect, these should be answered. However, an extended delay is counterproductive and just increases the fear. The examiner should be mindful of this and be firm about doing the exam to complete it.

With an adult, a nasopharyngoscopy examination can be done in a matter of a few minutes. When working with young children, however, nasopharyngoscopy takes more time and a lot more patience. If the child is prepared in advance and the examiner commits to spending whatever time is necessary, an adequate nasopharyngoscopy study can usually be obtained with most children, even those as young as 3 years of age.

Positioning the Patient

For best results in inserting the scope, the individual should be seated upright in a chair in front of the examiner. Ideally, the individual should be positioned so that he or she can watch the procedure on the monitor (Figure 17–7). (A supine position is not recommended because gravity may affect the typical function of the velopharyngeal valve.)

For a young child, the patient may need to be stabilized. It can be helpful to have the

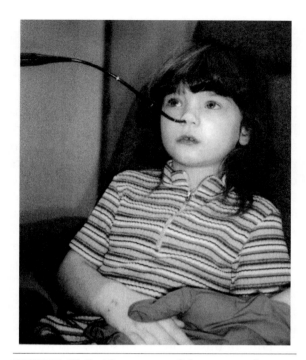

FIGURE 17–7   The position of the scope and patient during the nasopharyngoscopy procedure.

child seated on the parent's lap. The parent is then instructed to "hug" the child around the arms and hold the child's hands. This prevents the child from grabbing the scope during the procedure. It is also helpful to have another person gently hold the child's head to be sure that it does not move erratically during the exam. At times, it is also necessary for the parent to wrap his or her legs around the child's legs to keep the child from kicking.

NASOPHARYNGOSCOPY PROCEDURE

Who Performs the Procedure?

The nasopharyngoscopy procedure can be done by either a physician, such as a plastic surgeon or otolaryngologist, or by a speech pathologist who has been trained in the procedure. The speech pathologist should consult the ASHA training guidelines for endoscopic evaluations (ASHA, 1997). Adequate training and experience are important so that the procedure can be performed with good results and without causing discomfort for the individual.

Although some speech pathologists are performing this procedure around the country, the numbers probably remain few. In 1993, Pannbacker and colleagues (Pannbacker, Lass, Hansen, Mussa, & Robison, 1993) conducted a survey regarding nasopharyngoscopy. The survey was sent to speech-language pathologists who were randomly selected from the *Directory of the American Cleft Palate Craniofacial Association* (ACPA, 1504 East Franklin Street, Suite 102, Chapel Hill, NC, 27504-2820). Although the majority of respondents rated nasopharyngoscopy as important in the assessment of velopharyngeal function and said they also believed that it should be performed by speech-language pathologists, the majority did not perform nasopharyngoscopy examinations. Moreover, 40% had no academic preparation in the procedure and 20% had no clinical experience in nasopharyngoscopy. It is probable that, even today, those who are currently performing nasopharyngoscopy evaluations were trained by a mentor or another professional on the job. On-the-job training is not necessarily inappropriate in this case. It is impractical to train all graduate students in speech pathology in the procedure, because only a few will ever have the need or opportunity to perform nasopharyngoscopy. In addition, training is usually more effective if it is done in a clinical setting by someone who has clinical experience in both performing and interpreting nasopharyngoscopy.

For speech pathologists who are performing endoscopy evaluations, whether it's to evaluate velopharyngeal function, feeding, or the anatomic and physiological correlates of voice, it is important that they are skilled in basic competencies. The needed competencies to perform endoscopy evaluations are listed in the *Training Guidelines for Laryngeal Videoendoscopy/Stroboscopy*, which has been developed by a committee of the American Speech-Language-Hearing Association (1997). This report also outlines educational modalities that can be used to prepare interested professionals to perform these studies. These activities include didactic or classroom learning, mentoring through a one-on-one relationship with another speech pathologist or otolaryngologist, supervised clinical experience, continuing education courses, videotape reviews of previous evaluations, and direct experience that ultimately leads to expertise.

Passing the Scope

A deviated septum, narrow nasal passage, stenotic nasal passage, choanal atresia, or even bone spurs make passage of the scope more challenging. Therefore, the examiner should determine the most patent side of the nose for passage of the scope. To determine which side has a larger opening, the examiner can put the scope at the entrance of each nostril to view the passageway. This can also be determined by having the individual close one nostril at a time and then inspire deeply through the other. The nostril with the higher pitch during inspiration is probably the one with the smallest passageway; therefore, the other nostril would be chosen for passage of the scope (Shprintzen, 1996). For individuals with a history of cleft lip, this is usually the noncleft side. Once the largest side is determined and the end of the scope is coated with lidocaine gel, the exam can begin.

The best way to hold the scope is to place the viewing or camera end in one hand (usually the dominant hand) with the tip control lever on top for manipulation with either the thumb or the index finger. The thumb and fingers of the other hand should grasp the insertion end of the scope and gently pass it into the nostril (Figure 17–8). The examiner can rest his or her hand against the patient's nasal bridge or forehead for maximum control during insertion. If a camera is being used, the examiner may need to turn it slightly (usually with the cord down) to be sure the image is upright. At this point, it is best to direct the individual's attention to the television monitor, which can serve as a distraction to some extent.

The scope is usually guided into the middle nasal meatus and then back to the nasopharynx where it periscopes down to view the velum (Figure 17–9). If it goes through the inferior nasal meatus, which is on the floor of the nose, it will be on top of the velum when it reaches the port. In this position, the scope will usually bounce up and down with velar movement during speech, thus obscuring the examiner's vision of velopharyngeal function. The superior nasal meatus is too narrow for comfortable passage of the scope. Therefore, the middle nasal meatus is the passage of choice. The middle meatus is large enough to allow the scope to fit through easily, and due to its position, it allows an unobstructed view of the port from above. During insertion of the scope, the field of view may periodically appear to be totally white. This is due to the light bouncing off a close object. If there is only white light in the field of view or if contact occurs, the examiner should withdraw the scope slightly and then reposition it before advancing the scope through the meatus.

Because the nasal septum can be sensitive to pressure, the examiner should avoid contact with it as much as possible. This can be done by carefully observing the passage of the scope through the meatus and adjusting the position of the scope accordingly. If contact occurs, it

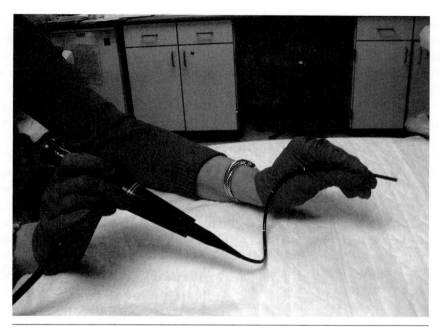

FIGURE 17–8 The best way to hold the scope is to place the viewing end in one hand (usually the dominant hand) with the tip control lever on top for manipulation with either the thumb or the index finger. The thumb and fingers of the other hand should grasp the insertion end of the scope and gently pass it into the nostril.

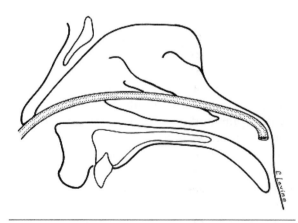

FIGURE 17–9 The scope is usually guided into the middle nasal meatus and then back to the nasopharynx where it periscopes down to view the velum.

will be felt by the examiner as resistance against the scope, and it will be felt by the individual as pressure or mild pain. It is especially important to avoid hitting a bone spur, which can be painful. The back of the nose, just in front of the choana, is the narrowest part of the canal and is the area that is usually the most sensitive, even with good anesthetic coverage. As the scope passes through this area, it may cause minor discomfort. It can also cause the individual's eyes to water and will often elicit a sneeze. To avoid unnecessary discomfort, it is always a good idea to tell the individual to let you know if it hurts or is especially uncomfortable so that appropriate adjustments can be made in the position of the scope.

Once the scope reaches the choana, the area opens up and there is less discomfort for the individual. At this point, the velopharyngeal port can be visualized. If the eyepiece only is being used to view the port, the velum will be seen at the bottom of the screen and the posterior pharyngeal wall will be seen at the top of the screen. Because the patient is facing the examiner, the left side of the screen will show the individual's right lateral pharyngeal wall and vice versa. If a camera is attached to the eyepiece, however, the entire view may be turned sideways or even upside down. When this occurs, the camera needs to be turned until the velum is seen at the bottom of the screen.

When the scope is first passed through the choana, it may be oriented in a horizontal position so that the view is of the nasopharyngeal wall rather than of the velopharyngeal port. To look down on the velopharyngeal port, the end of the scope needs to be turned down. This is done with control apparatus (lever or wheel) on the scope near the eyepiece. It is important that the end of the scope is perpendicular to the port so that the examiner can look down into the port rather than across the port. If the scope is not perpendicular to the port, it can cause significant error in interpretation because the examiner is not viewing the appropriate area (Henningsson & Isberg, 1991). Even if the scope is in good vertical position, the entire port may not be seen at one time. To examine the entire area, the instrument is rotated slightly from one side to the other so that each lateral border can be seen completely. Therefore, by moving the lever of the scope up and down, or by turning the entire scope from side to side, the examiner can view all areas of the velopharyngeal port from just one nostril.

Because the velopharyngeal mechanism is a three-dimensional valve, it is important to assess its entire length. The best view is usually from well above the valve. However, what is observed at the superior end of the valve may not accurately reflect what is occurring farther down in the valve. Therefore, the scope should be moved down for an additional view. The examiner should be careful not to place the scope too far down so that it is below the area of closure, however. This would give the false impression of velopharyngeal dysfunction, when the true closure is occurring above the level of view.

Once the velopharyngeal valve has been adequately assessed, the scope can be passed down to the hypopharynx to observe the vocal folds. The individual is asked to prolong an "eeee" as long as possible so that vocal fold movement can be observed. If stroboscopy is also available, the examiner can view the waveform of the vocal folds. Some children have difficulty with the concept of prolonging the sound. When this occurs and the child is not prolonging the sound, the speech pathologist can help by producing the sound simultaneously with the child in a contest to see who can hold it the longest.

During some examinations, the end of the scope will become very foggy and obscured by secretions. When this occurs, the first course of action is to ask the individual to sniff hard and then swallow to try to get rid of the secretions. If that does not work, then the scope is advanced into the oropharynx and the individual is asked to swallow. This is often sufficient to clear the scope. If the secretions in the nasopharynx persist and interfere with the view of the sphincter area, then the most effective course of action is to suction the individual's nose, if suction equipment is available. Suctioning can be done with the scope in place by putting the suction catheter in the same or opposite naris along the floor of the nose. If that still does not help, despite frequent swallows and suctioning, then it is necessary to remove the scope, wipe the end with alcohol or dip it in hot water, and then try again.

It is important to try to keep the child from crying during the examination so that an adequate assessment can be obtained. Crying during the exam can give a false impression of the status of velopharyngeal function for speech. When the child begins crying, all the adults in the room have the tendency to try to talk to the child at once, and everyone ends up yelling over each other to the child. This can have the opposite effect of the one intended. It is best for one person, preferably the speech pathologist who will be eliciting the speech sample, to primarily communicate with the child. It is important to talk softly and calmly to the child. Asking the child to open his or her eyes to look at you often helps to break the fear. Even distraction techniques can be useful. This might include a stuffed animal, puppet, or a bottle of bubbles. If the child will agree to blow some bubbles while the scope is in place, the act of blowing will necessarily stop the crying.

A successful examination is one in which there has been painless insertion of the scope and good patient cooperation. There must be good light saturation and good optical quality. There must be appropriate positioning of the scope so that there is good visualization of the airway and the velopharyngeal port. Finally, because the scope of view is limited to a portion of the velopharyngeal area, there must be good manipulation of the scope so that the entire sphincter has been adequately viewed (Shprintzen, 1995). For more information on the endoscopic procedure, please refer to the excellent book by Karnell entitled *Videoendoscopy: From Velopharynx to Larynx* (Karnell, 1994).

Speech Sample

Once the scope is in place, the velopharyngeal port should first be visualized at rest so that all the structures can be observed and the patency of the airway can be noted. The individual is then asked to repeat syllables or sentences so that velopharyngeal function can be directly observed. As with videofluoroscopy, the speech pathologist should determine the speech sample based on the observations in the perceptual evaluation. However, unlike videofluoroscopy, there is no inherent danger to the individual with this procedure; therefore, there is no need to restrict the length of the speech sample, unless the individual's cooperation is limited.

A combination of sentences loaded with pressure-sensitive phonemes (see Table 12–3), rote speech such as counting numbers and reciting the alphabet, and repetition of syllables can be used. It is particularly helpful to have the individual count from 60 to 70 to evaluate velopharyngeal function, because that combination of sibilants and plosives in blends with high vowels is particularly taxing on the velopharyngeal mechanism. Having the individual prolong an /s/ can be informative as, in some cases, the velopharyngeal closure that is initially achieved may break down with this task. Finkelstein and colleagues (Finkelstein, Talmi, Kravitz, Bar-Ziv, Nachmani, Hauben, & Zohar, 1991) recommend using the "forced sucking test (FST)" as an additional and complementary part of the endoscopic examination of the velopharyngeal valve. When the individual is asked to forcibly suck, it increases the appearance of some of the abnormal velopharyngeal characteristics, which can help in the analysis of velopharyngeal morphology.

If verbal apraxia is suspected, having the individual repeat multisyllabic words with a combination of placement points can be helpful (i.e., baseball bat, kitty cat, puppy dog, teddy bear, patty cake, basketball, ice cream cone, etc.). To isolate phoneme-specific nasal emission or phoneme-specific hypernasality, individuals syllables can be tested (i.e., pa, pa, pa; pee, pee, pee; sa, sa, sa; see, see, see; etc.). To test the effect of the fistula on the velopharyngeal valve, the speech sample can be done with the fistula open first and then it can be repeated with the fistula occluded (with an obturator or gum) so that a comparison can be made.

If hyponasality or upper airway obstruction is a concern, the examiner should assess the patency of the velopharyngeal port during nasal breathing and during the production of nasal sounds. This can be done by having the individual repeat sentences with nasal phonemes, count from 90 to 100, repeat nasal syllables (e.g., ma, ma, ma) and then prolong an /m/ as long as possible. The examiner should also have the individual close the mouth and breathe as normally as possible through the nose for at least 30 seconds. Keeping the lips closed, the individual should then be asked to inspire deeply through the nose. During all of these activities, the relative opening of the pharyngeal port should be assessed. If a pharyngeal flap is in place, the patency of each lateral port should be examined.

Occasionally, a child will cry and refuse to talk with the scope in the nose. In these cases, "desperate measures" are needed. For testing velopharyngeal function, a sentence like "Stop sticking this thing in my nose!" may be used. If nasal phonemes are needed, the child can repeat "No, no, no!" or "Not now!"

Potential Complications

Complications with nasopharyngoscopy occur very rarely. They include a vasovagal event, causing fainting. Fainting is usually the result of individual anxiety and can be avoided by watching the individual carefully and giving the individual a great deal of reassurance if needed. If the patient appears ashen, the procedure should be terminated immediately. The fainting response is not limited to the patient. The parent may actually be the one to faint. If fainting occurs, the individual should be placed in a reclining position with the head lower than the legs, or in a sitting position with the head below the knees.

Another rare complication is *epistaxis*, which is a nosebleed. Even when this occurs, the bleeding usually is slight and resolves quickly. Afrin and a little pressure may help to control the bleeding, but in most cases, it will stop on its own (J. Paul Willging, personal communication, May 12, 2006). Although the risk of medical complication is very slight, this procedure should be performed in a setting where medical support is available.

INTERPRETATION

Team Interpretation of the Results

Once the individual has been trained in nasopharyngoscopy, it is not difficult to pass the scope through the nose. The biggest challenge is the analysis and interpretation of the findings, and the formulation of appropriate recommendations. For this part of the evaluation, a team approach is definitely preferable. The team approach is advocated by most craniofacial professionals for the evaluation and treatment of craniofacial anomalies. The team approach is equally important for the evaluation and management of velopharyngeal dysfunction (D'Antonio et al., 1986, Willging, 2003).

The most appropriate team for nasopharyngoscopy evaluations is the speech pathologist and a pediatric otolaryngologist (or plastic surgeon). Because speech, resonance, and phonation are highly dependent on the structures of the vocal tract, and many of the problems seen through nasopharyngoscopy are related to the ear, nose, or throat, it is especially helpful to have an otolaryngologist as part of the team. Speech pathologists are trained to evaluate the velopharyngeal structures and function as they relate to the acoustic characteristics of speech, voice, and resonance. The gold standard for determining the need for intervention remains the perceptual quality of the speech. The speech pathologist can also determine if the individual is stimulable, which may suggest correction with speech therapy, or if the problem is functional, which definitely suggests correction with speech therapy. The speech pathologist is essential during the examination to determine the appropriate stimuli to emphasize the velopharyngeal closure defects. Finally, the speech pathologist can assist in determining the appropriate recommendations for treatment. The physician can assess the structural aspects of the oral cavity, pharynx, and nasal cavity with respect to the velopharyngeal valve and airway. Physicians are trained to assess the anatomy and physiology with a focus on disease and abnormality. They can determine the appropriate medical or surgical approaches to treatment for any abnormalities that are found. The physician can also identify associated problems, such as middle ear effusion, vocal nodules, and adenotonsillar hypertrophy.

The nasopharyngoscopy assessment is most valuable when it is not just viewed by both professionals, but when it is done live by both professionals working together as a team. It makes no difference who passes the scope, as long as both professionals take a part in the interpretation of the results and formulation of the recommendations. In this way, a separate referral and evaluation are often avoided, and recommendations for treatment can be made on the spot.

Clinical Observations

With the endoscope in place in the nasopharynx, the examiner can view the velopharyngeal structures with the velum at the bottom of the screen and the posterior pharyngeal wall at the top of the screen. The opening to the eusta-

chian tube can often be seen in the view (Figure 17–10). As noted previously, the view through the scope is from the patient facing the examiner. Therefore, the left side of the screen is the individual's right side and vice versa. This is particularly important to keep in mind when reporting the location of an opening or growth, or reporting asymmetrical movement.

Nasopharyngoscopy shows the nasal surface of the velum, which can be scrutinized for signs of a submucous cleft palate or occult submucous cleft (Figure 17–11). This might include a hypoplastic musculus uvula, which appears as a flattening or concavity in the area where there should be a convex shape. There may also be a depression or a notch near the posterior border of the velum. A velopharyngeal opening during speech often corresponds to this area of deficiency in the midline (Gosain, Conley, Marks, & Larson, 1996; Lewin, Croft, & Shprintzen,

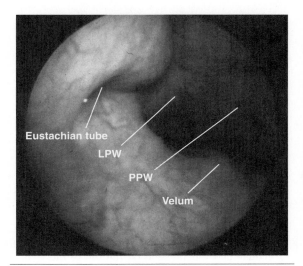

FIGURE 17–10 A nasopharyngoscopy view of normal velopharyngeal structures. The nasal surface of the velum is always at the bottom of the screen and the posterior pharyngeal wall is always at the top of the screen. The opening to the eustachian tube can be seen on the left side of the view.

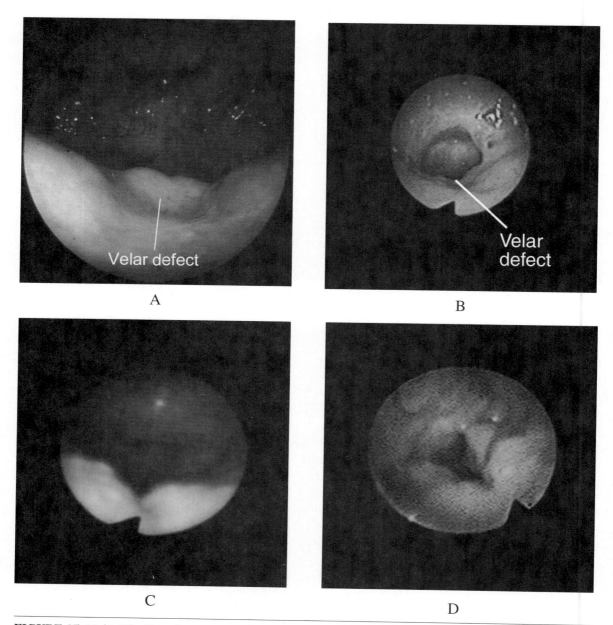

FIGURE 17–11 (A–D) Nasopharyngoscopy view of four submucous clefts. Note that in all cases, there is a notch in midline and a depression on the top of the velum where there should be a bulge from the musculus uvulae muscles. In example D, note the large tonsils that are intruding into the oropharynx.

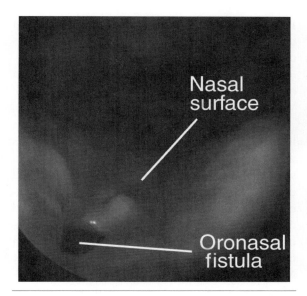

FIGURE 17–12 View of an oronasal fistula as seen through nasopharyngoscopy.

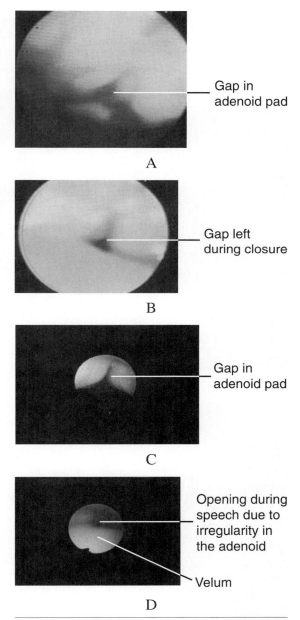

FIGURE 17–13 (A–D) A and C. View of an irregular adenoid pad. B and D. View during veloadenoidal closure. Note that the irregularity in the adenoid causes a small opening.

1980; Peterson-Falzone, 1985; Shprintzen, 1995; Shprintzen, 1996; Shprintzen & Golding-Kushner, 1989). If there is an oronasal fistula in the hard palate, even this can be seen through the endoscope (Figure 17–12).

The posterior pharyngeal wall can be examined from this perspective. The adenoid pad is evaluated for its size, surface, and location. The adenoid tissue may be large and blocking the nasopharynx, the opening of the choanal (see Figure 8–8), or the opening to one or both eustachian tubes. It may also have an irregular surface or fissures in the surface that prohibit the velum from achieving a tight veloadenoidal seal (Figure 17–13). This is a particular concern in children who often achieve velar contact against the adenoids (Finkelstein, Berger, Nachmani, & Ophir, 1996; Gereau & Shprintzen, 1988; Mason, 1973; Morris, 1975; Siegel-Sadewitz & Shprintzen, 1986; Williams, Preece, Rhys, & Eccles, 1992).

If there is a Passavant's ridge during speech, this can often be observed if there is a velopharyngeal opening (Figure 17–14). With complete or nearly complete closure, the

Passavant's ridge usually cannot be seen through nasopharyngoscopy because it appears only with velopharyngeal closure and is usually located below the area of closure (Finkelstein et al., 1991; Finkelstein, Lerner, et al., 1993; Witzel & Posnick, 1989).

The posterior pharyngeal wall should always be observed at rest, particularly in individuals who have velopharyngeal insufficiency due to a submucous cleft of unknown origin. It is well documented that individuals with velocardiofacial syndrome often have medially displaced carotid arteries (Figure 17–15). In this case, one or both of the arteries may be seen pulsating on the posterior pharyngeal wall (D'Antonio & Marsh, 1987; Finkelstein, Zohar, et al., 1993; MacKenzie-Stepner, Witzel, Stringer, Lindsay, et al., 1987; Ross, Witzel, Armstrong, & Thomson, 1996; Witt, Miller, Marsh, Muntz, & Grames, 1998). There may even be unusual findings on the pharyngeal wall, such as the scar band noted in Figure 17–16.

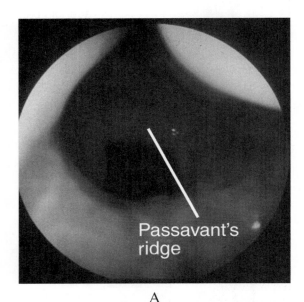

A

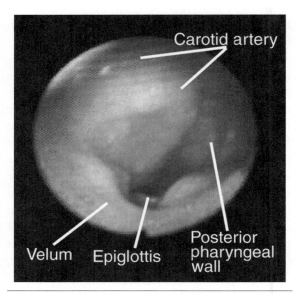

FIGURE 17–15 View of a medially displaced carotid artery, which is commonly seen in patients with velocardiofacial syndrome.

B

FIGURE 17–14 (A and B) Passavant's ridge as seen from above through nasopharyngoscopy.

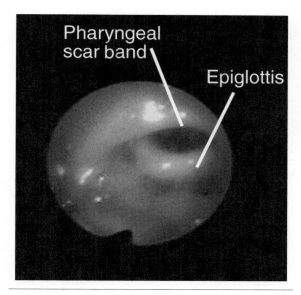

FIGURE 17–16 Scar band on the pharyngeal wall following an aggressive tonsillectomy.

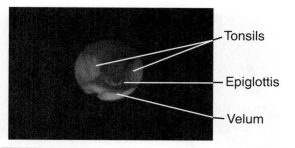

FIGURE 17–17 Tonsillar hypertrophy. Note both tonsils in the oropharynx as seen from above.

If the tonsils are large and intrude into the oropharynx or nasopharynx, this can be seen through nasopharyngoscopy (Figure 17–11D and Figure 17–17). At times, the tonsils are noted to be so large that they extend up to the area of velopharyngeal closure where they may interfere with closure because of their placement between the velum and posterior pharyngeal wall (see Figures 7–15A and 7–15B). They can also interfere with lateral pharyngeal wall movement (Finkelstein, Nachmani, & Ophir, 1994; Henningsson & Isberg, 1988; Kummer, Billmire, & Myer, 1993; MacKenzie-Stepner, Witzel, Stringer, & Laskin, 1987). Although a rare finding, this mechanical interference with velopharyngeal closure can be corrected with a tonsillectomy.

The degree of velar, lateral pharyngeal, and posterior pharyngeal wall movement should be observed and the symmetry of lateral wall movement should be noted. The relative contribution of all of these structures to closure should be assessed to determine the basic closure pattern (coronal, circular, or

sagittal) (Croft et al., 1981; Finkelstein, Lerner, et al., 1993; Igawa, Nishizawa, Sugihara, & Inuyama, 1998; Shprintzen, Rakof, Skolnick, & Lavorato, 1977; Siegel-Sadewitz & Shprintzen, 1982; Skolnick, Shprintzen, McCall, & Rakoff, 1975; Witzel & Posnick, 1989).

The adequacy of closure of the velopharyngeal sphincter should be directly assessed during connected speech. If there is a velopharyngeal opening, the size, shape, and location of the opening are important to determine. These observations can determine the type of surgical management and the placement of the correction (Shprintzen et al., 1979). Figure 17–18 shows various openings with different patterns of closure and therefore, different shapes.

A very small opening may not be seen immediately through nasopharyngoscopy. With connected speech, however, there will be bubbling of the secretions (Figure 17–18F). Whenever bubbling is noted, the examiner can be sure that it is due to a velopharyngeal opening, which is usually small in size. This bubbling is due to air pressure being forced through a small velopharyngeal opening. If the opening were larger, there would be less friction and less bubbling. This bubbling, and the friction that goes with it, correspond to the perception of a nasal rustle, also called nasal turbulence (Kummer, Curtis, Wiggs, Lee, & Strife, 1992). Often, the opening will be to the

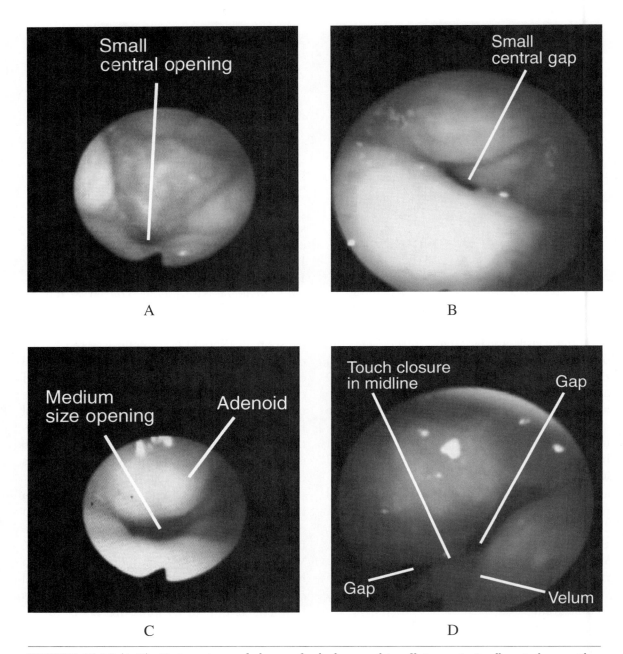

FIGURE 17–18 (A–L) Various sizes and shapes of velopharyngeal insufficiency. A. Small central gap with a circular pattern of closure. B. Small central gap with a coronal pattern of closure. C. Moderate-sized opening with a circular pattern of closure. D. Narrow coronal opening with touch closure in midline. (*continues*)

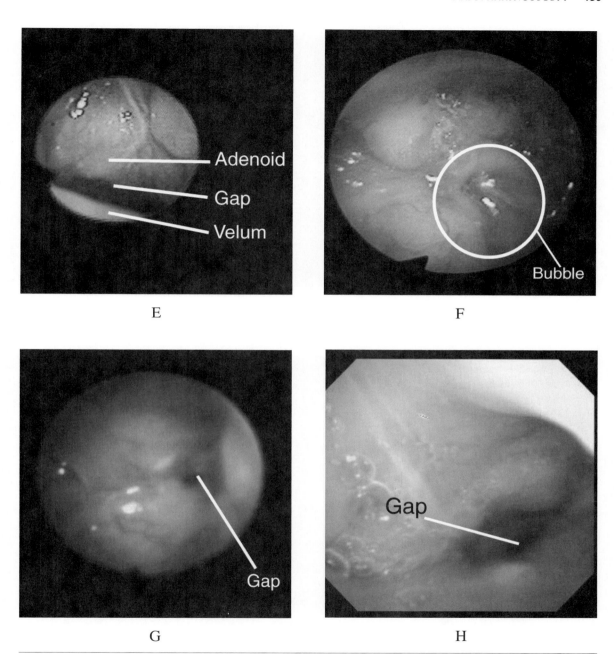

FIGURE 17–18 (A–L) (*continued*)   E. Wide coronal opening. F. Very small gap on the (patient's) left of midline. This is most easily noted by the bubbling in that area during speech. G. Small opening to the left of midline. H. Larger opening to the left of midline. (*continues*)

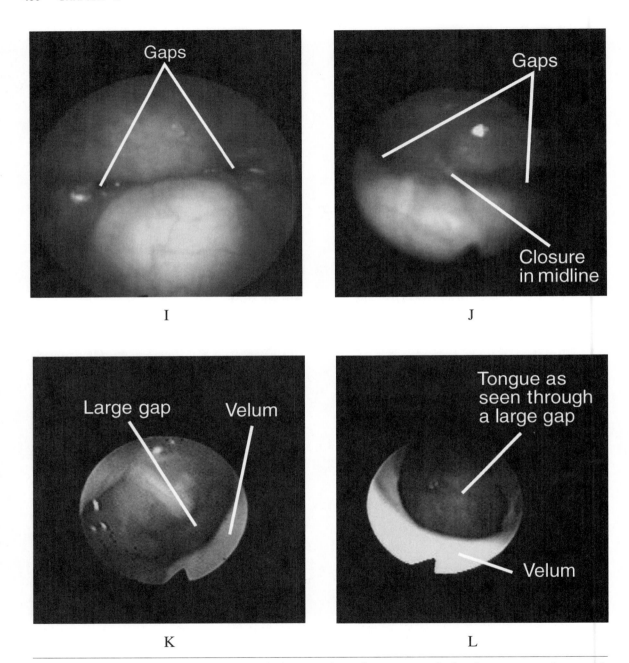

FIGURE 17–18 (A–L) (*continued*)   I. Bowtie closure with small openings on both sides. J. Bowtie closure with moderate size openings on both sides. K. Large velopharyngeal opening due to short velum. L. Very large velopharyngeal opening showing the tongue base and epiglottis.

left or right of midline. This is important to document because it has implications for surgical management.

If there is inconsistent closure, the examiner should analyze whether the opening occurs only on certain phonemes. If it is phoneme-specific (i.e., occurs only on certain sounds), this is usually due to faulty articulation (Peterson-Falzone & Graham, 1990). Therefore, the examiner should attempt to elicit closure on those phonemes using the monitor for biofeedback. Inconsistent closure may also be due to fatigue with connected speech or prolonged speaking. In this case, the individual may be able to achieve closure, but is not able to maintain it over time. The examiner can assess this by having the patient count or produce a form of rote speech. Closure should be maintained throughout the utterance unless there is a nasal phoneme within the utterance. The examiner should observe whether the closure occurs at the beginning of an utterance and then begins to break down toward the end. Inconsistent closure can also be due to abnormal timing of closure in relation to the production of oral phonemes. The examiner should watch for this with the production of connected speech or the repetition of multisyllabic words. Longer or more complex utterances will test the timing and coordination of all of the articulators, including those for velopharyngeal closure.

Nasopharyngoscopy is a good procedure for evaluation of velopharyngeal function if the patient has undergone a surgical procedure, such as an adenoidectomy, pharyngeal flap (Figure 17–19), sphincteroplasty (Figure 17–20), or pharyngeal augmentation (see Chapter 18). Because nasopharyngoscopy allows direct visualization of the pharynx, the structural and functional results of the surgery can be accurately assessed through this procedure.

In all cases, the examiner should keep in mind that the closure that is seen through nasopharyngoscopy represents what the individual does with speech, not what the individual is capable of doing. For example, if glottal stops are used, the velopharyngeal valve may not close. The speech pathologist should try to determine the patient's true potential for velopharyngeal closure before making assumptions that an opening is due to a structural problem. This is particularly true with individuals who have had surgical correction of velopharyngeal insufficiency. The examiner should keep in mind that changing structure does not change function. Therefore, surgical correction of velopharyngeal insufficiency may give the individual the structure to achieve closure, but he or she may require speech therapy to learn how to use the structure to achieve closure during speech.

Because of the high incidence of vocal nodules or voice disorders in individuals with velopharyngeal dysfunction (D'Antonio et al., 1988; Hirschberg et al., 1995; Lewis, Andreassen, Leeper, Macrae, & Thomas, 1993; Zajac & Linville, 1989), an evaluation of the larynx and vocal folds should also be performed, particularly if dysphonia was noted in the perceptual evaluation. By viewing the vocal folds, the examiner can determine the presence of vocal nodules (Figure 17–21), a laryngeal web (Figure 17–22), or whether there is thickening or edema of the folds. The movement of the folds can be observed and the use of ventricular folds during phonation should be noted if it occurs. Any other anomalies of the vocal folds or their movement should also be noted.

With nasopharyngoscopy, it is important to determine the cause of the opening (VPI versus mislearning). This information will help to determine the type of treatment indicated (i.e., surgery versus speech therapy).

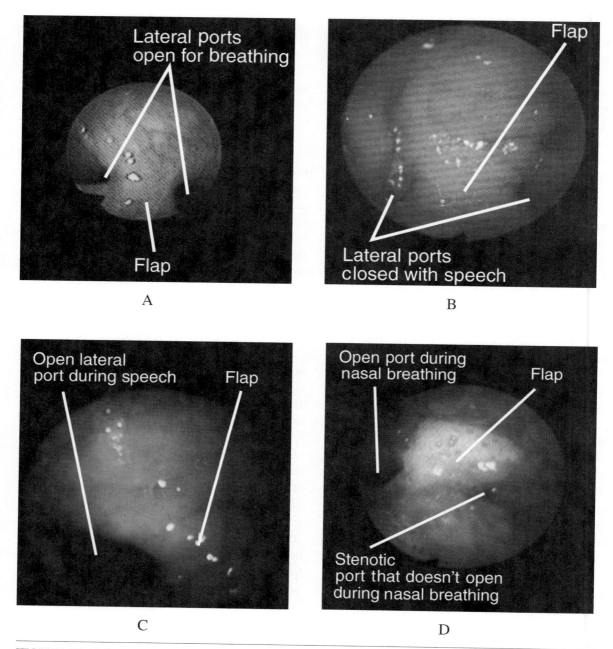

FIGURE 17–19 (A–D) Nasopharyngoscopy of a pharyngeal flap. A. Pharyngeal flap during rest. Note the lateral ports on each side are patent for normal nasal breathing. B. Pharyngeal flap during speech with both ports closed. C. Pharyngeal flap with a persistent opening in the right port during speech. D. Pharyngeal flap at rest with the right port open for normal nasal breathing, but the left port stenosed, causing upper airway obstruction.

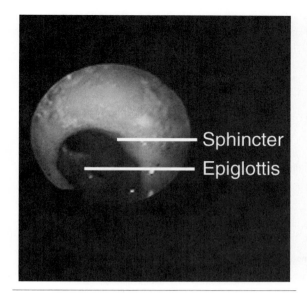

FIGURE 17–20 Sphincter pharyngoplasty. Although the sphincter is noted on the pharyngeal wall, it is not deep enough to completely close the port during speech in this case.

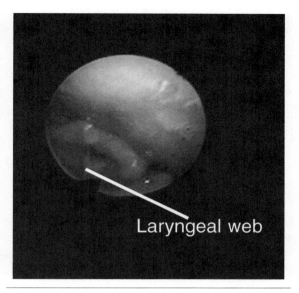

FIGURE 17–22 A laryngeal web in a patient with velocardiofacial syndrome.

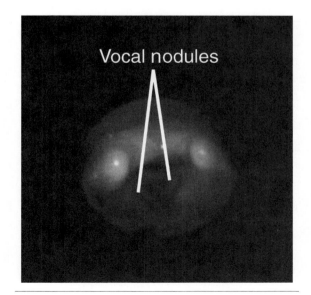

FIGURE 17–21 Bilateral vocal fold nodules.

If surgery is indicated, it is important to note the size, location, and shape of the opening in order to select the type of procedure that is most likely to be effective. For a simple checklist of observations through nasopharyngoscopy, see (Table 17–1).

Reporting the Results

As with videofluoroscopic speech studies, some centers report nasopharyngoscopy results with a narrative report. Several authors have suggested using either a numeric scale or a particular form to rate various parameters of structure and function (D'Antonio, Marsh, Province, Muntz, & Phillips, 1989; D'Antonio et al., 1988; Karnell, Ibuki, Morris, & Van Demark, 1983; Sinclair, Davies, & Bracka, 1982; Zwitman, Sonderman, & Ward, 1974). What is most important is that there is consistency in the observations that are made in each study and in the way that the studies are reported.

TABLE 17–1 Nasopharyngoscopy Checklist

Velopharyngeal Function

☐ **Normal** ☐ **Abnormal:** ☐ borderline ☐ mild ☐ moderate ☐ severe ☐ very severe

Velopharyngeal Opening

Size: ☐ pinhole ☐ small ☐ medium ☐ large ☐ very large

Shape: ☐ circular ☐ sagittal ☐ coronal ☐ bowtie

Location:

☐ midline ☐ right of midline ☐ right corner ☐ left of midline ☐ left corner ☐ both corners

Consistency: ☐ consistent ☐ inconsistent

☐ phoneme-specific-sounds affected: _____

Effect of Stimulation: ☐ improved closure ☐ no change

Previous Secondary Surgery: ☐ **None**

Type: ☐ pharyngeal flap   ☐ sphincter pharyngoplasty

☐ pharyngeal augmentation   ☐ Furlow palatoplasty

Status: ☐ intact ☐ too low   ☐ too narrow

Ports during Speech:

Left Port: ☐ open ☐ stenosed **Right Port:**   ☐ open   ☐ stenosed

Both Ports: ☐ open ☐ stenosed **Central (Sphincter) Port:** ☐ open ☐ stenosed

Comments:_____

Additional Findings: (occult submucous cleft, bubbling of secretions, tonsils in oropharynx, large tonsils, irregular adenoids, medialized carotid arteries, Passavant's ridge, fistula, vocal nodules, laryngeal web, etc.)

_____

_____

Probable Cause of the Problem

☐ VP insufficiency (short or abnormal velum, deep pharynx, etc.)

☐ VP incompetence: ☐ poor velar movement ☐ poor lateral wall movement

Adenoids: ☐ irregular ☐ protruding

☐ Misarticulations: ———————————————————————————————

Other: ————————————————————————————————————

Recommendations

☐ Surgical Intervention

☐ pharyngeal flap   ☐ sphincter pharyngoplasty

☐ pharyngeal augmentation   ☐ palatoplasty

☐ adenoidectomy   ☐ tonsillectomy

☐ Prosthetic Intervention

☐ palatal lift ☐ palatal obturator ☐ speech bulb

☐ Speech Therapy

As noted previously, a multidisciplinary group of clinicians was assembled in 1990 by the American Cleft Palate-Craniofacial Association to address the question of standardizing reporting techniques for multiview videofluoroscopy and nasopharyngoscopy. Their report was an attempt to develop standards in the methodology for reporting results (Golding-Kushner et al., 1990). The proposed system was to rate the movement of the velum, the posterior pharyngeal wall, and each lateral wall in relation to the structure that it is moving toward. The resting position of the structure is rated as 0.0 and the resting position of the opposing structure is 1.0. Using a ratio, the movement of the structure is scored according to the degree of its movement toward the resting position of the opposing structure. It is unclear how many centers are currently using this system, but its use may be somewhat limited due to its complexity.

The reliability of judgments from nasopharyngoscopy, regardless of the procedure used to report the results, seems to be greatly dependent on the experience of the evaluator (D'Antonio et al., 1989). Therefore, working with another experienced examiner initially is important to help the novice evaluator to develop the necessary skills. After that, practice is important for honing the skills required for observation and analysis.

Although results are reported to other professionals, they also need to be reported to the family. It is very important that the person who counsels the family uses clear, easy to understand language. All medical terms should be clearly defined. When discussing the function of the velopharyngeal mechanism, pictures and diagrams must be used. After the initial explanation, it may also be helpful to play the videotape of the procedure and point out the structures and their function.

CLEANING AND STORING THE ENDOSCOPE

Once the endoscope has been used, care should be taken so that the scope is not placed on a surface that will be touched by others. Instead, the scope should be taken for immediate cleaning and disinfection. Guidelines for disinfection of the scope have been developed by the Association of Professionals in Infection Control and Epidemiology and also by the Association for the Advancement of Medical Instrumentation (American National Standard Institute, 1996; Rutala, 1996). However, each medical facility should have a specific policy on how endoscopes are reprocessed. Cleaning and high-level disinfection or sterilization is easier and more complete for endoscopes that are immersible. Therefore, this should be considered when purchasing a new scope.

There are nine steps to reprocessing an endoscope, as noted in the following list (J. Paul Willging, personal communication, May 12, 2006):

1. **Precleaning:** Prior to disinfection and sterilization, the scope should be carefully cleaned of visible residue with a cloth and enzymatic detergent solution. "Sterile dirt" can still cause infection (Catalone & Koos, 2005).

2. **Transportation to the cleaning facility:** The scope should be placed in a closed, rigid container for the protection of patients, healthcare workers, and the scope. The cleaning facility must have a separate dirty area to receive the contaminated scope.

3. **Leakage testing:** The scope is tested for leakage to insure the integrity of the external skin. If cleaning materials leak in to the core of the scope, the fiberoptic bundles will be severely damaged. If

there is a leak, the scope is removed from service until it is repaired.

4. **Manual cleaning:** The scope is immersed in an enzymatic solution and cleaned manually to remove retained debris that can interfere with the capability of germicides to effectively kill microorganisms.

5. **Rinsing:** The endoscope is rinsed to remove residual debris and detergent. The endoscope is then dried to prevent dilution of the chemical germicide during disinfection.

6. **High-level disinfection:** A liquid chemical germicide is used with the required exposure time. These are toxic substances, so personal protection equipment is important (gloves, mask, eye protection, and impervious gown).

7. **Rinsing:** The scope is moved to a designated clean area and thoroughly rinsed in sterile, filtered water. It is important to remove the chemical residue to prevent injury to the skin and mucous membranes of the next patient.

8. **Drying:** The endoscope is dried with a lint-free towel. This inhibits the growth of waterborne organisms.

9. **Storage:** The scope is then hung in a storage cabinet with adequate ventilation to prevent moisture buildup or physical damage (Figure 17–23). The scope should not be stored in the case provided by the manufacturer.

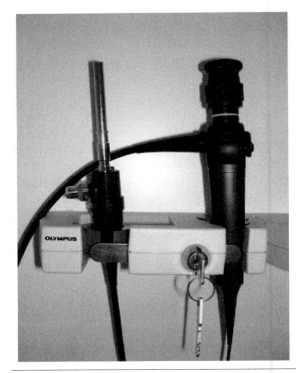

FIGURE 17–23 The scope should ideally be hung when stored for adequate ventilation to prevent moisture buildup and to prevent physical damage.

ADVANTAGES AND LIMITATIONS OF NASOPHARYNGOSCOPY

The most commonly used methods for direct visualization of the velopharyngeal mechanism are nasopharyngoscopy and videofluoroscopy (Rowe & D'Antonio, 2005). There are differences in opinion as to the best method of assessment in all cases. The examiner should consider what is more important to visualize in each patient's case, and the relative benefits and risks of each procedure before determining which type of assessment to use.

One advantage of nasopharyngoscopy over videofluoroscopy is that all structures of the velopharyngeal mechanism can be seen in great detail. In addition, small openings that cannot be seen with videofluoroscopy can be seen with nasopharyngoscopy. With nasopharyngoscopy, the structures and defects of the velum can be clearly seen in "living color." The location, size and shape of the opening can be determined more easily through nasopharyngoscopy than through videofluoroscopy. Of course, nasopharyngoscopy is done without radiation; therefore, there is no risk of harmful physical effects to the individual. Because there is no radiation involved, the examiner can take as much time as needed to determine the problem and the appropriate intervention. The procedure can also be repeated as often as needed for pre- and posttreatment assessments.

Nasopharyngoscopy can be used as a biofeedback tool. The speech pathologist can give the individual instructions on placement and the patient can watch the velopharyngeal results on the monitor as he or she tries to follow the instructions. This is a particularly powerful procedure for the treatment of certain learned causes of velopharyngeal dysfunction (Brunner et al., 1994; D'Antonio et al., 1988; Kunzel, 1982; Rich, Farber, & Shprintzen, 1988; Shelton et al., 1978; Siegel-Sadewitz & Shprintzen, 1982; Witzel et al., 1988; Witzel, Tobe, & Salyer, 1989; Yamaoka, Matsuya, Miyazaki, Nishio, & Ibuki, 1983; Ysunza et al., 1997). For more information on the use of nasopharyngoscopy in therapy, please see Chapter 21.

The risks or limitations associated with nasopharyngoscopy are minimal. The biggest disadvantage of nasopharyngoscopy is that the examiner cannot see the entire length of the pharyngeal wall during speech. In addition, some clinicians argue that videofluoroscopy is less invasive than nasopharyngoscopy. However, introduction of barium in the nasopharynx for videofluoroscopy is also invasive and the large machinery can be just as frightening to a child as nasopharyngoscopy.

Nasopharyngoscopy requires a moderate degree of cooperation from the individual to successfully complete the study. Getting the scope through to the right place is not difficult. However, getting a child to talk and repeat sentences with the scope in place and without crying can be a challenge. Although nasopharyngoscopy should not be a painful procedure, it can cause some discomfort, especially if the scope hits a nasal spur or the base of the nasal septum. However, with a good coating of topical anesthesia and with previous preparation as to what to expect, the nasopharyngoscopy procedure is usually well tolerated by children, even as young as 3 years of age. A final disadvantage is that the nasopharyngoscopy equipment is expensive to purchase and maintain.

SUMMARY

Instrumental assessment is not required for identification of velopharyngeal dysfunction in most cases because it can be determined through a perceptual assessment of resonance. However, nasopharyngoscopy is a very effective procedure for determining both the cause of velopharyngeal dysfunction, and the size and location of the opening. Nasopharyngoscopy can be used to determine the presence of obstruction in the vocal tract, which can also affect resonance. This information is very important in determining the most effective type of surgical management. Therefore, in many centers across the country, nasopharyngoscopy has become a standard evaluation procedure for individuals who exhibit resonance disorders or characteristics of velopharyngeal dysfunction.

FOR REVIEW, DISCUSSION, AND CRITICAL THINKING

1. What equipment is absolutely necessary for a nasopharyngoscopy examination? What additional components are preferable and why?

2. Why is it important to do a perceptual evaluation of speech prior to the nasopharyngoscopy exam?

3. Discuss the methods for nasal anesthesia and decongestion.

4. Describe the procedure for passing the scope. What conditions can make passing the scope more challenging? Why is the scope usually passed through the middle nasal meatus rather than the inferior nasal meatus or the superior nasal meatus? What

should you do if the scope lens becomes cloudy?

5. What determines the appropriate speech samples to use in the exam? Why is it preferable to get a sample without the child crying?

6. What are potential complications during the exam and how should they be handled?

7. What structures can be viewed through nasopharyngoscopy? What clinical observations can be seen that could affect resonance?

8. What are the advantages of nasopharyngoscopy? What are some of the limitations?

REFERENCES

American National Standard Institute. (1996). *Safe use and handling of flutaraldehyde-based products in health care facilities.* New York: Author.

American Speech-Language-Hearing Association. (1990, December). Report update. AIDS/HIV: Implications for speech-language pathologists and audiologists. *ASHA, 32*(Suppl. 9), 46–48.

American Speech-Language-Hearing Association. (1992a). Code of ethics of the American Speech-Language-Hearing Association. *ASHA, 34*(Suppl. 9), 1–2.

American Speech-Language-Hearing Association. (1992b). Sedation and topical anesthetics in audiology and speech-language pathology. *ASHA, 34*(Suppl. 7), 41–42.

American Speech-Language-Hearing Association. (1997). Training guidelines for laryngeal

videoendoscopy/stroboscopy. *ASHA desk reference.* Rockville, MD: Author.

American Speech-Language-Hearing Association. (1998). Training guidelines for laryngeal videoendoscopy/stroboscopy. *ASHA, 40* (Suppl. 18), 154–154.

Aviv, J. E., Kim, T., Thomson, J. E., Sunshine, S., Kaplan, S., & Close, L. G. (1998). Fiberoptic endoscopic evaluation of swallowing with sensory testing (FEESST) in healthy controls [see Comments]. *Dysphagia, 13*(2), 87–92.

Bastian, R. W. (1991). Videoendoscopic evaluation of patients with dysphagia: An adjunct to the modified barium swallow. *Otolaryngology—Head & Neck Surgery, 104*(3), 339–350.

Bastian, R. W. (1993). The videoendoscopic swallowing study: An alternative and partner to the videofluoroscopic swallowing study. *Dysphagia*, 8(4), 359–367.

Bastian, R. W. (1998). Contemporary diagnosis of the dysphagic patient. *Otolaryngology Clinics of North America*, 31(3), 489–506.

Brunner, M., Stellzig, A., Decker, W., Strate, B., Komposch, G., Wirth, G., & Verres, R. (1994). Video-feedback therapy with the flexible nasopharyngoscope. The potentials for modifying velopharyngeal closure and phonation deficiencies in cleft patients. *Fortschritte de Kieferorthopadei*, 55(4), 197–201.

Cain, A. J., Murray, D. P., & McClymont, L. G. (2002). The use of topical nasal anaesthesia before flexible nasendoscopy: A double-blind, randomized, controlled trial comparing cophenylcaine with placebo. *Clinical Otolaryngology & Allied Sciences*, 27(6), 485–488.

Catalone, B. & Koos, G. (2005). Beyond cleaning: Reprocessing flexible GI endoscopes successfully. *Heathcare Purchasing News*, 29(11), 38–39.

Centers for Disease Control and Prevention. (1987). Recommendations for prevention of HIV transmission in health-care settings. *Morbidity and Mortality Weekly Review*, 36 (Suppl. 25).

Centers for Disease Control and Prevention. (1988). Perspectives in disease prevention and health promotion. *Morbidity and Mortality Weekly Review*, 37, 377–388.

Croft, C. B., Shprintzen, R. J., Daniller, A. I., & Lewin, M. L. (1978). The occult submucous cleft palate and the musculus uvulae. *Cleft Palate Journal*, 15, 150–154.

Croft, C. B., Shprintzen, R. J., & Rakoff, S. J. (1981). Patterns of velopharyngeal valving in normal and cleft palate subjects: A multiview videofluoroscopic and nasendoscopic study. *Laryngoscope*, 91(2), 265–271.

D'Antonio, L. D., & Marsh, J. L. (1987). Abnormal carotid arteries in the velocardiofacial syndrome [Letter]. *Plastic and Reconstructive Surgery*, 80(3), 471–472.

D'Antonio, L. L., Achauer, B. M., & Vander Kam, V. M. (1993). Results of a survey of cleft palate teams concerning the use of nasendoscopy. *Cleft Palate-Craniofacial Journal*, 30(1), 35–39.

D'Antonio, L. L., Chait, D., Lotz, W., & Netsell, R. (1986). Pediatric videonasoendoscopy for speech and voice evaluation. *Otolaryngology–Head & Neck Surgery*, 94(5), 578–583.

D'Antonio, L. L., Marsh, J. L., Province, M. A., Muntz, H. R., & Phillips, C. J. (1989). Reliability of flexible fiberoptic nasopharyngoscopy for evaluation of velopharyngeal function in a clinical population. *Cleft Palate Journal*, 26(3), 217–225; Discussion 225.

D'Antonio, L. L., Muntz, H. R., Marsh, J. L., Marty-Grames, L., & Backensto-Marsh, R. (1988). Practical application of flexible fiberoptic nasopharyngoscopy for evaluating velopharyngeal function. *Plastic and Reconstructive Surgery*, 82(4), 611–618.

David, D. J., White, J., Sprod, R., & Bagnall, A. (1982). Nasendoscopy: Significant refinements of a direct-viewing technique of the velopharyngeal sphincter. *Plastic and Reconstructive Surgery*, 70(4), 423–428.

Douglas, R., Hawke, L., & Wormald, P. J. (2006). Topical anaesthesia before nasendoscopy: A randomized controlled trial of co-phenylcaine compared with lignocaine. *Clinical Otolaryngology*, 31(1), 33.

Federal Register. (1991). Occupational exposure to bloodborne pathogens: Final rule.

Occupational and Safety Health Administration, 29 CFR Part 1910.1030, 64175.

Finkelstein, Y., Berger, G., Nachmani, A., & Ophir, D. (1996). The functional role of the adenoids in speech. *International Journal of Pediatric Otorhinolaryngology, 34*(1/2), 61–74.

Finkelstein, Y., Lerner, M. A., Ophir, D., Nachmani, A., Hauben, D. J., & Zohar, Y. (1993). Nasopharyngeal profile and velopharyngeal valve mechanism. *Plastic and Reconstructive Surgery, 92*(4), 603–614.

Finkelstein, Y., Nachmani, A., & Ophir, D. (1994). The functional role of the tonsils in speech. *Archives of Otolaryngology—Head & Neck Surgery, 120*(8), 846–851.

Finkelstein, Y., Talmi, Y. P., Kravitz, K., Bar-Ziv, J., Nachmani, A., Hauben, D. J., & Zohar, Y. (1991). Study of the normal and insufficient velopharyngeal valve by the "Forced Sucking Test." *Laryngoscope, 101*(11), 1203–1212.

Finkelstein, Y., Zohar, Y., Nachmani, A., Talmi, Y. P., Lerner, M. A., Hauben, D. J., & Frydman, M. (1993). The otolaryngologist and the patient with velocardiofacial syndrome. *Archives of Otolaryngology—Head & Neck Surgery, 119*(5), 563–569.

Frosh, A. C., Jayaraj, S., Porter, G., & Almeyda, J. (1998). Is local anaesthesia actually beneficial in flexible fibreoptic nasendoscopy? *Clinics in Otolaryngology, 23*(3), 259–262.

Georgalas, C., Sandhu, G., Frosh, A., & Xenellis, J. (2005). Cophenylcaine spray vs. placebo in flexible nasendoscopy: A prospective double-blind randomized controlled trial. *International Journal of Clinical Practice, 59*(2), 130–133.

Gereau, S. A., & Shprintzen, R. J. (1988). The role of adenoids in the development of normal speech following palate repair. *Laryngoscope, 98*(3), 299–303.

Golding-Kushner, K. J., Argamaso, R. V., Cotton, R. T., Grames, L. M., Henningsson, G., Jones, et al. (1990). Standardization for the reporting of nasopharyngoscopy and multiview videofluoroscopy: A report from an International Working Group. *Cleft Palate Journal, 27*(4), 337–347; Discussion 347–348.

Gosain, A. K., Conley, S. F., Marks, S., & Larson, D. L. (1996). Submucous cleft palate: Diagnostic methods and outcomes of surgical treatment. *Plastic and Reconstructive Surgery, 97*(7), 1497–1509.

Henningsson, G., & Isberg, A. (1988). Influence of tonsils on velopharyngeal movements in children with craniofacial anomalies and hypernasality. *American Journal of Orthodontics and Dentofacial Orthopedics, 94*(3), 253–261.

Henningsson, G., & Isberg, A. (1991). Comparison between multiview videofluoroscopy and nasendoscopy of velopharyngeal movements. *Cleft Palate-Craniofacial Journal, 28*(4), 413–417; Discussion 417–418.

Hirschberg, J., Dejonckere, P. H., Hirano, M., Mori, K., Schultz-Coulon, H. J., & Vrticka, K. (1995). Voice disorders in children. *International Journal of Pediatric Otorhinolaryngology, 32*(Suppl.), S109–S125.

Hung, C. H., & Cheng, S. Y. (1989). Application of nasopharyngoscopy and videofluoroscopy in the fabrication of a speech aid for soft palate defects. *Journal of the Formosan Medical Association, 88*(8), 812–818.

Igawa, H. H., Nishizawa, N., Sugihara, T., & Inuyama, Y. (1998). A fiberscopic analysis of velopharyngeal movement before and after primary palatoplasty in cleft palate infants. *Plastic and Reconstructive Surgery, 102*(3), 668–674.

Karnell, M. P. (1994). *Videoendoscopy: From velopharynx to larynx.* San Diego, CA: Singular Publishing Group.

Karnell, M. P., & Langmore, S. (1998). Videoendoscopy in speech and swallowing for the speech-language pathologist. In A. F. Johnson & B. H. Jacobson (Eds.), *Medical speech-language pathology: A practitioner's guide* (pp. 563–584). New York: Thieme.

Karnell, M. P., Ibuki, K., Morris, H. L., & Van Demark, D. R. (1983). Reliability of the nasopharyngeal fiberscope (NPF) for assessing velopharyngeal function: Analysis by judgment. *Cleft Palate Journal, 20*(3), 199–208.

Karnell, M. P., Rosenstein, H., & Fine, L. (1987). Nasal videoendoscopy in prosthetic management of palatopharyngeal dysfunction. *Journal of Prosthetic Dentistry, 58*(4), 479–484.

Kidder, T. M., Langmore, S. E., & Martin, B. J. (1994). Indications and techniques of endoscopy in evaluation of cervical dysphagia: Comparison with radiographic techniques. *Dysphagia, 9*(4), 256–261.

Kummer, A. W., Billmire, D. A., & Myer, C. M. (1993). Hypertrophic tonsils: The effect on resonance and velopharyngeal closure. *Plastic and Reconstructive Surgery, 91*(4), 608–611.

Kummer, A. W., Curtis, C., Wiggs, M., Lee, L., & Strife, J. L. (1992). Comparison of velopharyngeal gap size in patients with hypernasality, hypernasality, and nasal emission, or nasal turbulence (rustle) as the primary speech characteristic. *Cleft Palate-Craniofacial Journal, 29*(2), 152–156.

Kunzel, H. J. (1982). First applications of a biofeedback device for the therapy of velopharyngeal incompetence. *Folia Phoniatrica, 34*(2), 92–100.

Langmore, S. E., Schatz, K., & Olsen, N. (1988). Fiberoptic endoscopic examination of swallowing safety: A new procedure. *Dysphagia, 2*(4), 216–219.

Lennox, P., Hern, J., Birchall, M., & Lund, V. (1996). Local anaesthesia in flexible nasendoscopy. A comparison between cocaine and co-phenylcaine. *Journal of Laryngology & Otology, 110*(6), 540–542.

Lewin, M. L., Croft, C. B., & Shprintzen, R. J. (1980). Velopharyngeal insufficiency due to hypoplasia of the musculus uvulae and occult submucous cleft palate. *Plastic and Reconstructive Surgery, 65*(5), 585–591.

Lewis, J. R., Andreassen, M. L., Leeper, H. A., Macrae, D. L., & Thomas, J. (1993). Vocal characteristics of children with cleft lip/palate and associated velopharyngeal incompetence. *Journal of Otolaryngology, 22*(2), 113–117.

Lotz, W. K., D'Antonio, L. L., Chait, D. H., & Netsell, R. W. (1993). Successful nasoendoscopic and aerodynamic examinations of children with speech/voice disorders. *International Journal of Pediatric Otorhinolaryngology, 26*(2), 165–172.

MacKenzie-Stepner, K., Witzel, M. A., Stringer, D. A., & Laskin, R. (1987). Velopharyngeal insufficiency due to hypertrophic tonsils: A report of two cases. *International Journal of Pediatric Otorhinolaryngology, 14*(1), 57–63.

MacKenzie-Stepner, K., Witzel, M. A., Stringer, D. A., Lindsay, W. K., Munro, I. R., & Hughes, H. (1987). Abnormal carotid arteries in the velocardiofacial syndrome: A report of three cases. *Plastic and Reconstructive Surgery, 80*(3), 347–351.

Mason, R. M. (1973). Preventing speech disorders following adenoidectomy by preoperative examination. *Clinics in Pediatrics, 12*(7), 405–414.

McWilliams, B. J., Glaser, E. R., Philips, B. J., Lawrence, C., Lavorato, A. S., Beery, Q. C., & Skolnick, M. L. (1981). A comparative study of four methods of evaluating velopharyngeal adequacy. *Plastic and Reconstructive Surgery, 68*(1), 1–10.

Miyazaki, T., Matsuya, T., & Yamaoka, M. (1975). Fiberscopic methods for assessment of velopharyngeal closure during various activities. *Cleft Palate Journal, 12,* 107–114.

Morris, H. L. (1975). The speech pathologist looks at the tonsils and the adenoids. *Annals of Otology, Rhinology, and Laryngology, 84*(2, Suppl. 19, Pt. 2), 63–66.

Olympus America Inc. P.O. BOX 90582, Corporate Center Dr., Melville, NY, 11747.

Osberg, P. E., & Witzel, M. A. (1981). The physiologic basis for hypernasality during connected speech in cleft palate patients: A nasendoscopic study. *Plastic and Reconstructive Surgery, 67*(1), 1–5.

Pannbacker, M. D., Lass, N. J., Hansen, G. G., Mussa, A. M., & Robison, K. L. (1993). Survey of speech-language pathologists' training, experience, and opinions on nasopharyngoscopy. *Cleft Palate-Craniofacial Journal, 30*(1), 40–45.

PENTAX Medical Company. A Division of PENTAX of America, Inc. 102 Chestnut Ridge Road, Montvale, NJ, 07645-1856.

Peterson-Falzone, S. J. (1985). Velopharyngeal inadequacy in the absence of overt cleft palate. *Journal of Craniofacial Genetics and Developmental Biology* (Suppl. 1), 97–124.

Peterson-Falzone, S. J., & Graham, M. S. (1990). Phoneme-specific nasal emission in children with and without physical anomalies of the velopharyngeal mechanism. *Journal of Speech and Hearing Disorders, 55*(1), 132–139.

Pigott, R. W., Bensen, J. F., & White, F. D. (1969). Nasendoscopy in the diagnosis of velopharyngeal incompetence. *Plastic and Reconstructive Surgery, 43*(2), 141–147.

Pigott, R. W., & Makepeace, A. P. (1982). Some characteristics of endoscopic and radiological systems used in elaboration of the diagnosis of velopharyngeal incompetence. British *Journal of Plastic Surgery, 35* (1), 19–32.

Pothier, D. D., Awad, Z., Whitehouse, M., & Porter, G. C. (2005). The use of lubrication in flexible fibreoptic nasendoscopy: A randomized controlled trial. *Clinical Otolaryngology, 30*(4), 353–356.

Ramamurthy, L., Wyatt, R. A., Whitby, D., Martin, D., & Davenport, P. (1997). The evaluation of velopharyngeal function using flexible nasendoscopy. *Journal of Laryngology & Otology, 111*(8), 739–745.

Rich, B. M., Farber, K., & Shprintzen, R. J. (1988). Nasopharyngoscopy in the treatment of palatopharyngeal insufficiency. *International Journal of Prosthodontics, 1*(3), 248–251.

Ross, D. A., Witzel, M. A., Armstrong, D. C., & Thomson, H. G. (1996). Is pharyngoplasty a risk in velocardiofacial syndrome? An assessment of medially displaced carotid arteries. *Plastic and Reconstructive Surgery, 98*(7), 1182–1190.

Rowe, M. R., & D'Antonio, L. L. (2005). Velopharyngeal dysfunction: Evolving developments in evaluation. *Current Opinion in Otolaryngology & Head & Neck Surgery, 13*(6), 366–370.

Rutala, W. A. (1996). APIC guideline for selection and use of disinfectants. *American Journal of Infectious Disease Control, 24,* 313–342.

Sadek, S. A., De, R., Scott, A., White, A. P., Wilson, P. S., & Carlin, W. V. (2001). The efficacy of topical anaesthesia in flexible nasendoscopy: A double-blind randomized controlled trial. *Clinical Otolaryngology & Allied Sciences, 26*(1), 25–28.

Shelton, R. L., Beaumont, K., Trier, W. C., & Furr, M. L. (1978). Videoendoscopic feedback in training velopharyngeal closure. *Cleft Palate Journal, 15*(1), 6–12.

Shprintzen, R. J. (1979). The use of multiview videofluoroscopy and flexible fiberoptic nasopharyngoscopy as a predictor of success with pharyngeal flap surgery. In R. Ellis & F. C. Flack (Eds.), *Diagnosis and treatment of palato-glossal malfunction* (pp. 6–14). London: College of Speech Therapists.

Shprintzen, R. J. (1995). Instrumental assessment of velopharyngeal valving. In R. J. Shprintzen & J. Bardach (Eds.), *Cleft palate speech management: A multidisciplinary approach* (Vol. 4, pp. 221–256). St. Louis: Mosby.

Shprintzen, R. J. (1996). Nasopharyngoscopy. In K. R. Bzoch (Ed.), *Communicative disorders related to cleft lip and palate* (Vol. 4, pp. 387–409). Austin, TX: Pro-Ed.

Shprintzen, R. J., & Golding-Kushner, K. J. (1989). Evaluation of velopharyngeal insufficiency. *Otolaryngology Clinics of North America, 22*(3), 519–536.

Shprintzen, R. J., Lewin, M. L., Croft, C. B., Daniller, A. I., Argamaso, R. V., Ship, A. G., & Strauch, B. (1979). A comprehensive study of pharyngeal flap surgery: Tailor-made flaps. *Cleft Palate Journal, 16*(1), 46–55.

Shprintzen, R. J., Rakof, S. J., Skolnick, M. L., & Lavorato, A. S. (1977). Incongruous movements of the velum and lateral pharyngeal walls. *Cleft Palate Journal, 14*(2), 148–157.

Siegel-Sadewitz, V. L., & Shprintzen, R. J. (1982). Nasopharyngoscopy of the normal velopharyngeal sphincter: An experiment of biofeedback. *Cleft Palate Journal, 19*(3), 194–200.

Siegel-Sadewitz, V. L., & Shprintzen, R. J. (1986). Changes in velopharyngeal valving with age. *International Journal of Pediatric Otorhinolaryngology, 11*(2), 171–182.

Sinclair, S. W., Davies, D. M., & Bracka, A. (1982). Comparative reliability of nasal pharyngoscopy and videofluorography in the assessment of velopharyngeal incompetence. *British Journal of Plastic Surgery, 35*(2), 113–117.

Skolnick, M. L., Shprintzen, R. J., McCall, G. N., & Rakoff, S. (1975). Patterns of velopharyngeal closure in subjects with repaired cleft palate and normal speech: A multi-view videofluoroscopic analysis. *Cleft Palate Journal, 12,* 369–376.

Smith, J. C., & Rockley, T. J. (2002). A comparison of cocaine and "co-phenylcaine" local anaesthesia in flexible nasendoscopy. *Clinical Otolaryngology & Allied Sciences, 27*(3), 192–196.

Storz Medicaal. 1000 Cobb Place Blvd., Bldg. 400, Suite 450, US-Kennesaw, GA, 30144.

Taub, S. (1966). The Taub oral panendoscope: A new technique. *Cleft Palate Journal, 3,* 328–346.

Willging, J. P. (2003). Velopharyngeal insufficiency. *Current Opinion in Otolaryngology & Head & Neck Surgery, 11*(6), 452–455.

Williams, R. G., Preece, M., Rhys, R., & Eccles, R. (1992). The effect of adenoid and tonsil surgery on nasalance. *Clinics in Otolaryngology, 17*(2), 136–140.

Witt, P. D., Miller, D. C., Marsh, J. L., Muntz, H. R., & Grames, L. M. (1998). Limited value of preoperative cervical vascular imaging in patients with velocardiofacial syndrome. *Plastic and Reconstructive Surgery, 101*(5), 1184–1195; Discussion 1196–1199.

Witzel, M. A., & Posnick, J. C. (1989). Patterns and location of velopharyngeal valving problems: Atypical findings on video nasopharyngoscopy. *Cleft Palate Journal, 26*(1), 63–67.

Witzel, M. A., Tobe, J., & Salyer, K. (1988). The use of nasopharyngoscopy biofeedback therapy in the correction of inconsistent velopharyngeal closure. *International Journal of Pediatric Otorhinolaryngology, 15*(2), 137–142.

Witzel, M. A., Tobe, J., & Salyer, K. E. (1989). The use of videonasopharyngoscopy for biofeedback therapy in adults after pharyngeal flap surgery. *Cleft Palate Journal, 26*(2), 129–134; Discussion 135.

Yamaoka, M., Matsuya, T., Miyazaki, T., Nishio, J., & Ibuki, K. (1983). Visual training for velopharyngeal closure in cleft palate patients: A fibrescopic procedure (preliminary report). *Journal of Maxillofacial Surgery, 11*(4), 191–193.

Ysunza, A., Pamplona, M., Femat, T., Mayer, I., & Garcia-Velasco, M. (1997). Videonasopharyngoscopy as an instrument for visual biofeedback during speech in cleft palate patients. *International Journal of Pediatric Otorhinolaryngology, 41*(3), 291–298.

Zajac, D. J., & Linville, R. N. (1989). Voice perturbations of children with perceived nasality and hoarseness. *Cleft Palate Journal, 26*(3), 226–231; Discussion 231–232.

Zwitman, D. H., Sonderman, J. C., & Ward, P. H. (1974). Variations in velopharyngeal closure assessed by endoscopy. *Journal of Speech and Hearing Disorders, 39*(3), 366–372.

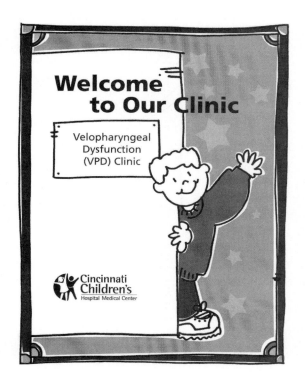

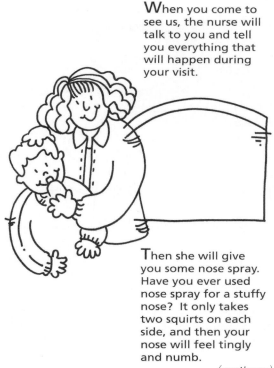

When you come to see us, the nurse will talk to you and tell you everything that will happen during your visit.

Then she will give you some nose spray. Have you ever used nose spray for a stuffy nose? It only takes two squirts on each side, and then your nose will feel tingly and numb.

(continues)

(continued)

Once the scope is in your nose, the speech pathologist will ask you to repeat some sentences again.

When you are talking, you can watch the inside of your nose on TV. There are parts in there that move... almost like magic.

It is very important to hold still so the tube doesn't bump around inside. If you want, you can sit on someone's lap to help you hold still.

Next it will be time to see your nose on TV. The doctor will put a long, skinny tube inside your nose. This is called a scope and here is what it looks like.

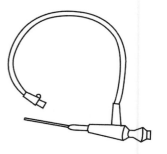

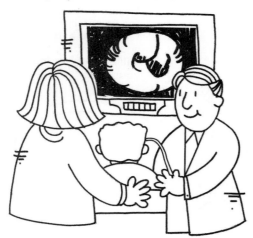

The scope only goes in a little bit.

It doesn't hurt because your nose will be numb from the nose drops.

Sometimes it seems a little scary though... so be brave!

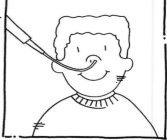

Coloring book pages to help prepare the child for the exam.

C H A P T E R

18

SURGICAL MANAGEMENT OF CLEFTS AND VELOPHARYNGEAL DYSFUNCTION

DAVID A. BILLMIRE, M.D.

CHAPTER OUTLINE

INTRODUCTION

Cleft lip and palate occur in a spectrum from the abortive form, such as a form fruste of the lip or an asymptomatic submucous cleft of the palate, to complete bilateral clefts of the lip and palate. Regardless of the degree of involvement, the surgical principals remain the same. The correction must take into account the anatomical and physiological derangement of a complete disruption in embryological development. For example, in a form fruste of the lip, the overlying skin is intact but the underlying muscle, nasal cartilage, and oral sphincter function usually are significantly affected. Therefore, correction requires a complete lip repair. For the same reason, correction of a symptomatic submucous cleft of the palate requires the same type of repair as if it were a complete cleft. (For those who would like more information about the actual surgical procedures, Virtual Surgery Videos are available free of charge through Smile Train at http://www.smiletrain.org.)

While surgical concepts and approaches have become more standardized in the last few years, there is a wide range of interpretation of these "standards" throughout the world, across the country, and even within a single treatment team. Treatment options, timing, surgical techniques, and philosophies are presented in this chapter solely as broad general guidelines.

It is important to remember that clefts of lip and palate involve much more than the obvious defect to the lip and roof of the mouth. Their sphere of influence extends to other aesthetic areas, such as the nose and midface; to other anatomical areas, such as the jaws, teeth, the oral sphincter and velopharyngeal sphincter; to the functional aspects of the airway, hearing, speech and feeding; and psychologically to the individual's identity. Surgical repair should seek to achieve a normal anatomical and physiological state as much as possible, which usually results in an improved psychological state as well. The successful treatment of the patient with cleft lip and palate hinges on the treatment team's adherence to and completion of a comprehensive program with well-defined goals and objectives.

CLEFT LIP REPAIR

Timing of the Cleft Lip Repair

There has been considerable debate over the years among surgeons about the appropriate timing for the cleft lip repair, also know as a *cheiloplasty*. At one time, the repair of the cleft lip was often done shortly after birth and before the child was sent home. It was felt that neonatal repair was appropriate since it allowed the mother to better bond to the infant. In addition, from an anesthetic standpoint, neonates were felt to be most physiologically sound immediately after birth before their own physiological systems became more active. Modern pediatric anesthesia has negated the later argument, while the former remains debatable. Although there are a few cleft palate centers that are reintroducing the concept of repair within the first week of life, most centers currently advocate delaying repair and following some variation of the *rule of 10s*. This "rule" is a guideline which says that the infant should be at least 10 weeks of age, weigh at least 10 pounds, and have a hemoglobin of 10 gm prior to the lip repair.

There are several reasons for delaying this initial surgery. These include the fact that cleft lip and palate are often associated with other abnormalities, a number of which are not readily apparent at birth. Delaying surgery allows a longer time for investigation of other potentially serious problems. In addition, an acceptable feeding technique must be established and weight gain assured prior to taking on extensive surgery. Finally, many teams use some form of active or passive presurgical orthopedics, often referred to as nasoalveolar molding devices (NAMs), to align the cleft. In incomplete clefts and those with a *Simonart's band* (a band of skin without underlying muscle bridging the cleft just below the nose) this option is usually unnecessary. Delaying surgery allows time for these devices to narrow or better position the cleft segments and reposition the nasal cartilages prior to repair so that a better result can be achieved. Despite the presence of the cleft lip, bonding will occur with the caregivers, which is crucial to the child's development. Given these considerations, in most cleft palate centers at this time, the initial repair of cleft lip is usually accomplished between 4 weeks and 12 weeks of age.

Presurgical Management

In wide clefts of the lip, whether they are unilateral or bilateral, it is not uncommon to narrow the gap prior to performing the formal repair. Aligning the segments prior to surgical repair can improve the ultimate outcome and can result in less tension on the lip repair once it is repaired.

With a unilateral cleft lip, there are number of options for aligning the segments. The simplest procedure is to tape the lip with adhesive tape (see Figure 9–22). This may also be used in conjunction with *dental elastics,* which are small rubber bands to add a dynamic component. In some centers, this technique may be used with a palatal molding plate to help guide the segments as they move. This method is usually used over a four- to six-week period. It relies heavily on parent cooperation and input, and therefore, should be carefully monitored.

A second option for aligning the segments is using an active dental appliance, sometimes referred to as a *Latham appliance* (Georgiade & Latham, 1975; Latham, 1980; Latham, Kusy, & Georgiade, 1976; Millard & Latham, 1990; Millard, Latham, Huifen, Spiro, & Morovic, 1999) (see Figure 9–21). This method uses a two-piece acrylic dental appliance pinned to the greater and lesser segments of the palate. On a daily basis, a screw is turned slowly, which draws the two segments together in order to close the gap. This usually takes about three to four weeks to accomplish.

Both the passive molding plate and the Latham appliance can also be combined with an acrylic extension to help form the nostril. These combined devices are called *nasal alveolar molding* devices or NAM (Da Silveira et al., 2003). They are labor intensive and require the skills of a pedodontist or orthodontist.

The third option for pulling the segments together is a surgical procedure called a *lip adhesion*. This is a simple straight-line lip repair that is performed so that the subsequent lip pressure will draw the segments together. This can also be used with a molding plate and/or NAM. The lip adhesion is usually done at 6 weeks of age followed by the formal lip repair three or four months later. The decision to use any of the above methods is highly dependent on the experience of the surgeon and the facilities available.

Presurgical treatment options in bilateral cleft lip are similar to those of unilateral clefts. The first is simple taping. In bilateral clefts of the lip, use of a headgear (bonnet) with Velcro elastic bands to draw the premaxilla back into position is a common and long-standing technique. Both the taping and the bonnet methods may be used with a passive molding plate to guide the segments into position. An active Latham appliance may also be used. Like the unilateral device, it is also pinned to the maxilla and dental chain elastics are used to pull the premaxilla back into position. With this appliance, there is also the possibility of expanding the two lateral segments, which are often collapsed together. The chain elastics are usually adjusted by the pediatric dentist. Again, acrylic extensions can be used to help mold the nose. Last, there is the surgical adhesion similar to the unilateral procedure, which uses the pressure of the "repaired" lip to draw the premaxilla back into position. One is more apt to see some type of technique used on bilateral lips, as the protrusion of the unrestrained premaxilla and prolabium puts tremendous pressure on the repaired lip.

Techniques for Unilateral Cleft Lip Repair

By examining an unrepaired unilateral cleft lip deformity, one can see that all the structures are present, including the philtral dimple and both of the philtral ridges. The cleft passes just to the lateral side of the philtral ridge. On the cleft side, the lip is short and the Cupid's bow is twisted up into the cleft. Early surgical techniques to repair this cleft lip deformity were simple straight-line repairs. This type of repair resulted in a lip that was characteristically short and notched.

Currently, there are two major methods for repairing the unilateral cleft lip: the Millard technique (Trier, 1985b) and the Tennison-Randall technique (Brauer, & Cronin, 1983; Lazarus, Hudson, van Zyl, Fleming, & Fernandes, 1998; Leon-Valle, 1980). Figure 18–1 shows the basic technique for the Millard lip

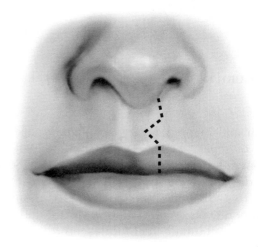

A. Randall-Tennison

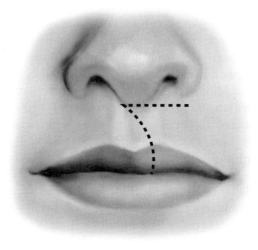

B. Millard

FIGURE 18–1 (A and B) Techniques of unilateral cleft lip repairs. A. Randall-Tennison repair. B. Millard repair.

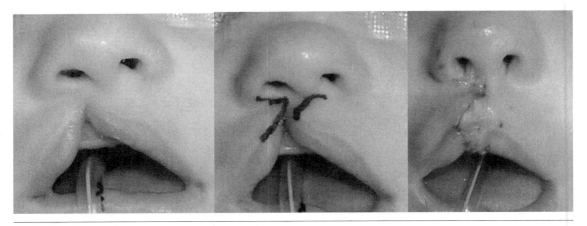

FIGURE 18–2   Photograph of a unilateral Millard lip repair.

repair and Figure 18–2 is a photograph of this type of repair. Figure 18–3A shows a patient preoperatively, Figure 18–3B shows the patient one day following a Millard repair, and Figure 18–3C shows the patient six months postoperatively. With both the Millard and the Tennison-Randall techniques, the philtral ridge is lengthened by inserting a "patch" of tissue into the ridge on the cleft side. This brings the ridge down to match the unaffected side. Since plastic surgeons are not able to do scarless surgery, an attempt is made to place the scars in normally occurring lines and anatomical breaks, such as the philtral ridges.

The Millard technique, or rotation advancement flap, is used in approximately 80% of cases and is perhaps the most anatomical of the repairs. It is known as a "cut as you go" technique because adjustments are constantly made during this procedure to bring the lip into balance. In this technique, the extra tissue or "patch" is inserted at the top of the lip, just beneath the nose. The initial incision is placed along the philtral ridge on the cleft side. As the incision is carried up along the ridge and beneath the nose in a curvilinear manner, the lip opens up and "rotates" down until the

Cupid's bow is level, hence the rotation part of the name. As the philtrum rotates into the correct position, it leaves a gap at the top of the lip, beneath the nose. Into this gap, tissue is inserted to maintain the length and fill the defect. This is done by advancing tissue from the lateral portion of the lip again beneath the nose (alae in this case) into this gap, hence the advancement portion of the name. By increasing or decreasing the amount of rotation, the lip length may be adjusted. Tissue, which is lateral to the incision on the philtral ridge, is used to lengthen the shortened columella on the cleft side.

The Millard repair, with its "cut as you go" philosophy, is thought by some to be the more difficult of the repairs. Additionally, the tissue is inserted at the point of maximum tension where the underlying structures are relatively fixed to the maxilla. In inexperienced hands, this can often lead to a lip that is too short. In very wide clefts, some will not consider this repair at all or will resort to a lip adhesion prior to formal repair. On the plus side, the normal philtral dimple is preserved, the scar follows and mimics the philtral ridge, and by inserting the tissue at the top of the lip, the result is a

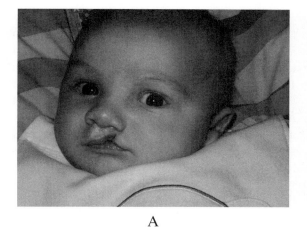

A

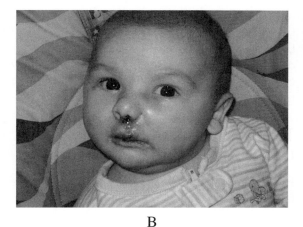

B

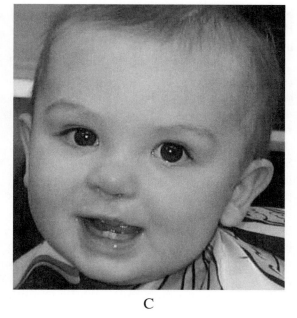

C

FIGURE 18–3 (A–C) A. Patient preoperatively. B. Patient one day postoperatively following a Millard repair. C. Patient six months postoperatively.

better nasal configuration (Becker, Svensson, McWilliam, Sarnas, & Jacobsson, 1998). Revisions when necessary are relatively easy. The most common problem is that the lip may be too short. If this is the case, the lip can simply be rerotated and lengthened in a second procedure. Its advantages far outweigh its disadvantages, and this explains why it is the most widely used repair today.

The Tennison-Randall procedure, or triangular flap technique, is used in about 20% of cases, and follows from an older technique, the LeMesurier repair or quadrilateral flap technique. The Tennison-Randall procedure is

precise and measured and therefore, it is often referred to as a "cookie cutter" technique. Many surgeons like the security of this type of fixed technique. In the Tennison-Randall method, an incision is placed about half way up through the philtral ridge on the cleft side. This opens a triangular opening (hence the name "triangular flap technique") in the inferior portion of the lip and the point of the Cupid's bow drops into position. A triangular-shaped flap from the lateral portion of the lip is inserted into this triangular-shaped gap. This "patch" of tissue is inserted in the bottom and most mobile portion of the lip.

Significant mobilization in the upper portion of the lip, where tension is the greatest, is thereby avoided.

Despite violating both the philtral ridge and philtral dimple, the results from this procedure can be quite good, with good lip configuration and a symmetrical Cupid's bow. The nasal results are usually not as good, however, since the alar base usually remains somewhat splayed. Subsequent nasal reconstruction is compromised because the tissue in the upper part of the lip will tend to bunch up as the alar base is brought into its proper position, and there is little possibility of creating a nostril sil. However, since the extra tissue is inserted in the most mobile portion of the lip, this repair, as previously stated, is often popular in wide clefts.

It is important to remember that the mouth is a sphincter and that clefts can affect both the oral and velopharyngeal sphincters. Just as it is important to reconstruct the velopharyngeal sphincter, it is important to reconstruct the oral sphincter. While this may seem intuitively obvious, historically this was ignored. When there is a cleft lip, the orbicularis oris muscles of the oral sphincter are divided. Instead of creating a complete ring around the mouth, they are discontinuous and the divided ends are abnormally inserted. In unilateral clefts the orbicularis oris inserts along the *piriform aperture* (the opening at the base of the ala) laterally and along the anterior nasal spine (at the base of the columella) medially. In the bilateral cleft, there is no muscle in the prolabial portion and the orbicularis oris abnormally inserts on either side of the piriform aperture at the alar bases. Regardless of the type of repair chosen, these abnormal insertions should be taken down and the muscles realigned into the correct orientation. Failure to do so will result in distortion of the lip on activation, noticeable depressions, and a poor aesthetic result.

In the past, and to a certain extent even today, there has been debate over whether to address the accompanying nasal deformity of the unilateral cleft lip with the initial lip repair. Historically, it was felt that the nose should not be operated on in infancy due to a concern that its growth potential would be adversely affected. In the last few decades, several surgeons have demonstrated that not only is this concern unfounded, but better long-term results can be achieved by early correction of the nasal deformity at the time of initial lip repair (Salyer, 1986). Therefore, all lip repair techniques involve some method of repositioning the distorted lower lateral cartilage of the nose and malpositioned alar base. While these early repairs on the lip and nose do not obviate the need for secondary surgery, they greatly reduce the initial deformity and lessen the extent of subsequent reconstruction.

Techniques for Bilateral Cleft Lip Repair

Repair of a bilateral cleft lip deformity is a more frustrating and a less successful endeavor when compared to the contemporary unilateral repair. The magnitude of the lip and nasal deformities can present formidable challenges to even the most experienced surgeons. A bilateral complete cleft of the primary palate can result in the unrestrained protrusion of the premaxillary complex. With the premaxilla protruding anteriorly, it is not uncommon for the two lateral segments to collapse behind it. Expansion of the lateral segments is sometime required in order to allow the premaxilla to drop back into position. The *prolabium* (the lip portion of the premaxilla) has no muscle in it and this lack of muscle tension across this portion of the lip results in an appearance of significant "shrinkage."

In the past, the appearance of a diminutive prolabium led to the incorrect assumption that there was a need for extra tissue in this area. This led to a whole host of repairs directed toward adding tissue to the prolabium. This tissue was added beneath the prolabium from the lateral lip elements. The resulting scars were shaped either like a "Y" or a goal post. This was hardly in keeping with the concept of hiding scars in naturally occurring lines. What became evident over time was that the prolabium, when exposed to muscle tension, would stretch. As a result, the lip ended up being tight transversely and very long vertically. The transverse tightness applied significant pressure on an already compromised maxilla, resulting in often dramatic retrusion of the upper jaw. In the 1960s, the shortcomings of this type of repair were realized and it was abandoned.

Currently, all contemporary bilateral cleft lip repairs are some variation of a modified straight-line repair. While each repair may boast of having a Z-plasty-type component, they all achieve about the same result. The prolabium forms the entire philtral area. Even though the prolabium is small, it is routinely made narrower and the lateral portions or parings are used in some form for eventual columellar lengthening. Immediately after the repair, the lip looks tight and bunched up. Within several weeks, the prolabium begins to stretch out and achieve a more normal size. If care is not taken to initially trim the prolabial segment down, it will be too large once the lip matures.

The two major methods of bilateral cleft lip repair are the Millard and some form of the modified Broadbent-Manchester repair. These repairs are illustrated in Figure 18–4. The major difference between the two procedures is the method in which the white roll of the philtrum is created. In the Millard repair, the white roll comes from the white roll of the lateral elements. In the modified

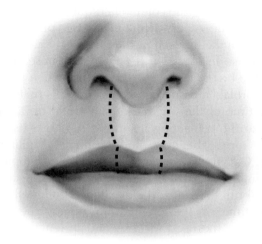

A. Modified Manchester

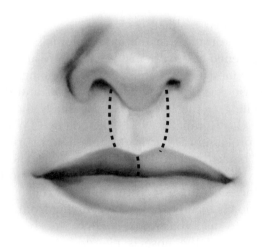

B. Millard Bilateral Cleft

FIGURE 18–4 (A and B) Techniques of bilateral lip repairs. A. Modified Manchester repair. B. Millard bilateral cleft repair.

Broadbent-Manchester repair, the white roll from the prolabium is preserved.

While most surgeons now feel that nasal repair in the unilateral lip can be accomplished with the initial lip repair, there is some controversy in bilateral lips. Traditional methods of lengthening the columella require banking or storing the excess tissue from the prolabium either in the lip itself or the floor of the nose for later use in elevating the tip of the nose. This had to be done in a staged manner when using the prolabial tissue because to use this tissue at the time of the original repair would devascularize the remaining necessary prolabial tissue that forms the new philtril dimple. Mulliken and Cutting have been successful in developing techniques that use tissue from the elongated nasal rim to form and elongate the columella at the time of the original lip repair, thereby negating the need for a secondary lengthening (Cutting & Grayson, 1993; Cutting et al. 1998; Kohout, Aljaro, Farkas, & Mulliken, 1998). This technique may be enhanced by the use of a nasoalveolar molding device.

In the event that the nasal columella is not lengthened at the original repair, there are two major methods of columellar lengthening that are widely used. The initial lip repair and the handling of the lateral parings usually dictate how the columella will be lengthened. When the prolabium is narrowed, the lateral parings are "banked" or stored in the floor of the nose. They appear as bumps in the floor of the nose. At the second stage on the bilateral repair, an incision is made transversely, curving from alar base to alar base just below the banked parings. As the nose is elevated, two things happen. The floor of the nose (the banked parings) is drawn up into the columella, thereby lengthening it. As the nose moves up, the alae move closer together, narrowing the base of the nose. This type of secondary lip repair is referred as a Cronin columellar lengthening procedure.

If no parings were created in the original repair and the full width of the prolabium was used to make the philtral dimple, the resulting dimple will be quite wide once the scars mature. In a sense, the parings were banked

in the lip, not the floor of the nose. When this is the case, a forked flap lengthening is used. At the time of the second surgery, the lateral parings are created and raised from the lip. This tissue is then used to lengthen the columella. This is usually the case in a Millard-type approach. Either approach can be used, depending on the configuration of the lip and the site of the excess tissue. Timing of this secondary procedure varies with each surgeon, but it is usually done between 9 months and 5 years of age.

Cleft Palate Repair: Palatoplasty

Timing of the Cleft Palate Repair

The timing of the *palatoplasty* (cleft palate repair) has been even more controversial than timing of the lip repair. There are a few teams that advocate palate repair in the first week of life, but this is extremely controversial. Most centers fall into two major philosophies—early and late. Early is defined as between 6 months and 15 months of age. Late is defined as between 15 months and 24 months of age.

In general, it is acknowledged that the earlier the palate repair is done, the lower the incidence will be of velopharyngeal insufficiency and development of compensatory articulation productions (Hardin-Jones & Jones, 2005; Witzel, Salyer, & Ross, 1984). However, early repair of the hard palate has raised concerns about the potential effect on the growth of the maxilla, which affects the appearance of the midface. Patients with a history of cleft palate and surgical repair often demonstrate midface retrusion and Class III malocclusion due to a lack of adequate midfacial and maxillary growth. Over the last

50 years, there has been a debate in the literature as to whether this is caused by the inherent nature of the cleft, or if it is the result of the surgical repair of the palate. One school of thought has been that midface deficiency is the direct result of the surgical repair of the palate. To avoid the potential adverse effect on facial growth, Schweckendiek (1955) advocated closing the velum (soft palate) only at an early age, usually around 6 months. The hard palate was closed at a later time, usually at 4 or 5 years of age, to avoid scarring of the growing hard palate. Until it was finally surgically closed, the hard palate was usually obturated for speech. The basic philosophy of this technique was that it promoted velopharyngeal closure while avoiding restriction in maxillary growth (Blocksma, Leuz, & Mellerstig, 1975; Dingman & Grabb, 1971; Perko, 1979; Schweckendiek, 1966, 1968, 1983; Schweckendiek & Doz, 1978).

In subsequent studies, the results of this two-stage approach have been found to be less than impressive. Several studies have shown that a high percentage of the patients treated with this method fail to develop acceptable speech and a large number require pharyngeal flaps (Bardach, Morris, & Olin, 1984; Cosman & Falk, 1980; Fara & Brousilova, 1988; Fara, Brousilova, Hrivnakova, & Tvrdek, 1992; Jackson, McLennan, & Scheker, 1983; Witzel et al., 1984). The hard palate has been found to be difficult to close when repaired at a later time (Cosman & Falk, 1980; Jackson et al., 1983). Finally, there is virtually no difference in facial group between patients who have early palate repair and those who have the two-stage procedure with delayed palate repair (Fara, Brousilova, Hrivnakova, & Tvrdek, 1992; Smahel & Horak, 1993). They also found that a greater orthodontic effort is needed to achieve an aligned dentoalveolar arch with the two-stage palatoplasty. Ross (1987) reported the results of cephalometric radiographs of 538 males with unilateral cleft lip and palate and compared the results to age of palate repair. The results of this study showed that the best facial outcome was for patients repaired in the teenage years or later. However, the next-best outcome was for those patients repaired by 11 months or earlier. The worst outcome was with patients who had palate repairs after 20 months. Given these findings, the possible advantages of the two-stage approach in relationship to maxillofacial growth remain difficult to prove and it is generally accepted that this delay in hard palate closure has a negative effect on speech. Despite these findings, there are some centers that still promote some variation of this practice.

In addition to the concern about midface growth, there is an additional factor that may delay the palate repair. When there is an extremely wide cleft, some inexperienced surgeons may not be comfortable closing the palate in a single stage. Some feel that closing the velum only will narrow the remaining cleft of the hard palate. As with the classic Schweckendiek technique, the speech results with this delay are less than desirable.

Techniques for Palatoplasty

While the cleft lip repair dates back to antiquity, successful palatal repair dates only from the early nineteenth century. With the advent of anesthesia and specialized instrumentation, success rates have improved dramatically.

Achieving a good result in palatal surgery is much more difficult than achieving a good result in lip surgery. While it may appear that a palate repair is simple in comparison to a lip repair, palate surgery can be quite challenging for several reasons. First, it is technically more demanding than a lip repair. In addition, there is a greater risk of postoperative problems, such as dehiscence, fistula formation, or excessive scarring. If these problems occur, they are difficult to correct. There is a potential for airway compromise or excessive bleeding, which may put the patient's life in jeopardy. Finally, merely closing the palate is not enough. The palate not only serves as a physical barrier between the mouth and nose, but also must function dynamically for normal speech.

The von Langenbeck repair is one of the oldest and most successful means of palatal closure and is still popular today (Murison & Pigott, 1992; Trier & Dreyer, 1984). Approximately 60% of palatoplasties performed today are of this type. This repair is illustrated in Figure 18–5. In this repair, an incision is made just inside the gum line, starting just behind the teeth and extending up to the area of the canine tooth. The mucoperiosteum over the bone is carefully raised off the bone and, in conjunction with the velum, separated in one large layer. The cleft margin is incised and the raw edges are brought together and sewn down the middle. The incisions along the gum line are usually left open. This operation was the procedure of choice until the 1930s. However, there was a high incidence of velopharyngeal insufficiency with this procedure. In addition, the levator muscle was typically not addressed with this repair. This set off a search for a procedure that not only closed the opening, but also actively lengthened the palate.

A number of approaches for lengthening the palate have been tried (Bae, Kim, Lee, Hwang, & Kim, 2002). Some have caused problems with growth, wound healing, and airway obstruction. One technique that is still commonly used is the Wardill-Kilner "V" to "Y," or pushback, procedure, which is illustrated in Figure 18–6. In this procedure, the initial incisions are similar to that of the von Langenbeck—except instead of leaving the mucoperiosteum attached in the front of the mouth, it is cut across as a "V." This frees up the mucoperiosteum of the whole palate and allows it to be pushed back in an attempt to lengthen it. The resulting open area is "Y" shaped. The levator muscle is not addressed with this procedure and a high incidence of anterior fistulae has been reported with this procedure (Moore, Lawrence, Ptak, & Trier, 1988).

Just as a cleft lip disrupts the oral sphincter in the lip and alters the insertion of the sphincteric muscles, a cleft palate also changes the velopharyngeal sphincter. In the patient with cleft palate, the levator veli palatini inserts onto the back of the hard palate instead of fusing together in the midline of the velum to form the levator sling. Initial palate repairs ignored this muscle and did nothing to correct its orientation. More recently, *intravelar veloplasty (IVVP)* or reconstruction of this sling has been advocated (Brown, Cohen, & Randall, 1983; Dreyer & Trier, 1984). The IVVP can be done in conjunction with any type of palate repair. Two contemporary repairs promote the reconstruction of this sling; the two-flap palatoplasty and the Furlow palatoplasty.

The Furlow palatoplasty (Furlow, 1986, 1990) (Figure 18–7) involves reconstruction of the levator sling, but it also lengthens the velum by closing it with a double opposing Z-plasty. The two-flap palatoplasty allows retro positioning of the levator sling, but does not incorporate a Z-plasty in the velum. Despite the more thorough approach advocated by these two repairs, there is still a 10% to 20% rate of VPI in patients with a history of palate repair. Intravelar veloplasty, whether as an isolated procedure in the treatment of submucous cleft or in conjunction with any type of palatoplasty, has not been as successful as was hoped (Brothers, Dalston, Peterson, & Lawrence, 1995; Coston, Hagerty, Jannarone,

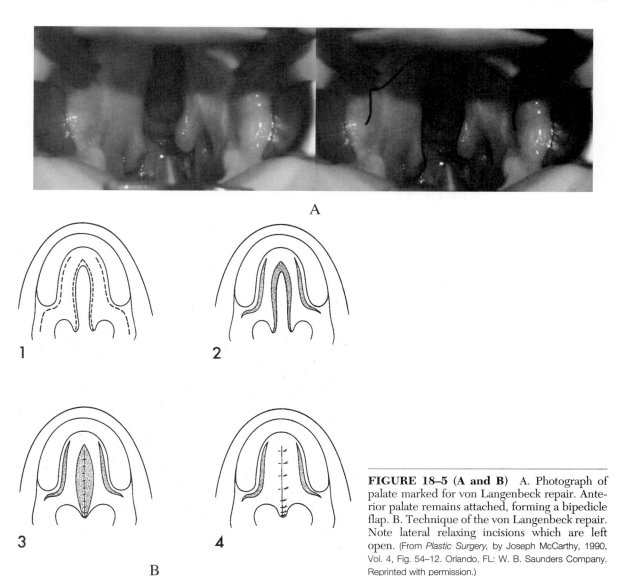

FIGURE 18–5 (A and B)   A. Photograph of palate marked for von Langenbeck repair. Anterior palate remains attached, forming a bipedicle flap. B. Technique of the von Langenbeck repair. Note lateral relaxing incisions which are left open. (From *Plastic Surgery,* by Joseph McCarthy, 1990, Vol. 4, Fig. 54–12. Orlando, FL: W. B. Saunders Company. Reprinted with permission.)

McDonald, & Hagerty, 1986; Jarvis & Trier, 1988). Gunther, Wisser, Cohen, and Brown (1998) reported a better speech outcome with the Furlow palatoplasty than with the intravelar veloplasty. Marsh, Grames, and Holtman (1989) found no difference in velopharyngeal function between palatoplasty with and with-

out intravelar veloplasty. These results suggest that either there is no beneficial effect of intravelar veloplasty or the effect is minimal.

Interpreting the data regarding the effect of each palatoplasty technique on speech is very difficult. There are many variables to consider, including the timing of surgery, the experience

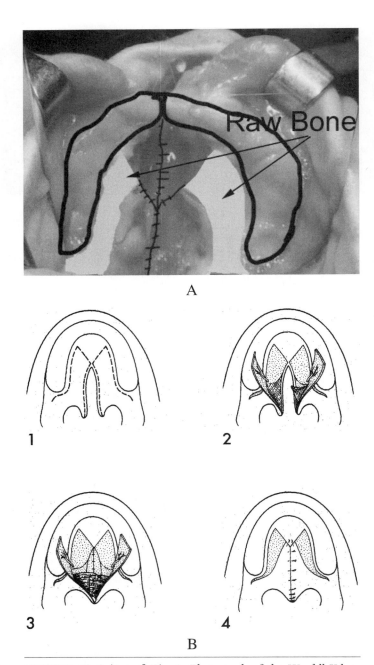

FIGURE 18–6 (A and B)   A. Photograph of the Wardill-Kilner repair. B. Technique of the Wardill-Kilner repair. Palate is lengthened by "pushing" back the mucoperiosteum. The raw area is allowed to fill by secondary healing (scarring). (From *Plastic Surgery*, by Joseph McCarthy, 1990, Vol. 4, Fig. 54–11. Orlando, FL: W. B. Saunders Company. Reprinted with permission.)

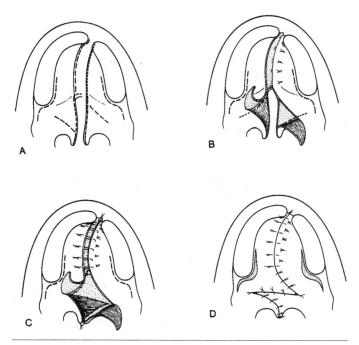

FIGURE 18–7 (A–D) Technique of the Furlow palatoplasty. Note Z-plasty closure of both nasal side and mirror image on the oral side. (From *Plastic Surgery*, by Joseph McCarthy, 1990, Vol. 4, Fig. 54–9. Orlando, FL: W. B. Saunders Company. Reprinted with permission.)

and skill of the surgeon, the experience and skill of the speech-language pathologist, and the very definition of success (normal, acceptable, or improved). However, there is general agreement that early repair is clearly better than late repair when considering speech results. In addition, experienced surgeons have a lower incidence of growth disturbance. Most experienced cleft palate centers report an incidence of between 17% and 20% of VPI requiring secondary surgery following the palate repair.

Fistula Repair Techniques

Fistulas are persistent openings between the nasal and oral cavity that occur when the palate fails to heal after a palatoplasty. In most cases, a fistula is deliberately left in the alveolus (under the lip) at the time of the primary palatoplasty. This *intentional fistula* results in less restriction of anterior facial growth. This fistula is usually closed in early-to-mid mixed dentition with a bone graft from the rib or iliac crest. This completes the dental arch and allows eruption of the permanent dentition.

Unintentional fistulas occur in between about 5% and 30% of reported series. While fistulas can be asymptomatic, they can also cause significant hypernasality and nasal air emission during speech, as well as regurgitation, of food and fluids into the nasal cavity during eating. Closure of a fistula can be a daunting task and traditionally carries a 37% or more recurrence risk (Cohen, Kalinowski, LaRossa, & Randall, 1991). Fistulas are often blamed on expansion of the dental arch or growth of the patient. However, growth and expansion do not cause fistulas, but they commonly reveal ones that already exist.

Closure of fistulas is usually attempted with the use of local autogenous tissue first. If there is not adequate local tissue, or if this has failed in a previous closure attempt, more complex and difficult procedures may be necessary. Techniques include using turbinates, flaps of tissue from the buccal surface based on the facial artery, and frequently a tongue flap (Figure 18–8) (Argamaso, 1990; Assuncao, 1993; Barone & Argamaso, 1993; Busic, Bagatin, & Boric, 1989; Coghlan, O'Regan, & Carter, 1989; Pigott, Rieger, & Moodie, 1984; Posnick & Getz, 1987; Thind, Singh, & Thind, 1992). With the tongue flap procedure, the dorsum of the tongue is sutured into the fistula and left for about two to three weeks to develop its blood supply. At that point, the tongue flap is severed from the rest of the tongue. Although this leaves scarring on the top of the tongue, it does not adversely affect the movement of the tongue for speech or feeding. The scar on the tongue is usually not well received by patients.

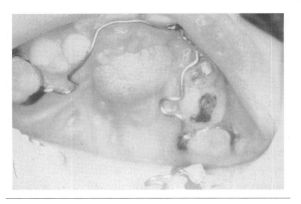

FIGURE 18–8 Fistula repair with a tongue flap. Note the tongue tissue in the anterior portion of the palate.

SURGERY FOR VELOPHARYNGEAL INSUFFICIENCY/ INCOMPETENCE (VPI)

VPI following a palatal repair can be due to a number of factors. There may be velopharyngeal insufficiency due to scarring from the initial palatoplasty. This can shorten the velum, making it impossible for it to reach the posterior pharyngeal wall during speech. In other cases, the nasopharynx can be deep relative to the position of the velum. There may also be velopharyngeal incompetence, where the velum has adequate length, but there is poor movement due to inadequate muscle insertion or neuromuscular dysfunction.

Successful surgical management of VPI has been a relatively recent accomplishment. In fact at one time, VPI was primarily treated with prosthetic obturation. In the 1970s, the use of both videofluoroscopy and nasopharyngoscopy led to a better understanding of the velopharyngeal valve and therefore, better methods of surgical correction have evolved. At this point, surgical correction of VPI is the norm and prosthetic devices are rarely used for this purpose with children.

Any surgical procedure of the pharynx that is designed to correct VPI is called a *pharyngoplasty*. Whether the problem is anatomical, neurological, or both, the surgical correction involves introducing something into the velopharyngeal opening to reduce the size of the gap and to take advantage of the velopharyngeal movement that is present.

Timing of Secondary Surgery

The diagnosis of VPI cannot be made until the child begins to produce connected speech and can adequately cooperate with the speech-language pathologist. This is typically around the age of 3. In addition to assessing speech and velopharyngeal function in the preschool years, longitudinal follow-up of patients with a history of cleft is critical, since there are those individuals who will present with velopharyngeal insufficiency as the adenoid pad shrinks.

Evaluation of velopharyngeal function may include nasopharyngoscopy and/or videofluoroscopy, in addition to the speech-language pathologist's examination. The speech-language pathologist's evaluation is the most critical since surgical decisions are based on the auditory perception of the speech rather than instrumental measures.

Once an assessment is completed, surgery can be performed, if indicated. The earliest this is done is usually around 3½ to 4 years of age. Pharyngoplasty procedures can technically be performed earlier than age 3; at one time, one group advocated simultaneous palatal repair and pharyngeal flap. This is no longer an acceptable practice since this resulted in significant morbidity in many of these patients and the procedure was done before it was determined that it was really needed for speech.

If the patient has a history of Pierre Robin sequence with micrognathia and upper airway obstruction, secondary surgery may be delayed for a time until the mandible grows or the size of the airway increases. If the child has any signs of obstructive sleep apnea, this must be resolved before proceeding with any procedure to correct VPI. In patients with Pierre Robin sequence, this may require a mandibular advancement procedure, a tongue base reduction, or removal of enlarged lymphoid tissue in the nasopharyngeal area (or any combination of the procedures).

Intervention should occur as soon as possible after the diagnosis of velopharyngeal insufficiency or incompetence is made, since a successful outcome is less likely in the older individual who has had VPI for a long period of time. Generally early intervention at age 4 to 5 years can result in success in greater than 90% of cases, but as the child ages and persists in using compensatory productions, the chance of success decreases. By adulthood, the chance of success or even improvement is significantly reduced so that surgical intervention should be carefully considered, especially in the face of potential complications, such as obstructive sleep apnea.

Whether it is due to an anatomical or neurological cause, *VPI is a surgical disorder*. Therefore, therapeutic endeavors, such as speech therapy, and especially blowing and sucking exercises, are ineffective. However, it is important to institute speech therapy as soon as possible in order to avoid the development of compensatory productions, which can be difficult to eliminate, even after surgical correction. Speech therapy for improvement of articulation placement can be done before the surgery and again after the surgery until these errors are corrected.

Surgical Preparation

Prior to the surgical procedure to correct VPI, the patient should undergo a thorough head and neck examination. Particular attention should be paid to the size of the tonsils and the adenoid pad, and the presence of micrognathia (small jaw), as is common in Pierre Robin sequence. Enlarged tonsils, adenoid hypertrophy, or micrognathia may portend towards airway obstruction in the immediate postoperative period, as well as long-term problems with sleep apnea. Some centers advocate routine tonsillectomy prior to pharyngoplasty, although this is usually not necessary unless the tonsils are enlarged. If tonsillectomy is indicated, it should precede the pharyngoplasty by at least six weeks.

While adenoidectomy is usually not recommended for patients with repaired cleft palate, an adenoidectomy prior to pharyngoplasty may allow the surgeon to position the flap higher in the nasopharynx for better speech results and to avoid port obstruction postoperatively. Therefore, since enlargement of the tonsils is often accompanied by enlargement of the adenoids, a conservative adenoidectomy at the time of tonsillectomy is often appropriate. The characteristics of VPI will worsen until the pharyngoplasty is done.

If the patient has velocardiofacial syndrome, a careful examination of the posterior pharyngeal wall may be indicated. One of the phenotypic features of this syndrome is tortuosity of the carotid arteries (D'Antonio & Marsh, 1987; Finkelstein et al., 1993; MacKenzie-Stepner et al., 1987; Ross, Witzel, Armstrong, & Thomson, 1996). As a result, they often course medially beneath the posterior wall of the pharynx, rather than on the lateral side of the pharyngeal wall, putting them in harm's way with the placement of a pharyngeal flap. This can often be seen through nasopharyngoscopy (Ysunza et al., 2004). Some advocate preoperative magnetic resonance angiography (MRA) studies or nasopharyngoscopy to identify the position of the carotid arteries (Krugman & Brant-Zawadski, 1997; Lai, Lo, Wong, Wang, & Yun, 2004; Mitnick, Bello, Golding-Kushner, Argamaso, & Shprintzen, 1996). Others feel that this is unnecessary because the vessels can usually be found by palpating the pharyngeal walls when the patient is in surgery (Mehendale & Sommerlad, 2004; Witt, Miller, Marsh, Muntz, & Grames, 1998).

Choice of Procedure

The choice of a surgical procedure to treat VPI involves a number of factors, including the etiology, pattern of closure, and size and location of the opening (Armour, Fischbach, Klaiman, & Fisher, 2005; Seagle, Mazaheri, Dixon-Wood, & Williams, 2002; Ysunza et al., 2002). Therefore, the differential diagnosis of the speech-language pathologist is important (Witt & D'Antonio, 1993). The selected procedure also depends on the experience and skill of the surgeon, the patient's medical condition, the size of the airway, and previous surgeries. In its simplest form, the treatment may involve augmentation of the posterior pharyngeal wall or repeat palatoplasty. Larger gaps require some type of flap- or sphincter-type procedure.

As any of these procedures may fail, it is important that surgical correction be performed with this possibility in mind. For instance, while the superiorly based pharyngeal flap is the gold standard and provides the highest chance of success, it carries with it a higher incidence of complications (i.e., obstructive sleep apnea and airway obstruction). However, if it needs to be taken down due to airway obstruction, it can be converted to simple augmentation or sphincteroplasty, and does not interfere with redo palatoplasty. If a sphincteroplasty operation is done and fails to correct the VPI, it is not possible to convert to the superiorly based pharyngeal flap. Posterior wall augmentations can usually be "upgraded" to either a flap- or sphincter-type operation, while rolled flaps can only be changed to a sphincter.

There is not yet a consensus regarding the specific choice of one procedure versus the other for surgical management of VPI (Sloan, 2000). Further research on the outcomes of each procedure for different patient populations is greatly needed. However, centers vary in their criteria for determining success. In some cases, the surgery in considered a success only when the postoperative speech is normal. In some centers (including ours at Cincinnati Children's

Hospital), the surgery is considered a success only when the postoperative speech is normal (aside, that is, from articulation errors). In other cases, success is defined as either "acceptable" speech or improved speech (Lauck, Lee, Kummer, Billmire, & Bandaranayake, 2006). Centers also vary in who determines success (the surgeon, the speech-language pathologist, or the family) and the procedures for measuring success (perceptual judgment or instrumental assessment). Until there is standardization of the measurement of success, it will be impossible to compare studies of surgical efficacy.

Surgical Techniques: Redo Palatoplasty

The apparent success of the Furlow palatoplasty in reducing the incidence of VPI when used as a primary procedure has led to its use in the treatment of VPI. It has become the initial treatment of VPI secondary to submucous cleft palate. In addition, it is now used in some cases for treatment of mild VPI; a rerepair is done of the palate with the Furlow technique when the original repair was done with another approach (Deren et al., 2005; Lindsey & Davis, 1996; Perkins, Lewis, Gruss, Eblen, & Sie, 2005; Sie & Gruss, 2002; Sie, Tampakopoulou, Sorom, Gruss, & Eblen, 2001). This repair has two advantages. It lengthens the palate by virtue of the Z-plasty technique used and it guarantees reconstruction of the levator sling. A similar approach advocated by several centers promotes the "radical" retro displacement of the levator muscles to accomplish the same effect.

Surgical Techniques: Pharyngeal Wall Augmentation

The velopharyngeal opening that occurs as a result of VPI has led to the search for some type of internal obturation. When the velopharyngeal opening is small, no more than 10 mm in diameter, posterior *pharyngeal wall augmentation* has been used by some surgeons. With this procedure, an implant is surgically placed or injected in the posterior pharyngeal wall in the area of the velopharyngeal opening. The implant is placed deep in the superior pharyngeal constrictors, but superficial to the prevertebral fascia. Figure 18–9 illustrates velopharyngeal insufficiency prior to the implant and then the closure that occurs with the augmented posterior pharyngeal wall as a result of the implant. Various materials have been reported for posterior pharyngeal wall (and sometimes velar) augmentation including cartilage, fascia, fat, silicone, proplast, and polytetrafluoroethylene (Teflon) (Dejonckere & van Wijngaarden, 2001; Denny, Marks, & Oliff-Carneol, 1993; Furlow, Williams, Eisenbach, & Bzoch, 1982; Gray, Pinborough-Zimmerman, & Catten, 1999; Remacle, Bertrand, Eloy, & Marbaix, 1990; Terris & Goode, 1993; Trigos, Ysunza, Gonzalez, & Vazquez, 1988; Witt et al., 1997; Wolford, Oelschlaeger, & Deal, 1989). Initially, overcorrection is required for all injectable augmentation material because the vehicle solution becomes absorbed. Complications from implantation of foreign materials in the posterior pharyngeal wall include infections, extrusion, reabsorption, and even migration of the material after insertion. Granuloma formation and migration of the material leading to embolus has been associated with Teflon implantation, and therefore, it is no longer used. These implants are not always effective due to the fact that they are often too small or in the wrong location to completely fill the opening. On the other hand, overcorrection can occur, which may result in hyponasality and upper airway obstruction.

Another procedure for pharyngeal wall augmentation is the use of a *rolled flap*. In

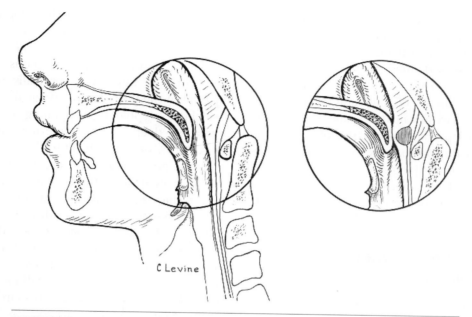

C Levine

FIGURE 18–9 This drawing illustrates velopharyngeal insufficiency prior to the implant—and then the closure that occurs with the augmented posterior pharyngeal wall as a result of the implant.

this case, a flap of tissue is raised from the posterior pharyngeal wall and is rolled up onto itself. This roll forms a bulge on the posterior pharyngeal wall that fills in the velopharyngeal gap (Gray et al., 1999). Some of these techniques have worked with careful patient selection, but their overall success rates have been disappointing.

Surgical Techniques: Pharyngoplasty

There are currently two *pharyngoplasty* techniques that are most commonly used to correct velopharyngeal dysfunction: the pharyngeal flap and the sphincter pharyngoplasty. Both of these techniques are designed to reduce the size of the pharyngeal port so that during speech, the movement that is present is sufficient for closing the entire port.

A *pharyngeal flap* is the most commonly used procedure for correction of VPI (Figure 18–10) (Cable, Canady, Karnell, Karnell, & Malick, 2004). It is designed to be a passive, soft tissue obturator that is placed in the middle of the velopharyngeal port (Tharanon, Stella, & Epker, 1990; Trier, 1985a; Vedung, 1995; Wu & Epker, 1990; Yoshida, Stella, Ghali, & Epker, 1992). As such, it is effective in the management of midline gaps (as is most common following a cleft repair) and large gaps in the anterior-posterior dimension. With this procedure, a flap of tissue is dissected from the pharyngeal wall by an incision that begins at the top of the nasopharynx and then goes down to the area near the base of the tongue. The incision then goes across the width of the pharynx between the tonsillar pillars, and then up again so that the base of the flap is connected at the very top of the nasopharynx.

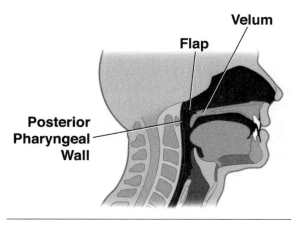

FIGURE 18–10 A lateral view of a pharyngeal flap. The flap is raised from the posterior pharyngeal wall, and then sutured into the velum. Ports are left on both sides of the flap for normal nasal breathing.

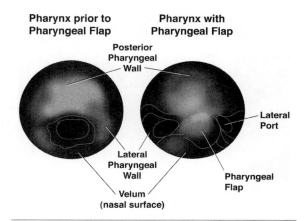

FIGURE 18–11 A superior view (as would be seen through nasopharyngoscopy) of a normal pharynx during nasal breathing, and the same view of a pharynx with a pharyngeal flap during nasal breathing. Note the pharyngeal flap in midline and the open lateral ports on either side.

The pharyngeal flap includes the mucosal surface and the underlying musculature all the way down to the prevertebral fascia of the spinal column. The blood supply comes in through the attached portion of the flap at the base of the skull. The velum is split up to the hard palate and the flap from the posterior pharyngeal wall is then elevated and sutured into the velum. A port or opening is left on each side of the flap to allow normal nasal breathing, drainage of nasal secretions, and normal nasal resonance. Stents may be placed in the ports over night to keep them patent, but are removed the next day.

Figure 18–11 shows a superior view (as would be seen through nasopharyngoscopy) of a normal pharynx during nasal breathing, and the same view of a pharynx with a pharyngeal flap during nasal breathing. Note the pharyngeal flap in midline and the open lateral ports on either side for normal nasal breathing. Figure 18–12 A and B shows a pharyngeal flap as it would be viewed through nasopharyngoscopy. The pharyngeal flap can be seen in midline and the lateral ports are viewed on

either side of the flap. With the flap in place, the lateral pharyngeal walls move medially to close against the flap during speech, thus closing the lateral pharyngeal ports and the entire pharyngeal opening.

There are several factors that will determine the success of the flap in correcting characteristics of VPI. One factor is the vertical position in the nasopharynx (Skolnick & McCall, 1972). As a general rule, it is important that the flap is set as high as possible, preferably at the level of the skull base and level with the hard palate, because this is usually the area of maximum lateral pharyngeal wall movement and is also the normal point of contact for the velum. Although the inferiorly based pharyngeal flap was used at one time, it was found to result in a position that was too low in the nasopharynx. In addition, it often tethered the movement of the velum, preventing closure with either the posterior or lateral walls of the pharynx. A properly set superiorly based flap is positioned behind the velum. Therefore, it usually cannot

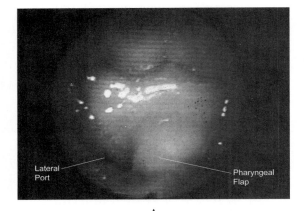

A

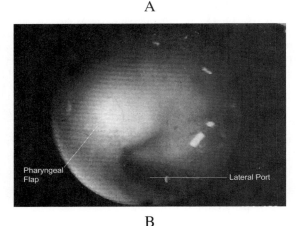

B

FIGURE 18–12 (A and B) A pharyngeal flap as viewed through nasopharyngoscopy. A. This photo shows the pharyngeal flap in midline and the lateral ports on either side. B. This photo shows a better view of the patient's left lateral port.

be seen through an intraoral examination. This is not to say that a low set flap cannot work, but it is more likely to cause problems with persistent VPI and possibly with airway obstruction. Readvancing a flap like this will often solve these problems.

The extent of lateral pharyngeal wall movement is also a primary factor in the success of the flap. The role of lateral pharyngeal wall movement in determining the success of a pharyngeal flap was studied by Argamaso et al. (1980). They evaluated 202 patients with pharyngeal flaps through nasopharyngoscopy and multiview videofluoroscopy. Through these studies they found that where there was no evidence of VPI following placement of the flap, the sole determiner of velopharyngeal closure was the medial movement of the lateral pharyngeal walls to meet the flap. In cases where the flap failed to correct the VPI, there was an inappropriate degree, level, or symmetry of the lateral pharyngeal wall motion in relation to the position and width of the flap. Lewis and Pashayan (1980) looked for an increase in the degree of lateral pharyngeal wall motion following placement of a pharyngeal flap in 20 patients. They found that there was no significant difference in the lateral wall motion of their patients postoperatively. On the other hand, Karling, Henningsson, Larson, and Isberg (1999) found a potential for adaptation of pharyngeal wall adduction to different flap widths. They reported that in patients with limited preoperative lateral pharyngeal wall adduction, pharyngeal wall activity increased in the presence of a narrow flap. When preoperative adduction was pronounced, however, the postoperative activity decreased because of mechanical hindrance of the flap, and the degree of impediment was correlated to the width of the flap. Although this study suggests that there is some adaptation of lateral pharyngeal wall movement to the width of the flap, if the flap is too narrow so that the lateral pharyngeal walls do not close against it, there will be persistent hypernasality or nasal air emission postoperatively.

Because lateral pharyngeal wall motion is the key to the function of the velopharyngeal mechanism following the placement of the flap, patients with a sagittal pattern of closure or good lateral pharyngeal wall movement preoperatively have the best prognosis for total correction of VPI with a pharyngeal flap. Patients with poor lateral wall motion require a wider flap for total correction. The challenge in these cases is to make the flap wide enough so that the lateral walls can close against it on both sides during speech, yet not so wide that it causes upper airway obstruction with hyponasality and sleep apnea. When there is hypotonia, as in velocardiofacial syndrome, or a compromised airway due to retrognathia, the surgeon may need to compromise perfect speech results for a functional airway.

A wide flap is preferable to a narrow flap, not only because it increases the possibility of lateral port closure during speech, but also because the pharyngeal flap receives its blood supply from its base. Therefore, the wider the base, the greater the blood supply will be. Flaps should also be made as long as possible because if they are too short, they will be under greater tension. If there is tension or limited blood supply, this can result in more scarring and contraction, which will adversely affect the function of the flap. In general, pharyngeal flaps should be wide, long, and set as high as possible.

The *Orticochea sphincteroplasty* (Orticochea, 1970, 1983, 1997, 1999), also referred to as just a *sphincter pharyngoplasty*, was designed to create a sphincter that encircles the velopharyngeal port (Figure 18–13). Initially, it was felt that this procedure would create a dynamic sphincter as opposed to a passive obturator. However, recent studies have shown that the muscle fibers in the sphincter are actually passive and that all movements seen postoperatively are caused by the contraction of the superior constrictor muscles (Ysunza, 2005). The sphincter pharyngoplasty procedure has undergone a series of modifications and in its most current and widely used form, it now exists with the Jackson modification (Jackson, 1985; Jackson,

McGlynn, Huskie, & Dip, 1980; Jackson & Silverton, 1977; Losken, Williams, Burstein, Malick, & Riski, 2003; Sie et al., 1998).

In this procedure, bilateral superiorly based myomucosal flaps are raised from the posterior faucial pillars, which include the palatopharyngeus muscles. These flaps are rotated posteriorly and inset into a transverse incision in the nasopharynx, just at the level of velopharyngeal closure. This effectively narrows the pharynx. A small, superiorly based pharyngeal flap is then raised and attached to the lateral flaps. This leaves a single round opening of about 1 centimeter in diameter in the center of the pharynx. A sphincter pharyngoplasty is usually done bilaterally, but it can also be done unilaterally if the opening is just on one side.

Since this procedure results in a narrowing of the lateral border of the velopharyngeal sphincter, it has been advocated for use with coronal gaps that include poor lateral pharyngeal wall motion, or gaps due to deep lateral pharyngeal recesses, with better closure in the center of the port. A sphincter pharyngoplasty is useful in the treatment of VPI secondary to unilateral palatal paralysis, as occasionally seen in hemifacial microsomia.

Surgical Complications and Follow-Up

Immediately after placement of the pharyngeal flap or sphincter, there is significant *edema* or swelling in the pharynx. As a result, most patients will exhibit hyponasality and loud snoring during the immediate postoperative period. Snoring is the most common consequence of pharyngoplasty, especially after the pharyngeal flap, and many patients will snore to some extent for the rest of their lives.

Sleep apnea is another possible sequela of the surgery. Temporary sleep apnea is common,

**Small superiorly based
pharyngeal flap**

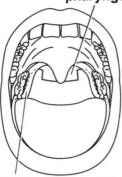

**Posterior tonsilar pillar
containing palatopharyngeous
muscle**

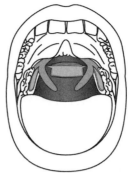

**Palatopharyngeous flaps
and pharyngeal flap elevated**

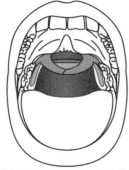

**Palatopharyngeous flaps
interdigitated**

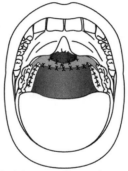

**Sphincter flaps inset
into pharyngeal flaps and
donor sites closed**

FIGURE 18–13 A sphincter pharyngoplasty. In this procedure, bilateral myocutaneous flaps are raised from the posterior faucial pillars, which include the palatopharyngeus muscles. These muscles are rotated posteriorly and inset into a transverse incision on the posterior pharyngeal wall, just at the level of velopharyngeal closure. A small superiorly based flap may also be raised and attached to the lateral flaps. This effectively narrows the velopharyngeal port for speech. (From *Plastic Surgery,* by Joseph McCarthy, 1990, Vol. 4, Fig. 58–11. Orlando, FL: W. B. Saunders Company. Reprinted with permission.)

but this usually resolves within two to six weeks postoperatively, or after the swelling has gone down. Chronic sleep apnea can occur in a small number of patients, however (Tharanon et al., 1990; Trier, 1985a; Vedung, 1995; Ysunza, Garcia-Velasquez, Garcia-Garcia, Haro, & Valencia, 1993). Chronic sleep apnea is a serious problem and cannot be ignored since it can cause serious health problems if left to continue. Some authors have reported a prevalence of sleep apnea of as high as 10% following pharyngeal flap surgery, but a prevalence of 5% or less is probably more common (personal data). At one time, it was thought that the sphincter pharyngoplasty did not cause sleep apnea, so this procedure was recommended for patients at high risk. Recent studies have shown that sleep apnea can also occur following the sphincter pharyngoplasty (Abyholm et al., 2005; de Serres et al., 1999; Saint Raymond et al., 2004; Witt, Marsh, Muntz, Marty-Grames, & Watchmaker, 1996). Sleep apnea is the greatest risk for patients who have micrognathia, such as those with Pierre Robin sequence (Abramson, Marrinan, & Mulliken, 1997; Wells, Vu, & Luce, 1999), or for patients with neurological impairment.

The cause of sleep apnea can often be difficult to determine. For example, the source of the obstruction in a patient with a pharyngeal flap might be due to micrognathia, glossoptosis, or hypotonia rather than the flap, which seems the most obvious cause. If sleep apnea persists beyond the initial postoperative period, it is usually evaluated with *polysomnography*, which is a diagnostic test during which a number of physiologic variables are recorded during a sleep study. Nasopharyngoscopy is also done to help identify the source of obstruction. Finally, a sleep MRI can be helpful in determining the cause of obstruction in complex cases.

If treatment for sleep apnea is indicated, this usually involves *continuous positive air pressure* (CPAP), which is a device that delivers air pressure into the airway during sleep through a specially designed mask. This positive air pressure keeps the pharynx patent during sleep. Patients with sleep apnea are restudied about every six months and in most cases, the problem will resolve within one to two years. In refractory cases however, the flap is taken down. Fortunately, taking down the flap does not necessary cause deterioration in speech. The bulk of tissue from the flap, which remains in the posterior pharyngeal wall, continues to provide a pad to assist with velopharyngeal closure. In addition, the speech patterns that the patients learned with the flap in place are often maintained after flap division (Agarwal et al., 2003).

In addition to airway obstruction and sleep apnea, the surgical procedure may fail in a number of ways. First and foremost, it can fail to completely correct the VPI. This may be due to several reasons, including dehiscence, low-lying flaps, and hypotonicity of the velopharyngeal mechanism (Kasten et al., 1997; Witt, Marsh, Marty-Grames, & Muntz, 1995). In addition, the pharyngoplasty can fail by over-correcting the VPI, leading to hyponasality. Evaluation of postoperative results begins with a good history and speech evaluation, followed by a nasopharyngoscopy. The nasopharyngoscopy gives essential information regarding the location of the persistent gap and the function of the port(s); the function of the velum; the position and integrity of the flap or sphincter; and the airway. Armed with this information, the surgeon can do a revision as needed.

Revisions may be indicated within the first year following surgery. In other cases, there may be many years of normal function and then a sudden change in resonance due to a growth spurt. With the pharyngeal flap procedure, one or both lateral ports can become stenosed due to scarring. This can result in hyponasality, upper airway obstruction, and, in the severe cases, sleep apnea. For correction, one or both ports need to be opened. More commonly, a port needs to be augmented or closed down for correction of persistent or recurrent hypernasality or nasal air emission. If one port is not closing after the flap is in place, an auxiliary flap can be raised to augment the primary flap on the side of the leaking port.

With pharyngeal flaps, secondary revisions are relatively uncommon. An appropriately placed pharyngeal flap has a greater than 90% chance for normal speech when accompanied by speech therapy (our series). The sphincter pharyngoplasty has a fairly high incidence of secondary revision and the overall success rate has been reported to be less than that of the pharyngeal flap. The success rate with sphincteroplasty for the elimination of hypernasality and nasal air emission has been reported as between 60% to 80% (James, Twist, Turner, & Milward, 1996; Kasten, Buchman, Stevenson, & Berger, 1997; Riski, Ruff, Georgiade, & Barwick, 1992; Riski, Ruff, Georgiade, Barwick, & Edwards, 1992; Roberts & Brown, 1983; Sie et al., 1998; Witt, D'Antonio, Zimmerman, & Marsh, 1994). One problem may be patient selection. The sphincteroplasty procedure results in a narrowing of the lateral borders of the velopharyngeal port, but there is often a remaining gap in the anterior-posterior dimension (Ren & Wang, 1993). Therefore, it is more appropriate for patients with poor lateral wall movement yet good velar movement. It is unlikely to be successful in cases where there is a short velum or a gap that is primarily in the midline.

Regardless of the pharyngoplasty procedure chosen, the surgery must be followed by a reassessment of the speech so that an appropriate plan of speech therapy can be instituted. Since it takes about three months for most of the swelling to resolve and the flap or sphincter to begin to function, this is the best time for the reevaluation. Patients and parents must realize

that treating VPI is a two-stage process. The surgery is done first in order to correct the anatomical defect. Following the surgery, speech therapy is required to help the child to eliminate compensatory productions and learn how to use the new mechanism effectively.

SUMMARY

The goals of surgical correction of cleft lip and palate are to normalize feeding, speech, dentition, facial profile, and aesthetics. There are several surgical approaches that can be used to correct each type of deformity. The success of the surgery is dependent upon many factors, including the location, size and severity of the cleft, type of procedure used, and experience of the surgeon. With the improvement in surgical techniques in recent years, the functional and aesthetic outcomes of surgery have also improved.

VPI continues to be a risk in the patient with cleft palate, even after successful palate repair. It should be remembered that VPI requires surgery for correction of the structures. However, the successful treatment of VPI requires close cooperation and teamwork between the surgeon and the speech-language pathologist. Failure to work cooperatively may result in unnecessary additional surgery, unnecessary speech therapy, or both.

FOR REVIEW, DISCUSSION, AND CRITICAL THINKING

1. What is the "rule of 10s" and how does it relate to cleft lip repair?

2. Discuss the general timing of cleft lip repair. What are the potential advantages and disadvantages of early versus late lip repair?

3. What are the reasons for aligning the maxillary segments prior to cleft lip

surgery? Why is this not done in all cases? What are the different methods?

4. What procedures are done for a unilateral cleft lip repair? What are done for a bilateral cleft lip repair?

5. Discuss the general timing of cleft palate repair. What are the potential advantages

and disadvantages of early versus late repair of the palate?

6. Describe the difference between the von Langenbeck, the Wardill-Kilner V-Y push-back, and the Furlow palatoplasty as if you were explaining it to a parent.

7. List the types of surgeries that can be done for velopharyngeal dysfunction and describe the basic procedures for each as

if you were explaining it to a parent. What factors influence the choice of procedure for the patient?

8. Discuss the potential complications of surgery for velopharyngeal dysfunction. Which patients may be at particular risk? How would you counsel the family about the risk and benefits of the surgery?

REFERENCES

Abramson, D. L., Marrinan, E. M., & Mulliken, J. B. (1997). Robin sequence: Obstructive sleep apnea following pharyngeal flap. *Cleft Palate-Craniofacial Journal, 34*(3), 256–260.

Abyholm, F., D'Antonio, L., Davidson Ward, S. L., Kjoll, L., Saeed, M., Shaw, W., et al. (2005). Pharyngeal flap and sphincterplasty for velopharyngeal insufficiency have equal outcome at 1 year postoperatively: Results of a randomized trial. *Cleft Palate-Craniofacial Journal, 42*(5), 501–511.

Agarwal, T., Sloan, G. M., Zajac, D., Uhrich, K. S., Meadows, W., & Lewchalermwong, J. A. (2003). Speech benefits of posterior pharyngeal flap are preserved after surgical flap division for obstructive sleep apnea: Experience with division of 12 flaps. *Journal of Craniofacial Surgery, 14*(5), 630–636.

Argamaso, R. V. (1990). The tongue flap: Placement and fixation for closure of postpalatoplasty fistulae. *Cleft Palate Journal, 27*(4), 402–410.

Argamaso, R. V., Shprintzen, R. J., Strauch, B., Lewin, M. L., Daniller, A. I., Ship, A. G., & Croft, C. B. (1980). The role of lateral pharyngeal wall movement in pharyngeal flap surgery. *Plastic and Reconstructive Surgery, 66*(2), 214–219.

Armour, A., Fischbach, S., Klaiman, P., & Fisher, D. M. (2005). Does velopharyngeal closure pattern affect the success of pharyngeal flap pharyngoplasty? *Plastic and Reconstructive Surgery, 115*(1), 45–52; Discussion, 53.

Assuncao, A. G. (1993). The design of tongue flaps for the closure of palatal fistulas. *Plastic and Reconstructive Surgery, 91*(5), 806–810.

Bae, Y. C., Kim, J. H., Lee, J., Hwang, S. M., & Kim, S. S. (2002). Comparative study of the extent of palatal lengthening by different methods. *Annals of Plastic Surgery, 48*(4), 359–362; Discussion 362–354.

Bardach, J., Morris, H. L., & Olin, W. H. (1984). Late results of primary veloplasty: The Marburg Project. *Plastic and Reconstructive Surgery, 73*(2), 207–218.

Barone, C. M., & Argamaso, R. V. (1993). Refinements of the tongue flap for closure of difficult palatal fistulas. *Journal of Craniofacial Surgery, 4*(2), 109–111.

Becker, M., Svensson, H., McWilliam, J., Sarnas, K. V., & Jacobsson, S. (1998). Millard repair of unilateral isolated cleft lip: A 25-year follow-up. *Scandinavian Journal of Plastic and Reconstructive Surgery and Hand Surgery, 32*(4), 387–394.

Blocksma, R., Leuz, C. A., & Mellerstig, K. E. (1975). A conservative program for managing cleft palates without the use of mucoperiosteal flaps. *Plastic and Reconstructive Surgery, 55*(2), 160–169.

Brauer, R. O., & Cronin, T. D. (1983). The Tennison lip repair revisited. *Plastic and Reconstructive Surgery, 71*(5), 633–642.

Brothers, D. B., Dalston, R. W., Peterson, H. D., & Lawrence, W. T. (1995). Comparison of the Furlow double-opposing Z-palatoplasty with the Wardill-Kilner procedure for isolated clefts of the soft palate. *Plastic and Reconstructive Surgery, 95*(6), 969–977.

Brown, A. S., Cohen, M. A., & Randall, P. (1983). Levator muscle reconstruction: Does it make a difference? *Plastic and Reconstructive Surgery, 72*(1), 1–8.

Busic, N., Bagatin, M., & Boric, V. (1989). Tongue flaps in repair of large palatal defects. *International Journal of Oral Maxillofacial Surgery, 18*(5), 291–293.

Cable, B. B., Canady, J. W., Karnell, M. P., Karnell, L. H., & Malick, D. N. (2004). Pharyngeal flap surgery: Long-term outcomes at the University of Iowa. *Plastic and Reconstructive Surgery, 113*(2), 475–478.

Coghlan, K., O'Regan, B., & Carter, J. (1989). Tongue flap repair of oronasal fistulae in cleft palate patients. A review of 20 patients. *Journal of Craniomaxillofacial Surgery, 17*(6), 255–259.

Cohen, S. R., Kalinowski, J., LaRossa, D., & Randall, P. (1991). Cleft palate fistulas: A multivariate statistical analysis of prevalence, etiology, and surgical management. *Plastic and Reconstructive Surgery, 87*(6), 1041–1047.

Cosman, B., & Falk, A. S. (1980). Delayed hard palate repair and speech deficiencies: A cautionary report. *Cleft Palate Journal, 17*(1), 27–33.

Coston, G. N., Hagerty, R. F., Jannarone, R. J., McDonald, V., & Hagerty, R. C. (1986). Levator muscle reconstruction: Resulting velopharyngeal competence—A preliminary report. *Plastic and Reconstructive Surgery, 77*(6), 911–918.

Cutting, C., & Grayson, B. (1993). The prolabial unwinding flap method for one-stage repair of bilateral cleft lip, nose, and alveolus. *Plastic and Reconstructive Surgery, 91*(1), 37–47.

Cutting, C., Grayson, B., Brecht, L., Santiago, P., Wood, R., & Kwon, S. (1998). Presurgical columellar elongation and primary retrograde nasal reconstruction in one-stage bilateral cleft lip and nose repair. *Plastic and Reconstructive Surgery, 101*(3), 630–639.

Cutting, C., Grayson, B., McCarthy, J. G., Thorne, C., Khorramabadi, D., Haddad, B., et al. (1998). A virtual reality system for bone fragment positioning in multisegment craniofacial surgical procedures. *Plastic and Reconstructive Surgery, 102*(7), 2436–2443.

Cutting, C., LaRossa, D., McComb, H., Millard, D. R., Mulliken, J., Noordhoff, S., & Sommerlad, B. (2001). *Virtual surgery videos*. New York: Smile Train. http://www.smiletrain.org.

D'Antonio, L. D., & Marsh, J. L. (1987). Abnormal carotid arteries in the velocardiofacial syndrome [Letter]. *Plastic and Reconstructive Surgery, 80*(3), 471–472.

Da Silveira, A. C., Oliveira, N., Gonzalez, S., Shahani, M., Reisberg, D., Daw, J. L., Jr., et al. (2003). Modified nasal alveolar molding appliance for management of cleft lip defect. *Journal of Craniofacial Surgery, 14*(5), 700–703.

Dejonckere, P. H., & van Wijngaarden, H. A. (2001). Retropharyngeal autologous fat transplantation for congenital short palate: A nasometric assessment of functional results. *Annals of Otology, Rhinology, & Laryngology, 110*(2), 168–172.

Denny, A. D., Marks, S. M., & Oliff-Carneol, S. (1993). Correction of velopharyngeal insufficiency by pharyngeal augmentation using autologous cartilage: A preliminary report. *Cleft Palate-Craniofacial Journal, 30*(1), 46–54.

Deren, O., Ayhan, M., Tuncel, A., Gorgu, M., Altuntas, A., Kutlay, R., et al. (2005). The correction of velopharyngeal insufficiency by Furlow palatoplasty in patients older than 3 years undergoing Veau-Wardill-Kilner palatoplasty: A prospective clinical study. *Plastic and Reconstructive Surgery, 116*(1), 85–93; Discussion 94–86.

De Serres, L. M., Deleyiannis, F. W., Eblen, L. E., Gruss, J. S., Richardson, M. A., & Sie, K. C. (1999). Results with sphincter pharyngoplasty and pharyngeal flap. *International Journal of Pediatric Otorhinolaryngology, 48*(1), 17–25.

Dingman, R. O., & Grabb, W. C. (1971). A rational program for surgical management of bilateral cleft lip and cleft palate. *Plastic and Reconstructive Surgery, 47*(3), 239–242.

Dreyer, T. M., & Trier, W. C. (1984). A comparison of palatoplasty techniques. *Cleft Palate Journal, 21*(4), 251–253.

Fara, M., & Brousilova, M. (1988). Long-term experience with 2-stage surgery of cleft palate in total unilateral and bilateral clefts from the aspect of maxillary development. *Rozhledy v Chirugii, 67*(11), 729–741.

Fara, M., Brousilova, M., Hrivnakova, J., & Tvrdek, M. (1992). Long-term experiences with the two-stage palatoplasty with regard to the development of maxillary arch. *Acta Chirurgiae Plasticae, 34*(3), 138–142.

Finkelstein, Y., Zohar, Y., Nachmani, A., Talmi, Y. P., Lerner, M. A., Hauben, D. J., & Frydman, M. (1993). The otolaryngologist and the patient with velocardiofacial syndrome. *Archives of Otolaryngology—Head & Neck Surgery, 119*(5), 563–569.

Furlow, L. T., Jr. (1986). Cleft palate repair by double opposing Z-plasty. *Plastic and Reconstructive Surgery, 78*(6), 724–738.

Furlow, L. T., Jr. (1990). Flaps for cleft lip and palate surgery. *Clinics in Plastic Surgery, 17*(4), 633–644.

Furlow, L. T., Jr., Williams, W. N., Eisenbach, C. R. D., & Bzoch, K. R. (1982). A long-term study on treating velopharyngeal insufficiency by Teflon injection. *Cleft Palate Journal, 19*(1), 47–56.

Georgiade, N. G., & Latham, R. A. (1975). Maxillary arch alignment in the bilateral cleft lip and palate infant, using pinned coaxial screw appliance. *Plastic and Reconstructive Surgery, 56*(1), 52–60.

Gray, S. D., Pinborough-Zimmerman, J., & Catten, M. (1999). Posterior wall augmentation for treatment of velopharyngeal insufficiency. *Otolaryngology—Head & Neck Surgery, 121*(1), 107–112.

Gunther, E., Wisser, J. R., Cohen, M. A., & Brown, A. S. (1998). Palatoplasty: Furlow's double reversing Z-plasty versus intravelar veloplasty. *Cleft Palate-Craniofacial Journal, 35*(6), 546–549.

Hardin-Jones, M. A., & Jones, D. L. (2005). Speech production of preschoolers with cleft palate. *Cleft Palate-Craniofacial Journal, 42*(1), 7–13.

Jackson, I. T. (1985). Sphincter pharyngoplasty. *Clinics in Plastic Surgery, 12*(4), 711–717.

Jackson, I. T., McGlynn, M. J., Huskie, C. F., & Dip, I. P. (1980). Velopharyngeal incompetence in the absence of cleft palate: Results of treatment in 20 cases. *Plastic and Reconstructive Surgery, 66*(2), 211–213.

Jackson, I. T., McLennan, G., & Scheker, L. R. (1983). Primary veloplasty or primary palatoplasty: Some preliminary findings. *Plastic and Reconstructive Surgery, 72*(2), 153–157.

Jackson, I. T., & Silverton, J. S. (1977). The sphincter pharyngoplasty as a secondary procedure in cleft palates. *Plastic and Reconstructive Surgery, 59*(4), 518–524.

James, N. K., Twist, M., Turner, M. M., & Milward, T. M. (1996). An audit of velopharyngeal incompetence treated by the Orticochea pharyngoplasty [see Comments]. *British Journal of Plastic Surgery, 49*(4), 197–201.

Jarvis, B. L., & Trier, W. C. (1988). The effect of intravelar veloplasty on velopharyngeal competence following pharyngeal flap surgery. *Cleft Palate Journal, 25*(4), 389–394.

Karling, J., Henningsson, G., Larson, O. & Isberg, A. (1999). Adaptation of pharyngeal wall adduction after pharyngeal flap surgery. *Cleft Palate-Craniofacial Journal, 36*(2), 166–172.

Kasten, S. J., Buchman, S. R., Stevenson, C., & Berger, M. (1997). A retrospective analysis of revision sphincter pharyngoplasty. *Annals of Plastic Surgery, 39*(6), 583–589.

Kohout, M. P., Aljaro, L. M., Farkas, L. G., & Mulliken, J. B. (1998). Photogrammetric comparison of two methods for synchronous repair of bilateral cleft lip and nasal deformity. *Plastic and Reconstructive Surgery, 102*(5), 1339–1349.

Krugman, M. E., & Brant-Zawadski, M. (1997). Magnetic resonance angioplasty for prepharyngoplasty assessment in velocardiofacial syndrome. *Cleft Palate-Craniofacial Journal, 34*(3), 266–267.

Lai, J. P., Lo, L. J., Wong, H. F., Wang, S. R., & Yun, C. (2004). Vascular abnormalities in the head and neck area in velocardiofacial syndrome. *Chang Gung Medical Journal, 27*(8), 586–593.

Latham, R. A. (1980). Orthopedic advancement of the cleft maxillary segment: A preliminary report. *Cleft Palate Journal, 17*(3), 227–233.

Latham, R. A., Kusy, R. P., & Georgiade, N. G. (1976). An extraorally activated expansion appliance for cleft palate infants. *Cleft Palate Journal, 13*, 253–261.

Lauck, L., Lee, L. Kummer, A. W., Billmire, D., & Bandaranayake, D. (2006, April). Speech outcomes following surgical management of velopharyngeal dysfunction. Paper presented at the Annual Meeting of the American Cleft Palate-Craniofacial Association, Vancouver, Canada.

Lazarus, D. D., Hudson, D. A., van Zyl, J. E., Fleming, A. N., & Fernandes, D. (1998). Repair of unilateral cleft lip: A comparison of five techniques. *Annals of Plastic Surgery, 41*(6), 587–594.

Leon-Valle, C. (1980). The use of a cutaneous-musclar flap for primary nasolabial repair with a modified Tennison-Randall technique. *British Journal of Plastic Surgery, 33*(2), 266–269.

Lewis, M. B., & Pashayan, H. M. (1980). The effects of pharyngeal flap surgery on lateral pharyngeal wall motion: A videoradiographic evaluation. *Cleft Palate Journal, 17*(4), 301–308.

Lindsey, W. H., & Davis, P. T. (1996). Correction of velopharyngeal insufficiency with Furlow palatoplasty. *Archives of Otolaryngology—Head & Neck Surgery, 122*(8), 881–884.

Losken, A., Williams, J. K., Burstein, F. D., Malick, D., & Riski, J. E. (2003). An outcome evaluation of sphincter pharyngoplasty for the management of velopharyngeal insufficiency. *Plastic and Reconstructive Surgery, 112*(7), 1755–1761.

MacKenzie-Stepner, K., Witzel, M. A., Stringer, D. A., Lindsay, W. K., Munro, I. R., & Hughes, H. (1987). Abnormal carotid arteries in the velocardiofacial syndrome: A report of three cases. *Plastic and Reconstructive Surgery, 80*(3), 347–351.

Marsh, J. L., Grames, L. M., & Holtman, B. (1989). Intravelar veloplasty: A prospective study. *Cleft Palate Journal, 26*(1), 46–50.

Mehendale, F. V., & Sommerlad, B. C. (2004). Surgical significance of abnormal internal carotid arteries in velocardiofacial syndrome in 43 consecutive Hynes pharyngoplasties. *Cleft Palate-Craniofacial Journal, 41*(4), 368–374.

Millard, D. R., Jr., & Latham, R. A. (1990). Improved primary surgical and dental treatment of clefts. *Plastic and Reconstructive Surgery, 86*(5), 856–871.

Millard, D. R., Latham, R., Huifen, X., Spiro, S., & Morovic, C. (1999). Cleft lip and palate treated by presurgical orthopedics, gingivoperiosteoplasty, and lip adhesion (POPLA) compared with previous lip adhesion method: A preliminary study of serial dental casts. *Plastic and Reconstructive Surgery, 103*(6), 1630–1644.

Mitnick, R. J., Bello, J. A., Golding-Kushner, K. J., Argamaso, R. V., & Shprintzen, R. J. (1996). The use of magnetic resonance angiography prior to pharyngeal flap surgery in patients with velocardiofacial syndrome. *Plastic and Reconstructive Surgery, 97*(5), 908–919.

Moore, M. D., Lawrence, W. T., Ptak, J. J., & Trier, W. C. (1988). Complications of primary palatoplasty: A twenty-one-year review. *Cleft Palate Journal, 25*(2), 156–162.

Murison, M. S., & Pigott, R. W. (1992). Medial Langenbeck: Experience of a modified von Langenbeck repair of the cleft palate. A preliminary report. *British Journal of Plastic Surgery, 45*(6), 454–459.

Orticochea, M. (1970). Results of the dynamic muscle sphincter operation in cleft palates. *British Journal of Plastic Surgery, 23*(2), 108–114.

Orticochea, M. (1983). A review of 236 cleft palate patients treated with dynamic muscle sphincter. *Plastic and Reconstructive Surgery, 71*(2), 180–188.

Orticochea, M. (1997). Physiopathology of the dynamic muscular sphincter of the pharynx. *Plastic and Reconstructive Surgery, 100*(7), 1918–1923.

Orticochea, M. (1999). The timing and management of dynamic muscular pharyngeal sphincter construction in velopharyngeal incompetence. *British Journal of Plastic Surgery, 52*(2), 85–87.

Perkins, J. A., Lewis, C. W., Gruss, J. S., Eblen, L. E., & Sie, K. C. (2005). Furlow palatoplasty for management of velopharyngeal insufficiency: A prospective study of 148 consecutive patients. *Plastic and Reconstructive Surgery, 116*(1), 72–80; Discussion 81–74.

Perko, M. A. (1979). Two-stage closure of cleft palate (Progress report). *Journal of Maxillofacial Surgery, 7*(1), 46–80.

Pigott, R. W., Rieger, F. W., & Moodie, A. F. (1984). Tongue flap repair of cleft palate fistulae. *British Journal of Plastic Surgery, 37*(3), 285–293.

Posnick, J. C., & Getz, S. B., Jr. (1987). Surgical closure of end-stage palatal fistulas using anteriorly based dorsal tongue flaps.

Journal of Oral Maxillofacial Surgery, 45(11), 907–912.

Remacle, M., Bertrand, B., Eloy, P., & Marbaix, E. (1990). The use of injectable collagen to correct velopharyngeal insufficiency. *Laryngoscope, 100*(3), 269–274.

Ren, Y. F., & Wang, G. H. (1993). A modified palatopharyngeous flap operation and its application in the correction of velopharyngeal incompetence. *Plastic and Reconstructive Surgery, 91*(4), 612–617.

Riski, J. E., Ruff, G. L., Georgiade, G. S., & Barwick, W. J. (1992). Evaluation of failed sphincter pharyngoplasties. *Annals of Plastic Surgery, 28*(6), 545–553.

Riski, J. E., Ruff, G. L., Georgiade, G. S., Barwick, W. J., & Edwards, P. D. (1992). Evaluation of the sphincter pharyngoplasty. *Cleft Palate-Craniofacial Journal, 29*(3), 254–261.

Roberts, T. M., & Brown, B. S. (1983). Evaluation of a modified sphincter pharyngoplasty in the treatment of speech problems due to palatal insufficiency. *Annals of Plastic Surgery, 10*(3), 209–213.

Ross, D. A., Witzel, M. A., Armstrong, D. C., & Thomson, H. G. (1996). Is pharyngoplasty a risk in velocardiofacial syndrome? An assessment of medially displaced carotid arteries. *Plastic and Reconstructive Surgery, 98*(7), 1182–1190.

Ross, R. B. (1987). Treatment variables affecting facial growth in complete unilateral cleft lip and palate. Part 1–Part 7. *Cleft Palate Journal, 24*(1), 5–77.

Saint Raymond, C., Bettega, G., Deschaux, C., Lebeau, J., Raphael, B., Levy, P., et al. (2004). Sphincter pharyngoplasty as a treatment of velopharyngeal incompetence in young people: A prospective evaluation of effects on sleep structure and sleep respiratory disturbances. *Chest, 125*(3), 864–871.

Salyer, K. E. (1986). Primary correction of the unilateral cleft lip nose: A 15-year experience. *Plastic and Reconstructive Surgery, 77*(4), 558–568.

Schweckendiek, W. (1955). Zur zweiphasigen Gauimenspalten-operation bei primarem Velumerschluss. *Fortschritte Kiefer- und Gesichtschts-chirurgie, 1,* 73–76.

Schweckendiek, W. (1966). The technique of early veloplasty and its results. *Acta Chirurgiae Plasticae, 8*(3), 188–194.

Schweckendiek, W. (1968). Early veloplasty and its results. *Acta Oto-Rhino-Laryngologica Belgica, 22*(6), 697–703.

Schweckendiek, W. (1983). Primary closure of cleft lip and cleft palate. *Zahnarztl Prax, 34*(8), 317–320.

Schweckendiek, W., & Doz, P. (1978). Primary veloplasty: Long-term results without maxillary deformity. A twenty-five year report. *Cleft Palate Journal, 15*(3), 268–274.

Seagle, M. B., Mazaheri, M. K., Dixon-Wood, V. L., & Williams, W. N. (2002). Evaluation and treatment of velopharyngeal insufficiency: The University of Florida experience. *Annals of Plastic Surgery, 48*(5), 464–470.

Sie, K. C., & Gruss, J. S. (2002). Results with Furlow palatoplasty in the management of velopharyngeal insufficiency [Comment]. *Plastic and Reconstructive Surgery, 109*(7), 2588–2589; Author reply 2590–2581.

Sie, K. C., Tampakopoulou, D. A., de Serres, L. M., Gruss, J. S., Eblen, L. E., & Yonick, T. (1998). Sphincter pharyngoplasty: Speech outcome and complications. *Laryngoscope, 108*(8, Pt. 1), 1211–1217.

Sie, K. C., Tampakopoulou, D. A., Sorom, J., Gruss, J. S., & Eblen, L. E. (2001). Results with Furlow palatoplasty in management of velopharyngeal insufficiency. *Plastic and Reconstructive Surgery, 108*(1), 17–25; Discussion 26–19.

Skolnick, M. L., & McCall, G. N. (1972). Velopharyngeal competence and incompetence following pharyngeal flap surgery: Videofluoroscopic study in multiple projections. *Cleft Palate Journal, 9*(1), 1–12.

Sloan, G. M. (2000). Posterior pharyngeal flap and sphincter pharyngoplasty: The state of the art. *Cleft Palate-Craniofacial Journal, 37*(2), 112–122.

Smahel, Z., & Horak, I. (1993). The effect of two-stage palatoplasty on facial development in unilateral cleft lip and palate. *Acta Chirurgiae Plasticae, 35*(1/2), 67–72.

Terris, D. J., & Goode, R. L. (1993). Costochondral pharyngeal implants for velopharyngeal insufficiency. *Laryngoscope, 103*(5), 565–569.

Tharanon, W., Stella, J. P., & Epker, B. N. (1990). The modified superior-based pharyngeal flap. Part III. A retrospective study. *Oral Surgery, Oral Medicine, Oral Pathology, and Endodontics, 70*(3), 256–267.

Thind, M. S., Singh, A., & Thind, R. S. (1992). Repair of anterior secondary palate fistula using tongue flaps. *Acta Chirurgiae Plasticae, 34*(2), 79–91.

Trier, W. C. (1985a). The pharyngeal flap operation. *Clinics in Plastic Surgery, 12*(4), 697–710.

Trier, W. C. (1985b). Repair of bilateral cleft lip: Millard's technique. *Clinics in Plastic Surgery, 12*(4), 605–625.

Trier, W. C., & Dreyer, T. M. (1984). Primary von Langenbeck palatoplasty with levator reconstruction: Rationale and technique. *Cleft Palate Journal, 21*(4), 254–262.

Trigos, I., Ysunza, A., Gonzalez, A., & Vazquez, M. C. (1988). Surgical treatment of borderline velopharyngeal insufficiency using homologous cartilage implantation with videonasopharyngoscopic monitoring. *Cleft Palate Journal, 25*(2), 167–170.

Vedung, S. (1995). Pharyngeal flaps after one- and two-stage repair of the cleft palate: A 25-year review of 520 patients. *Cleft Palate-Craniofacial Journal, 32*(3), 206–215; Discussion 215–206.

Wells, M. D., Vu, T. A., & Luce, E. A. (1999). Incidence and sequelae of nocturnal respiratory obstruction following posterior pharyngeal flap operation. *Annals of Plastic Surgery, 43*(3), 252–257.

Witt, P. D., & D'Antonio, L. L. (1993). Velopharyngeal insufficiency and secondary palatal management. A new look at an old problem. *Clinics in Plastic Surgery, 20*(4), 707–721.

Witt, P. D., D'Antonio, L. L., Zimmerman, G. J., & Marsh, J. L. (1994). Sphincter pharyngoplasty: A preoperative and postoperative analysis of perceptual speech characteristics and endoscopic studies of velopharyngeal function. *Plastic and Reconstructive Surgery, 93*(6), 1154–1168.

Witt, P. D., Marsh, J. L., Marty-Grames, L., & Muntz, H. R. (1995). Revision of the failed sphincter pharyngoplasty: An outcome assessment. *Plastic and Reconstructive Surgery, 96*(1), 129–138.

Witt, P. D., Marsh, J. L., Muntz, H. R., Marty-Grames, L., & Watchmaker, G. P. (1996). Acute obstructive sleep apnea as a complication of sphincter pharyngoplasty. *Cleft Palate-Craniofacial Journal, 33*(3), 183–189.

Witt, P. D., Miller, D. C., Marsh, J. L., Muntz, H. R., & Grames, L. M. (1998). Limited value of preoperative cervical vascular imaging in patients with velocardiofacial syndrome. *Plastic and Reconstructive Surgery*, *101*(5), 1184–1195; Discussion 1196–1189.

Witt, P. D., O'Daniel, T. G., Marsh, J. L., Grames, L. M., Muntz, H. R., & Pilgram, T. K. (1997). Surgical management of velopharyngeal dysfunction: Outcome analysis of autogenous posterior pharyngeal wall augmentation. *Plastic and Reconstructive Surgery*, *99*(5), 1287–1296; Discussion 1297–1300.

Witzel, M. A., Salyer, K. E., & Ross, R. B. (1984). Delayed hard palate closure: The philosophy revisited. *Cleft Palate Journal*, *21*(4), 263–269.

Wolford, L. M., Oelschlaeger, M., & Deal, R. (1989). Proplast as a pharyngeal wall implant to correct velopharyngeal insufficiency. *Cleft Palate Journal*, *26*(2), 119–126; Discussion 126–128.

Wu, J., & Epker, B. N. (1990). The modified superiorly based pharyngeal flap technique. Part II. An anatomic study. *Oral Surgery, Oral Medicine, Oral Pathology*, *70*(3), 251–255.

Yoshida, H., Stella, J. P., Ghali, G. E., & Epker, B. N. (1992). The modified superiorly based pharyngeal flap. Part IV. Position of the base of the flap. *Oral Surgery, Oral Medicine, Oral Patholology*, *73*(1), 13–18.

Ysunza, A. (2005). Fisiologia de musculos faringeos posterior a la restauracion quirurgica del esfinter velofaringeo. *Gaceta Medica de Mexico*, *141*(3), 195–199.

Ysunza, A., Garcia-Velasco, M., Garcia-Garcia, M., Haro, R., & Valencia, M. (1993). Obstructive sleep apnea secondary to surgery for velopharyngeal insufficiency. *Cleft Palate-Craniofacial Journal*, *30*(4), 387–390.

Ysunza, A., Pamplona, M. C., Molina, F., Drucker, M., Felemovicius, J., Ramirez, E., et al. (2004). Surgery for speech in cleft palate patients. *International Journal of Pediatric Otorhinolaryngology*, *68*(12), 1499–1505.

Ysunza, A., Pamplona, C., Ramirez, E., Molina, F., Mendoza, M., & Silva, A. (2002). Velopharyngeal surgery: A prospective randomized study of pharyngeal flaps and sphincter pharyngoplasties. *Plastic and Reconstructive Surgery*, *110*(6), 1401–1407.

CHAPTER

19

ORTHOGNATHIC SURGERY FOR CRANIOFACIAL DIFFERENCES

JULIA CORCORAN, M.D.

CHAPTER OUTLINE

INTRODUCTION

Craniofacial differences, including cleft and craniosynostosis syndromes, affect not only soft tissues, but they also affect underlying bony tissues. The craniofacial skeleton can be viewed as scaffolding for the soft tissue envelope of the face. If alveolar, palatal, maxillary, or mandibular segments are missing, unstable, or in poor anatomic relationship to one another, the functions of breathing, swallowing, speaking, and chewing can be impaired. Furthermore, the overlying face appears abnormal, drawing unfavorable attention to the patient.

Orthognathic surgery, which involves the bones of the upper jaw (the maxilla) and the lower jaw (the mandible), can address several different problems that occur in these patients. Congenital absence of bone in cleft patients can be corrected by bone grafting to improve the alveolar arch and occlusion. Lack of midfacial growth in patients with a cleft or craniosynostosis can be compensated for by repositioning the maxilla in a more normal occlusal relationship to the mandible with Le Fort osteotomies (surgical cuts made within bone). An inadequate mandible associated with airway collapse in Pierre Robin sequence, or facial asymmetry in facioauriculovertebral syndrome (hemifacial microsomia), can be addressed by mandibular advancement through multiple techniques, including distraction osteogenesis, osteotomy, or reconstruction with bone grafting. All of these techniques aim to improve both the function of the scaffolding as well as the appearance of the facial soft tissue. This chapter will briefly explain these procedures and their potential effects on articulation, resonance, and airway function.

ALVEOLAR BONE GRAFTING

One of the greatest improvements in care of the patient with cleft lip and palate has been the routine implementation of alveolar bone grafting. While *cheiloplasty* (lip repair) restores the continuity of the lip muscular sphincter, and palatoplasty restores the continuity of the velopharyngeal sphincter, the alveolus is not addressed routinely by either of these procedures. This situation leaves the lesser and greater palatine segments floating free, which usually leads to lateral crossbite on the side of the cleft (the lesser segment). Furthermore, the anterior gap in the arch can lead to loss of the permanent lateral incisor and cuspid teeth because of lack of supporting bone for the periodontal ligament that secures the tooth within the alveolus. This gap is usually associated with an oronasal fistula with its concomitant problems of discomfort and liquid loss into the nasal cavity (Waite & Waite, 1996).

The crossbite, anterior alveolar gap, and the loss of teeth potentially set the patient up for articulation errors in the production of fricatives and affricates, especially the sibilants. These problems can be addressed by positioning the two alveolar segments in a normal arch alignment and then securing them with a bone graft which, when healed, provides a stable scaffold for the permanent dentition and the upper lip. Figure 19–1 is a preoperative photo of a patient just prior to the bone graft. Figure 19–2 is a

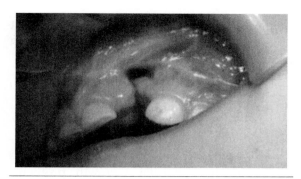

FIGURE 19–1 The bony cleft in the alveolus can be seen as the dark gap between the teeth. (Photograph courtesy of Delmar Halak, D.D.S.)

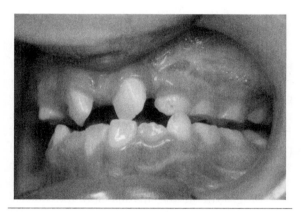

FIGURE 19–2 The gap has been closed and the gingiva has healed after a successful bone graft. (Photograph courtesy of Delmar Halak, D.D.S.)

postoperative photo of the same patient following the bone graft.

Timing and Technique of Bone Grafting

The timing of bone grafting is controversial. Repair of the alveolus can be done prior to the eruption of teeth either at the time of palatoplasty or in a separate operation—so-called primary bone grafting. It also can be delayed until the age of mixed dentition when the permanent teeth that will erupt into the grafted area are ready to descend—so-called delayed or intermediate bone grafting. The timing of bone grafting is debated, sometimes quite vigorously, between adherents of each philosophy.

Primary bone grafting can be done in one of two ways. A procedure called a *gingivoperiosteoplasty* opens alveolar soft tissues; that is, the gingiva and the underlying periosteum on each edge of the cleft. These raw surfaces are advanced and sewn together. This technique allows the bone progenitor cells found in the gingivoperiosteum to lay down bone as the patient grows. Bone need not be harvested from elsewhere in the body. Sometimes, this procedure will provide adequate bonestock to support the permanent dentition. Another technique for primary bone grafting is to use a piece of rib graft as a strut across the alveolar cleft and then cover the repair with the gingivoperiosteum.

Surgeons who favor this early, or primary, approach point out that the maxillary arch is aligned appropriately from almost the beginning. The disadvantage of primary bone grafting is that, while bone often will form across the alveolar cleft, it may not be of sufficient quantity or quality to support the permanent dentition—necessitating a delayed or secondary bone graft (Dado, 1993; Santiago et al., 1998). This situation becomes tricky, as the success of bone grafting is directly dependent on the surrounding soft tissues having good blood flow. Scar tissue from the previous primary procedure has a poorer blood supply, hindering the bone engraftment.

Other surgeons favor delaying bone grafting of the alveolus until the permanent dentition begins erupting, the stage of mixed dentition. Delayed or intermediate bone grafting of this type occurs between 6 to 10 years of age when the permanent lateral incisor or the cuspid tooth roots are about one-third developed. These teeth are the ones located at the edges of the cleft. If unsupported by adequate bone, the teeth will be lost. Timing of the delayed bone graft depends on which tooth is more at risk, the lateral incisor or the cuspid, although the lateral incisor erupts earlier than the cuspid. Therefore, the actual age of bone grafting is patient-specific, depending on the anatomy and the child's dental development (Cohen, Polley, & Figueroa, 1993).

The pediatric dentist/orthodontist follows the child through serial radiographs to determine when the tooth roots are mature. While waiting for maturation, the dentist/orthodontist uses an expanding device to put the arch segments into correct alignment. Once aligned, a holding device, such as a retainer or a lingual holding arch of wire, is placed.

For the graft, bone is harvested from the marrow cavity of the skull or the hip (iliac crest). The edges of the cleft are opened as in a gingivoperiosteoplasty. The floor of the nose is sewn closed and the bone graft is packed into the space. The gingiva is then repaired over the bone graft. This approach also helps build up the bone deficiency in the nasal base and para-alar areas as well.

Postoperative Complications and Management of Bone Grafting

Certain complications can occur with bone grafting. Bleeding and infection are possible, and are probably the most common adverse occurrences. Inadequate bone graft take and breakdown of the repair can also happen. During the healing phase, the first six weeks after the surgery, the patient's palatal segments are held steady by an orthodontic device. Mastication is limited by placing the patient on a diet of soft and pureed foods. Brushing the teeth is replaced by using antimicrobial mouth rinses and a Waterpik® appliance. About three months later, when the bone is solidly healed, the orthodontist can then direct the teeth into the appropriate positions along a complete maxillary alveolar arch.

MAXILLARY ADVANCEMENT

Patients with cleft lip and palate, facioauriculovertebral syndrome, and craniosynostosis syndromes have maxillary growth problems that lead to concave profiles and malocclusion. In patients with clefts or synostosis, the maxillary arch sits behind the mandibular arch, an Angle's Class III occlusion. A review of the growth patterns of the maxilla and mandible explain why the malocclusion develops.

Children with clefts initially can be placed into a fairly normal occlusal relationship but revert to a Class III relationship. Mandibular growth continues later into life than maxillary growth, which is the normal growth pattern. However, frequently maxillary growth in cleft patients is inhibited, presumably because of scar tissue and disturbances to the growth centers from previous surgeries. Eventually the lack of growth in the maxilla and the normal growth in the mandible place the jaws in Class III malocclusion. Children with craniosynostosis syndromes fail to grow normally because the sutures between the facial bones and the skull bones have closed prematurely and stunted the growth.

In addition to these problems, the patient with facioauriculovertebral syndrome also has a *cant* (slant in occlusion) to the maxilla, presumably caused by the relationship of the maxilla to the affected hemimandible. Normally, the maxilla continues its downward growth until the maxillary teeth meet the mandibular teeth. In the case of facioauriculovertebral syndrome, the shortened mandible on the affected side leaves inadequate room for the maxilla on that side to grow.

Common problems with a retrodisplaced or small maxilla include articulation errors, sleep apnea, and hyponasality. The crowding of the maxillary teeth and the relatively narrow arch of the palate in these situations create a constricted oral cavity space. The anatomy of this situation can lead to articulation errors, such as the palatal-dorsal production of consonants and frontal or lateral lisping. The relative posterior displacement of the maxilla leads to a small pharyngeal space, which allows the tongue to obstruct the entire cavity in the recumbent position, explaining the sleep apnea and hyponasality. A less common problem is a shallow orbit because the cheeks are underdeveloped. The bones affected include not only the maxilla but also the zygoma, as found in syndromic synostosis (Apert and Crouzon syndromes), or complex clefting (Treacher Collins syndrome). Because the orbit is essentially too small, *proptosis* (protrusion) of the globe, with exposure of the cornea, can result in the potential loss of sight. Orthognathic surgery to advance the maxilla can improve these situations. In addition to bringing the midface forward, the maxilla can be rotated to match midlines and tilted to correct cant with the various Le Fort osteotomies.

Maxillary Osteotomies

Le Fort (1901) originally described the naturally occurring fracture planes in the facial skeleton. These lines of natural weakness in the facial skeleton collapse or break during trauma and are used to describe midfacial fracture patterns. His three labeled levels have been translated so that the surgeon can use these areas to create *osteotomies* (surgical cuts) in the maxilla and then position the bone in a more functional and pleasing position. Figure 19–3 illustrates the levels of the three Le Fort osteotomies.

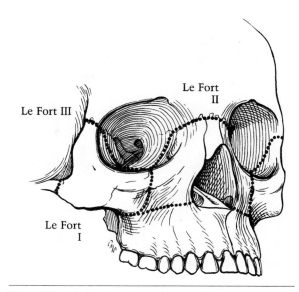

FIGURE 19–3 This line drawing demonstrates the level of the various Le Fort osteotomies. The Le Fort II osteotomy includes the territory of the Le Fort I osteotomy as well. The Le Fort III osteotomy includes the territory of the Le Fort I and Le Fort II osteotomies as well. (From *Grabb and Smith's Plastic Surgery,* 4th ed., edited by James W. Smith and J. Sherrell, 1991, Fig. 12–24, p. 374. Boston: Aston, Little, Brown and Company. Reprinted with permission.)

The most common of these osteotomies is the Le Fort I that transversely cuts the maxilla just above the tooth roots and the base of the nose, in essence allowing the surgeon to move the alveolar arch and palate as a single unit. One can imagine this movement as an edentulous individual being able to move his denture plate forward and out of his mouth. Figure 19–4 demonstrates the dramatic results of moving this segment of maxilla forward. If the surgeon needs to reposition the bridge of the nose as well as the teeth, as might be true in the case of patients with Treacher Collins, a Le Fort II osteotomy would include both the nasal pyramid and the alveolar arch. When the cheeks need to be brought forward to correct proptosis, as might be true in the case of patients with Apert's syndrome, a Le Fort III

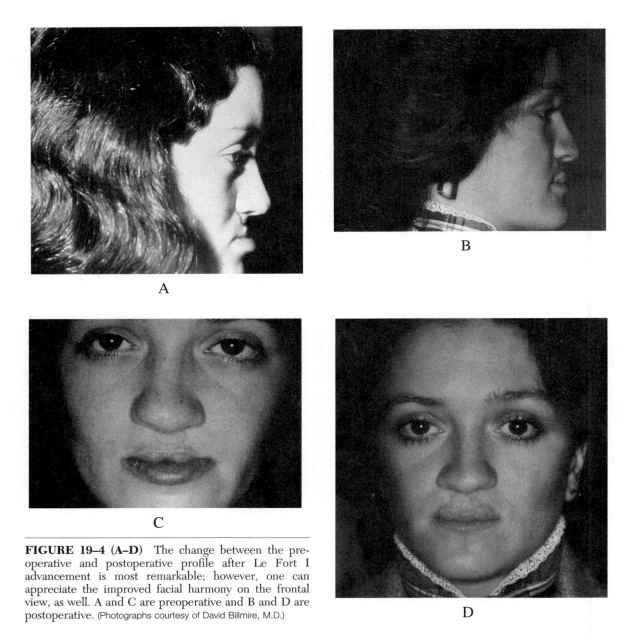

A

B

C

FIGURE 19–4 (A–D) The change between the preoperative and postoperative profile after Le Fort I advancement is most remarkable; however, one can appreciate the improved facial harmony on the frontal view, as well. A and C are preoperative and B and D are postoperative. (Photographs courtesy of David Billmire, M.D.)

D

osteotomy that includes cheek bones, orbital rims, nasal pyramid, and alveolar arch can be used. Figure 19–5A and 19–5C show preoperative proptosis and open bite, and Figures 19–5B and 19–5D show the postoperative improvement in a patient with Crouzon's syndrome.

The goals of maxillary repositioning include normal occlusion, normal-sized oral and

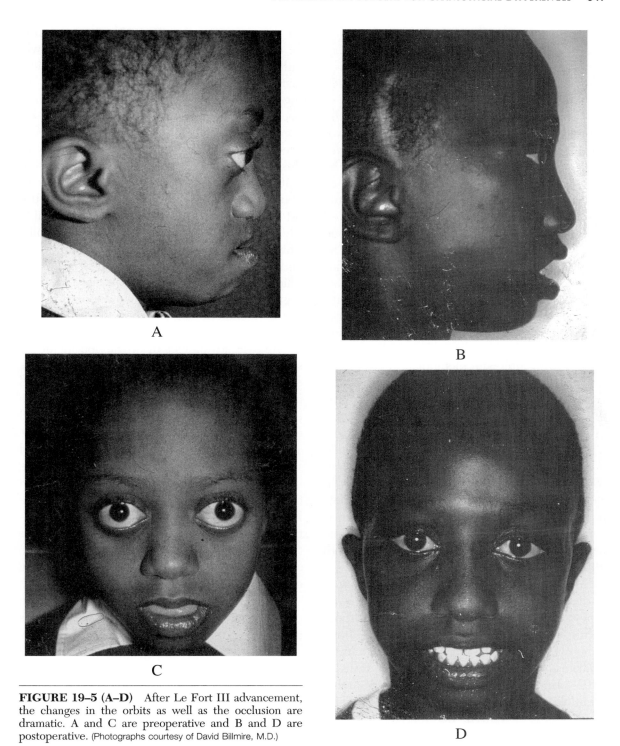

FIGURE 19–5 (A–D) After Le Fort III advancement, the changes in the orbits as well as the occlusion are dramatic. A and C are preoperative and B and D are postoperative. (Photographs courtesy of David Billmire, M.D.)

pharyngeal resonance cavities, and improved facial proportions. Orthognathic surgery of this magnitude requires careful planning between the orthodontist, surgeon, and speech pathologist.

The orthodontist and surgeon compare the patient's maxillary placement against known normative values by evaluating the *cephalogram*, which is a lateral radiograph of the craniofacial skeleton. Using these values, they determine how far and at what angle the maxilla must be moved to achieve the desired occlusion and profile. The orthodontist then places the teeth into position using braces. The final planning comes with performing the surgery on plaster cast models to assure the surgeon, orthodontist, and patient of the outcome. Splints to be used in the operating room are made from the cast. The osteotomies are made. At this point, the surgeon can choose to fix the maxilla into the advanced position with metal plates and screws. If the advancement is unstable or greater than 10 mm, bone grafts are necessary to support the maxilla and to prevent relapse back into its original position.

Postoperatively, these patients may be held in occlusion with wire bands temporarily and then in rubber band ligatures for six to eight weeks while the maxilla heals in its new position. During this period the patient is kept on pureed and soft diets. Afterwards, final orthodontia can be applied to move the teeth into the most ideal position.

Another method for maxillary advancement is distraction osteogenesis. *Distraction osteogenesis* is a recent development in orthognathic surgery and is used to lengthen bone (Cheung, & Chua, 2006; Cohen, Burstein, & Williams, 1999; Denny, Kalantarian, & Hanson, 2003; Imola & Tatum, 2002; McCarthy, Stelnicki, Mehrara, & Longaker, 2001; Mofid et al., 2001; Swennen, Schliephake, Dempf, Schierle, & Malevez, 2001). This technique involves making a *corticotomy* (a partial cut) in the middle of a bone, and then slowly pulling apart the cut ends with a mechanical distraction device. New bone is able to regenerate between the cut ends and in time becomes normal bone, obviating the need for bone grafts. When distraction osteogenesis is used, the presurgical planning and surgery to this point are identical. Rather than using plates and screws however, the surgeon can place a distraction device after making the osteotomies. This framework provides stability while the maxilla is moved forward gradually. This slow, deliberate advancement allows the body to lay down new bone growth, which solidly bolsters the maxilla in its new position. Figure 19–6 shows a patient preoperatively, in her distraction device, and then shows the result postoperatively.

Surgical advantages of distraction include a shorter surgery with less blood loss and less postoperative swelling. New bone is generated in the process of distraction. Therefore, there is no need for bone grafting of open spaces and no need to harvest donor bone. Because the advancement is gradual, it can be adjusted somewhat to the dynamic situation of the individual rather than to the static moment in the operating room. The gradual nature of the bone repositioning allows soft tissue adaptation to occur over time, which often increases the amount of advancement which can be achieved. The living bone formation in the distraction path prevents relapse.

Disadvantages include the obvious nature of the hardware, although this aspect is improving as portions of the device can now be buried beneath the soft issue—so-called *internal distraction devices*. There may be pain, sleeping difficulty, speech and eating problems, and disturbance of recreational activities (Primrose, Broadfoot, Diner, Molina, Moos, & Ayoub, 2005). There is the potential

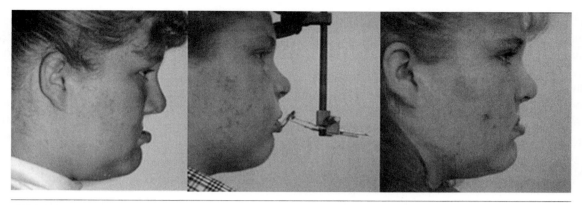

FIGURE 19–6 Distraction osteogenesis as applied to the midface. The left panel demonstrates the preoperative profile. The middle panel shows the patient at the end of distraction in her halo device. The right panel shows the postoperative results.

for hardware to fail and require replacement during the distraction period; sometimes this also requires a return to the operating room. The majority of external devices can be removed in the office setting, but internally based hardware may require surgical removal in the operating room.

Timing of Orthognathic Surgery

Orthognathic surgery of the maxilla cannot be performed readily until the maxillary sinus is well developed. In the young child, the sinus area of the maxilla is the storehouse for the permanent dentition. Once a child enters mixed dentition, suitable space exists to introduce the surgical saw and allow Le Fort III advancement. These procedures are used most commonly in the patients with synostosis syndromes to improve the airway, close the anterior open bite, increase the oral cavity size and, most importantly, protect the proptotic globes. Because of the shorter operations and lower blood loss, maxillary distraction as a method of midface advancement is well suited to the younger patient. Any surgery done at this age will not hold up to future growth however. Therefore, the patient will likely need a Le Fort I advancement, or possibly a repeat Le Fort III, in the teenage years to balance the occlusion, improve facial harmony, and create a convex profile.

Secondary orthognathic surgery for patients with craniosynostosis and primary orthognathic surgery for patients with cleft lip and palate are usually delayed until after facial skeletal maturity and complete eruption of the permanent dentition. The last bone to mature in the facial skeleton is the mandible. Waiting until mandibular growth is complete assures that new maxillary placement will be adequate for facial maturity. Consequently, this type of surgery is delayed to age 15–16 in girls and age 17–18 in boys. Prior to Le Fort I maxillary advancement, impacted third molars usually are addressed, although in some cases they can be removed at the time of maxillary advancement. Presurgical orthodontia must be completed before maxillary advancement.

Maxillary Advancement and the Velopharyngeal Mechanism

Advancement of the maxilla, and thus the velum, changes the dimensions of the pharyngeal cavity.

This can be beneficial for patients with craniosynostosis syndromes who are likely to have hyponasality and even airway obstruction due to the stenotic suture lines between the facial bones and the cranial base. For these patients, the increased diameter of the pharynx and the reduction of nasal airway resistance often improves or eliminates the hyponasality and upper airway obstruction (Dalston, 1996; Maegawa et al., 1998; McCarthy et al., 1979).

For patients with a repaired cleft palate or submucous cleft, maxillary advancement, even through distraction, can have a negative effect on velopharyngeal function. With the anterior movement of the velum, there is an increase in the anterior-posterior depth that the velopharyngeal sphincter must close during speech. If the velum is unable to stretch sufficiently to make up the difference, this will result in the development of or worsening of velopharyngeal insufficiency (Dalston, 1996; Dalston & Vig, 1984; Haapanen, Kalland, Heliovaara, Hukki, & Ranta, 1997; Heliovaara, Hukki, Ranta, & Haapanen, 2004; Heliovaara, Ranta, Hukki, & Haapanen, 2002; Janulewicz, Costello, Buckley, Ford, Close, & Gassner, 2004; Kummer, Strife, Grau, Creaghead, & Lee, 1989; Maegawa, Sells, & David, 1998; Mason, Turvey, & Warren, 1980; Okazaki et al., 1993; Satoh et al., 2004; Watzke, Turvey, Warren, & Dalston, 1990). It would seem that the gradual nature of maxillary advancement through distraction might allow for the velopharyngeal mechanism to adapt to its new situation and minimize postadvancement hypernasality. Studies have shown, however, that even with distraction, patients with borderline velopharyngeal closure can develop velopharyngeal insufficiency (Guyette, Polley, Figueroa, & Smith, 2001; Ko, Figueroa, Guyette, Polley, & Law, 1999; Trindade, Yamashita, Suguimoto, Mazzottini, & Trindade, 2003).

Postoperative hypernasality and nasal emission are most likely to occur in patients with tenuous velopharyngeal closure initially, or with maxillary advancements that are greater than 10 mm. Some patients have a temporary period of hypernasality that corrects itself as the velopharyngeal structures accommodate to their new anatomic relationships. Other patients will require either a pharyngeal flap or pharyngoplasty to ameliorate the situation.

Prior to maxillary advancement by either method, at least an informal speech assessment is essential to predict the consequences of the procedure on the velopharyngeal sphincter. This is important in order to properly inform the patient and family of the risks and benefits of such surgery (Phillips, Klaiman, Delorey, & MacDonald, 2005). In elective orthognathic cases done for improvement of facial harmony, a simple interview with a sampling of speech suffices. Clues to tenuous velopharyngeal closure in speech samples include nasal emission during connected speech. Patients with craniofacial differences, however, require more sophisticated evaluations. In this case, a speech pathologist should evaluate articulation, resonance, and velopharyngeal function. In some cases, nasopharyngoscopy should be done to assess the anatomy of the velopharyngeal sphincter in this group of patients.

The second velopharyngeal situation affecting maxillary advancement is the presence of a pharyngeal flap. Because these patients already have a history of velopharyngeal insufficiency (VPI), they are at increased risk for recurrent VPI postoperatively. Another problem is that from a technical point of view, the flap causes more difficulty in bringing the maxilla forward because of soft tissue tethering. Also, over time, patients with pharyngeal flaps prior to maxillary advancement seem to have increased incidence of relapse (retropositioning of the maxilla toward its original location), which is presumably due to the pull of the flap. Therefore, in order to achieve enough maxillary advancement and reduce the risk of relapse, some flaps may require division prior to the advancement procedure. Fortunately, if the flap has been in place for some time, division of the flap does not always cause a deterioration in velopharyngeal function. This is probably due to the residual flap tissue and possibly changes in the inclination of the pharyngeal wall that would have occurred with growth.

Maxillary Advancement and Articulation

A primary purpose of maxillary advancement is to normalize the occlusal relationship between the maxillary and mandibular arches. Since malocclusion is a common cause of articulation errors, it stands to reason that the correction of the malocclusion could improve the articulation errors (Ward, McAuliffe, Holmes, Lynham, & Monsour, 2002). In fact, several studies have reported improved articulation following maxillary advancement, without intervening speech therapy (Guyette, Polley, Figueroa, & Smith, 2001; Kummer et al., 1989; Lee, Whitehill, Ciocca, & Samman, 2002; Maegawa et al., 1998; Mason et al., 1980; McCarthy, Coccaro, & Schwartz, 1979; Trinadade, 2003; Vallino, 1990). This improvement is only noted in cases of obligatory errors—where tongue position was normal during production, but the structure was abnormal, causing the distortions. When there are compensatory errors resulting in abnormal tongue position, the maxillary advancement does not improve speech. Instead, speech therapy is required postoperatively for correction of these articulation errors.

Complications of Maxillary Advancement

Complications associated with maxillary advancement include major blood loss requiring massive transfusion, infection of the facial soft tissues, relapse of the maxilla, decreased sensation in the upper lip and midface, loss of teeth, loss of gingiva, persistent malocclusion not correctable with orthodontia, and, most significant to this topic, velopharyngeal insufficiency.

To correct relapse of the maxilla and persistent malocclusion not correctable with orthodontia, maxillary advancement must be performed again, including the presurgical orthodontia. Loss of gingiva can be improved by periodontal correction. Loss of teeth can be masked with bridgework or other prosthetic replacement. Changes in sensation may correct over time or, more likely, the patient becomes used to the new situation and compensates. Velopharyngeal insufficiency may correct over time or may require a pharyngeal flap or pharyngoplasty.

MANDIBULAR RECONSTRUCTION

Management of the mandible can be a significant challenge for surgeons caring for patients with craniofacial differences. Micrognathia is associated with many of the craniofacial differences including the Pierre Robin sequence, Treacher Collins syndrome, and bilateral facioauriculovertebral syndrome. A normal mandible appearing prognathic is problematic for patients with craniosynostosis syndromes and with cleft lip and palate. An asymmetric mandible with hypoplastic or absent portions occurs in hemifacial microsomia. An asymmetric mandible and relative prognathism rarely influences the airway or alimentation. However, malocclusion of this type can cause problems with tooth erosion and with articulation.

Many infants with Pierre Robin sequence have significant airway obstruction due to the small, retrognathic mandible. The problems can range from desaturation during feeding and sleep apnea when supine, to complete airway obstruction regardless of position. The initial management of these infants is to provide an adequate airway for vegetative respiration and a method for alimentation. Simple temporizing measures include prone positioning of the baby while sleeping and feeding. More complex methods include placement of a nasal-pharyngeal airway (a so-called trumpet) and gavage feedings through an intermittently placed nasogastric tube. Severe cases may require tracheostomy for airway management and gastrostomy for feeding.

Children with severe micrognathia requiring tracheostomy may require some sort of mandibular advancement to allow for decannulation. The earlier decannulation can be done in life, the better the prognosis will be for speech development. This is because the presence of the tracheostomy circumvents subglottic airflow which is necessary for speech production. The inability to produce speech normally also affects the development of expressive language skills.

Mandibular reconstruction options for these infants are as varied as the surgeons who attempt to solve these problems. The more common methods include distraction osteogenesis, rib graft reconstruction, free tissue microsurgical reconstruction (free-flap), and mandibular osteotomies, the most versatile being the sagittal split osteotomy.

Advancement by Distraction Osteogenesis

Prior to the technique of mandibular distraction, the surgical advancement of the mandible in young patients was rare and fraught with difficulties. Such reconstruction was delayed until later in life and usually performed at 5 to 6 years of age when the ribs were sufficiently developed to use as struts and grafts. Mandibular distraction osteogenesis has allowed decannulation of patients as young as toddlers (Williams, Maull, Grayson, Longaker, & McCarthy, 1999). McCarthy, Schreiber, Karp, Thorne, and Grayson (1992) presented the first reports of mandibular distraction in children in 1992. Since that time, many different approaches to mandibular distraction have been tried and the technique has gained widespread acceptance. Devices can now have multiple planes of distraction, can be internal or external, and since its inception only 15 years ago, have been applied to all of the facial bones. Mandibular distraction can be applied to the hemimandible to improve symmetry in situations such as facioauriculovertebral syndrome (hemifacial microsomia)—or can be applied bilaterally to patients with micrognathia, such as those with Pierre Robin sequence.

All of the distraction techniques take advantage of the fact that the body will heal a fractured bone by laying down new bone. If the ends of a fracture are gradually separated, the body will create new bone in this gap as well. All distraction procedures produce a fracture— either complete (osteotomy) or partial (corticotomy). To advance the mandible, these cuts are made bilaterally in the non-tooth-bearing area of the mandibular body, in the mandibular angle, or in the *ramus*, which is the upturned, perpendicular extremity of the mandible on both sides. After several days of rest, the so-called latent period, the distraction device is activated and the cut ends of the bone are separated gradually, usually one to two millimeters daily (the active period). Once the desired advancement is achieved, the device is left in place as a scaffold until the new bone has solidified, the so-called resting period. This period is usually equal to or longer than the period of active distraction. The device is then removed. Variations on this procedure include whether the surgeon approaches the patient externally or intraorally, whether the device is external or internal, whether one or more osteotomies are used, and whether the device can move the mandible in one, two, or three dimensions.

When applied bilaterally to micrognathic patients, the distractors can pull the base of the tongue as well as the mandible forward, in effect opening the pharyngeal space. For this reason, it has been used to help decannulate micrognathic children who have required tracheostomy. Some centers are distracting infants primarily to reduce the need for tracheostomy. Whether this practice will hold up to scrutiny is actively being debated at this time.

In order to determine whether advancement has been sufficient to allow decannulation of the patient, the patient is examined prior to end of the active period of distraction. Lateral cephalograms can demonstrate the increased dimensions of the nasopharyngeal cavity.

A more certain evaluation is laryngoscopy and bronchoscopy. This is performed in the operating room by a pediatric otolaryngologist who can attend to the other issues which surround chronic airway cannulation, including subglottic stenosis, laryngomalacia, and granulation tissue.

A more physiologic test of airway adequacy is blocking the cannula temporarily with a valve to see if the child can maintain his airway. Figure 19–7 shows a tracheostomy-dependent child with micrognathia prior to, during, and after distraction.

One of the beauties of distraction osteogenesis is the versatility of the technique. Distraction can be repeated on the same patient should mandibular advancement be needed again as the midface grows. The technique can also be applied unilaterally to rotate the canted, hypoplastic side of the mandible in the patient with facioauriculovertebral syndrome. Rib graft used to reconstruct a mandible can also be distracted as if it were native mandible (Corcoran, Hubli, & Salyer, 1997).

Complications with distraction are many, but usually minor in nature (Corcoran et al., 1997).

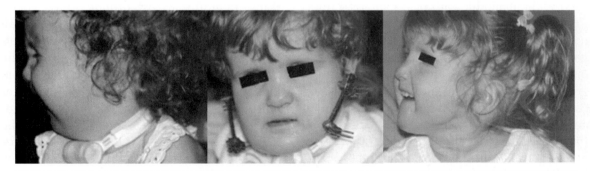

FIGURE 19–7   Distraction osteogenesis as applied to the mandible. In this case an external distractor was applied through and intraoral approach. The left panel demonstrates the degree of preoperative micrognathia. The middle panel shows the patient in her distractor. The right panel shows the amount of advancement obtained. Note that the patient has her tracheostomy successfully decannulated. (Photographs courtesy of David Billmire, M.D.)

The skin surrounding the device can become infected, and on occasion the device can fail. Unusual complications include facial nerve palsies and fibrous malunion. Distraction, however, has stood the test of time. In the decade since its inception, problems with relapse have not been reported despite frequent application of this technique (McCarthy, Stelnicki, & Grayson, 1999).

The changes in velopharyngeal function and articulation, as the mandibular height and relationships change, have been reported by Guyette, Polley, Figueroa, and Cohen (1996). Initially, articulation and resonance may become worse; however, with time resonance can normalize and articulation improves.

Rib Graft Reconstruction

Reconstructive surgeons have taken advantage of the natural structure of the rib with its bony shaft and cartilaginous tip to recreate hypoplastic and absent mandibles, especially in facioauriculovertebral syndrome. The child must have adequate-sized ribs, which precludes doing this type of reconstruction prior to 5 to 6 years of age. The cartilage tip is used to mimic the condyle of the mandible and the shaft of the rib to recreate the ramus and body. The graft is fixed to the mandible with plates and/or screws.

This technique has been mainstay of mandibular reconstruction for several surgical generations. A unique problem with rib grafting is the inability to predict postoperative growth patterns. The graft can partially or completely resorb, leaving the patient without any advancement. Alternatively, it can remain the same size, so that as the child's other facial bones grow, the asymmetry reproduces itself. Rarely, the rib graft can overgrow and create a secondary asymmetry requiring resection of a portion of the graft. Another drawback to rib graft reconstruction of the hypoplastic mandible is its lack of soft tissue replacement. While a rib graft can replace the missing facial height and mandibular length, the soft tissue fullness and contour is not provided by this technique, leaving the patient with an asymmetric appearance.

Free Tissue Transfer (Free-Flap) Reconstruction

One of the more elegant solutions to the lack of soft tissue and lack of growth in a rib graft has been the use of free tissue transfer (free-flap) to reconstruct the mandible and overlying soft tissues. The surgeon can harvest bone or bone and soft tissue with their blood vessels and transfer this flap to the mandible, hooking the donor blood vessels into the recipient blood vessels of the face. These small vessels are sewn together with the aid of the operating microscope. The scapula and its overlying soft tissue can be used to transfer bone and soft tissue to the mandible. It also provides a reliable growth center. If only soft tissue is necessary, many donor sites have been used, including the greater omentum from the abdomen.

Mandibular Osteotomies

Many mandibular osteotomies have been designed. The most versatile is the sagittal split osteotomy which allows advancement, setback, and rotation. The surgeon splits the ramus of the mandible between its inner and outer tables, separating the condyle and outer table of the ramus from the body and the inner table (Figure 19–8). The unique advantage of the sagittal split is the large contact area it leaves for the two ends of the mandible to heal, allowing the surgeon to advance, set back, or rotate the segment. The pieces of the mandible are put into their new positions with the aid of splints, as described for maxillary advancement. The

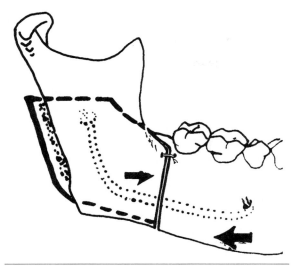

FIGURE 19–8 This line drawing demonstrates the anatomy of a sagittal split osteotomy and the versatility of either advancement, rotation, or set-back that can be obtained. (From *Grabb and Smith's Plastic Surgery*, 4th ed., edited by James W. Smith and J. Sherrell, 1991, Fig. 7–6, p. 233. Boston: Aston, Little, Brown and Company. Reprinted with permission.)

surgeon can then secure the segments with wires, screws, or plates.

Postoperatively the patient must comply with a physical therapy regimen to prevent stiffness of the temporomandibular joint. Proper interoperative positioning of the mandibular segments is essential to prevent temporomandibular joint problems. Depending on the stability of the mandibular movement, the patient may require *intermaxillary fixation*, which involves wiring the mandible against the maxilla to keep it closed, or elastic

band therapy. Frequently the patient will be uncomfortable with how the maxillary and mandibular teeth meet. This malocclusion, whether subjective or objective, can usually be improved by postoperative orthodontia.

The technique of sagittal split osteotomy with a rib graft or free-flap reconstruction can be applied unilaterally (as in facioauriculovertebral syndrome) or bilaterally. It can be done in conjunction with a maxillary advancement to improve facial harmony when advancement is limited by soft tissue constraints. It is the work horse osteotomy of craniofacial reconstruction.

The horizontal mandibular osteotomy for chin advancement, also called a *genioplasty*, is another frequent osteotomy of the mandible. Chin advancement can be done in conjunction with other mandibular or maxillary osteotomies or alone. While it does not change airway or speech considerations, it does greatly improve facial aesthetics.

SUMMARY

The success of reconstruction of children with craniofacial differences is the sum of its parts. With manipulation of the facial bones, significant improvements can be made in the soft tissue contours and the appearance of the child. These bone improvements can also have profound influences on the speech of the child, affecting both articulation and resonance.

FOR REVIEW, DISCUSSION, AND CRITICAL THINKING

1. What is orthognathic surgery? What is the goal of this type of surgery? Why do you think it is commonly done for patients with cleft lip and palate?

2. Discuss the reason for alveolar bone grafting and describe how it is done as if

   you were explaining it to a parent. Discuss the controversy regarding timing. What are potential complications?

3. Explain the origin of the Le Fort classification system. What is the difference between Le Fort I, Le Fort II, and Le

Fort III osteotomies? When is this type of surgery usually done and why?

4. Why do children with a history of cleft lip and palate often benefit from maxillary advancement? What are the potential effects of maxillary advancement on speech and resonance? What are the concerns of maxillary advancement when there is a preexisting pharyngeal flap? Discuss the appropriate timing of this surgery.

5. You have done a speech evaluation on a 17-year-old boy who is scheduled to undergo maxillary advancement. Speech is characterized by obligatory articulation errors due to occlusion and barely audible, inconsistent nasal emission. Describe the potential risks and benefits of this surgery as if you were explaining it to the boy and his family. What kind of follow-up should be done postoperatively?

6. Describe the process of distraction osteogenesis as if you were explaining it to a parent. At what age can this be done? What are the potential advantages of this technique? What are potential complications?

7. In what cases would mandibular advancement be appropriate? What are the potential benefits of this surgery?

8. What are the purposes the following: rib graft reconstruction, free tissue transfer, and mandibular osteotomy?

REFERENCES

Cheung, L. K., & Chua, H. D. (2006). A meta-analysis of cleft maxillary osteotomy and distraction osteogenesis. *International Journal of Oral & Maxillofacial Surgery, 35*(1), 14–24.

Cohen, M., Polley, J. W., & Figueroa, A. A. (1993). Secondary (intermediate) alveolar bone grafting. *Clinics in Plastic Surgery, 20*(4), 691–705.

Cohen, S. R., Burstein, F. D., & Williams, J. K. (1999). The role of distraction osteogenesis in the management of craniofacial disorders. *Annals of the Academy of Medicine, Singapore, 28*(5), 728–738.

Corcoran, J., Hubli, E. H., & Salyer, K. E. (1997). Distraction osteogenesis of costochondral neomandibles: A clinical experience. *Plastic and Reconstructive Surgery, 100*(2), 311–315; Discussion 316–317.

Dado, D. V. (1993). Primary (early) alveolar bone grafting. *Clinics in Plastic Surgery, 20*(4), 683–689.

Dalston, R. M. (1996). Velopharyngeal impairment in the orthodontic population. *Seminars in Orthodontics, 2*(3), 220–227.

Dalston, R. M., & Vig, P. S. (1984). Effects of orthognathic surgery on speech: A prospective study. *American Journal of Orthodontics, 86*(4), 291–298.

Denny, A. D., Kalantarian, B., & Hanson, P. R. (2003). Rotation advancement of the midface by distraction osteogenesis. *Plastic and Reconstructive Surgery, 111*(6), 1789–1799; Discussion 1800–1783.

Guyette, T. W., Polley, J. W., Figueroa, A. A., & Cohen, M. N. (1996). Mandibular distraction osteogenesis: Effects on articulation and velopharyngeal function. *Journal of Craniofacial Surgery, 7*(3), 186–191.

Guyette, T. W., Polley, J. W., Figueroa, A., & Smith, B. E. (2001). Changes in speech following maxillary distraction osteogenesis. *Cleft Palate-Craniofacial Journal, 38*(3), 199–205.

Haapanen, M. L., Kalland, M., Heliovaara, A., Hukki, J., & Ranta, R. (1997). Velopharyngeal function in cleft patients undergoing maxillary advancement. *Folia Phoniatrica et Logopedica*, 49(1), 42–47.

Heliovaara, A., Hukki, J., Ranta, R., & Haapanen, M. L. (2004). Cephalometric pharyngeal changes after Le Fort I osteotomy in different types of clefts. *Scandinavian Journal of Plastic and Reconstructive Surgery and Hand Surgery*, 38(1), 5–10.

Heliovaara, A., Ranta, R., Hukki, J., & Haapanen, M. L. (2002). Cephalometric pharyngeal changes after Le Fort I osteotomy in patients with unilateral cleft lip and palate. *Acta Odontologica Scandinavica*, 60(3), 141–145.

Imola, M. J., & Tatum, S. A. (2002). Craniofacial distraction osteogenesis. *Facial Plastic Surgery Clinics of North America*, 10(3), 287–301.

Janulewicz, J., Costello, B. J., Buckley, M. J., Ford, M. D., Close, J., & Gassner, R. (2004). The effects of Le Fort I osteotomies on velopharyngeal and speech functions in cleft patients. *Journal of Oral & Maxillofacial Surgery*, 62(3), 308–314.

Ko, E. W., Figueroa, A. A., Guyette, T. W., Polley, J. W., & Law, W. R. (1999). Velopharyngeal changes after maxillary advancement in cleft patients with distraction osteogenesis using a rigid external distraction device: A 1-year cephalometric follow-up. *Journal of Craniofacial Surgery*, 10(4), 312–320; Discussion 321–312.

Kummer, A. W., Strife, J. L., Grau, W. H., Creaghead, N. A., & Lee, L. (1989). The effects of Le Fort I osteotomy with maxillary movement on articulation, resonance, and velopharyngeal function. *Cleft Palate Journal*, 26(3), 193–199; Discussion 199–200.

Lee, A. S., Whitehill, T. L., Ciocca, V., & Samman, N. (2002). Acoustic and perceptual analysis of the sibilant sound /s/ before and after orthognathic surgery. *Journal of Oral & Maxillofacial Surgery*, 60(4), 364–372; Discussion 372–363.

Le Fort, R. (1901). Etude experimental sur les fractures de la machoire superieure. Parts I, II, III. *Revue de Chirurgie de Pari*, 23, 201, 360, 479.

Maegawa, J., Sells, R. K., & David, D. J. (1998). Speech changes after maxillary advancement in 40 cleft lip and palate patients. *Journal of Craniofacial Surgery*, 9(2), 177–182; Discussion 183–184.

Mason, R., Turvey, T. A., & Warren, D. W. (1980). Speech considerations with maxillary advancement procedures. *Journal of Oral Surgery*, 38(10), 752–758.

McCarthy, J. G., Coccaro, P. J., & Schwartz, M. D. (1979). Velopharyngeal function following maxillary advancement. *Plastic and Reconstructive Surgery*, 64(2), 180–189.

McCarthy, J. G., Schreiber, J., Karp, N., Thorne, C. H., & Grayson, B. H. (1992). Lengthening the human mandible by gradual distraction [see Comments]. *Plastic and Reconstructive Surgery*, 89(1), 1–8; Discussion 9–10.

McCarthy, J. G., Stelnicki, E. J., & Grayson, B. H. (1999). Distraction osteogenesis of the mandible: A ten-year experience. *Seminars in Orthodontics*, 5(1), 3–8.

McCarthy, J. G., Stelnicki, E. J., Mehrara, B. J., & Longaker, M. T. (2001). Distraction osteogenesis of the craniofacial skeleton. *Plastic and Reconstructive Surgery*, 107(7), 1812–1827.

Mofid, M. M., Manson, P. N., Robertson, B. C., Tufaro, A. P., Elias, J. J., & Vander Kolk, C. A. (2001). Craniofacial distraction osteogenesis: A review of 3,278 cases.

Plastic and Reconstructive Surgery, 108(5), 1103–1114; Discussion 1115–1107.

Okazaki, K., Satoh, K., Kato, M., Iwanami, M., Ohokubo, F., & Kobayashi, K. (1993). Speech and velopharyngeal function following maxillary advancement in patients with cleft lip and palate. *Annals of Plastic Surgery, 30*(4), 304–311.

Phillips, J. H., Klaiman, P., Delorey, R., & MacDonald, D. B. (2005). Predictors of velopharyngeal insufficiency in cleft palate orthognathic surgery. *Plastic and Reconstructive Surgery, 115*(3), 681–686.

Primrose, A. C., Broadfoot, E., Diner, P. A., Molina, F., Moos, K. F., & Ayoub, A. F. (2005). Patients' responses to distraction osteogenesis: A multicentre study. *International Journal of Oral & Maxillofacial Surgery, 34*(3), 238–242.

Santiago, P. E., Grayson, B. H., Cutting, C. B., Gianoutsos, M. P., Brecht, L. E., & Kwon, S. M. (1998). Reduced need for alveolar bone grafting by presurgical orthopedics and primary gingivoperiosteoplasty. *Cleft Palate-Craniofacial Journal, 35*(1), 77–80.

Satoh, K., Nagata, J., Shomura, K., Wada, T., Tachimura, T., Fukuda, J., et al. (2004). Morphological evaluation of changes in velopharyngeal function following maxillary distraction in patients with repaired cleft palate during mixed dentition. *Cleft Palate-Craniofacial Journal, 41*(4), 355–363.

Swennen, G., Schliephake, H., Dempf, R., Schierle, H., & Malevez, C. (2001). Craniofacial distraction osteogenesis: A review of the literature: Part 1: Clinical studies.

International Journal of Oral & Maxillofacial Surgery, 30(2), 89–103.

Trindade, I. E., Yamashita, R. P., Suguimoto, R. M., Mazzottini, R., & Trindade, A. S., Jr. (2003). Effects of orthognathic surgery on speech and breathing of subjects with cleft lip and palate: Acoustic and aerodynamic assessment. *Cleft Palate-Craniofacial Journal, 40*(1), 54–64.

Vallino, L. D. (1990). Speech, velopharyngeal function, and hearing before and after orthognathic surgery. *Journal of Oral and Maxillofacial Surgery, 48*(12), 1274–1281; Discussion 1281–1282.

Waite, P. D., & Waite, D. E. (1996). Bone grafting for the alveolar cleft defect. *Seminars in Orthodontics, 2*(3), 192–196.

Ward, E. C., McAuliffe, M., Holmes, S. K., Lynham, A., & Monsour, F. (2002). Impact of malocclusion and orthognathic reconstruction surgery on resonance and articulatory function: An examination of variability in five cases. *British Journal of Oral & Maxillofacial Surgery, 40*(5), 410–417.

Watzke, I., Turvey, T. A., Warren, D. W., & Dalston, R. (1990). Alterations in velopharyngeal function after maxillary advancement in cleft palate patients. *Journal of Oral and Maxillofacial Surgery, 48*(7), 685–689.

Williams, J. K., Maull, D., Grayson, B. H., Longaker, M. T., & McCarthy, J. G. (1999). Early decannulation with bilateral mandibular distraction for tracheostomy-dependent patients. *Plastic and Reconstructive Surgery, 103*(1), 48–57; Discussion 58–59.

C H A P T E R

20

PROSTHETIC MANAGEMENT

INTRODUCTION

Individuals with a history of cleft lip, cleft palate, or other craniofacial anomalies often have anatomical problems that affect facial aesthetics, dental arch stability, speech, mastication, and swallowing. These physical and functional problems can also affect the social, emotional, and psychological well-being of the patient in a very negative way.

Historically, patients with cleft lip and palate underwent multiple surgical and habilitative procedures in order to achieve an acceptable aesthetic and functional outcome. Surgical repairs were done later in life than they are today and the success level of the surgical procedures was not as high as it is currently. Despite the best efforts of the surgeon, the patient often had remaining dental and maxillary arch deficiencies and also speech problems due to occlusal anomalies and velopharyngeal insufficiency. Because of these residual problems, prosthetic management was often the most effective form of treatment and therefore, was commonly used. In recent years, however, there has been an increase in the understanding of the nature of craniofacial growth and development. In addition, advancements and improvements in surgical techniques have resulted in greatly improved outcomes. Therefore, prosthetic devices are no longer needed to achieve optimum results in most patients, particularly those who received early and appropriate surgical intervention (Delgado, Schaaf, & Emrich, 1992; Reisberg, 2000).

Although surgery is usually the option of choice for correction or improvement of many of these structural and functional problems, there still is a need for prosthetic treatment in certain cases. The overall goal of management, whether it is through surgical or prosthetic treatment, is to obtain the optimum results. However, in choosing a treatment option for the patient, the patient, family, and health care providers must consider not only the expected outcome with each option, but also the total amount of time necessary for achieving results, the risks to the patient, the cost of treatment, and the desires of the patient. A successful treatment option is one that meets the particular needs and expectations of the patient and the family.

The purpose of this chapter is to discuss the various types of prosthetic devices available for individuals with a history of cleft lip/palate or other craniofacial conditions. Speech-language pathologists should be well informed about the options for prosthetic management and when it is appropriate for the patient.

PROSTHETIC DEVICES

A *prosthesis*, also called a prosthetic device or appliance, is a fabricated substitute for a body part that is missing or malformed. This substitute may be fixed, so that it is essentially permanent, or it can be removable so that the patient can take it out for eating, sleeping, and cleaning. Prosthetic management can be done on a temporary basis prior to surgical correction or on a permanent basis.

Construction of a prosthetic device may be done by an orthodontist or pediatric dentist. However, this work is most often done by a prosthodontist who specializes in the construction of these devices. A *prosthodontist* is a dental professional who not only deals with the restoration of teeth, but also deals with the development of appliances to improve the appearance of oral and facial structures and to assist with feeding and velopharyngeal closure. The prosthodontist can be a very important member of a craniofacial team, because regardless of the surgical results, prosthodontists often can further improve the speech and appearance of individuals with significant anomalies.

Dental Appliances

Patients with a history of cleft lip that includes the entire primary palate often have missing teeth, particularly in the line of the cleft. Individuals with other craniofacial anomalies are also at risk for missing and malformed teeth, in addition to malocclusion. In these cases, prosthetic management is appropriate. Facial aesthetics, the function of mastication, and even speech can be improved significantly by the replacement of missing teeth or the correction of malocclusion and other forms of deviant dental anatomy.

There are significant challenges when attempting to replace teeth for individuals with a history of cleft of the primary palate. These challenges may include a shortened upper lip, decreased upper lip mobility due to scarring, protrusion of the premaxilla, spaces created by missing teeth, and supernumerary teeth. Additional problems include jaw discrepancies, an occlusal cant, distortion of the midline of the dentition and face, or scar tissue in the alveolar and palatal areas (Ramstad, 1998). Added to these challenges may be poor dental hygiene, which is common in this population due to neglect as a result of psychological factors.

Replacement of teeth can be done in several ways. A *fixed bridge* is typically used to replace dental segments and complete *dentures* are used when all of the teeth need to be replaced. If some of the teeth are to be retained but are not functional, *overlay dentures* are often used. Overlay dentures fit over the existing teeth and usually provide more vertical dimension. The long-term use of this type of denture can place the remaining teeth at risk for decay and periodontal disease due to the forms of retention and the accumulation of plaque. However, some individuals can benefit from overlay dentures. These are individuals who have overclosure of the vertical dimension, resulting in a deep bite. Overlay dentures can increase the vertical dimension to improve function and appearance. These dental appliances also can be combined with any type of speech appliance, if this is also needed.

Although malaligned teeth can make the fabrication of dentures a challenge, tooth extractions are typically avoided unless required for orthodontic purposes. The tooth may serve a purpose in the future, such as providing an anchor for a prosthetic device. Tooth extraction in the cleft area must be especially avoided because it usually results in resorption of the alveolar bone, which will widen and deepen the cleft. This tissue and bone loss may exceed that which can be replaced by a fixed partial prosthesis. Therefore, correction would result in a more complex reconstruction than if the tooth is preserved (McKinstry, 1998a).

Facial Prostheses

Individuals with craniofacial anomalies often demonstrate significant facial defects that affect the person's overall appearance to such a degree that their quality of life is greatly affected. Although surgical intervention often leads to correction, or at least improvement, this is not always the case. Acquired facial defects, due to an injury or ablative surgery for cancer, can be even more challenging to improve with surgery. In these cases, a facial prosthesis can result in a dramatic improvement in appearance (Grisius, 1991; Lundgren, Moy, Beumer, & Lewis, 1993; Schaaf, 1984). Figure 20–1 shows the type of person who can benefit from a facial prosthesis. This type of rehabilitation can make a major difference in the person's life, allowing the person to function normally in society.

A facial prosthesis can be used to replace any missing or disfigured parts of the facial anatomy. For example, individuals with an aural atresia can benefit from the fabrication of a prosthetic ear. Although the ear will not be functional, it will appear very much like a real ear and thus, the anomaly is not noted by others. The same can be done for the eyes or nose, and even for the cheek (Singh, Bharadwaj, & Nair, 1997). The skilled prosthodontist is able to match skin color, skin tone, skin texture, and overall appearance so that the prosthesis blends in with the natural tissue. Even glossectomy patients can benefit from a specially designed prosthesis for the tongue (Aramany, Downs, Beery, & Aslan, 1982; Davis, Lazarus, Logemann, & Hurst, 1987).

Retention of the prosthesis is often accomplished through the use of *osseointegrated implants* (implants that are drilled in the bone) (Beumer, Roumanas, & Nishimura, 1995; Parel, Holt, Branemark, & Tjellstrom, 1986). With the implants in place, the prosthesis can be secured through the use of mechanical clips, magnetic bars, or implants (Chang, Garrett, Roumanas, & Beumer,

2005). Because of what is involved to secure the device, facial prostheses work best for adults who are responsible and motivated. They do not work as well for young children who may be less motivated and are certainly less responsible. In addition, periodic modifications and replacement are necessary for children as they grow.

Feeding Obturators

A feeding obturator is a prosthetic appliance that can be used in the first few months of life to assist the infant with cleft palate in feeding normally (see Figure 5–8A) (Nagda, Deshpande, & Mhatre, 1996; Osuji, 1995; Savion & Huband, 2005). The obturator serves to cover the infant's unrepaired cleft palate during feeding. With the obturator in place, the nasal cavity is separated from the oral cavity, which helps to eliminate the regurgitation of liquids into the nose (see Figure 5–8B). The feeding appliance keeps the tongue from resting inside the cleft, and it provides a solid surface so that the tongue can achieve compression of the nipple in order to express the milk. The appliance does not obturate the soft palate, however, so it does not help the infant to achieve suction, which would require complete closure (McKinstry, 1998b).

The feeding obturator is fabricated using plaster molds and is made of light-cured resins or acrylic. It is made so that it fits tightly against the roof of the mouth during feeding. Because the infant does not have teeth to anchor the appliance in place, suction against the palate and a tight fit are particularly important. One or two holes are drilled in the appliance and dental floss is then tied to the appliance through the holes. These "strings" are attached to the appliance to make it easy for the caregiver to remove it following the feeding.

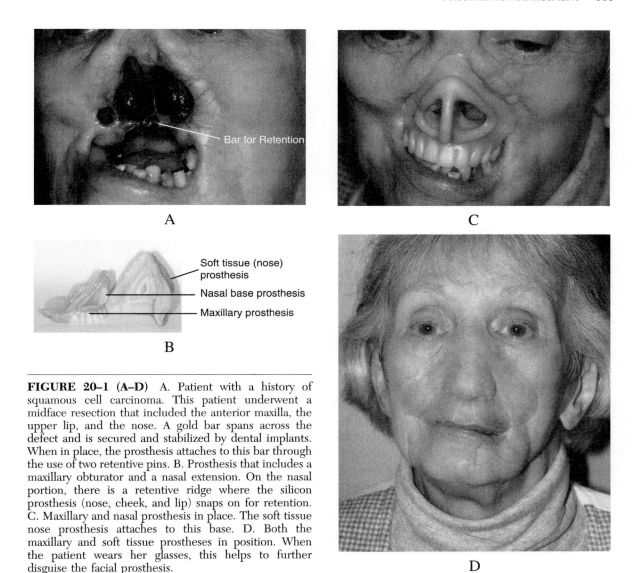

A

B

Soft tissue (nose) prosthesis
Nasal base prosthesis
Maxillary prosthesis

C

D

FIGURE 20–1 (A–D) A. Patient with a history of squamous cell carcinoma. This patient underwent a midface resection that included the anterior maxilla, the upper lip, and the nose. A gold bar spans across the defect and is secured and stabilized by dental implants. When in place, the prosthesis attaches to this bar through the use of two retentive pins. B. Prosthesis that includes a maxillary obturator and a nasal extension. On the nasal portion, there is a retentive ridge where the silicon prosthesis (nose, cheek, and lip) snaps on for retention. C. Maxillary and nasal prosthesis in place. The soft tissue nose prosthesis attaches to this base. D. Both the maxillary and soft tissue prostheses in position. When the patient wears her glasses, this helps to further disguise the facial prosthesis.

Although obturators are recommended and used in some centers across the country, many other centers feel that they are usually unnecessary. With other simple modifications, infants with cleft palate can feed adequately and gain weight appropriately (see Chapter 5).

Usually, only infants with multiple structural anomalies of the airway or severe brain abnormalities require special feeding devices (Sidoti & Shprintzen, 1995). In fact, there are some obvious disadvantages of using feeding obturators. These include the expense of construction and the increased effort needed to train the parents and the infant in its use.

SPEECH APPLIANCES

When surgical correction of velopharyngeal dysfunction or a symptomatic fistula is not an option, prosthetic management is a very good alternative (Gallagher, 1982; Gardner & Parr, 1996). In a position statement of the American Speech-Language-Hearing Association, it was stated that "[P]articipation in the evaluation and treatment of individuals being considered for oral and oropharyngeal prostheses to facilitate speech and swallowing is within the scope of practice of the certified speech-language pathologist" (American Speech-Language-Hearing Association, 1993). Typically, an interdisciplinary team does an assessment to determine if the patient is a good candidate for an appliance. The role of the speech-language pathologist is to identify the aspects of speech that may be impacted by the appliance and determine the potential benefit on speech intelligibility. The speech-language pathologist also actively participates in the designing of the appliance to achieve the best speech outcomes (American Speech-Language-Hearing Association, 1993). The knowledge and skills necessary for the speech-language pathologist to assist in the design of a speech prosthesis are outlined in this position statement.

Three types of speech appliances can be used to assist with speech production: a palatal obturator, a *palatal lift*, and a speech bulb obturator. The palatal obturator is used to close defects of the hard palate or velum. The palatal lift is used for velopharyngeal incompetence and the speech bulb obturator is used for velopharyngeal insufficiency. Each of these speech appliances is described separately in the following sections.

Palatal Lift

A palatal lift prosthesis is a removable device that elevates the velum and holds it in place against the posterior pharyngeal wall for speech (Figure 20–2). This device is positioned so that it elevates the velum at the point of its natural bend. A palatal lift is indicated in cases of velopharyngeal incompetence, where the

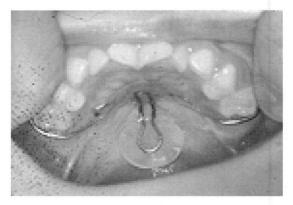

A

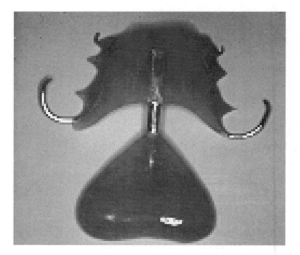

B

FIGURE 20–2 (A and B)   A palatal lift. This device is positioned so that it elevates the velum at the point of its natural bend.

velum is of sufficient length to achieve closure but does not move well enough to accomplish closure. A palatal lift is not useful if the cause of velopharyngeal dysfunction is a short velum because it does not add to the length or fill in the gap. This prosthesis works best if the velum is very flaccid because when the palate raises, it can cause the prosthesis to become dislodged (Reisberg, 2000).

Neurological disorders account for the largest number of acquired conditions causing velopharyngeal dysfunction (Posnick, 1977). A palatal lift is very effective in the treatment of individuals with neurological impairment that prevents proper movement, timing, and coordination of velopharyngeal structures. It can be particularly effective for dysarthric patients when hypernasality is the primary contributor to the unintelligibility of speech, and when articulation, phonation, and respiration are not severely compromised (Bedwinek & O'Brien, 1985; Dworkin & Johns, 1980; Esposito, Mitsumoto, & Shanks, 2000; La Velle & Hardy, 1979; Marshall & Jones, 1971; Riski & Gordon, 1979; Schweiger, Netsell, & Sommerfeld, 1970; Shifman, Finkelstein, Nachmani, & Ophir, 2000; Yorkston, Beukelman, & Traynor, 1988). A palatal lift has even been used successfully with apraxia (Hall, Hardy, & LaVelle, 1990).

The palatal lift device consists of an anterior base that is retained and stabilized by the teeth, and a fingerlike *tail piece* that extends to the velum. When treatment is first initiated, the tail piece may reach to the anterior portion of the velum only. As the patient learns to tolerate the device, this extension is gradually lengthened until it reaches the area of the velar dimple at the very least. The extension exerts an upward force against the velum to displace it in a superior and posterior direction. It is important that this tail piece is positioned correctly so that it can push the velum against the posterior pharyngeal wall in the area of maximum lateral pharyngeal wall movement. With the palatal lift in place, the velum is held against the posterior pharyngeal wall at all times. Because this is the appropriate position for speech, additional velar movement during speech is essentially unnecessary. However, the lateral pharyngeal walls must move against the velum to complete closure for speech.

Individuals who have a hyperactive gag reflex or those who are hypersensitive to touch in the area of the soft palate may require desensitization of the area before a palatal lift can be effective. Gentle massage of the soft palate with the index finger can help to increase the person's tolerance for touch in this area. The finger should massage the velum from side to side and then gradually move posteriorly (Daniel, 1982).

One disadvantage of a palatal lift is that, since the velum is held against the posterior pharyngeal wall at all times, it can potentially interfere with the production of nasal sounds and nasal breathing. Nasal breathing often can be accomplished through openings on either side of the velum, because usually only the middle portion of the velopharyngeal port remains closed. However, hyponasality is often a necessary side effect of forced velopharyngeal closure for adequate oral speech. Fortunately, the palatal lift can be removed during sleep, so sleep apnea is not a concern.

Palatal Obturator

As noted above, a palatal obturator is a prosthetic device that can be used to cover an open palatal defect (Walter, 2005). Figure 20–3A shows a large palatal defect as a result of a maxillectomy for the treatment of cancer. Figure 20–3B shows the palatal obturator in place. Figure 20–3C shows another obturator

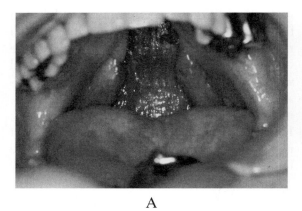

A

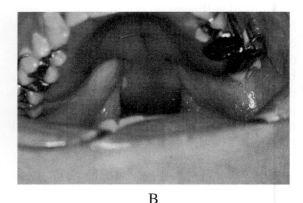

B

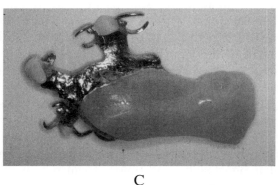

C

FIGURE 20–3 (A–C) A. This is a patient with a large palatal defect following a maxillectomy for a malignancy. B. A palatal obturator. This is a prosthetic device that can be used to cover even a very large open palatal defect. It is appropriate if surgical correction is not indicated or will be delayed and the palatal opening is large enough to be symptomatic during speech or feeding. C. Palatal obturator to fill a large defect. Note the tooth replacements on the body of the appliance.

that was made to cover a large palatal defect. The use of a palatal obturator is appropriate if the palatal opening is symptomatic during speech or causes nasal regurgitation during feeding, and if surgical correction is not planned, at least not in the near future. This prosthetic appliance functions by closing off the nasal cavity from the oral cavity. For speech, this can normalize resonance and improve the ability to impound intraoral pressure for the production of speech.

The most common use of palatal obturators is to cover a palatal fistula. Although palatal fistulas do not occur as frequently as they did in the past, they still are a problem to be dealt with in caring for individuals with a history of

cleft palate. When a fistula is present, the surgical closure is often delayed so that it can be done as part of another surgery. With either a delay in surgical correction or a decision not to surgically correct the fistula, obturation can be considered for temporary or permanent correction (Pinborough-Zimmerman, Canady, Yamashiro, & Morales, 1998).

At one time, some treatment centers subscribed to the theory that early cleft palate closure contributed to a reduction in midfacial growth, causing the high incidence of maxillary deficiency in this population (Schweckendiek, 1966, 1968). To counter this effect, these centers opted to close only the velum at an early age and leave the hard palate open until facial growth was complete (around age 14 for girls and age 18 for boys). Therefore, obturators were commonly used to close the clefts of the palate until the palate was ultimately repaired. More recent research has suggested that it is not the early repair that affects maxillary growth, but rather the inherent deficiency in the maxilla. As a result, surgical correction of hard palate and velum are now done at the same time, usually at around 10 months of age.

Certainly early surgery is the preferred method of treatment to permit normal articulation development. However, when early surgery is not planned for medical reasons, prosthetic management can provide an alternative treatment for the promotion of more normal articulation development, especially if the child receives some speech stimulation (Berkowitz, 1985; Lohmander-Agerskov, Soderpalm, Friede, & Lilja, 1990). The prosthesis should be placed prior to development of meaningful speech to avoid the development of compensatory articulation productions (Dorf, Reisberg, & Gold, 1985).

Although obturators are used less frequently with children, they remain a very important method of treatment for adult patients. They can be effective in covering defects for patients who have undergone ablative surgery due to cancer or other maxillary tumors (Bohle et al., 2005; Myers & Aramany, 1977). They also can be used for those who have had traumatic injuries to the palate where surgical correction is not an option.

A palatal obturator consists of an acrylic body that looks similar to a dental retainer. However, it has additional acrylic on the top of the appliance, which should fit perfectly into the area of deficiency. The obturator is made to tightly fill in the area of the defect to prevent a leak of air pressure or fluid into the nasal cavity. If the obturator has to be large in order to fill in the defect, it can be hollowed

out so that its weight does not cause a problem for retention (Blair & Hunter, 1998).

Speech Bulb Obturator

A *speech bulb obturator*, also known as a *speech aid appliance*, is also a removable device that is used for the treatment of velopharyngeal insufficiency. When the velum is short relative to the depth of the posterior pharyngeal wall, the bulb serves to fill in the pharyngeal space. A speech bulb appliance is particularly applicable for patients with oral cancer who have had ablative surgery (Bohle et al., 2005; Chambers, Lemon, & Martin, 2004; Keyf, Sahin, & Aslan, 2003). Figure 20–4A shows a speech bulb obturator. Figure 20–4B shows the same speech bulb in place. The bulb sits in the nasopharynx to occlude the velopharyngeal port for speech and eliminate nasal regurgitation during swallowing. A speech bulb obturator, as with any other type of appliance, can be combined with partial or complete dentures. Figure 20–5A shows a patient with a very short velum and posterior teeth with gold crowns. A speech bulb that is combined with an anterior dental overlay is seen in Figure 20–5B. This same prosthesis, with the overdenture, is seen in place in Figure 20–5C. In Figure 20–5D, the placement of the speech bulb in the pharynx can be seen through the X–ray tracing.

The speech bulb obturator usually has an oral base section that clasps to the teeth and then a posterior palatal strap with the bulb on the end. The bulb courses upward to fit behind the velum in the nasopharynx. When it is in place, the speech bulb is not visible from an intraoral perspective.

Speech bulb appliances must be removable for several reasons. First, breathing and sleeping could potentially be difficult with the bulb

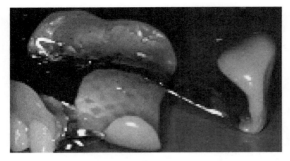

A

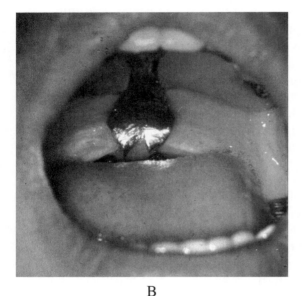

B

FIGURE 20–4 (A and B) A. A speech bulb obturator. B. The speech bulb obturator in place. The bulb sits in the nasopharynx to occlude the velopharyngeal port during speech. This improves speech and can also improve swallowing, since it eliminates nasal regurgitation.

in place. Removal of the appliance at night allows breathing to be normalized and eliminates the risk of sleep apnea. Although the appliance can help to improve swallowing and eliminate nasal regurgitation, some individuals prefer to remove the appliance during meals.

Finally, removal of the bulb is necessary so that it can be cleaned for good oral hygiene.

Fabrication of a Speech Appliance

Speech appliances are individually designed to meet the specific needs of the patient. Therefore, there is considerable variation. In addition, dental professionals may differ in some of the techniques and materials that are used. However, there are many commonalties among speech devices in the way that they are designed.

Most speech appliances have an anterior palatal section, which is the body portion of the appliance. In some cases, this part of the prosthesis may appear similar to a common orthodontic retainer. The palatal section is designed to fit snugly against the contours of the individual's teeth and hard palate so that it can resist movement during oral activity. The purpose of this section is to hold the appliance in place against the roof of the mouth. It can also serve as an obturator to close off a defect in the palate.

The *palatal section* is usually made of either acrylic resins or metal, and is formed from a plaster model of the roof of the mouth. Artificial palatal rugae can also be added to assist with tongue tip orientation and articulation (Gitto, Esposito, & Draper, 1999). This part of the appliance must be made thick enough to avoid easy breakage, but not so thick as to interfere with speech production. The palatal section is held in place by metal wires, which are attached around the teeth for anchorage. The teeth may need to be prepared with buccal lugs on soldered bands, special caps, crowns, or undercuts to adequately retain the wires and the appliance.

The palatal lift and speech bulb appliances are designed to close the middle portion of the

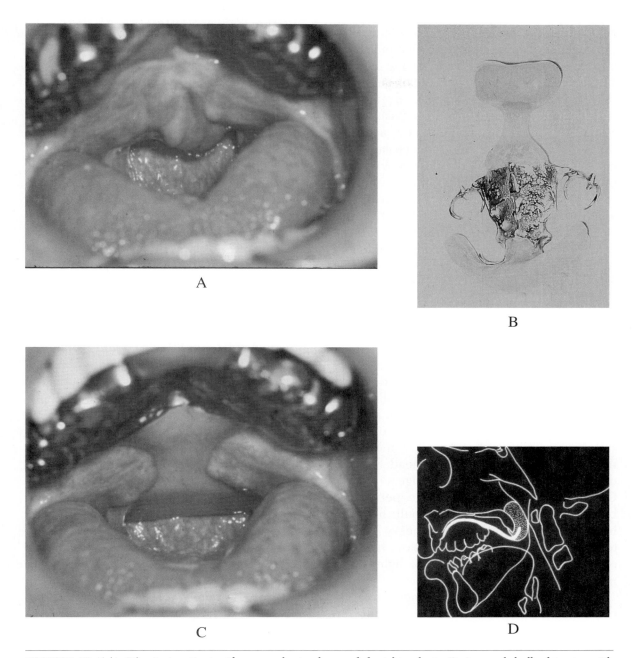

FIGURE 20–5 (A–D)   A. A patient with a very short velum and dental implants. B. A speech bulb obturator with dentures. C. The speech bulb obturator in place with the overdentures. D. The placement of the speech bulb in the pharynx can be seen through this X–ray tracing.

velopharyngeal port so that the lateral pharyngeal walls can be more effective in achieving closure against this area during speech. These devices have an extension, or tail piece, that projects posteriorly. The palatal appliance is fabricated first, as it forms the basis of the rest of the prosthesis. In designing a palatal lift or speech bulb, the speech-language pathologist should work closely with the prosthodontist by providing information on speech changes that occur as a result of modifications to the device.

In fabricating a speech bulb obturator, the prosthodontist starts with a small bulb and then slowly adds a thin layer of thermoplastic wax compound until the appropriate size and shape are achieved. This is usually done by putting it in the individual's mouth and having the patient move the head up and down, and back and forth, to mold the bulb appropriately. Wax is gradually added to the bulb until it fits comfortably and works effectively in the pharynx. The challenge is to make the bulb fill the space, while keeping it from causing undue pressure against the soft tissue of the pharynx. The individual must be able to move the head without discomfort or irritation of pharyngeal mucosa. Once the form is finalized, the permanent bulb is made of acrylic. If the bulb needs to be large, it may become too heavy for the teeth to bear. When this is the case, the bulb can be hollowed out to make it lighter and more stable.

One of the biggest challenges for the prosthodontist is when a patient with an edentulous maxilla requires a speech aid appliance. Retention and stability of the appliance can be a significant problem without the use of teeth for anchors. Fortunately, recent advances in implant prosthodontics have greatly increased the ability to rehabilitate individuals with intraoral anomalies and an edentulous dental arch (Grisius, 1991; Hudson & Russell, 1994; Lundqvist & Haraldson, 1992; Lundqvist, Haraldson, & Lindblad, 1992; Parel, Branemark, & Jansson, 1986; Parel, Branemark, Tjellstrom, & Gion, 1986). Problems with retention due to a lack of teeth can now be minimized or even resolved with the use of *osseointegrated implants*. Osseointegrated implants are small cylinders (5 to 6 mm in diameter) that are usually made of titanium. They are fitted into a carefully prepared channel that is drilled into the alveolar bone. At least four implants of a minimum of 10 mm in length are usually recommended in the maxilla of patients with clefts (Ramstad, 1998). Once in place, the bone grows directly to the implant, resulting in osseointegration and a pseudo root. With these implants embedded in the bone, a speech appliance can be attached and retained. Implants can also be used to support dental restorations. A single implant can support a crown to replace an individual tooth. Multiple implants can be used to support restorations of a row of missing teeth or to secure dentures for an entire dental arch.

Depending on the needs of the patient, various combinations of appliances can be constructed. For example, the speech appliance may have an oral base section with partial or complete dentures. A *palatal obturator* can be combined with a palatal lift or speech bulb (Alpine, Stone, & Badr, 1990) (see Figure 20–3B) or it can be used with an expansion appliance (Hobson & Clasper, 1995). A maxillary prostheses and mandibular prostheses can also be combined if this results in increased function (Davis et al., 1987). Although these combinations are very beneficial to the patient, the mechanical design of prosthetic appliances should be kept as simple as possible. Wear and tear on the device should be expected and breakage will occasionally occur. Therefore, devices that are simple and easy to repair are best in the long term (Mazahari, 1996). It is also most important that the device is designed so that oral hygiene can be maintained.

Some children and adults learn to accept and tolerate the prosthetic appliance quickly and easily, especially those who are motivated to work for aesthetic or speech improvement. On the other hand, some patients, particularly young children, are less compliant and even resistant to wearing a prosthetic device. In these cases, working through the family is the best avenue for achieving compliance and the inherent benefits of the device. Close cooperation among the surgeon, speech-language pathologist, and prosthodontist is also necessary to ensure maximal benefits through prosthetic treatment.

Procedures for Assessment and Modification of a Speech Appliance

In comparison to a palatal lift or a speech bulb, a palatal obturator is very easy to fit because the fistula can and should be totally closed. However, for the other appliances, fine adjustments must be made to the appliance so that the velopharyngeal port is closed enough for speech, but not overly closed so that it causes upper airway problems. Achieving an appropriate balance of good speech and normal nasal breathing is the ultimate goal. Therefore, the speech-language pathologist should provide appropriate feedback to the prosthodontist so that the device can be adjusted for optimal function.

When perceptual measures are used to assess the effectiveness of the speech appliance, the examiner should test the production of pressure-sensitive phonemes, such as plosives, fricatives, and affricates. The examiner

could use a simple listening tube for further information regarding the closure of the velopharyngeal port. If pressure-sensitive sounds can be produced in words and sentences without nasal air emission and there is no evidence of hypernasality, then the velopharyngeal port is closed adequately for speech. The speech-language pathologist should then assess the ease of nasal breathing with the appliance in place and also test the production of nasal sounds (/m/, /n/, /ng/) in words and sentences. Based on this assessment, the appliance can be modified until an appropriate balance is achieved between closure for oral speech and patency for nasal breathing and the production of nasal phonemes (Rosen & Bzoch, 1997).

In addition to a perceptual assessment of the effect of the appliance, indirect instrumental measures can be used to evaluate the effectiveness of a prosthetic appliance. Aerodynamic measures (Reisberg & Smith, 1985; Riski, Hoke, & Dolan, 1989) and nasometry (Pinborough-Zimmerman et al., 1998; Scarsellone, Rochet, & Wolfaardt, 1999) are indirect instrumental procedures that can give objective information regarding the extent of improvement with the appliance, and the relative normalcy of the speech as a result. They also provide information regarding the patency of the airway while the appliance is in place.

Although a perceptual assessment and indirect instrumental assessment techniques are helpful in evaluating the effect of an appliance, these procedures do not give adequate information if the appliance needs to be adjusted. When adjustments are necessary, the prosthodontist needs to know where the appliance should be augmented and where it should be shaved down. For this information, a direct instrumental approach is needed so that the extent of closure can be visualized. Although a lateral cephalometric X-ray or videofluoroscopy could be used (Mazaheri & Hoffman, 1962; Turner & Williams, 1991), the best procedure for assessment of velopharyngeal function with the appliance in place is nasopharyngoscopy.

Using nasopharyngoscopy, the extent of velopharyngeal closure with the device in place can be easily determined (D'Antonio, Muntz, Marsh, Marty-Grames, & Backensto-Marsh, 1988; Karnell, Rosenstein, & Fine, 1987; Rich, Farber, & Shprintzen, 1988; Riski et al., 1989; Turner & Williams, 1991). An optimal fit often requires trial and error and several adjustments to the appliance. If one side of the velopharyngeal port is not closing adequately, then the appliance can be augmented on that side. The patency of the airway can also be evaluated with this technique. At times, the airway must be compromised slightly for the best speech benefit. At other times, perfect speech must be compromised for the sake of the airway. With the benefit of a nasopharyngoscopy view, the device can be modified until closure appears to be optimal for both speech and the airway.

CLINICAL INDICATIONS AND CONTRAINDICATIONS FOR PROSTHETIC MANAGEMENT

Although surgical correction is usually considered the best option for the treatment of structural defects, there are cases where prosthetic management is more appropriate or necessary. These include patients with a history of cleft for whom surgery must be delayed due to a medical condition or the need to do other procedures first. Prosthetic devices can be used effectively in the management of large soft palate perforations or palatal fistulas. They can also be appropriate for patients with persistent velopharyngeal insufficiency or incompetence after unsuccessful surgical repairs (Hoffman, 1985). For example, if a pharyngeal flap was done, but the lateral ports do not close sufficiently, a device can be made that has a bulb on each side of the flap to fill in the area of the ports (McKinstry, 1998a). They can even be used on a trial basis in cases where the outcome of surgical correction is unclear. If the prosthodontist is routinely consulted in the initial treatment planning, alternatives to surgical management might be considered for patients with high potential for postsurgical failure (McKinstry & Aramany, 1985).

Speech appliances are sometimes appropriate for patients with structural disorders not related to cleft palate. For example, in rare cases, individuals will develop velopharyngeal insufficiency following a uvulopalatopharyngoplasty (UPPP), which is done to alleviate snoring and sleep apnea. When this occurs, prosthetic management is often appropriate, because there is no risk of causing further sleep problems with this form of correction (Finkelstein, Shifman, Nachmani, & Ophir, 1995). Prosthetic management is particularly useful following cancer treatment, especially if the treatment involved ablative surgery of the maxilla or velum (Myers & Aramany, 1977; Ramsey & Quarantillo, 1977). Patients with oral carcinomas often require resection of other parts of the mouth as well, including the tongue, the floor of the mouth, or the bone of the mandible. Postoperatively, these patients often encounter problems with chewing, swallowing, and speech. In these cases, prosthetic treatment may include a tongue prosthesis or other prostheses, in addition to the palatal device. Prosthetic management of this type can help to improve articulation, resonance, and swallowing. Socialization is also enhanced through the improved appearance that these prosthetic devices can provide (Aramany et al., 1982).

Patients who exhibit normal velopharyngeal anatomy, but demonstrate velopharyngeal incompetence secondary to neuromotor disorders, may not be appropriate surgical candidates (La Velle & Hardy, 1979). However, as mentioned before, individuals with dysarthria (Bedwinek & O'Brien, 1985; Dworkin & Johns, 1980; Riski & Gordon, 1979) or apraxia (Hall et al., 1990) may derive significant benefit from a palatal lift. This allows the individual to concentrate on anterior articulation and not be concerned about velopharyngeal articulation.

Prosthetic management is usually most successful with individuals who have adequate dentition for retention of the device and good oral hygiene. Another consideration when trying to fit a palatal lift of speech bulb is the gag reflex. Although the prosthodontist can work to gradually desensitize the patient to the device, a strong gag reflex or oral sensitivity makes successful prosthetic management very difficult, if not impossible, to achieve. Finally, successful prosthetic management is somewhat dependent on good articulation because corrected velopharyngeal function for speech will not improve intelligibility significantly if the articulation is poor.

Although prosthetic devices have been used successfully by many patients for correction of velopharyngeal dysfunction, they have some distinct disadvantages. Unlike surgery, these devices do not result in a permanent correction. In fact, they usually need to be removed at night and during eating. With removal, the speech symptoms recur. They are expensive and may not be covered by insurance. They can be easily lost or damaged. Of course, manual dexterity or the assistance of others is important for proper insertion and removal of the device. They may be uncomfortable to wear and can cause ulceration of the surrounding mucosa. Retention of appliances can be a challenge for patients with a history of cleft palate or craniofacial anomalies due to irregularities in the dentition and missing teeth. In young children, appliances require frequent adjustments as the child grows and as deciduous teeth are lost and permanent teeth erupt, thus increasing the cost.

Because of these limitations, removable prosthetic devices are not well suited for patients who are very young, are developmentally delayed, or have significant physical handicaps. They do not work well for patients who have difficulty managing secretions, who have a strong gag reflex, or who have upper airway obstruction. In fact, most patients who are able to undergo surgical correction usually do opt for surgery after a period of prosthetic management (Marsh & Wray, 1980). Despite their limitations, prosthetic devices should always be considered for correction of a palatal defect or velopharyngeal dysfunction when surgery is not an option for medical reasons (McKinstry, 1998a).

PROSTHETIC MANAGEMENT AND SPEECH THERAPY

Speech therapy cannot correct velopharyngeal dysfunction or hypernasality. However, once there is sufficient improvement in velopharyngeal function with prosthetic treatment, speech therapy is often required to further improve the speech (Fletcher & Sooudi, 1973; Gallagher, 1982; La Velle & Hardy, 1979.) The presence of a speech appliance does not correct articulation, but it does improve the ability to impound intraoral air pressure, and thus produce oral sounds. Speech therapy is necessary to help the individual to learn to use this air pressure to produce sounds normally. Therapy is also needed to eliminate any compensatory articulation productions that developed prior to the prosthetic management. Finally, speech therapy can be effective in eliminating the nasal rustle (turbulence) that often occurs due to a very small or inconsistent opening with the prosthesis in place.

Prosthetic devices have also been used as a form of therapy to attempt to improve velopharyngeal function. This type of therapy, called *reduction therapy*, is done in hopes of stimulating increased movement of the velopharyngeal structures in order to avoid surgery or reduce the extent of the surgery that is needed. When a palatal lift is used in reduction therapy, the length of the lift is gradually reduced, or the wearing time of the lift is gradually decreased, in hopes of stimulating velar movement. However, it has been shown that the mechanical elevation of the velum actually reduces levator veli palatine muscle activity (Tachimura, Nohara, Fujita, Hara, & Wada, 2001).

If a speech bulb is used in reduction therapy, the size of the bulb is gradually reduced, in hopes of gradually increasing lateral wall movement. The ultimate goal is to improve velopharyngeal function so that surgical management is either not needed, or the extent of management, such as the size of the pharyngeal flap, is reduced. Some authors have reported some success in improving lateral wall motion with this procedure (Golding-Kushner, Cisneros, & LeBlanc, 1995). However, these results are not always maintained and most individuals still require surgical intervention for correction (Witt et al., 1995; Wolfaardt, Wilson, Rochet, & McPhee, 1993). Considering this fact, and the time and expense of the prosthesis and speech therapy, surgical correction may still be the most appropriate and effective option for correction of velopharyngeal dysfunction when possible.

SUMMARY

Prosthetic management is not required in the habilitation of individuals who have repaired clefts as frequently as in years past. With the advances in surgical procedures and improvement in the timing of surgery, the outcomes of surgical intervention are usually superior to those that can be obtained with prosthetic management. However, in certain cases, there is a definite need for prosthetic management, particularly when surgical intervention is not an option. Prosthetic management can be very effective in improving the individual's appearance, swallowing, and speech. The ultimate goal of prosthetic management is to meet the needs of the patient and to achieve the best possible outcome.

FOR REVIEW, DISCUSSION, AND CRITICAL THINKING

1. What types of patients could benefit from a facial or oral prosthetic device? Why do you think prosthetic devices are actually used less than they were 20 years ago? Which professionals are trained to construct these devices?

2. What is the purpose of a dental appliance? What are the different types? How do you think dental appliances could affect speech?

3. What is the purpose of a facial prosthesis? How is it retained?

4. Describe the construction and retention of a feeding obturator. Why is this not used for all children born with cleft palate?

5. Describe the three types of speech appliances that are used for improvement of resonance. What is the appropriate indication for each? Why is a palatal lift inappropriate for a child with velopharyngeal insufficiency?

6. What are the components of most speech appliances? What materials are used? How are they retained?

7. Describe ways that the speech pathologist should work with the prosthodontist (or dental professional) in order to achieve the best outcome with a speech appliance.

8. What are the clinical indications and contraindications for the use of prosthetic devices for speech?

9. How have prosthetic devices been used as part of the speech therapy process? Discuss the controversy regarding this practice.

REFERENCES

Alpine, K. D., Stone, C. R., & Badr, S. E. (1990). Combined obturator and palatal-lift prosthesis: A case report. *Quintessence International*, *21*(11), 893–896.

American Speech-Language-Hearing Association (1993). Position statement and guidelines for oral and oropharyngeal prostheses, *ASHA*, *35*(Suppl. 10), 14–16.

Aramany, M. A., Downs, J. A., Beery, Q. C., & Aslan, Y. (1982). Prosthodontic rehabilitation for glossectomy patients. *Journal of Prosthetic Dentistry*, *48*(1), 78–81.

Bedwinek, A. P., & O'Brien, R. L. (1985). A patient selection profile for the use of speech prostheses in adult dysarthria. *Journal of Communication Disorders*, *18*(3), 169–182.

Berkowitz, S. (1985). Timing cleft palate closure—Age should not be the sole determinant. *Journal of Craniofacial Genetics and Developmental Biology Supplement*, *1*, 69–83.

Beumer, J. III, Roumanas, E., & Nishimura, R. (1995). Advances in osseointegrated implants for dental and facial rehabilitation following major head and neck surgery. *Seminars in Surgical Oncology*, *11*(3), 200–207.

Blair, F. M., & Hunter, N. R. (1998). The hollow box maxillary obturator. *British Dental Journal*, *184*(10), 484–487.

Bohle, G., 3rd, Rieger, J., Huryn, J., Verbel, D., Hwang, F., & Zlotolow, I. (2005). Efficacy of speech aid prostheses for acquired defects of the soft palate and velopharyngeal inadequacy—Clinical assessments and cephalometric analysis: A Memorial Sloan-Kettering Study. *Head & Neck*, *27*(3), 195–207.

Chambers, M. S., Lemon, J. C., & Martin, J. W. (2004). Obturation of the partial soft palate defect. *Journal of Prosthetic Dentistry*, *91*(1), 75–79.

Chang, T. L., Garrett, N., Roumanas, E., & Beumer, J., 3rd. (2005). Treatment satisfaction with facial prostheses. *Journal of Prosthetic Dentistry*, *94*(3), 275–280.

Daniel, B. (1982). A soft-palate desensitization procedure for patients requiring palatal lift prostheses. *Journal of Prosthetic Dentistry*, *48*(5), 565–566.

D'Antonio, L. L., Muntz, H. R., Marsh, J. L., Marty-Grames, L., & Backensto-Marsh, R. (1988). Practical application of flexible fiberoptic nasopharyngoscopy for evaluating velopharyngeal function. *Plastic and Reconstructive Surgery, 82*(4), 611–618.

Davis, J. W., Lazarus, C., Logemann, J., & Hurst, P. S. (1987). Effect of a maxillary glossectomy prosthesis on articulation and swallowing. *Journal of Prosthetic Dentistry, 57*(6), 715–719.

Delgado, A. A., Schaaf, N. G., & Emrich, L. (1992). Trends in prosthodontic treatment of cleft palate patients at one institution: A twenty-one year review. *Cleft Palate-Craniofacial Journal, 29*(5), 425–428.

Dorf, D. S., Reisberg, D. J., & Gold, H. O. (1985). Early prosthetic management of cleft palate. Articulation development prosthesis: A preliminary report. *Journal of Prosthetic Dentistry, 53*(2), 222–226.

Dworkin, J. P., & Johns, D. F. (1980). Management of velopharyngeal incompetence in dysarthria: A historical review. *Clinics in Otolaryngology, 5*, 61–74.

Esposito, S. J., Mitsumoto, H., & Shanks, M. (2000). Use of palatal lift and palatal augmentation prostheses to improve dysarthria in patients with amyotrophic lateral sclerosis: A case series. *Journal of Prosthetic Dentistry, 83*(1), 90–98.

Finkelstein, Y., Shifman, A., Nachmani, A., & Ophir, D. (1995). Prosthetic management of velopharyngeal insufficiency induced by uvulopalatopharyngoplasty. *Otolaryngology—Head & Neck Surgery, 113*(5), 611–616.

Fletcher, S. G., & Sooudi, I. (1973). Joint prosthetics and speech treatment of hypernasality: Report of case. *Journal of the American Dental Association, 87*(7), 1418–1425.

Gallagher, B. (1982). Prosthesis in velopharyngeal insufficiency: Effect on nasal resonance. *Journal of Communication Disorders, 15*(6), 469–473.

Gardner, L. K., & Parr, G. R. (1996). Prosthetic rehabilitation of the cleft palate patient. *Seminars in Orthodontics, 2*(3), 215–219.

Gitto, C. A., Esposito, S. J., & Draper, J. M. (1999). A simple method of adding palatal rugae to a complete denture. *Journal of Prosthetic Dentistry, 81*(2), 237–239.

Golding-Kushner, K. J., Cisneros, G., & LeBlanc, E. (1995). Speech bulbs. In R. J. Shprintzen & J. Bardach (Eds.), *Cleft palate speech management* (pp. 352–363). St. Louis, MO: Mosby.

Grisius, R. J. (1991). Maxillofacial prosthetics. *Current Opinions in Dentistry, 1*(2), 155–159.

Hall, P. K., Hardy, J. C., & LaVelle, W. E. (1990). A child with signs of developmental apraxia of speech with whom a palatal lift prosthesis was used to manage palatal dysfunction. *Journal of Speech and Hearing Disorders, 55*(3), 454–460.

Hobson, R. S., & Clasper, R. (1995). A combined obturator and expansion appliance for use in patients with patent oral-nasal fistula. *British Journal of Orthodontics, 22*(4), 357–359.

Hoffman, S. (1985). Correction of lateral port stenosis following a pharyngeal flap operation. *Cleft Palate Journal, 22*(1), 51–55.

Hudson, J. W., & Russell, R., Jr. (1994). Contributions within dental science to cleft lip/palate management: A literature review. *Compendium, 15*(1), 116, 118–120, 122; Quiz 126.

Karnell, M. P., Rosenstein, H., & Fine, L. (1987). Nasal videoendoscopy in prosthetic management of palatopharyngeal dysfunction. *Journal of Prosthetic Dentistry*, 58(4), 479–484.

Keyf, F., Sahin, N., & Aslan, Y. (2003). Alternative impression technique for a speech-aid prosthesis. *Cleft Palate-Craniofacial Journal*, 40(6), 566–568.

La Velle, W. E., & Hardy, J. C. (1979). Palatal lift prostheses for treatment of palatopharyngeal incompetence. *Journal of Prosthetic Dentistry*, 42(3), 308–315.

Lohmander-Agerskov, A., Soderpalm, E., Friede, H., & Lilja, J. (1990). Cleft lip and palate patients prior to delayed closure of the hard palate: Evaluation of maxillary morphology and the effect of early stimulation on pre-school speech. *Scandinavian Journal of Plastic and Reconstructive Surgery and Hand Surgery*, 24(2), 141–148.

Lundgren, S., Moy, P. K., Beumer, J. III, & Lewis, S. (1993). Surgical considerations for endosseous implants in the craniofacial region: A 3-year report. *International Journal of Oral and Maxillofacial Surgery*, 22, 272–277.

Lundqvist, S., & Haraldson, T. (1992). Oral function in patients wearing fixed prosthesis on osseointegrated implants in the maxilla: A 3-year follow-up study. *Scandinavian Journal of Dental Research*, 100(5), 279–283.

Lundqvist, S., Haraldson, T., & Lindblad, P. (1992). Speech in connection with maxillary fixed prostheses on osseointegrated implants: A three-year follow-up study. *Clinics in Oral Implants Research*, 3(4), 176–180.

Marsh, J. L., & Wray, R. C. (1980). Speech prosthesis versus pharyngeal flap: A randomized evaluation of the management of velopharyngeal incompetency. *Plastic and Reconstructive Surgery*, 65(5), 592–594.

Marshall, R. C., & Jones, R. N. (1971, March). Effects of a palatal lift prosthesis upon the speech intelligibility of a dysarthric patient. *Journal of Prosthetic Dentistry*, 327–333.

Mazahari, M. (1996). Prosthetic speech appliances for patients with cleft palate. In S. Berkowitz (Ed.), *Cleft lip and palate with introduction to other craniofacial abnormalities: Perspectives in management* (Vol. 2, pp. 177–194). San Diego, CA: Singular Publishing Group.

Mazaheri, M., & Hoffman, F. A. (1962). Cineradiography speech appliance construction. *Journal of Prosthetic Dentistry*, 12, 571–575.

McKinstry, R. E. (1998a). Cleft palate prosthetics. In R. E. McKinstry (Ed.), *Cleft palate dentistry* (pp. 206–235). Arlington, VA: ABI Professional Publications.

McKinstry, R. E. (1998b). Presurgical management of cleft lip and palate patients. In R. E. McKinstry (Ed.), *Cleft palate dentistry* (pp. 33–66). Arlington, VA: ABI Professional Publications.

McKinstry, R. E., & Aramany, M. A. (1985). Prosthodontic considerations in the management of surgically compromised cleft palate patients. *Journal of Prosthetic Dentistry*, 53(6), 827–831.

Myers, E. N., & Aramany, M. A. (1977). Rehabilitation of the oral cavity following resection of the hard and soft palate. *Transactions of the American Academy of Ophthalmology and Otolaryngology*, 84(5), ORL941–951.

Nagda, S., Deshpande, D. S., & Mhatre, S. W. (1996). Infant palatal obturator. *Journal of the Indian Society of Pedodontics & Preventive Dentistry*, 14(1), 24–25.

Osuji, O. O. (1995). Preparation of feeding obturators for infants with cleft lip and palate. *Journal of Clinical Pediatric Dentistry*, 19(3), 211–214.

Parel, S. M., Branemark, P. I., & Jansson, T. (1986). Osseointegration in maxillofacial prosthetics: Part I. Intraoral applications. *Journal of Prosthetic Dentistry, 55*(4), 490–494.

Parel, S. M., Branemark, P. I., Tjellstrom, A., & Gion, G. (1986). Osseointegration in maxillofacial prosthetics: Part II. Extraoral applications. *Journal of Prosthetic Dentistry, 55*(5), 600–606.

Parel, S. M., Holt, G. R., Branemark, P. I., & Tjellstrom, A. (1986). Osseointegration and facial prosthetics. *International Journal of Oral and Maxillofacial Implants, 1*(1), 27–29.

Pinborough-Zimmerman, J., Canady, C., Yamashiro, D. K., & Morales, L., Jr. (1998). Articulation and nasality changes resulting from sustained palatal fistula obturation. *Cleft Palate-Craniofacial Journal, 35*(1), 81–87.

Posnick, W. R. (1977). Prosthetic management of palatopharyngeal incompetency for the pediatric patient. *Journal of Dentistry for Children, 44*(2), 117–121.

Ramsey, W. O., & Quarantillo, E. P. (1977). Prosthetic obturation subsequent to total resection of the soft palate. A comparison of two case histories. *Journal of the Baltimore College of Dental Surgery, 32*(1), 50–68.

Ramstad, T. (1998). Fixed prosthodontics. In R. E. McKinstry (Ed.), *Cleft palate dentistry* (pp. 236–262). Arlington, VA: ABI Professional Publications.

Reisberg, D. J. (2000). Dental and prosthodontic care for patients with cleft or craniofacial conditions. *Cleft Palate-Craniofacial Journal, 37*(6), 534–537.

Reisberg, D. J., & Smith, B. E. (1985). Aerodynamic assessment of prosthetic speech aids. *Journal of Prosthetic Dentistry, 54*(5), 686–690.

Rich, B. M., Farber, K., & Shprintzen, R. J. (1988). Nasopharyngoscopy in the treatment of palatopharyngeal insufficiency. *International Journal of Prosthodontics, 1* (3), 248–251.

Riski, J. E., & Gordon, D. (1979). Prosthetic management of neurogenic velopharyngeal incompetency. *North Carolina Dental Journal, 62*(1), 24–26.

Riski, J. E., Hoke, J. A., & Dolan, E. A. (1989). The role of pressure flow and endoscopic assessment in successful palatal obturator revision. *Cleft Palate Journal, 26*(1), 56–62.

Rosen, M. S., & Bzoch, K. R. (1997). Prosthodontic management of the individual with cleft lip and palate for speech habilitation needs. In K. R. Bzoch (Ed.), *Communicative disorders related to cleft lip and palate* (Vol. 4, pp. 153–168). Austin, TX: Pro-Ed.

Savion, I., & Huband, M. L. (2005). A feeding obturator for a preterm baby with Pierre Robin sequence. *Journal of Prosthetic Dentistry, 93*(2), 197–200.

Scarsellone, J. M., Rochet, A. P., & Wolfaardt, J. F. (1999). The influence of dentures on nasalance values in speech. *Cleft Palate-Craniofacial Journal, 36*(1), 51–56.

Schaaf, N. G. (1984). Maxillofacial prosthetics and the head and neck cancer patient. *Cancer, 54*(11, Suppl.), 2682–2690.

Schweckendiek, W. (1966). [The technique of early veloplasty and its results]. *Acta Chiruriae Plasticae, 8*(3), 188–194.

Schweckendiek, W. (1968). [Early veloplasty and its results]. *Acta Oto-Rhino-Laryngologica Belgica, 22*(6), 697–703.

Schweiger, J. W., Netsell, R., & Sommerfeld, R. M. (1970). Prosthetic management and speech improvement in individuals with dysarthria of the palate. *Journal of the*

American Dental Association, *80*(6), 1348–1353.

Shifman, A., Finkelstein, Y., Nachmani, A., & Ophir, D. (2000). Speech-aid prostheses for neurogenic velopharyngeal incompetence. *Journal of Prosthetic Dentistry*, *83*(1), 99–106.

Sidoti, E. J., & Shprintzen, R. J. (1995). Pediatric care and feeding of the newborn with a cleft. In R. J. Shprintzen & J. Bardach (Eds.), *Cleft palate speech management* (pp. 63–74). St. Louis, MO: Mosby.

Singh, V. P., Bharadwaj, G., & Nair, K. C. (1997). Direct observation of tongue positions in speech—A patient study. *International Journal of Prosthodontics*, *10*(3), 231–234.

Tachimura, T., Nohara, K., Fujita, Y., Hara, H., & Wada, T. (2001). Change in levator veli palatini muscle activity of normal speakers in association with elevation of the velum using an experimental palatal lift prosthesis. *Cleft Palate-Craniofacial Journal*, *38*(5), 449–454.

Turner, G. E., & Williams, W. N. (1991). Fluoroscopy and nasoendoscopy in designing palatal lift prostheses. *Journal of Prosthetic Dentistry*, *66*(1), 63–71.

Walter, J. D. (2005). Obturators for cleft palate and other speech appliances. *Dental Update*, *32*(4), 217–218.

Witt, P. D., Rozelle, A. A., Marsh, J. L., Marty-Grames, L., Muntz, H. R., Gay, W. D., & Pilgram, T. K. (1995). Do palatal lift prostheses stimulate velopharyngeal neuromuscular activity? *Cleft Palate-Craniofacial Journal*, *32*(6), 469–475.

Wolfaardt, J. F., Wilson, F. B., Rochet, A., & McPhee, L. (1993). An appliance-based approach to the management of palatopharyngeal incompetency: A clinical pilot project. *Journal of Prosthetic Dentistry*, *69*(2), 186–195.

Yorkston, K. M., Beukelman, D. R., & Traynor, C. D. (1988). Articulatory adequacy in dysarthric speakers: A comparison of judging formats. *Journal of Communication Disorders*, *21*(4), 351–361.

CHAPTER

21

SPEECH THERAPY: MAKING IT SIMPLE!

CHAPTER OUTLINE

INTRODUCTION

Individuals with a history of cleft lip/palate or craniofacial anomalies are at risk for certain speech and resonance disorders secondary to velopharyngeal dysfunction (VPD), oral anomalies, and dental malocclusion. Even with early surgical repair, the majority of preschoolers with a history of cleft palate demonstrate delays in speech sound development (Hardin-Jones & Jones, 2005). Velopharyngeal dysfunction can occur due to a variety of other reasons, in addition to cleft palate.

As has been discussed in other chapters, when the velopharyngeal valve is defective, speech may be characterized by hypernasality and nasal air emission. In addition, inadequate intraoral pressure as a result of nasal emission can result in weak articulation, short utterance length, and the development of compensatory articulation productions. It is important to determine the underlying cause of these speech characteristics through perceptual and instrumental methods, because the cause has a direct impact on the selection of the appropriate treatment method.

When speech therapy is appropriate for this population, the techniques are not complicated. The purpose of this chapter is to convey all needed information so that any speech-language pathologist can treat these patients with competence and confidence.

TIMETABLE FOR INTERVENTION AND GOALS

Infants and Toddlers

During the first few weeks of life, feeding is necessarily the first priority. Once effective feeding has been established, the next priority is language development. The parents should be counseled that during the first three years, they should concentrate on the *quantity* of speech (how much the child can understand, how many different words the child uses, and how many words are used in utterances), and not worry as much about the *quality* of speech (articulation, resonance, and intelligibility).

The speech-language pathologist for the cleft palate/craniofacial team is responsible for counseling families on methods of language stimulation during this critical period of time. The families should always be given written information, including a home language stimulation program, to use as a guide (Hardin, 1991) (see Appendix 6–1). Because the parents are the primary instructors of language for the child, they should be advised on how to be most effective in that job (Hahn, 1989; O'Gara & Logemann, 1990; Phillips, 1990). If language does not develop normally, or if there are feeding problems, therapy should be initiated immediately.

Although articulation and resonance are not the primary focus of the first three years, there are some things that parents should do to stimulate early phonemic development. Parents should be shown how to encourage vocalizations by imitating the child's cooing and babbling. If there is a cleft palate, they should be instructed on how to encourage the production of plosives once the cleft is repaired. (See Appendix 21–1 for a sample home program that shows how to stimulate speech production.) The speech-language pathologist should actively teach the parents ways to work with the child on normal sound production in order to try to prevent the development of compensatory articulation productions (Golding-Kushner, 2001). If there is hypernasality or nasal air emission during production, the parent can be shown how to gently pinch the child's nostrils during sound imitation to allow for more normal production.

Preschool Children

By the age of 3, most children are communicating with complete sentences, although errors in syntax and morphology are common. The child should be using nasal and plosive sounds, some fricatives, and even affricate phonemes. Therefore, this is an appropriate time to evaluate speech, resonance, and velopharyngeal function and, if indicated, begin treatment. If it is determined that secondary surgical intervention is needed, this is best done between the ages of 3 and 5. Speech therapy can be initiated prior to correction of the structure and work can begin on the correction of articulation placement errors. However, if the structure is corrected first, the therapy will be easier and less frustrating for the child. In addition, progress will be much faster, and as a result, the therapy will be more cost-effective.

Parents and even older siblings need to be active in the treatment process for the best results. Therefore, they should be encouraged to observe therapy and, if possible, one spouse should videotape the session for the other spouse to view at home. The parents should be actively taught to be the "therapist" at home. Progress will be much faster if the parent is involved and there is practice in between the therapy sessions (Pamplona & Ysunza, 2000; Pamplona, Ysunza, & Jimenez-Murat, 2001; Pamplona, Ysunza, & Uriostegui, 1996).

The goal of physical management and speech therapy in the preschool years is to attain age-appropriate speech, or close to it, by the time the child enters kindergarten. This is important for several reasons. Most importantly, preschool children are more receptive to acquiring new speech patterns and correcting abnormal speech patterns than older children. This is due to the fact that they are in a critical period of brain development so the brain is more receptive to learning these skills (Dowling, 2004). Also, during the first five years, speech patterns are not strongly habituated, and are therefore, easier to change. With early private therapy, parents are available so that they can be active partners in the therapeutic process. Finally, early correction avoids the social and emotional problems that come from teasing in the school-age years.

A practical reason for early intervention is that funding for private speech therapy through medical insurance is very limited for school-age children. Although older children are able to receive speech therapy through the schools, they are not able to receive the necessary intensity of treatment due to the size of school caseloads and the break in the summer. The school speech-language pathologists do not have frequent access to the parents, making work on carry-over difficult. Finally, school speech-language pathologists must be generalists, and therefore, they usually do not have the specialty expertise in this area.

School-Age Children

School-age children who continue to have speech problems typically receive therapy through their school. At this point, VPI should have been corrected, if it was present. If there is still hypernasality or nasal emission, the child should be referred to the craniofacial team for physical management.

When therapy is required for this age group, it is usually for the correction of any articulation errors that are either residual compensatory errors from VPI, or are errors related to dental malocclusion. These errors may be either compensatory (such as a glottal stop for plosives) or obligatory (such as nasal emission). Either way, correction is difficult, if not impossible, as long as the structural anomaly is still present. Speech therapy is not appropriate for obligatory errors, unless the structure cannot or will not be corrected. This is because correcting the structure will correct the speech. When there are compensatory errors, ideally the structure should be corrected before trying to correct these placement errors with speech therapy.

One dilemma is that Class III malocclusion usually requires surgical intervention (usually maxillary advancement), which cannot be done until after facial growth is complete. This is usually around age 14 for girls and age 18 for boys. In the meantime, the speech distortion persists. The speech-language pathologist should not be pressured into providing speech therapy for obligatory errors, since this would be very inappropriate in this case. In addition, speech therapy for compensatory errors is very difficult and usually ineffective until after the structural anomaly has been corrected.

Some cleft palate or craniofacial centers have offered summer camps or residential programs for their school-age patients who continue to demonstrate speech problems that are correctable with therapy (Nash, Stengelhofen, Toombs, Brown, & Kellow, 2001; Pamplona et al., 2005; Schendel, & Bzoch, 1979). The purpose of this type of program is to provide intensive speech therapy, while giving the children opportunities to interact with others who have similar problems and experiences. The biggest disadvantages of this mode of intervention are cost and logistics.

Adolescents and Adults

Occasionally, an older child or an adult with a history of cleft will decide to seek improvement in his or her speech. If the primary problem is uncorrected VPI, surgical or prosthetic intervention should be done first to correct the structural problem. If articulation errors are also noted, speech therapy could be initiated. However, the individual should be informed that the prognosis for normal speech at older ages is somewhat guarded after the critical period of speech development has passed; this is also due to habit strength. Therefore, to be successful, the patient needs to be highly motivated to improve his or her speech.

APPROPRIATE CANDIDATES FOR SPEECH THERAPY

Speech therapy is appropriate for the elimination of compensatory articulation productions that have developed secondary to VPI. If multiple compensatory articulation errors are noted or the patient is stimulable for improvement with a change in placement, then a trial period of speech therapy should be initiated prior to considering surgery. This is because velopharyngeal function may improve with a replacement of nasal sounds with oral sounds (Golding-Kushner, 2001; Hoch, Golding-Kushner, Siegel-Sadewitz, & Shprintzen, 1986; Tomes, Kuehn, & Peterson-Falzone, 1996; Ysunza, Pamplona, & Toledo, 1992; Ysunza-Rivera, Pamplona-Ferreira, & Toledo-Cortina, 1991). Speech therapy is also appropriate for correction of abnormal articulation (function) that causes phoneme-specific nasal emission or phoneme-specific hypernasality. Speech therapy is also appropriate when there is hypernasality or nasal emission due to oral-motor dysfunction, such as apraxia or dysarthria. Finally, speech therapy is indicated in many cases after the VPI has been treated surgically or prosthetically because changing structure through surgery does not change function (i.e., learned articulation patterns). In this case, the individual may need to learn appropriate articulatory placement and oral airflow.

If in doubt about whether the individual is a surgical candidate for VPI, a trial period of speech therapy should always be done (Hardin, 1991). The therapy should be short-term, no more than a few months, as it does not take long to determine whether the child will respond to therapy. If the individual continues to demonstrate hypernasality or nasal air emission, even with an improvement in articulation, then surgical intervention should be considered.

Speech therapy is not appropriate if the cause of the speech disorder is a structural defect (either VPI or malocclusion). It should be remembered that speech therapy cannot correct abnormal structure. In fact, for ethical reasons, the speech pathologist must refuse to offer speech therapy for an individual who does not have the structural or physiological ability to succeed with speech therapy. The only exception to the rule is if the structure cannot (or will not) be corrected. In that case, speech therapy may be appropriate in order to develop compensatory strategies to improve the intelligibility of speech. Because hyponasality and cul-de-sac resonance are due to a blockage somewhere in the vocal tract, this requires medical or surgical intervention and speech therapy is not appropriate. The only exception is if there is intermittent hyponasality due to the timing deficits of apraxia.

It may be tempting to try speech therapy with individuals who demonstrate a small or inconsistent velopharyngeal opening. These individuals may be able to achieve closure with extra effort (as in the therapy session). However, if the cause is a structural defect, they usually are not able to maintain this closure due to the extra effort that it requires. Therefore, surgical management is usually more appropriate, even though the opening is small. The decision to consider surgical management for a small opening should be made based on how much the defect affects the quality and intelligibility of speech. Only the family and patient can determine if its effect on speech warrants surgical intervention.

SPEECH THERAPY TECHNIQUES

The correction of misarticulations and other functional sequelae of velopharyngeal valving disorders and malocclusion is done through standard articulation therapy. The goal of therapy is to correct placement (and sometimes manner) of production, which often leads to a change in velopharyngeal closure and elimination of the nasality.

The speech therapy techniques used with this population are not very different from the techniques that are used in basic articulation/phonology therapy. Therefore, the basic steps of correction are as follows:

1. Using a phonological approach, which usually results in faster progress (Pamplona, Ysunza, & Espinosa, 1999), determine which category of phonemes needs to be targeted first, based on the child's stimulability and the sounds that will have the biggest impact on intelligibility.

2. Begin with anterior sounds because they are most visible.

3. Always start with the voiceless cognate and then add voicing.

4. Change one feature at a time when moving from one sound in a group to the next sound.

5. For each phoneme, develop auditory (and visual) discrimination of correct versus incorrect productions.

6. Establish correct placement (and manner) of productions in isolation.

7. Incorporate correct sounds in syllables, single words (initial, medial, and final positions), and then sentences.

8. Practice productions every day at home, preferably several times each day.

9. Complete carry-over of new sounds into spontaneous speech.

It is assumed that the reader understands the basic techniques of articulation therapy and therefore, this will not be reviewed in this text. However, the following section describes some specific therapy techniques that are helpful for this population.

Whenever possible, clinical decision making should incorporate the principles of evidence-based practice (EBP) (American Speech-Language-Hearing Association, 2005). EBP is the integration of practitioner expertise with current research to provide quality clinical care. The therapy techniques that are offered here are based primarily on this author's extensive experience and expertise. Research is always needed on the efficacy of specific techniques in comparison with others.

Hypernasality and Nasal Emission (with Weak Consonants)

Hypernasality and nasal emission are very difficult, and most often impossible, to correct with speech therapy because they are usually due to VPI, not velopharyngeal mislearning. Therefore, the speech pathologist will rarely, if ever, provide speech therapy for these characteristics. There are some techniques that can encourage oral resonance, however, and may be effective with hypernasality secondary to dysarthria or apraxia. If there is nasal emission on pressure-sensitive phonemes (plosives, fricatives, affricates), this will cause consonants to be very weak in intensity and pressure. Therefore, correction involves decreasing nasal emission in order to increase oral air pressure.

Because the therapy techniques are essentially the same for hypernasality and nasal air emission, they are included together under the general term of "nasality." The following sections describe various therapy techniques and offer suggestions for implementing them. The techniques described in the numbered lists involve following a sequential series of steps.

Auditory Feedback

- Increase awareness of the nasality by presenting different samples of normal speech and speech with nasality on audio clips or by simulating nasal and oral speech.

- Use audio recordings (tape recorder, computer, or even Nasometer) of the child's speech that demonstrate abnormal productions, and then attempts at normal productions. Have the child self-evaluate.

- Using a straw or listening tube, have the child put one end at the entrance of a nostril and the other end near his/her ear (Figure 21–1). When nasality occurs, it is very audible and even loud. The child is then asked to try to make adjustments in articulation to reduce or eliminate the nasality on oral sounds.

- Put the end of the listening tube in the front of the mouth and the other end at the child's ear (Figure 21–2). The child will

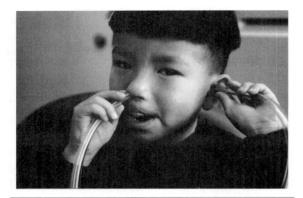

FIGURE 21–1 Use of a "listening tube." The child places one end of the tube at the entrance to a nostril and the other end by the ear. When hypernasality or nasal air emission occur, they can be heard loudly through the tube. This provides excellent auditory feedback. The child is instructed to eliminate the sound in his or her ear when producing the oral sounds.

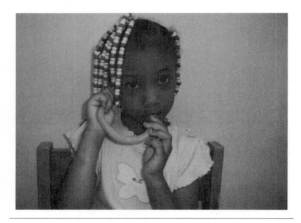

FIGURE 21–2 Use of a tube to provide feedback of oral pressure. The child is asked to produce the sound so that it is loud in his or her ear.

be able to hear the air pressure during the production of oral sounds. (The sound of air going through the tube can usually be heard, even without putting the tube in the ear.) Have the child try to increase the oral pressure.

- Although a simple tube will provide the child with feedback on resonance and

airflow, the placement of the tubing makes it harder for the clinician to hear the sound at the same time. This affects the clinician's ability to provide appropriate feedback and instruction. Therefore, for therapy, using the Oral & Nasal Listener™ (ONL) (Super Duper®, Inc. 5201 Pelham Road, P.O. Box 24997, Greenville, SC 29616) (Figure 21–3) is by far preferable to using a simple tube. With the ONL, both the speech-language pathologist and the child hear the nasal emission and hypernasality at the same time and at the same volume. This makes it much easier for the speech-language pathologist to give appropriate feedback to the child. The ONL is also very helpful to parents. Although daily practice at home is critical for success in therapy, parents are often unsure about what they are hearing and how they are giving feedback. With the Oral & Nasal Listener, the parent and the child can easily hear abnormal nasal emission and hypernasality. This makes the practice at home more effective.

- The Oral & Nasal Listener can also be used to provide feedback about oral resonance and oral airflow. This is done by placing the funnel in front of the mouth, instead of in front of the nostrils. During speech, the ONL amplifies the sound and allows the child to easily hear the difference between weak consonants or hypernasal vowels and those that are oral. With the ONL, the child can better compare his or her own productions with the models provided by the clinician or the parent.

Visual Feedback

- The Nasometer can provide visual feedback of the acoustic properties of speech

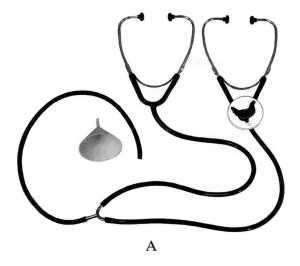

A

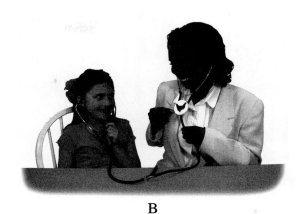

B

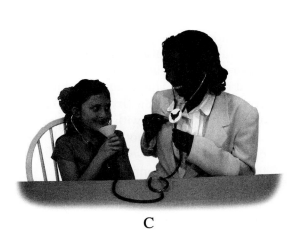

C

FIGURE 21–3 (A–C) A. The Oral & Nasal Listener (ONL). B. The Oral & Nasal Listener was designed to allow the child and the speech-language pathologist (or the parent) to hear the nasal emission or hypernasality in an amplified manner and at the same time. With this device, the adult is able to give the child appropriate feedback. Otherwise, it is hard for the adult to hear the nasal emission because the tube is in the child's nose. C. With the funnel, the oral pressure and sound is amplified for the child. Again, the adult can hear what the child hears. This device is useful for not only work on resonance and nasal emission, but it is also useful for working on articulation, particularly for children who need amplified feedback. (The Oral & Nasal Listener is available through Super Duper Publications [superduperinc.com]. It was developed by Jonathon Cross, Jessica Link, and Ann Kummer at Cincinnati Children's Hospital Medical Center and is patented under the name Nasoscope, 12/2/03, patent number: 6656128.)

and nasopharyngoscopy can provide visual feedback of velopharyngeal function. (See Chapter 14.)

- Place an air paddle in front of the child's mouth during the production of pressure-sensitive phonemes (Figure 21–4). Have the child try to produce the sounds with enough pressure to force the air paddle to move.

- Using a See-Scape, put the nasal olive in one nostril and ask the patient to try to produce pressure consonants repetitively without allowing the foam stopper to rise in the tube. (Note that the foam stopper will rise during the production of nasal phonemes and with nasal breathing at the end of the utterance.) (See Figure 21–5.)

- Using the See-Scape, put the nasal olive at the front of the mouth and have the child produce pressure-sensitive sounds (Figure 21–6). The goal is to make the stopper rise in the tube.

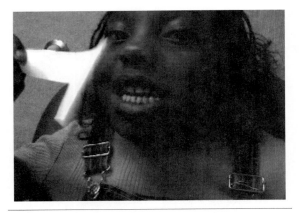

FIGURE 21–4 Use of an air paddle to encourage an increase in oral pressure during production of plosives. The child is instructed to try to make the paper move with each plosive production.

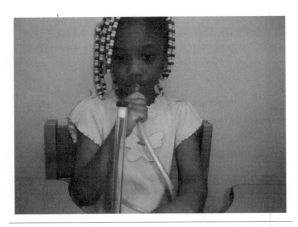

FIGURE 21–6 Use of the See-Scape. The child is asked to produce the sounds with a lot of oral air pressure so that the stopper will move.

Tactile-Kinesthetic Feedback

1. While the child is producing vowel sounds, preferably /ah/, raise the velum up and down with a tongue blade to produce oral-nasal contrasts. This should be done by gradually stimulating first the hard palate and then the velum with the tongue blade so the gag reflux is not activated. If the child has a very active gag reflex, this technique is not appropriate. (Note: If there is a significant difference in resonance with elevation using the tongue blade, the patient may be a good candidate for a palatal lift.)

2. Next, have the child try to raise and lower the velum independently during the production of vowel sounds to produce oral-nasal contrasts.

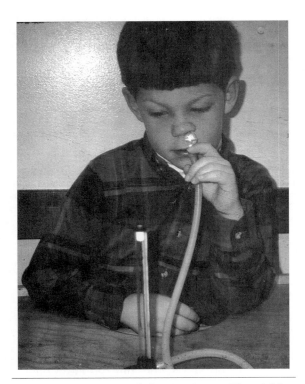

FIGURE 21–5 Use of the See-Scape. The child is instructed to put the nasal olive in one nostril. The child is then asked to try to produce pressure consonants repetitively without allowing the foam stopper to rise in the tube.

Tactile Feedback

- Have the child lightly touch the side of his/her nose and face to feel for vibration during the production of nasal phonemes versus oral phonemes (Figure 21–7). Ask the child to carefully produce oral sounds or sentences without the vibration.

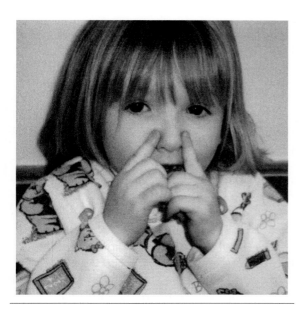

FIGURE 21–7 Tactile feedback for nasal air emission or hypernasality. By having the child lightly touch the side of his or her nose, the child will be able to feel the vibration that occurs with hypernasality or nasal air emission.

- Have the child place his/her hand in front of your mouth as you produce plosives in a forceful manner to feel the air pressure. Then have the child place his/her hand in front of his/her own mouth to do the same.

The following are some specific techniques that can be used to reduce nasality. All forms of feedback (auditory, visual, or tactile) can be used with these techniques. However, auditory feedback, particularly with the Oral & Nasal Listener (ONL), will be most effective.

Lower the Back of the Tongue

1. Get the back of the tongue down and the velum up by having the child yawn.

2. Have the child coarticulate the yawn with vowels and anterior sounds.

3. Have the child think of the yawn movements when articulating other sounds.

Increase Volume

- Have the child increase volume, which will increase respiratory support, velopharyngeal effort and therefore closure, oral air pressure, and the force of articulation (McHenry, 1997). The ultimate goal is a normal degree of volume, however.

Increase Oral Activity

- Have the child increase anterior oral activity, which will increase posterior oral (thus velar) movement at the same time. Increasing mouth opening can also reduce oral resistance and increase oral resonance. The ultimate goal is a normal degree of oral activity, however.

Nose Pinch (Cul-de-Sac) Technique

1. Begin with correct placement of the sound using the nasal cognate of the oral target (e.g., /m/ for bilabial, /n/ for lingual-alveolars, and /ng/ for velars). Have the child feel the placement while prolonging the sound.

2. Have the child achieve that placement and then silently open the lips or drop the tongue as appropriate.

3. Have the child pinch his/her nostrils and whisper while achieving the placement and then opening the lips or dropping the tongue (Figure 21–8). (A nose clip can be used during therapy and practice.) Have the child note the increase in oral airflow and pressure.

4. Have the child try to produce the sounds in the same way with the nostrils unoccluded.

Light, Quick Contacts

- Have the child produce pressure-sensitive sounds with light, quick contacts. This

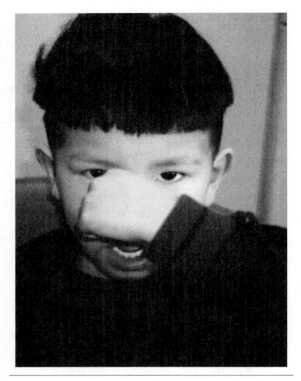

FIGURE 21–8 Nose pinch or cul-de-sac technique. The child is asked to pinch his or her nostrils during the production of pressure sounds to eliminate the nasal air emission. The child is told to feel the increase in oral airflow and pressure. The child is then instructed to produce the sounds in the same way with the nostrils unoccluded.

helps to eliminate the back-up of air pressure in the nasopharynx during oral cavity occlusion and reduces the occurrence of nasal air emission and a nasal rustle.

Misarticulations (Compensatory Productions and Phoneme-Specific Nasality)

Compensatory articulation productions usually develop because there is inadequate oral pressure for normal productions. Correcting

compensatory productions in the presence of persistent velopharyngeal dysfunction is not easy. It is usually better to wait until after the surgery before beginning therapy. If surgery needs to be delayed, therapy can still be done on placement by plugging the nose either manually, or with a nose clip, for better oral air pressure during therapy.

Phoneme-specific nasality occurs due to misarticulations that result in an open velopharyngeal port during production. These misarticulations, and thus the nasality, are corrected by normalizing articulation placement.

For all of the misarticulations noted below, the therapy can be augmented with a large mirror, so that the child can see his/her production and compare it with that of the speech-language pathologist. In addition, a lateral diagram of the tongue and palate allows the speech-pathologist to indicate the child's current placement and the desired placement (Peterson-Falzone, Trost-Cardamone, Karnell, Hardin-Jones, 2006). The diagram works best for older children, but is less effective with preschool children who often have difficulty understanding this concept. Again, auditory feedback is always important and can be augmented by the use of the Oral & Nasal Listener (ONL) for feedback of both resonance and airflow.

Glottal Stops

Glottal stops are usually compensatory errors due to VPI. After surgical correction of the VPI, speech therapy is indicated to correct the glottal stops.

1. Have the child place feel his/her hand on his/her neck during the production of a glottal stop to feel the "jerk" (Figure 21–9). Then have the child feel his/her neck during a prolonged vowel or nasal consonant in order to feel the difference in voice

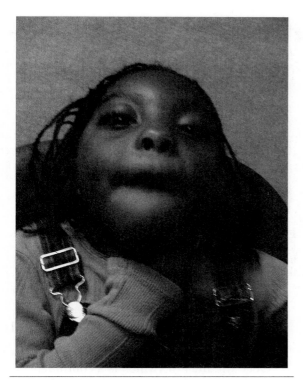

FIGURE 21–9 To eliminate glottal stops, have the child feel his or her neck for the "jerk" during production. Then have the child feel the difference with the production of /h/.

onset. Tell the child that you are going to eliminate the "jerk" during speech.

2. Have the child produce voiceless plosives slowly without the vowel. (The glottal stop does not occur until transition to the vowel.)

3. Have the child produce the voiceless plosive and then the vowel preceded by an /h/ (which keeps the vocal folds open and prevents the glottal stop) (i.e., "p... hhhha" for "pa," and "p...hhhho" for "po"). Gradually decrease the transition time from the consonant to the vowel until the syllable is produced without the glottal stop.

4. Once voiceless consonants can be produced, move to voiced plosives. Have the

child whisper the syllable slowly. Then gradually add "smooth" voicing, and transition to the vowel with an inserted /h/. Have the child feel his/her neck for feedback.

Nasalized Plosives

Nasalized plosives can persist after surgical correction of VPI and therefore, require therapy.

1. Work on the placement of bilabial and lingual-alveolar plosives first.

2. Ask the child to produce a big yawn, which pushes the back of the tongue down and the velum up.

3. Have the child be aware of the "stretch" in the back of the mouth.

4. Have the child coarticulate anterior articulation with a posterior yawn movement to produce the sounds. Once these are mastered, work on velar plosives.

5. Have the child alternately open and close the nose during production. He or she should try to produce the sound the same for both conditions.

Nasalized Vowels

Nasalized vowels can be obligatory errors due to VPI. In this case, therapy is inappropriate. They can also be learned errors that cause phoneme-specific hypernasality. This typically occurs on high vowels, particularly /eee/.

• Have the child alternately close and open the nose during production of the vowel. If he/she hears a difference in the two productions, have the child try to make them the same.

Or,

1. Ask the child to produce a big yawn, which pushes the back of the tongue down and the velum up.

2. Have the child be aware of the "stretch" in the back of the mouth.

3. Have the child coarticulate the vowel with the yawn.

ng/l Substitution

The ng/l substitution can be a compensatory production or a learned misarticulation.

1. Have the child produce a big yawn to get the base of the tongue down and the velum up.

2. Have the child be aware of the "stretch" in the back of the mouth.

3. With the yawn, have the child coarticulate the /l/.

4. Gradually eliminate the use of the yawn movement but tell the child to think of the movement during production.

Nasalized /r/ (ng/r Substitution or Incorrect /r/)

The final /r/ sound is produced by articulating the sides of the tongue against the gum behind the molars. The middle portion of the tongue forms a boat-like shape through which sound resonates. If the child raises the entire back of the tongue, the sound becomes an /ng/ sound, which results in nasal resonance.

1. Using your hand, show the child how the shape of the tongue forms a boat and that the back of the tongue must touch behind the back teeth.

2. With a tongue blade, stimulate both sides of the tongue towards the back. Then stimulate the upper gum ridge behind the molars. Tell the child to put the two together.

3. Assist the child with posterior tongue elevation by pushing up against the base of the chin with the middle finger while

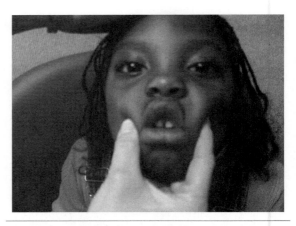

FIGURE 21–10 To encourage appropriate placement for final /r/, use your middle finger to push up firmly under the child's chin, near the neck. This pushes against the base of the tongue. With the index finger and thumb, squeeze the cheeks to promote lip rounding.

squeezing the cheeks with the thumb and forefinger (Figure 21–10).

4. Once the final /r/ (which is a continuant) is established, then demonstrate with your hand how the tongue tip moves forward for the initial /r/.

Or,

1. If the child continues to raise the entire back of the tongue for /r/, resulting in an /ng/, close the child's nose during production of the sound. That will make the /ng/ sound impossible to produce.

2. If necessary, place a tube in the middle of the tongue so that sound goes through, but the middle of the tongue cannot go up to articulate against the velum.

Pharyngeal Plosives (Substituted for the Velar Plosives)

Pharyngeal plosives are usually compensatory productions as a result of VPI.

1. Establish placement for velar plosives (/k/ and /g/) by starting with an /ng/. If the

child can't produce an /ng/, use an upside-down spoon (or tongue blade if necessary) to hold the tip of the tongue down. Then firmly press your thumb under the base of the chin, which is under the base of the tongue (just as when working on /r/). This promotes the velar production (and works in establishing /k/ and /g/ in other cases as well).

2. Starting with /ng/, have the child work on an up-and-down movement of the back of the tongue, rather than a back-and-forth movement which occurs with the pharyngeal plosive. This can be done silently.

3. Have the child take a breath, place his/her tongue in an /ng/ position, and then keeping the tongue position, release the air pressure slowly. This will result in a velar fricative (which is not a sound in English).

4. Once the child can produce the velar fricative, have the child start with the /ng/, build up air pressure, and then release it quickly with the downward movement to produce the velar plosive.

Pharyngeal Fricatives, Pharyngeal Affricates, and Posterior Nasal Fricatives

Pharyngeal fricatives, pharyngeal affricates, and posterior nasal fricatives can be compensatory productions that require therapy after surgical correction of VPI, or they can be mislearned productions that cause phoneme-specific nasal air emission. Regardless of the original cause, the methods for correction are the same.

For /s/:

1. Have the child produce a loud /t/ sound repetitively.

2. Then have the child produce the /t/ with the teeth closed, which will result in /ts/.

3. Increase the duration of the production until it becomes /tssss/.

4. Have the child note the position of the tongue and the airstream flowing over the tongue during production.

5. Finally, eliminate the tongue tip movement for the /t/ component.

For /sh/, /ch/ and /j/:

1. Start with /ch/ because this sound contains a /t/. Follow the same procedures as noted above for /s/, but keep the lips rounded. Also, have the child try to produce this sound as a loud sneeze with the teeth closed.

2. Once the /ch/ sound is mastered, work on the /j/ in the same way, but start with a /d/ sound.

3. Once /ch/ is mastered, follow steps (4) and (5) of the /s/ sound to achieve a /sh/.

Straw technique:

1. Place a straw at the point of your own central incisors during production of a sibilant sound. Note the sound of the airflow through the straw.

2. Have the child put the straw in front of his incisors and try to produce the sound until he/she can hear the airflow through the straw (Figure 21–11).

Or,

1. Have the child produce fricative sounds with the nostrils occluded and then open in order to get the feel for oral rather than pharyngeal airflow.

Middorsum Palatal Stops (Palatal-Dorsals)

Middorsum palatal stops are substituted for lingual-alveolars (/t/, /d/, /n/, or /l/) and velars (/k/, /g/, or /ng/). This placement is also used for sibilants (/s/, /z/, /sh/, /ch/, and /j/) and

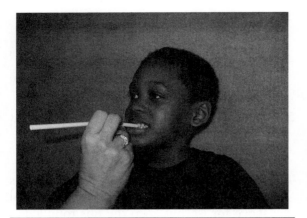

FIGURE 21–11 To promote anterior airflow during production of /s/ and other sibilants, put a straw in front of the child's incisors and have him or her try to produce the sound until he or she can hear the airflow through the straw. (This also works for correction of a lateral lisp.)

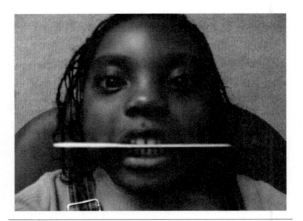

FIGURE 21–12 To eliminate palatal-dorsal articulation of lingual-alveolar sounds, have the child bite on a tongue blade. Then have the child try to produce the sounds with the tongue tip articulating on the tongue blade.

results in a lateral lisp. Middorsum palatal stops are often compensatory errors as a result of anterior crowding due to an anterior cross-bite and Class III malocclusion.

For lingual-alveolars or velars:

1. Have the patient bite on a tongue blade so that it is between the incisors (Figure 21–12).

2. Have the child produce lingual-alveolar sounds (/t/, /d/, and /n/) with the tongue tip touching the tongue blade.

Or,

1. Have the child prolong a nasal sound /n/ to establish placement for lingual-alveolars or /ng/ to establish placement for velars. If the child can't produce /ng/, have the child put his or her head way back and allow gravity to help, or use your thumb to push firmly under the chin (almost by the neck) to help push the base of the tongue up.

2. Have the child work on achieving that placement and then dropping the tongue. This can be done silently.

3. Have the child take a deep breath, then achieve that placement and hold it.

4. Have the child release some of the pressure while holding the placement. This will result in a fricative-type sound.

5. Then have the child repeat step (4), but drop the tongue to produce the plosive.

For sibilants:

1. Place a straw at the front of your own closed incisors and produce an /s/. Make sure that the airstream is heard through the straw.

2. Place the straw at the front of the child's closed incisors during production of the /s/ and note the lack of airstream through the straw (see Figure 21–11).

3. Move the straw to the side of the child's dental arch during production of the /s/, and find the place where the airstream can be heard through the straw (Figure 21–13).

4. Have the child put the straw at the front of his/her closed incisors and produce a /t/ while keeping the teeth closed. Tell the child to push the air into the straw.

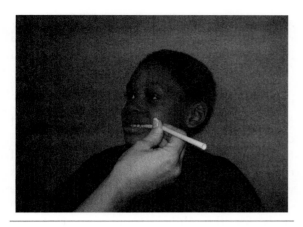

FIGURE 21–13 To eliminate a lateral distortion, put a straw on the side of the dental arch until you hear air going through the straw during a sustained /s/. Then place the straw in the front of the mouth and have the child work on articulation placement until the airstream is going through the straw during production of a sustained /s/.

5. Then have the child prolong the /t/ until it is a /tssssss/, while pushing the air through the straw. Because the /ch/ sound already contains the /t/ sound, in some cases it may be easier to work on /ch/ first using a /t/ and then a prolonged /sh/.

6. Have the child feel the air flow over the tongue and hear the air through the straw.

7. Then have the child achieve that position without the initial /t/ and prolong the /s/.

8. Once the /s/ is established, the same techniques can be used to achieve other sibilant sounds.

BIOFEEDBACK TECHNIQUES USING INSTRUMENTATION

Biofeedback is a technique for making unconscious or autonomic physiological processes perceptible to the senses in order to manipulate them by conscious mental control. Biofeedback techniques are based on the principle that a desired response can be learned when it is determined that a specific thought process can produce that physiological response.

Different types of biofeedback techniques have been used in medicine for years and have been found to be effective for certain uses, such as reducing tension, decreasing heart rate, and even decreasing pain. In recent years, biofeedback techniques have been applied in speech pathology, particularly in the area of voice (McGillivray, Proctor-Williams, & McLister, 1994; Prosek, Montgomery, Walden, & Schwartz, 1978; Rossiter, Howard, & DeCosta, 1996; Stemple, Weiler, Whitehead, & Komray, 1980), fluency (Davis & Drichta, 1980; Weiss, Carson, & Brady, 1979), and dysarthria (Gentil, Aucouturier, Delong, & Sambuis, 1994; Murdoch, Pitt, Theodoros, & Ward, 1999; Nemec & Cohen, 1984; Rubow, Rosenbek, Collins, & Celesia, 1984; Rubow & Swift, 1985).

There are several ways to provide biofeedback of velopharyngeal function. The feedback can be auditory, visual, or tactile-kinesthetic. The clinician must keep in mind, however, that biofeedback will only be successful if the individual is anatomically and physiologically capable of achieving normal velopharyngeal closure. In addition, the individual needs to be old enough to actively participate and cognitively understand the feedback, and to determine what needs to be done to achieve a desired result.

Aerodynamics

Pressure-flow instrumentation has numerous biofeedback applications. It can be used to provide feedback for phoneme-specific nasal air emission and can be very helpful in eliminating glottal stops and pharyngeal stops. With posterior compensatory productions, there is usually no oral pressure (see Figure 15–20). Pressure-flow instrumentation can provide visual feedback to help facilitate a change in placement of articulation for such compensations. The modification of a middorsum palatal stop, for example, may be facilitated by placement of a pressure catheter behind the alveolar ridge. A lingual-alveolar placement for stop production will result in the appearance of dramatic oral air pressure pulses. Negative practice may also be implemented by instructing the speaker to revert to the middorsum place of articulation once lingual advancement has been accomplished. Inappropriate nasal air emission may also be targeted in this fashion. Although the use of devices such as the See-Scape will also provide feedback, pressure-flow instrumentation has the advantage of providing objective documentation of therapy progress.

Aerodynamic instrumentation can also be useful for providing feedback regarding breath support. With the use of a mouthpiece and pneumotachograph, real-time feedback of respiratory parameters, such as inspiratory volume and maximum phonation volume, can be monitored by the patient. To isolate the effect of inadequate respiratory support from velopharyngeal dysfunction, the nostrils can be plugged for one measurement and then open for another. The prolongation of voiceless continuants, such as /s/, may be especially helpful for discriminating between respiratory and velopharyngeal factors.

Nasometry

Nasometry is an excellent biofeedback instrument because it provides the individual with visual feedback regarding the amount of nasal acoustic energy (nasalance) that is generated during speech. The Nasometer is particularly useful in remediating phoneme-specific nasal air emission. It can also be used to modify resonance in certain cases of velopharyngeal incompetence due to neuromotor dysfunction (Heppt, Westrich, Strate, & Mohring, 1991).

Using the Nasometer, visual feedback can be displayed in the form of either a bar graph (histogram) or a contour display. The type of display that is used in therapy depends on the type of speech sample. On both types of displays, the height of the graph increases with an increase in nasal acoustic energy. The speech-language pathologist can set tangible goals for the child during the treatment process and the child can receive immediate feedback on his or her success in attaining those goals.

The bar graph is best when working on individual phonemes, as it displays only one production at a time. The clinician can begin by having the child produce a prolonged /m/ and then a sustained "ah" in order to see the difference in the graphic display. The clinician can then determine an appropriate threshold line, which will serve as the child's visual target. If the child typically achieves around 30% nasalance on a particular phoneme, the examiner might place the bar at 25% and have the child repeat the phoneme without going over the bar. The target can be adjusted downward as the child becomes more proficient in reaching the goal.

The filled contour display is most appropriate for use with connected speech because it consists of a 4-second time axis. If left in the normal mode, the goal is to keep the contour as low as possible, which reflects a decrease in nasal energy and/or an increase in oral energy. Since most children naturally want to make the contour as high as possible, the clinician can invert the display so that 0% is at the top and 100% is at the bottom. This way, the child must produce the high "mountains" as the goal. The Nasometer software also includes games designed to be used as part of a therapy protocol. These games are fun for children of all ages and help to break the monotony of repetitive practice. They also provide visual rewards for success.

The Nasometer software includes lists of sentences that are useful in therapy. These sentences are grouped according to phoneme and degree of difficulty in achieving velopharyngeal closure. Since statistics regarding performance are automatically generated with each speech sample, the clinician can use these objective data for each group of sentences to determine the child's ability to achieve each goal. The clinician can also track the child's progress over time with serial records.

Nasopharyngoscopy

Nasopharyngoscopy can be a particularly useful tool in therapy because it can provide visual feedback regarding the actions of the velopharyngeal mechanism during speech (Brunner, Stellzig-Eisenhauer, Proschel, Verres, & Komposch, 2005; Hoch et al., 1986; Rich, Farber, & Shprintzen, 1988; Shelton, Beaumont, Trier, & Furr, 1978; Siegel-Sadewitz & Shprintzen, 1982; Witzel, Tobe, & Salyer, 1988, 1989; Ysunza, Pamplona, Femat, Mayer, & Garcia-Velasco, 1997). This can help the patient to develop a degree of active control of the velopharyngeal movements for opening and closing the valve. Nasopharyngoscopy is the only practical method for direct visualization of the velopharyngeal mechanism for therapy because it is well-tolerated by most patients, does not impede speech, and it can be repeated whenever necessary without any risk to the patient (Witzel et al., 1989).

As a biofeedback tool, nasopharyngoscopy is appropriate for patients who have the physical ability to achieve velopharyngeal closure, but demonstrate phoneme-specific nasal emission or hypernasality due to faulty articulation (Witzel et al., 1988). Nasopharyngoscopy may also be useful in helping patients to increase lateral pharyngeal wall movement following a pharyngeal flap procedure (Siegel-Sadewitz & Shprintzen, 1982; Witzel et al., 1989; Ysunza et al., 1997).

The biofeedback procedure begins by helping the patient to identify the velopharyngeal structures on the video monitor. The person is then instructed to swallow, blow, or produce a sound repetitively that results in complete closure. The action of the velopharyngeal mechanism is pointed out and the patient is encouraged to try to identify the sensation of the movement and closure of the port. Therapy then focuses on achieving velopharyngeal closure for the phonemes where closure is normally incomplete. This is done not only by using the visual feedback, but also by changing the place of production for these sounds.

Once the placement is changed and the patient is able to achieve closure on the target phoneme, it is sometimes helpful to have the patient go back and forth between the "good production" and the "bad production" to be able to feel, see, and hear the difference. This helps to develop voluntary control. Once the placement is achieved and the sound can be reproduced with correct placement easily, then the patient is ready for traditional speech therapy where the production is established first in syllables, then in words and sentences, and finally in connected speech.

OTHER SPECIAL PROCEDURES

Continuous Positive Airway Pressure (CPAP)

A *continuous positive airway pressure* (CPAP) device is an instrument that consists of a flow generator, a valve mechanism, a hose, and a nasal mask. Airflow and air pressure are delivered to the nasal cavity, and thus the pharynx, through the hose and nasal mask. CPAP has been found to be useful in the treatment of individuals with obstructive sleep apnea (OSA) because the positive pressure prevents the collapse of the pharyngeal airway during sleep.

In 1991, Kuehn (1991) described the use of CPAP as a means for treating hypernasality. He suggested that CPAP could provide resistance training for the velopharyngeal muscles by having them work actively against the positive air pressure. Based on the principles of exercise physiology, CPAP therapy is designed to overload the muscles by subjecting them to a greater level of resistance than usual during velar elevation for speech. Therefore, the muscles of the velum must work harder. Once the muscles adapt to a certain level of pressure, the pressure is increased. Through this progressive resistance training, the muscles are thought to gain strength and become more resistance to fatigue. This strengthening of the musculature could therefore improve velopharyngeal closure. This procedure has been found to reduce the degree of hypernasality in some patients (Kuehn et al., 2002).

Kuehn, Moon, and Folkins (1993) compared electromyographic activity of the levator veli palatini during the use of CPAP and with atmospheric air pressure only. There was a significant increase in the activity of the levator muscle with an increase in the intranasal pressure, suggesting that this muscle actively reacts to the resistance and possibly increases in strength.

Kuehn listed several advantages of the CPAP technique, including the fact that it is noninvasive, easy to use, and can be done at home (Kuehn, 1991, 1997; Kuehn et al., 2002). An important difference between this procedure and other muscle training procedures is that this is done during speech and for speech activities only.

Some caveats of this form of treatment might include the fact that patient selection is very important. This form of treatment is best suited for cases with velopharyngeal incompetence where there is poor velar movement, as in the traumatic brain injury population (Cahill et al., 2004). However, it is unlikely to be successful if there is more than mild to moderate velopharyngeal incompetence or there is a structural defect. Although this technique has promise, further research is needed to clearly define the effects of CPAP on individuals with mild velopharyngeal incompetence, and whether short-term improvements are sustained once the CPAP therapy is terminated.

Prosthesis Reduction Therapy

Some authors have described the use of a temporary speech prosthesis as a means of improving velopharyngeal function (Blakeley, 1964, 1969; Golding-Kushner, Cisneros, & LeBlanc, 1995; Harkins and Koepp-Baker; 1948; Israel, Cook, & Blakeley, 1993; McGrath & Anderson, 1990; Shelton, Lindquist, Arndt, Elbert, & Youngstrom, 1971; Shelton et al., 1968; Weiss, 1971; Wolfaardt, Wilson, Rochet, & McPhee, 1993). The procedure is to use a palatal lift or speech bulb for a period of time, and then gradually reduce its size in hopes of promoting an increase in velopharyngeal movement. However, research has not shown that the lift does not promote an increase in muscle function and neither device eliminates the need for further surgery (Tachimura, Nohara, Fujita, Hara, & Wada, 2001; Yorkston et al., 2001). Therefore, this type of management is still controversial, especially since prosthetic devices are expensive and compliance with children is difficult. (See Chapter 20 for more information.)

Oral-Motor Exercises (That Don't Work!)

In the past, clinicians used oral-motor "exercises," such as blowing, sucking, whistling, cheek puffing, swallowing, and even playing wind instruments, in hopes of strengthening the muscles of the velopharyngeal valve for improved function with speech (Berry & Eisenson, 1956; Kanter, 1947; Massengill, Quinn, Pickrell, & Levinson, 1968; Moser, 1942; Van Riper, 1946, 1963; Wells, 1945, 1948). Several investigators even tried to stimulate velopharyngeal movement through the use of electrical stimulation or "exercisors" (Cole, 1971, 1979; Lubit & Larsen, 1969, 1971; Massengill, Quinn, & Pickrell, 1971; Peterson, 1974; Tash, Shelton, Knox, & Michel, 1971; Weber, Jobe, and Chase, 1970; Yules and Chase, 1969). However, these exercises did not seem to be very effective (Powers & Starr, 1974; Ruscello, 1982; Shelton, Hahn, & Morris, 1968).

Later research showed significant differences in the velopharyngeal closure patterns of speech and nonspeech activities, suggesting that nonspeech "exercises" could not possibly be effective in improving velopharyngeal function for speech (Flowers & Morris, 1973; Golding-Kushner, 2001; McWilliams & Bradley, 1965; Moll, 1965; Peterson, 1973; Peterson-Falzone, Trost-Cardamone, Karnell, & Hardin-Jones, 2006; Shprintzen, Lencione, McCall, & Skolnick, 1974). In addition, patients with a history of cleft have a structural abnormality, not weakness of the musculature. Despite this information and the fact that there is no evidence in the literature to support the efficacy of nonspeech exercises in improving velopharyngeal function (Yorkston et al., 2001), some clinicians continue to incorporate these exercises in treatment due to a lack of knowledge.

Given current knowledge and the need to adhere to evidence-based practice, procedures to avoid in therapy for sequelae of cleft palate or velopharyngeal dysfunction include: blowing, sucking, gagging, swallowing, icing, stroking, palatal massage, electrical stimulation or any other type of oral-motor exercises. (Golding-Kushner, 2001)

CARRY-OVER

Successful carry-over of new speech productions into everyday conversational speech is the measure of the true success of therapy. However, carry-over is often the most frustrating aspect of therapy because it can be the most difficult to achieve. Carry-over success depends on several factors. First, the new speech production must be easy to produce, and therefore practice in drills can be helpful. Second, the child must be able to self-monitor and self-correct. Finally, there must be support from the family to encourage the use of the sound at home and to correct the misarticulations when necessary.

The best way to work on all of the above is to involve the family members as partners in the treatment process. Speech therapy is very much like taking piano lessons . . . if you only go for the lessons and don't practice at home, you don't make progress. Given the cost of therapy (to the parents, insurance providers, and taxpayers), each therapy session should be geared toward moving to the next step and learning new skills. Learned skills that are not yet habituated should be practiced every day at home in the natural environment.

For the parents to be active participants, they must be taught how to be the "therapist" at home. By being actively involved in the initial therapy process, they will be more aware of the child's speech and more helpful in monitoring and correcting the child's speech during the carry-over stage.

THE ULTIMATE GOAL

In past generations, the goal of treatment for individuals with a history of cleft palate was acceptable or intelligible speech, because normal speech was not always obtainable. With increased knowledge over the past few decades of the nature of the velopharyngeal mechanism, and with the advances in evaluation and surgical treatment techniques, most individuals now born with cleft palate can expect to ultimately attain normal speech. If there are uncorrectable structural problems or neurological problems, such as pharyngeal hypotonia, dysarthria, or apraxia, then the prognosis for perfect speech is more guarded. Regardless, all efforts should be made to achieve normal speech through appropriate treatment whenever possible.

SUMMARY

Speech therapy is appropriate for the correction of articulation errors that cause nasal emission and hypernasality (phoneme-specific errors) and also for articulation errors that are caused by VPI (compensatory errors). Therapy is rarely appropriate for hypernasality or nasal emission because these characteristics are usually caused by VPI, which requires physical management. In addition, therapy is not appropriate for obligatory errors because they will self-correct with normalization of the structure. When in doubt regarding the cause of the speech characteristics and appropriate recommendations, a trial period of speech therapy can be done to determine the individual's response to therapy.

The therapy procedures for speech errors of patients with a history of cleft or VPI are no different than those used for other placement errors. Oral-motor exercises, including those that involve blowing and sucking, are inappropriate because they are not effective in this population (Golding-Kushner, 2001).

Therapy should continue as long as the child is making progress. If the child is not responding to the therapy and continues to have characteristics of VPI, it is very important to refer the child to a craniofacial anomaly team or specialist for further evaluation of velopharyngeal function. Surgical intervention or revision may be necessary.

FOR REVIEW, DISCUSSION, AND CRITICAL THINKING

1. Discuss the appropriate focus and intervention strategies for the following developmental stage: infants and toddlers, preschool children, school-age children, adolescents and adults. Explain why early intervention and early stimulation are critically important.

2. In what cases is speech therapy appropriate for children with a history of cleft palate? When is speech therapy inappropriate for correction of abnormal speech in this population?

3. Why is speech therapy almost always ineffective in correcting hypernasality or nasal emission? Why do you think that clinicians still keep children in speech therapy for these problems? If a physician refers a child to you for correction of hypernasality, what would you do and why?

4. Under what circumstances is speech therapy appropriate for nasal emission or hypernasality? What would you do if no progress was made after two months of therapy?

5. Discuss methods of auditory, visual, and tactile feedback that can be used as part of therapy. Which methods would be the most effective and why?

6. What is the nose pinch (cul-de-sac) technique? How can that help in therapy?

7. Your patient has a history VPI which was corrected by a pharyngeal flap. Speech is characterized by ng/l and nasal emission on s/z only. All other speech sounds are produced normally without hypernasality or nasal emission. Why is there still nasality on the /l/ sound and nasal emission on s/z? What speech therapy techniques might be used for these misarticulations?

8. How can the straw be used to correct inconsistent nasal emission? How can it be used to correct a lateral lisp due to malocclusion?

9. Describe therapy approaches for correction of the following: a glottal stop, a pharyngeal fricative, lateral distortion, phoneme-specific nasal air emission, and ng/l substitution.

10. Describe various high-tech and low-tech methods of providing biofeedback as part of the therapy process. What are the advantages and disadvantages of each?

11. What is CPAP therapy? What is the theory behind it? Why would it be inappropriate with a patient with a submucous cleft and short velum?

12. Why are oral-motor exercises and blowing and sucking exercises ineffective in the treatment of velopharyngeal dysfunction? Why do you think some clinicians still use them?

13. How would you explain to parents why their involvement is critically important to the success of therapy?

REFERENCES

American Speech-Language-Hearing Association. (2005). *Evidence-based practice in communication disorders* [Position statement]. Retrieved April, 20, 2006 from the ASHA Web site: http://www.asha.org/members/deskref-journals/deskref/default.

Berry, M. F., & Eisenson, J. (1956). Speech disorders: Principles and practices of therapy. New York: Appleton-Century-Crofts.

Blakeley, R. W. (1964). The complementary use of speech prostheses and pharyngeal flaps in palatal insufficiency. *Cleft Palate Journal, 1*, 194.

Blakeley, R. W. (1969). The rationale for a temporary speech prosthesis in palatal insufficiency. *British Journal of Disorders in Communication, 4*(2), 134–139.

Brunner, M., Stellzig-Eisenhauer, A., Proschel, U., Verres, R., & Komposch, G. (2005). The effect of nasopharyngoscopic biofeedback in patients with cleft palate and velopharyngeal dysfunction. *Cleft Palate-Craniofacial Journal, 42*(6), 649–657.

Cahill, L. M., Turner, A. B., Stabler, P. A., Addis, P. E., Theodoros, D. G., & Murdoch, B. E. (2004). An evaluation of continuous positive airway pressure (CPAP) therapy in the treatment of hypernasality following traumatic brain injury: A report of 3 cases. *Journal of Head Trauma Rehabilitation, 19*(3), 241–253.

Cole, R. M. (1971). Direct muscle training for the improvement of velopharyngeal function. In K. Bzoch (Ed.), *Communicative disorders related to cleft lip and palate* (pp. 250–256). Boston: Little, Brown and Company.

Cole, R. M. (1979). Direct muscle training for the improvement of velopharyngeal activity. In K. Bzoch (Ed.), *Communicative disorders related to cleft lip and palate* (2nd ed., pp. 328–340). Boston: Little, Brown and Company.

Davis, S. M., & Drichta, C. E. (1980). Biofeedback theory and application in allied health: Speech pathology. *Biofeedback and Self-Regulation, 5*(2), 159–174.

Dowling, J. E. (2004). *The great brain debate: Nature or nurture?* Washington, DC: Joseph Henry Press.

Flowers, C. R., & Morris, H. L. (1973). Oral-pharyngeal movements during swallowing and speech. *Cleft Palate Journal, 10,* 181–191.

Gentil, M., Aucouturier, J. L., Delong, V., & Sambuis, E. (1994). EMG biofeedback in the treatment of dysarthria. *Folia Phoniatrica et Logopedia, 46*(4), 188–192.

Golding-Kushner, K. J. (2001). *Therapy techniques for cleft palate & related disorders.* Englewood Cliffs, NJ: Thomson Delmar Learning.

Golding-Kushner, K. J., Cisneros, G., & LeBlanc, E. (1995). Speech bulbs. In R. J. Shprintzen & J. Bardach (Eds.), *Cleft palate speech management* (pp. 352–375). St. Louis, MO: Mosby.

Hahn, E. (1989). Directed home language stimulation program for infants with cleft lip and palate. In K. R. Bzoch (Ed.), *Communicative disorders related to cleft lip and palate* (3rd ed., pp. 313–319). Boston: Little, Brown and Company.

Hardin, M. A. (1991). Cleft palate. Intervention. *Clinics in Communication Disorders, 1*(3), 12–18.

Hardin-Jones, M. A., & Jones, D. L. (2005). Speech production of preschoolers with cleft palate. *Cleft Palate-Craniofacial Journal, 42*(1), 7–13.

Harkins, C., & Koepp-Baker, H. (1948). Twenty-five years of cleft palate prosthesis. *Journal of Speech and Hearing Disorders, 13,* 23.

Heppt, W., Westrich, M., Strate, B., & Mohring, L. (1991). Nasalance: A new concept for objective analysis of nasality. *Laryngorhinootologie, 70*(4), 208–213.

Hoch, L., Golding-Kushner, K., Siegel-Sadewitz, V. L., & Shprintzen, R. L. (1986). Speech therapy. In B. J. McWilliams (Ed.), *Current methods of assessing and treating children with cleft palates* (pp. 313–326). New York: Thieme.

Israel, J. M., Cook, T. A., & Blakeley, R. W. (1993). The use of a temporary oral prosthesis to treat speech in velopharyngeal incompetence. *Facial and Plastic Surgery, 9*(3), 206–212.

Kanter, C. E. (1947). The rationale for blowing exercises for patients with repaired cleft palates. *Journal of Speech Disorders, 12,* 281.

Kuehn, D. P. (1991). New therapy for treating hypernasal speech using continuous positive airway pressure (CPAP). *Plastic and Reconstructive Surgery, 88*(6), 959–966; Discussion 967–969.

Kuehn, D. P. (1997). The development of a new technique for treating hypernasality: CPAP. *American Journal of Speech-Language Pathology, 6*(4), 5–8.

Kuehn, D. P., Imrey, P. B., Tomes, L., Jones, D. L., O'Gara, M. M., Seaver, E. J., et al. (2002). Efficacy of continuous positive airway pressure for treatment of hypernasality. *Cleft Palate-Craniofacial Journal, 39*(3), 267–276.

Kuehn, D. P., Moon, J. B., & Folkins, J. W. (1993). Levator veli palatini muscle activity in relation to intranasal air pressure variation. *Cleft Palate-Craniofacial Journal*, *30*(4), 361–368.

Lubit, E. C., & Larsen, R. E. (1969). The Lubit palatal exerciser: A preliminary report. *Cleft Palate Journal*, *6*, 120–133.

Lubit, E. C., & Larsen, R. E. (1971). A speech aid for velopharyngeal incompetency. *Journal of Speech and Hearing Disorders*, *36*(1), 61–70.

Massengill, R., Jr., Quinn, G. W., & Pickrell, K. L. (1971). The use of a palatal stimulator to decrease velopharyngeal gap. *Annals of Otology, Rhinology, and Laryngology*, *80*, 135–137.

Massengill, R., Jr., Quinn, G. W., Pickrell, K. L., & Levinson, C. (1968). Therapeutic exercise and velopharyngeal gap. *Cleft Palate Journal*, *5*, 44–47.

McGillivray, R., Proctor-Williams, K., & McLister, B. (1994). Simple biofeedback device to reduce excessive vocal intensity. *Medical and Biological Engineering Computing*, *32*(3), 348–350.

McGrath, C. O., & Anderson, M. W. (1990). Prosthetic treatment of velopharyngeal incompetence. In J. Bardach & H. L. Morris (Eds.), *Multidisciplinary management of cleft lip and palate* (pp. 809–815). Philadelphia: W. B. Saunders.

McHenry, M. A. (1997). The effect of increased vocal effort on estimated velopharyngeal orifice area. *American Journal of Speech-Language Pathology*, *6*(4), 55–61.

McWilliams, B. J., & Bradley, D. (1965). Ratings of velopharyngeal closure during blowing and speech. *Cleft Palate Journal*, *2*, 46.

Moll, K. L. (1965). A cinefluorographic study of velopharyngeal function in normals during various activities. *Cleft Palate Journal*, *2*, 112.

Moser, H. (1942). Diagnostic and clinical procedures in rhinolalia. *Journal of Speech Disorders*, *7*, 1.

Murdoch, B. E., Pitt, G., Theodoros, D. G., & Ward, E. C. (1999). Real-time continuous visual biofeedback in the treatment of speech breathing disorders following childhood traumatic brain injury: Report of one case. *Pediatric Rehabilitation*, *3*(1), 5–20.

Nash, P., Stengelhofen, J., Toombs, L., Brown, J., & Kellow, B. (2001). An alternative management of older children with persisting communication problems. *International Journal of Language & Communication Disorders*, *36*(Suppl.), 179–184.

Nemec, R. E., & Cohen, K. (1984). EMG biofeedback in the modification of hypertonia in spastic dysarthria: Case report. *Archives of Physical Medicine and Rehabilitation*, *65*(2), 103–104.

O'Gara, M. M., & Logemann, J. A. (1990). Early speech development in cleft palate babies. In J. Bardach & H. L. Morris (Eds.), *Multidisciplinary management of cleft lip and palate* (pp. 717–726). Philadelphia: W. B. Saunders.

Pamplona, M. C., & Ysunza, A. (2000). Active participation of mothers during speech therapy improved language development of children with cleft palate. *Scandinavian Journal of Plastic and Reconstructive Surgery and Hand Surgery*, *34*(3), 231–236.

Pamplona, M. C., Ysunza, A., & Espinosa, J. (1999). A comparative trial of two modalities of speech intervention for compensatory articulation in cleft palate children, phonologic approach versus articulatory approach. *International Journal of Pediatric Otorhinolaryngology*, *49*(1), 21–26.

Pamplona, M. C., Ysunza, A., & Jimenez-Murat, Y. (2001). Mothers of children with cleft palate undergoing speech intervention change communicative interaction. *International Journal of Pediatric Otorhinolaryngology*, 59(3), 173–179.

Pamplona, M. C., Ysunza, A., Patino, C., Ramirez, E., Drucker, M., & Mazon, J. J. (2005). Speech summer camp for treating articulation disorders in cleft palate patients. *International Journal of Pediatric Otorhinolaryngology*, 69(3), 351–359.

Pamplona, M. C., Ysunza, A., & Uriostegui, C. (1996). Linguistic interaction: The active role of parents in speech therapy for cleft palate patients. *International Journal of Pediatric Otorhinolaryngology*, 37(1), 17–27.

Peterson, S. J. (1973). Velopharyngeal closure: Some important differences. *Journal of Speech and Hearing Disorders*, 38, 89.

Peterson, S. J. (1974). Electrical stimulation of the soft palate. *Cleft Palate Journal*, 11, 72–86.

Peterson-Falzone, S. J., Trost-Cardamone, J. E, Karnell, M. P., Hardin-Jones, M. A. (2006). *The clinician's guide to treating cleft palate speech*. St. Louis, MO: Mosby Elsevier.

Phillips, B. J. (1990). Early speech management. In J. Bardach & H. L. Morris (Eds.), *Multidisciplinary management of cleft lip and palate* (pp. 732–736). Philadelphia: W. B. Saunders.

Powers, G. L., & Starr, C. D. (1974). The effect of muscle exercises on velopharyngeal gap and nasality. *Cleft Palate Journal*, 11, 28.

Prosek, R. A., Montgomery, A. A., Walden, B. E., & Schwartz, D. M. (1978). EMG biofeedback in the treatment of hyperfunctional voice disorders. *Journal of Speech and Hearing Disorders*, 43(3), 282–294.

Rich, B. M., Farber, K., & Shprintzen, R. J. (1988). Nasopharyngoscopy in the treatment of palatopharyngeal insufficiency. *International Journal of Prosthodontics*, 1(3), 248–251.

Rossiter, D., Howard, D. M., & DeCosta, M. (1996). Voice development under training with and without the influence of real-time visually presented biofeedback [Letter]. *Journal of the Acoustical Society of America*, 99(5), 3253–3256.

Rubow, R. T., Rosenbek, J. C., Collins, M. J., & Celesia, G. G. (1984). Reduction of hemifacial spasm and dysarthria following EMG biofeedback. *Journal of Speech and Hearing Disorders*, 49(1), 26–33.

Rubow, R., & Swift, E. (1985). A microcomputer-based wearable biofeedback device to improve transfer of treatment in parkinsonian dysarthria. *Journal of Speech and Hearing Disorders*, 50(2), 178–185.

Ruscello, D. M. (1982). A selected review of palatal training procedures. *Cleft Palate Journal*, 19(3), 181–193.

Schendel, L. L., & Bzoch, K. R. (1979). Advantages of intensive summer training programs. In K. R. Bzoch (Ed.), *Communicative disorders related to cleft lip and palate* (2nd ed., pp. 318–327). Boston: Little, Brown and Company.

Shelton, R. L., Beaumont, K., Trier, W. C., & Furr, M. L. (1978). Videoendoscopic feedback in training velopharyngeal closure. *Cleft Palate Journal*, 15(1), 6–12.

Shelton, R. L., Hahn, E., & Morris, H. L. (1968). Diagnosis and therapy. In D. R. Spriestersbach & D. Sherman (Eds.), *Cleft palate and communication* (pp. 225–268). New York: Academic Press.

Shelton, R. L., Lindquist, A. F., Arndt, W. B., Elbert, M., & Youngstrom, K. A. (1971). Effect of speech bulb reduction on movement of the posterior wall of the pharynx and posture of the tongue. *Cleft Palate Journal*, 8, 10–17.

Shelton, R. L., Lindquist, A. F., Chisum, L., Arndt, W. B., Youngstrom, K. A., & Stick, S. L. (1968). Effect of prosthetic speech bulb reduction on articulation. *Cleft Palate Journal*, 5, 195–204.

Shprintzen, R. J., Lencione, R. M., McCall, G. N., & Skolnick, M. L. (1974). A three-dimensional cinefluoroscopic analysis of velopharyngeal closure during speech and nonspeech activities in normals. *Cleft Palate Journal*, 11, 412–428.

Siegel-Sadewitz, V. L., & Shprintzen, R. J. (1982). Nasopharyngoscopy of the normal velopharyngeal sphincter: An experiment of biofeedback. *Cleft Palate Journal*, 19(3), 194–200.

Stemple, J. C., Weiler, E., Whitehead, W., & Komray, R. (1980). Electromyographic biofeedback training with patients exhibiting a hyperfunctional voice disorder. *Laryngoscope*, 90(3), 471–476.

Tachimura, T., Nohara, K., Fujita, Y., Hara, H., & Wada, T. (2001). Change in levator veli palatini muscle activity of normal speakers in association with elevation of the velum using an experimental palatal lift prosthesis. *Cleft Palate-Craniofacial Journal*, 38(5), 449–454.

Tash, E. L., Shelton, R. L., Knox, A. W., & Michel, J. F. (1971). Training voluntary pharyngeal wall movements in children with normal and inadequate velopharyngeal closure. *Cleft Palate Journal*, 8, 277–290.

Tomes, L., Kuehn, D., & Peterson-Falzone, S. (1996, April). Behavioral therapy for speakers with velopharyngeal impairment. *NCVS Status and Progress Report*, 9, 159–180.

Van Riper, C. (1946). *Speech correction: Principles and methods*. New York: Prentice-Hall.

Van Riper, C. (1963). *Speech correction: Principles and methods* (4th ed.). New York: Prentice-Hall.

Weber, J., Jobe, R. P., & Chase, R. A. (1970). Evaluation of muscle stimulation in the rehabilitation of patients with hypernasal speech. *Plastic and Reconstructive Surgery*, 46, 173–174.

Weiss, C. E. (1971). Success of an obturator reduction program. *Cleft Palate Journal*, 8, 291–297.

Weiss, T., Carson, L. F., & Brady, J. P. (1979). Effects of training schedule and biofeedback on speech dysfluency. *American Journal of Psychiatry*, 136(3), 342–344.

Wells, C. (1945). Improving the speech of the cleft palate child. *Journal of Speech Disorders*, 10, 162.

Wells, C. (1948). Practical techniques for speech training for cleft palate cases. *Journal of Speech and Hearing Disorders*, 13, 71.

Witzel, M. A., Tobe, J., & Salyer, K. (1988). The use of nasopharyngoscopy biofeedback therapy in the correction of inconsistent velopharyngeal closure. *International Journal of Pediatric Otorhinolaryngology*, 15(2), 137–142.

Witzel, M. A., Tobe, J., & Salyer, K. E. (1989). The use of videonasopharyngoscopy for biofeedback therapy in adults after pharyngeal flap surgery. *Cleft Palate Journal*, 26(2), 129–134; Discussion 135.

Wolfaardt, J. F., Wilson, F. B., Rochet, A., & McPhee, L. (1993). An appliance-based approach to the management of palatopharyngeal incompetency: A clinical pilot project. *Journal of Prosthetic Dentistry*, 69(2), 186–195.

Yorkston, K. M., Spencer, K. A., Duffy, J. R., Beukelman, D. R., Golper, L. A., Miller,

R. M., et al. (2001). Evidence-based practice guidelines for dysarthria: Management of velopharyngeal function. *Journal of Medical Speech-Language Pathology, 9*(4), 257–273.

Ysunza, A., Pamplona, C., & Toledo, E. (1992). Change in velopharyngeal valving after speech therapy in cleft palate patients. A videonasopharyngoscopic and multiview videofluoroscopic study. *International Journal of Pediatric Otorhinolaryngology, 24*(1), 45–54.

Ysunza, A., Pamplona, M., Femat, T., Mayer, I., & Garcia-Velasco, M. (1997). Videonasopharyngoscopy as an instrument for visual biofeedback during speech in cleft palate patients. *International Journal of Pediatric Otorhinolaryngology, 41*(3), 291–298.

Ysunza-Rivera, A., Pamplona-Ferreira, M. C., & Toledo-Cortina, E. (1991). [Changes in valvular movements of the velopharyngeal sphincter after speech therapy in children with cleft palate. A videonasopharyngoscopic and videofluoroscopic study of multiple incidence]. *Boletin Medico del Hospital Infantile de Mexico, 48*(7), 490–501.

Yules, R. B., & Chase, R. A. (1969). A training method for reduction of hypernasality in speech. *Plastic and Reconstructive Surgery, 43*(2), 180–185.

APPENDIX 21–1

SPEECH STIMULATION INFORMATION FOR PARENTS

The following suggestions are meant to assist you in working with your child on speech production:

Encourage your child to produce a variety of different sounds during cooing babbling, and vocal play by imitating his/her vocalizations.

Encourage your child to imitate specific speech sounds (consonants), then single words, phrases, and sentences. Speech sounds are learned in a general order of easiest to most difficult. A general order is: /p/, /b/, /m/, /t/, /d/, /n/, /k/, and /g/. Note: If there is a cleft palate, your child will only be able to produce nasal sounds (/m/, /n/, and /ng/) until the palate is closed. Once the palate is closed, concentrate on the rest of these sounds.

When your child can produce most of the first group of sounds easily, then start on more difficult sounds, such as: /f/, /v/, /l/, /s/, /z/, /sh/, /ch/, /j/. Sounds such as /r/ and /th/ are usually learned last.

When practicing the sound (in isolation, in words, or in sentences), use some sort of "token" for reinforcement. For example, each time your child says the sound correctly, he or she gets a token (penny, poker chip, small piece from a game, etc.). Hold the token up by your mouth so he/she is looking at your mouth. Produce the sound or word and have him/her imitate it. If he/she imitates the sound and it is close to correct, say "Good talking!" and put the token in a container (so he/she won't play with the tokens while you are working). A plastic bottle works well because the child can see the tokens and hear them go in, but can't get his/her hands in there to play with them. Having other children or adults play the "game" with the child can increase motivation. In addition, he/she can hear more correct (and purposefully incorrect at times) productions, which can affect progress. Tokens can be collected or traded in for little prizes, such as a sticker, balloon, gum, etc.

Play games, such as Go Fish or Candy Land, but have the child win five tokens (by saying five sounds) before he or she can make his/her move. All other players must do the same.

When working on certain speech sounds, use the following sequence:

- Practice the sound by itself. For example, with the sound /b/, have the child put his or her lips together, build up air pressure, and then release the sound. When your child can make this sound correctly at least 95% of the time, then you can move on to the next step.
- Practice the sound in syllables, with the sound being at the beginning of the

syllable (ba), at the end of the syllable (ab), and in the middle of the syllable (aba). When your child can do this correctly at least 95% of the time, move on to the next step.

- Practice the sound in words, with the sound being at the beginning of the word (bat), in the middle of the word (rabbit) and at the end of the word (tub). When your child can do this correctly at least 95% of the time, move on to the next step.
- Practice the sound in phrases or short sentences. It is most helpful to keep the same phrase or sentence for all of the words at first. For example: "I see the _____. I found the _____." When your child can do this correctly at least 95% of the time, then you can move on to the next step.
- Practice the sound in sentences. You can look in your child's books for some words that have the sounds that you are working on. Have him/her practice "reading" from the books. At this point, you can begin to point out the sound in situations other than practice situations. For example, practice the "b" when you are playing with bubbles or boats or when you have bubble gum.
- Once the child is producing the sound correctly in practice, you will find that he/she will start to use the sound spontaneously. Periodically comment when the child has produced the sound correctly, and periodically correct the child as well.

C H A P T E R

22

CLEFT LIP/PALATE MISSIONS TO DEVELOPING COUNTRIES

INTRODUCTION

Cleft lip and palate (CLP) is one of the most common of all birth defects, occurring in approximately 1 out of 700 live births. Considering the annual birth rates of the world, it is estimated that there are well over a quarter of a million babies born each year with cleft lip and palate (Lee, 1999). Several babies will be born with a cleft in the time that it takes to read this chapter.

Because cleft lip and palate affects facial appearance and speech, this birth defect has a major impact on a fundamental human need; that is, the need for social interaction and communication with others. Surgical repair is therefore necessary so that the individual is able to fulfill this basic need. Certainly, surgical repair of a cleft will result in improved quality of life for the individual.

In developed nations such as the United States, children born with cleft lip and palate receive surgical treatment at an early age. As a result, we are not accustomed to seeing individuals with open clefts in public. In developing countries, however, surgical services are often not available, especially to patients who live outside of the cities. In some cases, this is due to a lack of trained surgeons in the area. However, it is most often due to a lack of organization, inadequate funding for equipment and technology, and lack of focus on conditions that are not life threatening (Bermudez, 2004). Even when services are available, most families do not have the financial resources to pay for the surgery. Because of these problems and the fact that a cleft is not a fatal condition, many individuals in developing nations go through life with unrepaired clefts, and carry with them the aesthetic and functional problems that go with this condition.

This chapter will provide information on how some organizations are attempting to meet the needs of the world's population of individuals with cleft lip and palate through surgical missions. In addition, this chapter will provide information for clinicians who are interested in becoming speech-language pathology volunteers on international missions.

CLEFT PALATE MISSIONS

Purpose of Mission Organizations

To address the needs of children from around the world who are born with clefts or craniofacial conditions, several nonprofit or not-for-profit volunteer organizations have been formed in the United States (Interplast, Operation Smile, Operacion Esperanza, Rotoplast, Smile Train, etc.) and in other countries. These organizations send teams of professionals to countries with less-developed health care. Over a period of weeks, these teams provide services to individuals with cleft lip and palate who cannot otherwise obtain or afford the surgery.

Most organizations have two main goals. The first goal is to provide direct service for affected individuals. However, 100 surgeries will only help 100 patients (and their families). Most organizations recognize that to make a lasting impact, it is important to train in-country professionals to provide the same services. By teaching local surgeons cleft lip and palate repair techniques, these surgeons can then treat their own patients in their own countries and train others to do the same. Therefore, over time, there is less need for international support (Abenavoli, 2005; Lefevre, Stricker, Doan, & Stricker, 1999; Micheau & Lauwers, 1999; Ruiz-Razura, Cronin, & Navarro, 2000).

The need for education is not limited to the surgical team members. Many countries do not have speech-language pathologists, but have psychologists or other health care professionals who are interested in learning what they can to help children with speech disorders. Even when there are local speech-language pathologists (or similar professionals), these individuals may not be well trained in cleft management. Therefore, individual and group training, seminars, lectures, handouts, and books are greatly appreciated by the local professionals.

In 1997, the International Task Force on Volunteer Cleft Missions outlined recommendations for volunteer cleft missions based on (1) mission objectives, (2) organization, (3) personal health and liability, (4) funding, (5) use of trainees in volunteer cleft missions, and (6) public relations. They agreed that the main goals for these missions are "to provide top-quality surgical service, train local doctors and staff, develop and nurture fledgling cleft programs, and, finally, make new friends" (Yeow et al., 2002).

Concerns and Criticisms of Mission Organizations

Although most organizations subscribe to the above goals, some achieve these goals better than others. In addition, there have been criticisms about the way some of the missions operate (Silver, 2000). These criticisms include the following:

- Not using qualified local surgeons, which would be far less costly than sending surgeons from outside the country

- Using volunteers who are not qualified or not considered experts (i.e., using cosmetic surgeons who do not do cleft palate repairs in their practice)

- Using missions as training ground for residents who need more surgical experience

- Doing too many surgeries to keep numbers high

- Performing some cosmetic surgery during the mission

- Performing surgery on children who would not be considered healthy enough to qualify for surgery in the United States

- Not having records available for returning patients

- Not providing adequate follow-up after the team leaves

- Not providing enough training of in-country professionals

- Having a high rate of fistulas or velopharyngeal insufficiency after palate repair

- Spending too much money on administration and overhead, and not enough money on direct patient care

Another concern is that there are no studies of outcomes from these missions, so the actual success rates and complication rates are unknown. Because of this, there is an urgent need for more randomized clinical trials to evaluate both the outcomes of treatment and the complications so that clinical guidelines and protocols can be developed based on strong evidence (Lee, 1999).

Because some mission organizations are better than others, the prospective team member should learn as much as possible about the organization and also consider the following factors:

- Reputation of the organization

- Financial support of the organization

- Quality of procedures, policies, and structure

- Qualifications of the team members

- Method and priority systems for choosing cases

- Number of procedures typically done per surgeon

- Types of procedures done on a mission: cosmetic vs. reconstructive

- Method of record keeping

- Method for follow-up

- Involvement of team members in teaching and training in-country professionals

- Experience of others who have been on mission trips

Typical Team Members

Because cleft lip and palate is a complex condition and surgery requires a variety of professionals, mission teams can be very large. The professional members usually include the following:

1. Plastic surgeons and/or otolaryngologists

2. Anesthesiologists and/or nurse anesthetists

3. Medical students and/or residents

4. Nurses—surgical, post-anesthesia care, postoperative

5. Intensivist and/or pediatrician

6. Dentist and/or orthodontist and/or prosthodontist

7. Speech-language pathologist

In addition to the clinical professionals, many additional people are needed to provide coordination and support. These include the following:

1. Team coordinator

2. Biomedical technician

3. Child life specialist

4. Medical records workers

5. Education coordinator

6. Interpreters

7. Volunteers

In many cases, the team members do not know each other prior to the mission, and therefore have not developed the trust and respect that comes from working on a well-established team over time. However, all are committed to one purpose, and that is helping as many patients as possible. This is done by working very long days under less-than-ideal conditions. This shared dedication and experience actually helps the team to bond and work well together in a very short period of time.

Typical Schedules

Mission trips are at least a week in length, but most are two weeks or longer. During the first few days in the country, it is necessary to evaluate the patients and determine which ones are candidates for surgery, dental treatment, or prosthetic devices. During this time, the nurses are very busy setting up the operating and recovery rooms.

Once the screening of patients is complete and the operating rooms are ready, the rest of the days are devoted to direct treatment, including surgeries, dental and prosthodontic treatment, and speech counseling. Due to the sheer volume of patients who usually present for surgery, the majority of the surgeries tend to be primary lip and palate repairs. Therefore, if the palate is not sufficient after the primary surgery, many patients are not offered surgery again due to a lack of adequate resources. One mission group that was performing surgeries in the Philippines was concerned about the high rate of VPI with their palate repairs and the difficulty of doing secondary surgery. Therefore, they began doing a simultaneous Orticochea sphincteroplasty with the palate repair. They reported better speech outcomes as a result of this practice (Saboye, Chancholle, Tournier, & Maurette, 2004).

Education of in-country professionals occurs during both the diagnostic and treatment periods. A few of the nurses and physicians usually stay a few extra days after others have left to provide postoperative care for the last surgical patients.

Although mission trips are mostly work, there is also some play. Usually, there is a day or two off over the weekends for rest and relaxation. Some organizations will plan short trips or tours to entertain the team members. This is also a good time for shopping and for sampling the local culture and cuisine.

PREPARING TO GO

Know Your Stuff

Speech-language pathologists who work on cleft palate mission teams should all be able to meet at least the minimum requirements for practicing in the United States, and this includes having a master's degree in speech-language pathology. It is highly preferable that the person also has a Certificate of Clinical Competence (CCC) through the American Speech-Language-Hearing Association, as well as several years of clinical experience. Pediatric experience is particularly valuable.

Even with all the required qualifications and several years of experience, the speech-language pathologist can still be at a loss when it comes to working with the population of children with clefts and craniofacial anomalies. Therefore, those who are interested in serving on a mission team should seek additional specialty training in this area (D'Antonio & Landis, 1994; Ducote, 1998, 2005; Ducote & Juul, 1998).

It is important for the speech-language pathologist to have knowledge of and experience not only with cleft palate, but also with resonance disorders and velopharyngeal dysfunction. This knowledge is essential to have when being called upon to make decisions regarding candidates for secondary management of velopharyngeal insufficiency. The "Parameters" document of the American Cleft Palate-Craniofacial Association (1993a) can be a helpful resource for understanding basic standards of care. Finally, the speech-language pathologist can prepare for the trip by listening to the speech samples of nasal emission and hypernasality that can be found on the American Cleft Palate-Craniofacial Association Web site (ACPA, 2006b).

Learn about the Culture and Language

Prior to the mission trip, it is important to learn about the culture and language of the host country. As ambassadors of goodwill and humanitarian aid, the team members should make every effort to understand and respect the country's social customs and protocols (Yeow et al., 2002). Team members should know what behaviors are considered polite and what are considered impolite. The role of women in certain societies is important to consider when working with the families. Even if you do not speak the language, it is important to learn how to say "thank you," to memorize certain greetings and phrases, and to know the standard form of addressing children and adults (i.e., señor, señora, etc.).

On a practical note, it may be helpful for the prospective team member to learn about the food in the host country, especially if he/she has allergies or strong aversions to certain types of food. Knowledge about the currency and whether bargaining is expected is helpful when shopping.

Basic knowledge of the language and culture can help the team member to be more effective as a service provider and a good representative of his/her home country. It can also make trip more interesting and enjoyable.

Documents That You Need

Of course, all individuals must have a passport in order to travel to a foreign country. Some countries also require a visa. This should be determined months before the trip because it often takes that amount of time to obtain a visa. It is also wise to take a copy of your immunization records, written information regarding allergies or special medical issues, and the name and phone number of a contact person in case of emergency. It is always a good idea to keep copies of all travel documents in your suitcase and another set of copies at home.

Protect Your Health

Different parts of the world have different health risks for the traveler. Therefore, the team members should determine what the risks are and what precautions need to be taken prior to each mission trip. The Web site for the Centers for Disease Control and Prevention (2006) provides specific information, by geographic region, on risks for diseases, insect bites, and food and water contamination. Recommendations for prevention and treatment are also noted.

In general, the traveler should determine what vaccinations are recommended for that region of the world and receive them several weeks prior to the trip. Yellow fever and typhoid vaccinations are commonly recommended. Often the vaccinations are only available through a local health department.

If the mission will be in a tropical area, most authorities recommend using an insect repellent, particularly those containing DEET (N, N-diethylmetatoluamide), and malaria pills. Clothing to cover arms and legs is also suggested.

Water is often a risk in developing countries. If this is the case, it is best to avoid drinks with ice, as well as salads or raw vegetables (because they are rinsed in water). A toothbrush should be rinsed with bottled water rather than tap water. It is also wise to avoid swallowing water in the shower.

What to Pack

When packing for the mission trip, it is good to consider both comfort and culture. Because the days are usually very long, and there may be a lot of walking or standing in the hospital, comfortable shoes are a must. Many people retain water when traveling and therefore, loose shoes and clothes are preferable.

When selecting clothing, it helps to consider the climate and the probable lack of air conditioning or adequate heating. The cultural norms of dress should also be considered. For example, in Nicaragua, women do not wear pants. Therefore, loose fitting, comfortable, washable, and preferably inexpensive skirts and dresses should be worn by female team members when working with families.

For many countries, toilet paper is a luxury and not usually provided in public restrooms. Therefore, small packs of tissues should be taken because they fit well in a fanny pack or pocket.

In most cases, the speech-language pathologist must not only take clothing and personal items, but must also take everything that will be needed to work with the patients. A suggested list of items to take for clinical use is found in Table 22–1. A small rolling suitcase can be particularly useful for serving as a portable storage unit for all clinical supplies. It is best to take your "supply cabinet" back to the hotel at night because things that are left unattended usually disappear.

Expected Costs

As a volunteer, the team member is usually expected to cover some of the costs of travel. This may be done by paying a set amount up front, or by paying directly for a portion of airfare, hotel, and food. Typically, many meals are provided, particularly breakfast and lunch during screening and surgery days.

In addition to direct costs of travel, lodging, and food, there is also the cost of time for the volunteer team members. Most organizations require the employee to take vacation days for the time away from work for the mission trip.

THE SPEECH-LANGUAGE PATHOLOGIST ON A MISSION TEAM

It would seem that the speech-language pathologist would be a key member of the mission team, especially since the primary reason to repair a cleft palate is for speech.

TABLE 22–1 Items to Take for Clinical Use
• Tongue blades
• Dental mirror
• Pen lights and batteries
• Alcohol preps or cloths
• Hand sanitizer
• Box of gloves
• Tissues
• Plastic tubing—precut
• Bending straws
• Cleft palate bottles and nipples
• Therapy tokens
• Rewards (sticker sheets, safety pops, etc.)
• Handouts and diagrams of the anatomy (in the appropriate language)
• Lavaliere for pen and pen light
• Office supplies: pens, legal pad, paper clips, stapler, etc.
• Scrubs (for observing in surgery)
• Giveaways for parents (pens, hotel-sized toiletries, note cards, etc.)
• Camera
• Fanny pack
• Tote bag or small suitcase on rollers

In addition, a speech-language pathologist may be important because many individuals continue to have speech problems after the palate repair due to velopharyngeal insufficiency. The persistent speech problem can affect social, educational, and vocational opportunities. In some cultures, it can even exclude the individual from the mainstream of society (D'Antonio & Landis, 1994).

Despite these facts, not all mission organizations include a speech-language pathologist on their teams. One reason is that a speech evaluation is not needed to determine that a cleft needs to be repaired. In addition, secondary surgery for velopharyngeal dysfunction is often not done on these trips given the number of unrepaired clefts that need surgery, the risks of airway obstruction and sleep apnea with secondary surgery, and the lack of a means to follow these children postoperatively. Finally, despite the fact that speech therapy is usually needed following a palate repair, it cannot be done during the time of the mission trip.

Despite these limitations, the speech-language pathologist can be a very valuable member of the mission team because he or she can screen patients and determine which patients have the best chance of success with a palate repair and secondary surgery, if that is done. The speech-language pathologist can also serve to educate professionals and families on how to work with children after the surgery. The particular speech-language pathology activities are noted in the following sections.

Working with an Interpreter

Because speech-language pathologists work by interacting and talking with families and patients, a good interpreter is essential if the speech-language pathologist is not fluent in the country's language. The speech-language pathologist should meet with the interpreters as soon as possible after arriving at the mission site. Spending time with the interpreters prior to seeing patients will help the process to go more smoothly and save a great deal of time during screening. For specific tips in working with an interpreter, see Table 22–2.

Ideally, the interpreters should be given some written "scripts" of what will be asked or said during the evaluation and later, during the family counseling (Ducote, 1998, 2005; Ducote & Juul, 1998). It is important to make sure that the interpreter understands the information and the procedure that you want to follow.

TABLE 22–2 Tips for Working with an Interpreter
• Address remarks and questions directly to the listener, not to the interpreter.
• Use simple terms and short sentences.
• Avoid technical language, idioms, expressions, or slang.
• Pause frequently so that the interpreter can keep up.
• Use a positive tone and facial expression.
• Avoid body language or facial expressions that may be offensive or misconstrued.
• Periodically check the listener's understanding. Encourage him/her to request clarification when something is not understood.
• Reinforce understanding with visual diagrams and information written in the listener's language.

Note: The interpreter should interpret the information in the first person, as if you are talking directly to the person.
Source: Adapted from a handout of the Culture Competence Committee, Speech Pathology Department, Cincinnati Children's Hospital Medical Center, 2006.

In addition to reviewing what the interpreters will say, it is also good to learn some words and phrases from the interpreters. Knowing how to introduce yourself can enhance your interaction with the families. It helps to know the name of your profession in that country's language and to learn some basic words or sentences to use in the assessment (i.e., "Count to 20." "Open your mouth." "Stick out your tongue." "Say 'aaah.'").

Screening Procedures

On most mission trips, there are hundreds of children, including older children and even some adults, who need to be evaluated for possible surgery (Figure 22–1 A–H). These patients often travel long distances to be seen and are willing to wait for hours, and even days, in hopes of receiving treatment (Figure 22–2 A and B).

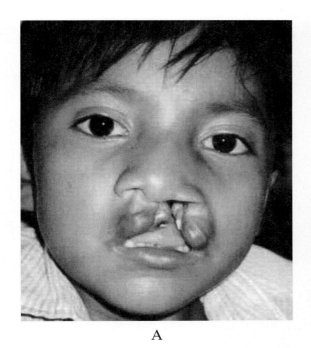

A

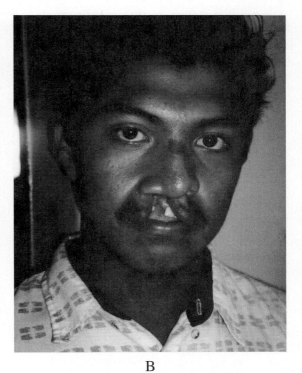

B

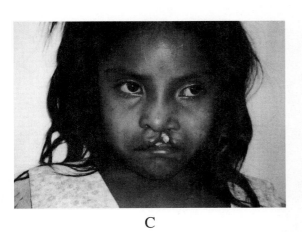

C

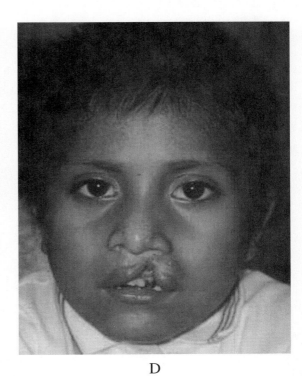

D

FIGURE 22–1 (A–H) Examples of older patients with
unrepaired clefts. (*continues*)

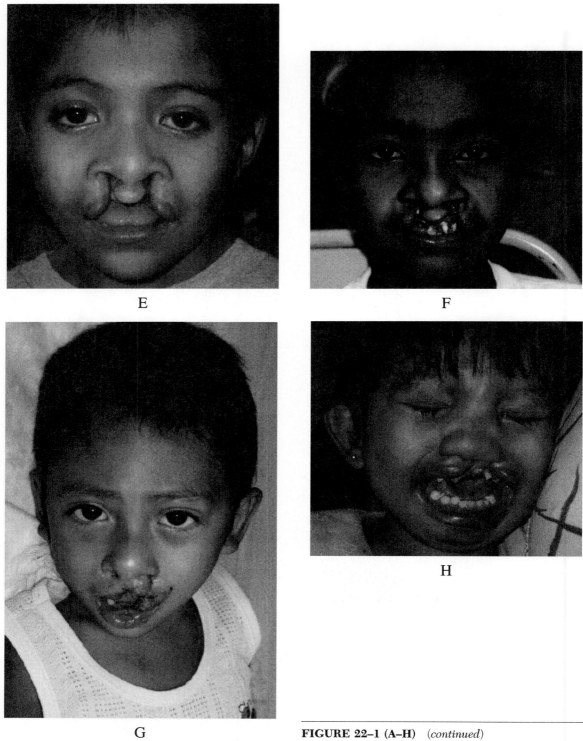

E

F

G

H

FIGURE 22–1 (A–H) *(continued)*

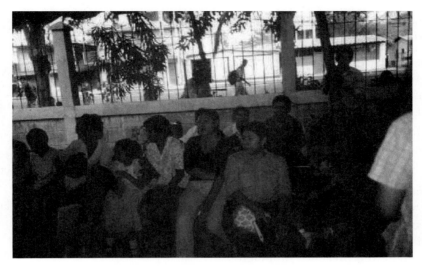

A

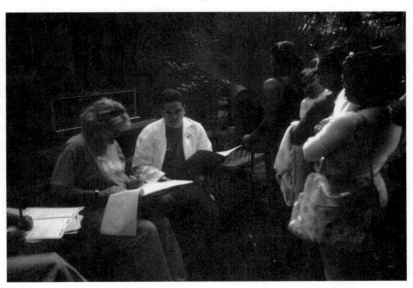

B

FIGURE 22–2 (A and B) Patients waiting for screening.

Because of the volume of patients that need to be seen, the screening has to be very fast and efficient. It's not uncommon to have to screen 100 patients or more in one day. Assuming a 10-hour day, this leaves six minutes per patient if there are no breaks for lunch or the restroom. Realistically, there may be no more than three to five minutes to do a speech assessment on each patient. This is particularly challenging if the speech-language pathologist is not fluent in the language and has to work through an interpreter.

To make the process as quick and efficient as possible, here are some suggestions:

- Before the patient comes to you, have a translator fill in identifying information and the answers to the screening questions on the screening form.

- Have a volunteer to manage the line and keep patients coming quickly, with their screening forms in hand.

- Do an intraoral examination first. (With an open cleft palate, you may not need to assess speech because you already know the individual needs a palate repair.) Particularly note the presence of a cleft, fistula, or previous surgery for velopharyngeal dysfunction.

- Ask the patient to count to 20 in his/her language. Have the patient repeat syllables with high pressure phonemes repetitively (i.e., pa, pa, pa; pi, pi, pi; sa, sa, sa; si, si, si, etc.).

- Evaluate for the presence of obligatory and compensatory articulation productions, hypernasality, and nasal emission.

- Complete the screening form and note additional comments in margins.

- Include recommendations for the following: surgery and type, prosthetic device and type, a more in-depth assessment, speech therapy, and parent counseling regarding speech-language stimulation techniques.

- For babies with open palates who are not yet candidates for a palate repair, give a written handout consisting of feeding instructions and suggestions for special bottles and nipples. Have a translator review the instructions. (Tell the parent to use boiled water for cleaning and for dry formula.)

Procedures During Surgery Days

Because therapy is not a quick fix and kids who are undergoing surgery cannot participate in therapy, speech therapy is not a primary focus during a mission. This does not mean that the speech-language pathologist has nothing to do.

During surgery week, the speech-language pathologist should (1) work with a dentist, orthodontist, or prosthodontist to determine those patients who are candidates for prosthetic devices; (2) make sure that the devices fit appropriately to maximize speech; and (3) help the patient learn to use the device. Surgery days are also an appropriate time to do lectures and in-service training for local professionals. It can be valuable to visit local schools for consultations or even have an open speech clinic for any children in the area with speech disorders.

Another important task during surgery days is to work with the families and counsel them regarding cleft issues (Figure 22–3). The families may have various beliefs regarding the cause of the cleft, including God's will, past sins, becoming pregnant during a full moon, or having hiccups during pregnancy (Weatherley-White, Eiserman, Beddoe, & Vanderberg, 2005). Therefore, counseling regarding the cause and the importance of good nutrition during pregnancy can be of benefit to the families. The speech-language pathologist should also counsel parents regarding methods of speech and language stimulation for children under the age of 3, and counsel parents regarding methods of speech stimulation for children over 3 or for those undergoing palate repair. Information should be given regarding normal velopharyngeal closure and the effects of a cleft palate on this closure. Diagrams and handouts are particularly important, and should be written in the parents' language.

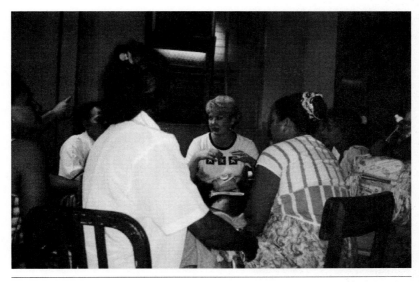

FIGURE 22–3 Counseling families in groups.

A procedure for doing the counseling is as follows:

- Set up a space near the surgical waiting area for group counseling.

- Obtain the surgery schedule for the day.

- Talk with parents in groups of five to seven while their children are in surgery.*

- Using the surgery schedule, check off the patient's name after the parents have been counseled.

- The day after surgery, meet in a group with all patients who have had a palate repair or flap/sphincter and their parents. Repeat counseling but direct it toward the older children. Demonstrate normal airflow and therapy correction techniques.

If there is any downtime between working on speech appliances, counseling families, and

teaching, it is expected that the clinician and all other team members will assist with other aspects of the team's work as needed (Ducote, 2005) (Figure 22–4).

Speech Pathology Follow-Up

The cleft palate mission concept works especially well for patients who require a lip repair, because the surgery is done primarily for aesthetic reasons and requires little follow-up. However, for children undergoing cleft palate repair, postoperative speech therapy is usually needed for the desired speech outcomes. This is because prior to the palate repair, the child cannot engage in typical oral-motor activities, such as sucking, cooing, and babbling. Speech therapy is often required after the palate has been repaired because these children have missed a critical period of sensorimotor speech learning and need help in gaining the necessary skills for speech. In addition, compensatory articulation productions often develop due to the open palate or persistent velopharyngeal

*For the counseling sessions, try to use the same interpreter. After doing the interpretation many times, some interpreters can then do the counseling on their own.

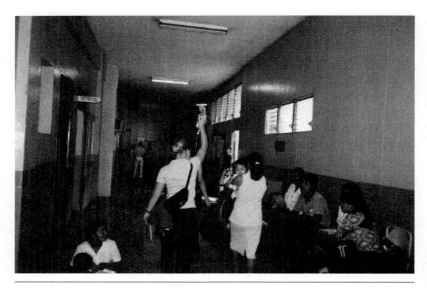

FIGURE 22–4 Helping out with other duties when necessary. In this case, the child needed someone to hold the IV bag while he walked to surgery because poles and gurneys were unavailable in the hospital.

insufficiency. Therefore, to maximize the outcome of the palate surgery, speech therapy is usually indicated as soon as possible after the palate repair.

Unfortunately, very few children in developing countries have the opportunity to receive speech therapy following a palate repair. This is due to the fact that speech-language pathologists are not available, or they are not affordable.

One organization that has been attempting to solve this problem is RSF-EARTHSPEAK. Cofounded by speech-language pathologist Andrea (Andi) Jobe, M.A., CCC, and her husband, plastic surgeon Richard Jobe, M.D., FACS, EARTHSPEAK provides programs in developing countries that train parents (or other caregivers) to work with their child after the palate is repaired (RSF-EARTHSPEAK, 2006). Training occurs in a week-long speech camp where both the child and trainer attend. At these camps, as many as 40 children receive group instruction with their caregivers (Jobe, 2005).

Of course, training parents in a week's time to provide "speech therapy" is not possible, especially since many are illiterate. Therefore, EARTHSPEAK has developed a method called "Corrective Babbling," which is a programmed approach that takes no clinical judgment. Trainers are taught how to follow a step-by-step program outlined for them in a training manual in their native language (RSF-EARTH-SPEAK, 2006). Speech sounds that are specific to the native language are presented in a developmental sequence in the training manual. The child learns to imitate the trainer in the production of early sounds in babbling sequences and then to produce later sounds in more complex phonemic combinations.

The theory of Corrective Babbling is that the sensorimotor learning that normally occurs through babbling during a time of cerebral neuroplasticity helps the child to build cortical pathways. With the Corrective Babbling approach, this sensorimotor learning is replicated so that new cortical pathways are established. Once the sounds are produced normally, they are carefully reconnected into meaningful language (Jobe, 2005). Essentially, the goal of Corrective Babbling is to extinguish old speech patterns and rebuild new ones through repetitions and success at each level.

This Corrective Babbling method is relatively new. Therefore, research is needed before generalizations can be made. However, the early outcomes have been very promising. This method is consistent with the second goal of most mission organizations, which is to teach the local people so that they become self-sufficient. Certainly, a system that can effectively provide speech treatment for children who have had cleft palate repair in developing nations would be a major contribution to those born with a cleft palate (Jobe, 2005).

SUMMARY

There are many organizations that send mission teams to do cleft repair in developing countries. Most organizations realize that educating in-country professionals is the best way to effect long-term change.

Speech-language pathologists can serve on these teams by providing input on which patients are best candidates for surgery. In addition, they can counsel families during the mission, and train local professionals. Speech therapy is not realistic on these trips given the limited time available. However, the Corrective Babbling method of training parents and caregivers holds promise for the future.

For those who have served on a mission team, most will say that it is a remarkable experience that can change your life. You have the opportunity to work with a group of people who may come from all around the world. All have a strong sense of purpose, dedication, and caring. They start out as strangers, but quickly become friends.

Perhaps the biggest joy, however, is working with children and families who have so little, but are so happy and grateful for what they have. By giving our time and efforts to them, we get so much more in return!

FOR REVIEW, DISCUSSION, AND CRITICAL THINKING

1. Why do you think that there is a need for surgical mission trips to various parts of the world for treatment of cleft lip and palate? Knowing what you do about the causes of clefts, why do you think the need is greater in some parts of the world than in others?

2. What are the typical goals of organizations that send teams to developing countries? Why do you think education is important?

3. List the typical clinical and support team members that would be needed on a mission trip. What would be the role for each? What would be the particular challenges for each professional on a mission team?

4. Other than the obvious, why is it particularly important to be knowledgeable about cleft palate management prior to going on a mission trip? Why is learning about the language and culture also important?

5. Pretend you are planning to go on your first mission trip. What would you need to do to prepare? What would you take?

6. Describe what you would do to screen a large number of patients who speak a language that you do not know.

7. What would you do on a mission trip while children are in surgery or in post-operative care? What can you do to maximize the long-term impact of your time and efforts?

8. What are the issues of palate repair at an older age when speech pathology services are not available? What are the challenges of obtaining postoperative speech therapy for patients who have a palate repair through one of these missions?

9. In lieu of regular speech pathology services, what can be offered to families of children following the palate repair? What is the theory behind "Corrective Babbling?" What are the potential advantages and disadvantages of parents being trained to work with the child following surgery?

REFERENCES

Abenavoli, F. M. (2005). Operation Smile humanitarian missions. *Plastic and Reconstructive Surgery, 115*(1), 356–357.

American Cleft Palate-Craniofacial Association. (1993a). Parameters for evaluation and treatment of patients with cleft lip/palate or other craniofacial anomalies. *American Cleft Palate-Craniofacial Journal, 30*(Suppl. 1), 1–16.

American Cleft Palate-Craniofacial Association. (1993b). *Parameters for evaluation and treatment of patients with cleft lip/palate or other craniofacial anomalies.* Retrieved on March 6, 2007 from http://cleftpalate-craniofacial.org/acpa/arecfrm.html

Bermudez, L. E. (2004). Humanitarian missions in the third world. *Plastic and Reconstructive Surgery, 114*(6), 1687–1689; Author reply 1689.

Centers for Disease Control and Prevention. (2006). *Travelers' health.* Retrieved on March 6, 2007 from http://www.cdc.gov/travel/vaccinat.htm

D'Antonio, L. L., and Landis, P. (1994). *Speech-language pathology services for the individual with cleft lip/palate: A training manual for volunteers to develop-ing nations.* Chapel Hill, NC: American Cleft Palate-Craniofacial Association.

Ducote, C. A. (1998). Speech-language pathology services for individuals with cleft lip/palate in less developed nations: The Operation Smile approach. American Speech-Language-Hearing Association Special Interest Division 5, *Speech Science and Orofacial Disorders, 8*(1),12–14.

Ducote, C. A. (2005). *Evaluation and treatment of cleft palate speech in developing countries: The Operation Smile approach.* Paper presented at the American Speech and Hearing Association Annual Convention, San Diego, CA.

Ducote, C. A., & Juul, A. M. (1998). *Guidelines for speech-language pathology volunteers on Operation Smile international missions.* New Orleans, LA: Operation Smile Speech Therapy Council.

Jobe, A. (2005). *Corrective babbling technique.* Paper presented at the American Speech and Hearing Association Annual Convention, San Diego, CA.

Lee, S. T. (1999). New treatment and research strategies for the improvement of care of cleft lip and palate patients in the new millennium. *Annals of the Academy of Medicine, Singapore, 28*(5), 760–767.

Lefevre, J. C., Stricker, M., Doan, G. D., & Stricker, C. (1999). Chirurgie des fentes labio-maxillo-palatines en mission humanitaire aux Philippines. *Annales de Chirurgie Plastique et Esthetique, 44*(1), 41–45.

Micheau, P., & Lauwers, F. (1999). Quels objectifs pour une mission humanitaire de chirurgie plastique reparatrice? *Annales de Chirurgie Plastique et Esthetique, 44*(1), 19–26.

RSF-EARTHSPEAK. (2006). RSF-EARTHSPEAK homepage. Retrieved March 6, 2007 from http://www.rsf-earthspeak.org/index.html

Ruiz-Razura, A., Cronin, E. D., & Navarro, C. E. (2000). Creating long-term benefits in cleft lip and palate volunteer missions. *Plastic and Reconstructive Surgery, 105*(1), 195–201.

Saboye, J., Chancholle, A. R., Tournier, J. J., & Maurette, I. (2004). Palatovelopharyngoplastie en un temps. Notre experience aux Philippines. *Annales de Chirurgie Plastique et Esthetique, 49*(3), 261–264.

Silver, L. (2000). Creating long-term benefits in cleft lip and palate volunteer missions. *Plastic and Reconstructive Surgery, 106*(2), 516–517.

Weatherley-White, R. C., Eiserman, W., Beddoe, M., & Vanderberg, R. (2005). Perceptions, expectations, and reactions to cleft lip and palate surgery in native populations: A pilot study in rural India. *Cleft Palate-Craniofacial Journal, 42*(5), 560–564.

Yeow, V. K., Lee, S. T., Lambrecht, T. J., Barnett, J., Gorney, M., Hardjowasito, W., et al. (2002). International Task Force on Volunteer Cleft Missions. *Journal of Craniofacial Surgery, 13*(1), 18–25.

Appendix A: Resources for Parent Information and Support

Resources for information regarding cleft lip and palate and craniofacial anomalies are available from a variety of sources. The following is a list of some of the national organizations that can be helpful in providing information and resources. This list is not inclusive by any means. In fact, there are many local and state organizations that can provide information and support. Information on other organizations and resources can be found on many of the Web sites listed.

AboutFace is an organization of individuals and families who have experienced the challenges of facial differences. This organization provides emotional support, information services, and educational programs about living with facial differences. AboutFace focuses on syndromes and conditions, psychosocial issues, public awareness, and integration issues. It provides a variety of resources, including newsletters, videotapes, and publications. There is a national chapter network for local access and networking. For further information:

Phone: (800) 665-FACE [800-665-3223] or (416) 597-2229
Fax: (416) 597-8494
E-mail: info@aboutfaceinternational.org
Web site: http://www.aboutfaceinternational.org
Address: 123 Edward Street, Suite 1003
    Toronto, ON, Canada M5G 1E2

The **American Cleft Palate-Craniofacial Association (ACPA)** is a professional organization, founded in 1943, which includes all disciplines involved in the care and treatment of cleft palate and craniofacial anomalies. Members are from the United States and from over 40 countries all over the world. Membership is open to individuals who are qualified to treat or conduct research in the areas of cleft lip, cleft palate, and other craniofacial anomalies. ACPA is dedicated to the study and treatment of all aspects of craniofacial anomalies, including cleft lip and palate. The organization has worked toward establishing standards of care for patients with craniofacial anomalies. Clinical and research information is shared through its quarterly *Cleft Palate-Craniofacial Journal.* Annual professional meetings are held at various locations around the country for the purpose of sharing and exchanging clinical information and the latest research findings. For further information:

Phone: (919) 933-9044

E-mail: info@acpa-cpf.org

Web site: http://www.acpa-cpf.org

Address: 1504 East Franklin Street, Suite 102

Chapel Hill, NC 27514-2820

The **Cleft Palate Foundation (CPF)** is a group that is associated with the American Cleft Palate-Craniofacial Association. The CPF has the mission of serving as a resource to families and professionals around the country. Services include a 24-hour toll-free phone number (CLEFT-LINE) that is available to both families and professionals who are seeking information about the evaluation or treatment of individuals with cleft lip, cleft palate, or other craniofacial birth defects. In addition, the CPF provides consumers with booklets on all aspects of cleft lip and palate (available in English and Spanish), craniofacial anomalies, and related syndromes. They provide a bibliography for parents of children with cleft lip/palate and a catalog of informational videocassettes. They can refer families to local and national support groups. Finally, the CPF provides consumers with a list of guidelines for choosing a medical team for cleft palate or craniofacial care, and also provides listings of qualified cleft and craniofacial anomaly teams in the patient's area. For further information:

Phone: (919) 933-9044

Fax: (919) 933-9604

E-mail: info@cleftline.org

Web site: http://www.cleftline.org

Address: 1504 East Franklin Street, Suite 102

Chapel Hill, NC 27514-2820

Children's Craniofacial Association offers assistance with doctor referrals and nonmedical assistance. There are annual family retreats and educational programs. The organization has publications about various craniofacial syndromes. For further information:

Phone: (800) 535-3643 or (214) 570-9099

Fax: (214) 570-8811

E-mail: contactCCA@ccakids.com

Web site: http://www.childrenscraniofacial.com

Address: 13140 Coit Road, Suite 307

Dallas, TX 75240

FACES: The National Craniofacial Association is a nonprofit organization that serves children and adults with craniofacial disorders by acting as a clearinghouse of information on specific disorders and available resources, providing networking opportunities with other families, publishing a quarterly newsletter, and providing financial assistance to families who cannot afford to travel away from home to a specialized craniofacial medical center. For further information:

    Phone: (800) 3FACES3 [800-332-2373]
    E-mail: faces@faces-cranio.org
    Web site: http://www.faces-cranio.org
    Address: P.O. Box 11082
        Chattanooga, TN 37401

Let's Face It is an information and support network for people with facial differences, their families, and professionals. Once a year, this organization publishes an extensive manual of organizations and resources for individuals with facial differences. To be placed on their mailing list, just send an e-mail address. For further information:

    University of Michigan
    School of Dentistry/Dentistry Library
    1011 N. University
    Ann Arbor, MI 48109-1078

Parents Helping Parents (PHP) is a parent-directed family resource center serving children with special needs, their families, and the professionals who serve them. This organization provides parent and professional training on how to begin and maintain a parent support network. Publications are available for training and information. For further information:

    Phone: (408) 727-5775
    Fax: (408) 727-0182
    E-mail: info@php.com
    Web site: http://www.php.com
    Address: 3041 Olcott Street
        Santa Clara, CA 95054

Smile Train has a free online library and links for articles from around the world on the cause and treatment of clefts. They also have informational booklets for families. For further information:

    Phone: (877) KID-SMILE [877-543-7645] or (212) 689-9199
    E-mail: info@smiletrain.org

Web site: http://www.smiletrain.org
Address: 245 Fifth Avenue, Suite 2201
New York, NY 10016

Wide Smiles is a nonprofit organization that is supported through contributions. Its purpose is to provide resources for individuals and family members with a history of cleft lip and palate. For further information:

Phone: (209) 942-2812
Fax: (209) 464-1497
E-mail: josmiles@yahoo.com
Web site: http://www.widesmiles.org
Address: P.O. Box 5153
Stockton, CA 95205-0153

Appendix B: Cleft Palate Foundation Publications

(Reprinted with permission from the Cleft Palate Foundation)
Available at http://cleftline.org

Fact Sheets (Full-Text Online Reports)

- *For Parents of Newborn Babies with Cleft Lip/Palate* (en español)
- *Answers to Common Questions about Scars* (en español)
- *Bonegrafting the Cleft Maxilla*
- *Choosing a Cleft Palate or Craniofacial Team* (en español)
- *Crouzon Syndrome*
- *Dealing With Your Insurance Company/HMO*
- *Dental Care for a Child with Cleft Lip and Palate* (en español)
- *Financial Assistance* (en español)
- *Letter to a Teacher*
- *Letter to the Parent of a Child with a Cleft* (en español)
- *Moebius Syndrome*
- *Pierre Robin Sequence*
- *Preparing Your Child for Social Situations*
- *Positional Plagiocephaly*
- *Replacing a Missing Tooth*
- *Selected Bibliography for Parents*
- *Speech Development* (en español)
- *Submucous Clefts*

- *Treacher Collins*
- *Treatment for Adults* (en español)

BOOKLET SUMMARIES (SUMMARIES OF DOCUMENTS AVAILABLE FOR ORDERING FROM THE CLEFT PALATE FOUNDATION)

These publications are provided free to families by the Cleft Palate Foundation. To receive a copy of any of the publications below, call the CLEFTLINE: 1-800-24CLEFT, or fill out an order form.

- *Cleft Lip and Palate: The First Four Years* (en español)
- *Cleft Lip and Palate: The School Aged Child* (en español)
- *As You Get Older: Information for Teens Born with Cleft Lip and Palate*
- *Cleft Lip and Palate: The Adult Patient*
- *Feeding an Infant with a Cleft* (en español)
- *Cleft Surgery* (en español)
- *Cleft Palate and Hearing Loss*
- *The Genetics of Cleft Lip and Palate: Information for Families*
- *Hemangiomas and Vascular Malformations*
- *Managing Speech Problems: Physical Treatment of Velopharyngeal Dysfunction*
- *Audiovisual and Supplemental Resource Catalog*
- *Parameters for Evaluation and Treatment of Patients with Cleft Lip/ Palate or Other Craniofacial Anomalies*: Summary of Recommendations, American Cleft Palate-Craniofacial Association, May, 1993, Rev. 2000

GLOSSARY

ablative surgery: surgery that involves removal of a part, such as a portion of the hard palate, due to a malignancy.

acrocentric: when the centromere of a chromosome is very close to one end of the chromosome.

active speech characteristics: see *compensatory errors*.

acute otitis media: bacterial infection of the middle ear.

adenoid: a normal collection of unencapsulated lymphoid tissue that is found on the posterior pharyngeal wall of the nasopharynx on the skull base; also called the *pharyngeal tonsil*.

adenoid facies: facial characteristics due to airway obstruction secondary to adenoid enlargement; characteristics include an open mouth posture, anterior tongue position, the mandible in a forward or downward position, facial elongation, suborbital coloring and puffy eyes, and the appearance of pinched nostrils.

adenoidectomy: surgical procedure to remove the adenoids; done to resolve recurrent infection, improve eustachian tube function, or eliminate upper airway obstruction.

adenotonsillectomy: a surgical procedure where both the tonsil and adenoid tissue are removed; done to resolve recurrent infection, improve eustachian tube function, or eliminate upper airway obstruction.

adipose: fat tissue.

aerodynamics: a branch of physics that deals with the mechanical properties of air and other gases in motion, the properties that set them in motion, and the results of that motion.

affricate sounds: pressure-sensitive consonants that require a build-up of intraoral air pressure and then slow release through a narrow opening; are produced as a combination of a plosive and fricative; includes /ch/ and /j/.

ala nasi: (pl. alae) Latin for "wing": the outside curved part of the nostril.

alar base: the area where the ala meets the upper lip.

alar rims: the part of the nose that surrounds the opening to the nostril on either side.

alleles: the alternative forms or variations of a given gene that are found at the same locus on an homologous chromosome.

almost-but-not-quite (ABNQ): a term used to refer to a small, yet consistent, velopharyngeal gap.

alveolar bone graft procedure: a surgical procedure of grafting bone, often from the iliac crest (hip bone), into the cleft site to stimulate new bone formation; this helps to repair the alveolar ridge, serves as the missing nasal floor and piriform (nasal) rim, and provides bone for eruption of teeth.

alveolar ridge: the portion of the maxilla and mandible that form the base and the bony support for the teeth; also called the *alveolus*, or simply the gum ridge.

alveolus: the socket of the tooth; also used as another word for *alveolar ridge*.

amnion: membrane surrounding the embryo and fetus.

amniotic bands: strands of tissue from the amnion that have ruptured and float in the amniotic cavity; these strands can attach to limbs, the head, or other body parts and act as tourniquets, cutting off blood supply to developing structures, resulting in amputations of limbs and digits, cleft lip, and encephalocele if the cranium is involved.

Angle's classification system: differentiates normal occlusion and three types of malocclusion.

ankyloglossia: a condition where the lingual frenulum is short or has an anterior attachment, resulting in restricted movement of the tongue tip; also known as *tongue-tie*.

anotia: absence of the external auditory canal.

anterior crossbite: a condition where a maxillary tooth or teeth are inside the mandibular arch; may involve any or all of the anterior teeth, such as the central incisors, lateral incisors, or canines; commonly seen in patients with dental or skeletal Class III malocclusion.

anterior nasal spine: the anterior point of the maxilla that corresponds to the base of the columella.

anterior-posterior (AP) view: see *frontal view*.

anticipation: in genetics, the tendency for a disorder to have earlier age of onset or more severe manifestations in successive generations.

antimongoloid slant: downward slant of the eyes.

apnea: see *sleep apnea*.

apraxia (of speech): (adj. apraxic) characterized by difficulty executing volitional oral movements and difficulty in sequencing oral movements for connected speech; can result in an inability to adequately coordinate velopharyngeal movement with the other subsystems of speech (respiration, phonation, and articulation); also called *dyspraxia* or *verbal apraxia*.

articulators: the oral structures that move to modify the airstream during speech; these include the lips, jaws (including the teeth), tongue, and velum.

association: in genetics, when two or more abnormalities appear together frequently but have not yet been classified together as a syndrome.

ataxia: an inability to coordinate muscle activity during voluntary movements; usually due to disorders of the cerebellum or posterior columns of the spinal cord.

atlas: the first cervical vertebrae; articulates with the occipital bone and rotates around the dens of the axis.

atresia: (adj. atretic) congenital absence or closure of any bodily orifice (opening, passage, or cavity); see *aural atresia*.

atrial septal defect (ASD): congenital discontinuity of the tissue that separates the upper chambers of the heart.

atrophy: shrinkage or degeneration of a structure.

attention deficit-hyperactivity disorder (ADHD): a cluster of behavioral characteristics involving impaired attention, distractibility, impulsivity, and hyperactivity; there appears to be a genetic basis to this disorder that affects the biochemical function in the brain.

attenuation: the combined absorption and scattering of radiation proton particles by the tissues.

audio: related to the sense of hearing.

audiologist: a professional who is responsible for testing hearing and middle ear function; the professional who works in conjunction with the otolaryngologist in the monitoring, evaluation, and treatment of hearing loss associated with middle ear disease, structural anomalies, or neurological anomalies that affect hearing recognition and perception.

auditory: pertaining to the sense of hearing or organs of hearing.

auditory atresia: see *aural atresia*.

auditory cortex: part of the brain that provides an awareness of sound.

auditory tube: see *eustachian tube*.

aural: related to the ear or hearing.

aural atresia: congenital closure of the auditory canal that usually results in a conductive hearing loss; also called *auditory atresia*.

auricle: the external ear; also known as *pinna* or *concha*.

autosomal recessive: traits that are manifest only when the trait is present in both copies of a gene.

autosome: (adj. autosomal) any chromosome that is not a sex chromosome.

backing of phonemes: a compensatory articulation strategy characterized by the production of most phonemes with the back of the tongue, and with the velum or with the posterior pharyngeal wall.

base view: X-ray view that allows the examiner to see the entire velopharyngeal sphincter during connected speech, as if looking up through the port; the relative contributions of the velum, the lateral pharyngeal walls, and posterior pharyngeal wall to closure can be determined; also called an *en face view*.

Bell's palsy: facial paralysis due to an infection.

Bernoulli effect: The low pressure created behind the fast-moving air column as it passes through the vocal folds. This causes the bottom of the folds to close, followed by the top. The closure of the vocal folds cuts off the air column and releases a pulse of air.

bicuspids: teeth that typically have two cusps.

bifid uvula: a congenital split or cleft in the uvula; a stigmata that is frequently associated with a submucous cleft palate.

biofeedback: a technique for making unconscious or autonomic physiological processes perceptible to the senses in order to manipulate them by conscious mental control; techniques are based on the learning principle that a desired response can be learned when it is determined that a specific thought process can produce the desired physiological response.

body section (of a prosthetic device): the anterior or palatal portion of a speech appliance that fits snugly against the contours of the individual's mouth and teeth; the purpose of the body section is to hold the appliance in place against the roof of the mouth or to serve as an obturator to close off a defect in the palate.

bone graft procedure: see *alveolar bone graft procedure*.

brachycephaly: a short skull.

brachydactyly: abnormally short digits (fingers or toes).

Brodie crossbite: occurs when the lingual cusps of all the maxillary posterior teeth are buccal to the mandibular teeth.

buccal (adj.): for the buccinator muscle of the cheeks; pertaining to, in the direction of, or adjacent to the cheek; the part of the dental arch that is posterior to the canine teeth and on the side of the teeth.

buccal crossbite: occurs when one or more maxillary teeth are positioned buccally such that the maxillary lingual cusps reside buccal to the mandibular cusps.

buccal sulcus: (pl. sulci) the area between the cheeks and teeth.

canines: teeth that have one point or cusp; also known as *cuspids.*

cant: a slant, as in dental occlusion.

canthus: (pl. canthi) the angle or corner of the eye.

caries: decay in the teeth, resulting in cavities.

cell cycle: the process of preparing for and undergoing cell division.

central fossa: (pl. fossae) the valley between the buccal cusp to lingual cusp of a tooth.

central sleep apnea: suspension of breathing during sleep due to medullary depression, which inhibits respiratory movement.

centromere: the area of constriction of a chromosome that divides the chromosome into two pairs of arms.

cephalogram: a lateral radiograph of the craniofacial skeleton; used in the planning of orthognathic surgery.

cephalometric radiographs: standardized lateral skull films used to measure the jaw relationship and the soft tissue profile of the forehead, nose, lips, and chin.

cheiloplasty: cleft lip repair.

choana: the opening on each side of the posterior part of the vomer that leads from the nasal cavity into the nasopharynx.

choanal atresia: congenital closure of the choana.

choanal stenosis: a narrowing of the choana.

cholesteatoma: a mass of keratinizing squamous epithelium and cholesterol in the middle ear, usually resulting from chronic otitis media.

chromosome: one of the bodies in the cell nucleus that contains genes; consists of a single linear double strand of DNA with associated proteins that function to organize and compact the DNA in a cell-for-cell division; the 46 chromosomes (23 pairs) contain the complete set of instructions for cell replication and differentiation.

cine study: see *cineradiography.*

cineradiography: radiography of an organ in motion; an old method for evaluating velopharyngeal function by recording multiple views on motion picture film in order to observe several dimensions; often referred to as a *cine study.*

circular pattern: pattern of velopharyngeal closure that occurs when all of the velopharyngeal structures contribute equally, and the closure pattern resembles a true sphincter.

circumvallate papilla: a line of prominent taste buds that makes an inverted "V" on the posterior tongue.

Class I occlusion: normal dental arch relationship, although the teeth may be misaligned; the mesiobuccal (front outside) cusp of the first maxillary molar fits in the buccal (outside) groove of the first mandibular molar.

Class II malocclusion: abnormal dental arch relationship where the mesiobuccal (front outside) cusp of the first maxillary molar is anterior to the buccal (outside) groove of the first mandibular molar; the maxillary arch is protrusive and too far in front of the mandibular arch.

Class III malocclusion: abnormal dental arch relationship where the mesiobuccal (front outside) cusp of the first maxillary molar is posterior to the buccal (outside) groove of the first mandibular molar; the maxillary arch is retrusive and too far behind the mandibular arch.

cleft: an abnormal opening or a fissure in an anatomical structure that is normally closed.

cleft lip: a congenital malformation that occurs in utero during the first trimester of pregnancy and involves a fissure of the lip and sometimes alveolus.

cleft muscle of Veau: refers to abnormal velar muscle insertion due to a cleft palate; the levator veli palatini muscle does not interdigitate in the midline and both this paired muscle and the palatopharyngeus muscles are inserted abnormally onto the posterior border of the hard palate, rendering them essentially nonfunctional.

cleft palate: a congenital malformation that occurs in utero during the first trimester of pregnancy and involves a fissure in the soft palate and sometimes the hard palate.

cleft palate team (CPT): a team of professionals that consists of a surgeon, an orthodontist, a speech-language pathologist, and one additional specialist according to the requirements of the American Cleft Palate-Craniofacial Association; other team members may include an audiologist, dentist, geneticist (dysmorphologist), nurse, oral surgeon (maxillofacial surgeon), and others.

clinodactyly: deflection or curvature of the digits (fingers or toes).

coarticulation: an abnormal consonant production characterized by one manner of production with simultaneous valving at two places of production.

cochlea: a part of the inner ear that is composed of a bony spiral tube that is shaped as a snail's shell and is responsible for hearing.

coding region: portions of a gene that determine the amino acid sequence for a polypeptide.

cognition: (adj. cognitive) refers to the individual's ability to engage in conscious intellectual activities, such as thinking, reasoning, imagining, or learning.

coloboma: a congenital defect, especially of the eye, which often involves a notch of the eyelid margin; usually affects the lower lid.

columella: the "little column" at the lower portion of the nose that separates the nostrils; cartilage and mucosa that are located under the nasal tip and at the lower end of the nasal septum.

compensatory errors: articulation gestures that are the individual's response to velopharyngeal dysfunction (or dental malocclusion), rather than the direct result of velopharyngeal dysfunction; also known as *active speech characteristics*.

complete cleft lip: involves the entire lip through the nostril sil and the alveolus (or dental arch) all the way to the area of the incisive foramen.

concha: (pl. conchae) a structure that is comparable to a shell in shape, such as the auricle or pinna of the ear or the turbinated bone within the nose; see *turbinates*.

conductive hearing loss: a type of hearing loss due to a blockage or problem with sound conduction to the inner ear.

condyle: the rounded articular surface of the bone, such as in the jaw joint.

congenital: a disease or deformity that is present at birth and may be the result of an inherited (genetic or chromosomal) condition, or may be due to something that occurred during the pregnancy (exogenous factors).

congenital palatal insufficiency (CPI): velopharyngeal dysfunction with no history of cleft palate, no apparent evidence of submucous cleft, or other known etiology.

conotruncal heart defects: also known as *outflow tract defects*; these are major abnormalities of the heart's chambers or blood vessels. They include truncus arteriosus, transposition of the great arteries, double outlet of the right ventricle, and tetralogy of Fallot.

consanguinity: mating between related individuals.

consulting team: a team of professionals whose members provide opinions regarding the total care of the patient; the opinions and recommendations are forwarded to the treating professionals for follow-up.

contiguous gene syndromes: syndromes caused by deletions large enough to contain several genes, but too small to be seen on routine cytogenetic analysis.

continuous positive airway pressure (CPAP): an instrument that delivers continuous airway pressure to the nasopharynx by means of a hose and nasal mask; used primarily in the treatment of sleep apnea to prevent pharyngeal collapse; has also been used to provide resistance training to strengthen the velopharyngeal musculature when there is velopharyngeal incompetence.

coronal pattern: a pattern of velopharyngeal closure that is accomplished primarily by the posterior movement of the velum against a broad area of the posterior pharyngeal wall and the possible anterior movement of the posterior pharyngeal wall; there is less contribution of the lateral pharyngeal walls during closure with this pattern.

corpus callosum: nerve fibers that allow communication between the left and right cerebral hemispheres. Consists mostly of contralateral axon projections. It appears as a wide, flat region just ventral to (below) the cortex.

corticotomy: a partial cut in the bone.

coupling: sharing of acoustic energy.

craniofacial anomaly: a structural or functional abnormality that affects the cranium or face.

craniofacial team (CFT): a team of professionals that consists of a craniofacial surgeon, an orthodontist, a mental health professional, and a speech-language pathologist according to the requirements of the American Cleft Palate-Craniofacial Association; other members may include a neurosurgeon, an ophthalmologist, and others.

craniosynostosis: abnormal development of the cranial skeleton due to premature ossification of one or more cranial sutures, resulting in malformation of the skull with growth; the shape of the skull depends on the sutures that are involved; can cause raised intracranial pressure (ICP) and mental retardation if not treated; can be syndromal, due to genetic factors, or nonsyndromal.

crossbite: a type of dental malocclusion where a maxillary tooth or teeth are inside the mandibular teeth; when the normal overlap of the upper teeth to the lower teeth is reversed, so that the lower teeth overlap the upper teeth buccally; can be anterior or lateral.

cryptorchidism: undescended testes.

cul-de-sac resonance: abnormal resonance during speech, which occurs when the transmission of acoustic energy is trapped in a blind pouch in the vocal tract with only one outlet; the speech is perceived as muffled due to the fact that the sound is contained in a cavity with no direct means of escape.

Cupid's bow: the shape of the top of the upper lip, which includes a rounded configuration with an indentation in the middle.

cusp: the point on a tooth.

cuspids: teeth that have one point or cusp; also known as *canines*.

cytogenetics: the branch of genetics that is concerned with the structure and function of the cell, particularly the chromosomes; molecular cytogenetics allows extremely small genetic abnormalities to be detected.

cytokinesis: the separation of the cell cytoplasm to form two distinct cells with separate cell membranes.

damping: to slow or stop the vibration or decrease the amplitude of an oscillating system.

deciduous teeth: primary or "baby" teeth.

deep bite: when the upper teeth overlap more than 25% of the lower teeth; the lower incisors may be in contact with the alveolar ridge of the palate.

deformation: (syn. deformity) birth defect that arises as a result of abnormal mechanical or physical forces in the fetal environment on an otherwise normal structure; usually results in the abnormal shape or form of a completely formed organ or structure, such as clubfoot.

deformity: see *deformation*.

dehiscence: breakdown of a surgical repair.

deletion: in genetics, absence of a piece of a chromosome or genetic material; often results in multiple malformations and developmental handicaps.

denasality: abnormal resonance due to a lack of vibration of the sound energy in the nasal cavity; total nasal airway obstruction and the resultant effect on resonance.

dental arch: the curved structure in the maxilla and mandible that consists of the alveolar ridge and teeth.

dental elastics: small rubber bands used to add a dynamic component for pulling teeth or bony segments together.

dental implants: cylindrical shaped pieces of titanium that can take the place of a missing tooth's root and are able to support crowns and prosthetic devices.

dental occlusion: the manner in which the maxillary teeth and mandibular teeth fit together, or the bite; in normal occlusion the upper arch overlaps the lower arch.

dentition: the teeth taken all together.

dentures: removable prosthetic teeth that replace an entire dental arch.

deoxyribonucleic acid (DNA): a nucleic acid made up of building blocks called nucleotides; contained in the nuclei of animal and vegetable cells and is the component of chromosomes; each DNA molecule contains many genes, which contain hereditary information; consists of two strands that wrap around each other in the shape of a twisted ladder or double helix.

dermatoglyphics: creases on the hands or changes in the fingerprints that can give clues to early developmental problems.

diastasis: a separation between two normally joined structures; as in separation of the levator veli palatini muscles when there is a submucous cleft palate.

diastema: a space or opening between the teeth, usually the upper central incisors.

differential pressure: the difference in pressure between the nasal cavity and the oral cavity during speech, as measured simultaneously through aerodynamic instrumentation.

direct measures: instrumental procedures that allow the examiner to visualize the anatomical and physiological defects that cause velopharyngeal dysfunction; includes videofluoroscopy and nasopharyngoscopy procedures.

disruption: a morphologic defect resulting from an extrinsic breakdown or interference with a normal developmental process.

distal (adj.): the direction away from the midline, following the curvature of the dental arch.

distraction osteogenesis: a method for increasing bone length; involves making a corticotomy in the middle of a bone, then slowly pulling the cut ends apart (distracting) with a mechanical device; new bone is able to regenerate between the cut ends, obviating the need for bone grafts; can be used for maxillary or mandibular advancement.

dolichocephaly: long, narrow skull seen with prematurity.

dominant inheritance: when only one gene is needed for expression of a trait (i.e., brown eyes); when one allele from one parent is expressed over a contrasting allele from the other parent.

dorsum: the top surface, as on the tongue.

double helix: coiled ladder of a DNA molecule that consists of two polymers of nucleotides.

duplication: when part of a chromosome is duplicated, often resulting in multiple malformations and developmental handicaps.

dysarthria: a motor speech disorder that affects the oral articulators and is characterized by abnormalities of muscular strength, range of motion, speed, accuracy, and tonicity due to a neurological injury or insult; speech is very slow and characterized by inaccurate movement of the articulators.

dysmorphogenesis: (adj. dysmorphic) the process of abnormal tissue formation, resulting in abnormally formed features.

dysmorphology: the study of abnormal shape or form.

dysphagia: abnormality or difficulty in swallowing.

dysphonia: (adj. dysphonic) refers to voice disorder that results in an alteration in the normal phonatory quality of the voice; characterized by breathiness, hoarseness, low intensity, and glottal fry.

dysplasia: an abnormal organization of cells into tissues and the outcome of the process.

dyspraxia: see *apraxia (of speech)*.

eardrum: see *tympanic membrane*.

ectopic tooth: a normal tooth that erupts in an abnormal position.

edema: an excessive amount of fluid in cells and tissues, causing swelling.

encephalocele: a congenital gap in the skull with herniation of brain tissue into the nose or palate.

endogenous: a factor from within the organism rather than from the environment, such as the genetic makeup of the organism.

endoscope: a specialized, flexible fiberoptic instrument that consists of an eyepiece at the end of a long tube or scope; used for examination of an internal canal or organ; can be used for evaluation of the velopharyngeal mechanism, pharynx, or larynx; a type of endoscope is a *nasopharyngoscope*.

endoscopy: a procedure that allows the visualization of the interior of a canal or hollow organ by means of a special instrument, usually called an *endoscope*.

en face view: see *base view*.

epibulbar dermoid: a cyst on the eyeball.

epicanthal folds: folds of tissue that extend from the upper eyelid to the lower part of the orbit at the inner canthus or corner of the eye.

epiphyseal dysplasia: underdevelopment or abnormality of the long bones of the extremities.

epitaxis: a nosebleed.

eustachian tube: the tube that connects the middle ear with the nasopharynx; usually closed at the pharyngeal end at rest, but opens with swallowing and yawning due to the action of the tensor veli palatini muscle; allows ventilation of the middle ear, equalization of air pressure on both sides of the tympanic membrane, and drainage of fluids; also known as the *auditory tube*.

exogenous: a factor that is outside an organism and is not indigenous to that organism, such as drugs or smoke.

exons: portions of the DNA in a gene function in the transcribed RNA template to direct the incorporation of amino acids into a protein.

exophthalmos: protrusion of one or both globes of the eye beyond the socket due to either congenital or pathological factors that provide pressure behind the eye; often associated with craniosynostosis involving the coronal suture.

exorbitism: excessive protrusion of the globe of the eye from its socket due to shallow orbits.

expressive language: the ability to generate and then transmit a message.

expressivity: the extent to which a gene is apparent in the phenotype.

external auditory canal: a skin-lined canal of the external ear that leads to the eardrum.

external ear: part of the ear that is comprised of the pinna and the external auditory canal.

fascia: a sheet of fibrous tissue that encloses muscles and muscle groups.

faucial pillars: bilateral curtainlike structures in the posterior portion of the oral cavity; the anterior faucial pillar is formed as the velum curves downward toward the tongue and the posterior faucial pillar is just behind the anterior pillar.

faucial tonsils: lymphoid tissue that is located on either side of the mouth between the anterior and posterior faucial pillars; also referred to as merely *tonsils*.

fiberoptic endoscopic evaluation of swallowing (FEES): a procedure where a flexible endoscope is used in the evaluation of swallowing disorders; involves the transnasal passage of an endoscope for viewing of the pharyngeal and laryngeal structures to study the integrity of airway protection during swallowing.

fistula: (pl. fistulae or fistulas) an abnormal hole or passage from one epithelialized cavity to another epithelialized cavity; examples included an oronasal (palatal) fistula or tracheoesophageal fistula.

fixed bridge: permanently placed prosthetic teeth typically used to replace dental segments.

fluorescent in situ hybridization (FISH): a procedure used in a cytogenetic laboratory that involves the use of a nucleic acid probe labeled with a fluorescent dye to localize a specified submicroscopic segment of DNA; used to determine deletion of parts of chromosomes, as in the diagnosis of velocardiofacial syndrome.

foramen: (pl. foramina) a normal hole or opening in a bony structure or membranous structure; often serves as a passageway to allow blood vessels and nerves to pass through to the area on the other side.

forme fruste: a partial or arrested form of a cleft lip where the overlying skin is intact, but the underlying muscle, nasal cartilage, and oral sphincter function usually are significantly affected; also called *microform cleft*.

fovea palati: (pl. foveae palati) one of the bilateral midline depressions at the junction of the hard and soft palate that are the openings to minor salivary glands.

frenulum: (pl. frenulae) a small frenum; see *frenum* and *lingual frenulum*.

frenum: (pl. frena or frenums) a narrow fold of mucous membrane or web that connects a fixed structure to a movable part and serves to check undue movement; see *frenulum* and *lingual frenulum*.

fricative sounds: pressure-sensitive sounds that require a gradual release of air pressure through a small opening; includes /f/, /v/, /s/, /z/, /sh/, /th/.

frontal view: an X-ray view that allows the examiner to visualize the lateral pharyngeal walls at rest and during speech; the orientation of this view is as if one is looking straight through the nose; also called the *anterior-posterior view* or simply the *AP view*.

gamete: a sex cell, either an ovum or sperm cell.

gastrostomy tube (G-tube) feeding: a method of parenteral feeding through the use of a tube that is place directly into the stomach through an opening that is surgically created.

gene: (adj. genetic) a functional unit of heredity that is submicroscopic, resides at a specific location or locus on a chromosome, and is capable of reproducing itself with each cell division; consists of a sequence of nucleotide bases in a molecule of deoxyribonucleic acid (DNA).

genetics: the science of patterns of heredity.

genioplasty: horizontal mandibular osteotomy for chin advancement.

genome: consists of chromosomes and DNA and contains a complete set of instructions for cell replication and differentiation for an organism; see *Human Genome Project*.

genotype: the genetic constitution of an individual.

gingivoperiosteoplasty: a procedure to close the cleft of the alveolus with raised gingival flaps and the underlying periosteum on each edge of the cleft; raw surfaces are advanced and sewn together to allow the bone progenitor cells to lay down bone as the patient grows.

glossopexy: a surgical procedure that involves suturing the tongue tip to the bottom lip to help to keep the airway open in patients with glossoptosis.

glossoptosis: the posterior displacement of the tongue in the pharynx; can cause airway obstruction.

glossus: related to the tongue.

glottal plosive: see *glottal stop*.

glottal stop: a compensatory articulation production characterized by forceful adduction of the vocal folds and the build-up and release of air pressure under the glottis, resulting in a grunt-type sound.

greater segment: palatal segment on the noncleft side.

hair cells: sensory cells, as in the organ of hearing, that have hair-like properties.

hard palate: a bony structure that serves as the roof of the mouth and floor of the nasal cavity and separates the oral cavity from the nasal cavity.

hemangioma: a congenital anomaly in which a proliferation of blood vessels results in a large mass.

hemifacial microsomia: lack of development of the bones on one side of the face; results in various degrees of both unilateral mandibular hypoplasia and facial weakness.

hemihypertrophy: where one side of the body grows faster than the other side.

hepatoblastoma: a malignant liver tumor; a risk for individuals with Beckwith-Wiedemann syndrome.

heterogeneity: the mutation of different genes leading to the same phenotype.

heterogeneous: a characteristic where more than one gene can cause the same clinical features.

heterozygous: having two different copies or alleles of a gene at the same locus on a pair of homologous chromosomes.

holoprosencephaly: failure of the forebrain to divide into the two hemispheres; often accompanied by a midline deficit in facial development or a midfacial cleft.

homozygotes: persons with two identical copies of a gene.

homozygous: when genes have two similar alleles.

horizontal plates: paired plates of the palatine bones located just behind the transverse palatine suture line; forms the posterior portion of the hard palate, ending with the protrusive posterior nasal spine.

Human Genome Project: an international initiative whereby researchers from all over the world are collaborating to compile a comprehensive map of the human genome.

hypernasality: a resonance disorder that occurs when sound enters the nasal cavity inappropriately during speech; the perceptual quality of speech is often described as just "nasal," muffled, or characterized by mumbling; is particularly perceptible on vowels.

hyperplasia: (adj. hyperplastic) overdevelopment of a structure; an increase in the number of cells in a tissue or organ, not related to tumor formation, whereby that body part is larger than normal.

hypertelorism: excessive distance between two paired organs, such as the eyes.

hypertrophy: (adj. hypertrophic) overgrowth of a structure.

hypoglycemia: low blood sugar.

hyponasality: a type of abnormal resonance that occurs when there is a reduction in nasal resonance during speech due to blockage in the nasopharynx or in the entrance to the nasal cavity; particularly affects the production of the nasal consonants (/m/, /n/, and /ng/).

hypopharynx: part of the pharynx, or throat, which is below the oral cavity and extends from the epiglottis inferiorly to the esophagus.

hypoplasia: (adj. hypoplastic) underdevelopment or defective formation of a tissue or organ, usually due to a decrease in the normal number of cells.

hypospadias: where the orifice of the penis is proximal to its normal location.

hypotelorism: narrow-spaced eyes.

hypotonia: (adj. hypotonic) a lack of adequate muscular tonicity or tension.

ideogram: a schematic drawing of the banding pattern of a chromosome.

idiopathic: a condition that appears without apparent cause or etiology.

imprinting: when some genes function differently, depending on whether they were inherited maternally or paternally.

incidence: in epidemiological terms, refers to the number of new cases of a disease or disorder in a given population, such as the number of persons becoming ill with a certain disease.

incisive foramen: a hole in the bone that is located in the alveolar ridge area of the maxillary arch, just behind the central incisors, and forms the tip of the premaxilla.

incisive papilla: the slight elevation of the mucosa at the anterior end of the raphe of the palate.

incisive suture lines: embryological suture lines in the hard palate that go between the lateral incisors and canines and meet posteriorly at the area of the incisive foramen; the suture lines that separate the premaxilla.

incisors: teeth that are somewhat shovel shaped; their biting surfaces are thin knifelike edges.

incomplete penetrance: the lack of a recognizable phenotype in an individual who carries a gene for an autosomal dominant trait.

incus (anvil): one of the ossicles in the middle ear; articulates with the malleus and the stapes.

indirect measures: instrumental procedures that provide object data regarding the results of velopharyngeal function, such as airflow, air pressure, or acoustic output, but do not allow visualization of the structures; includes nasometry and aerodynamic instrumentation.

infant oral orthopedics: see *palatal orthopedics*.

inner ear: part of the ear that consists of the cochlea and semicircular canals.

intelligence: relates to the ability to learn; a prerequisite for normal language development.

intentional fistula: a nasolabial fistula that is deliberately left in the alveolus (under the lip) at the time of the primary palatoplasty to allow unrestricted facial growth; it is closed with a bone graft at a later time.

interdisciplinary team: a group of professionals from various disciplines who work together to coordinate the care of a patient through collaboration, interaction, communication, and cooperation.

intermaxillary fixation: wiring the mandible against the maxilla to keep it closed and in place; often done for a period of time after orthognathic surgery.

intermaxillary palatine suture line: see *median palatine suture line.*

interosseous dental implants: implants that are imbedded in the bone so that a speech appliance or denture can be attached and retained.

interphase: the time between cell divisions.

intonation: refers to the frequent changes in pitch throughout an utterance, as controlled by subtle changes in vocal fold length and mass.

intraoral air pressure: a build-up of air pressure in the oral cavity that provides the force for the production of oral consonants, particularly plosives, fricatives and affricates.

intravelar veloplasty (IVVP): a surgical reconstruction of the levator veli palatini sling during palatoplasty for correction of a cleft of the velum.

introns: the portions of a gene's DNA sequence that are removed from the RNA transcript before it is transported to the cytoplasm for translation.

inversions: when a portion of a chromosome is turned 180° from its usual orientation; may not be associated with any abnormalities in the individual because the total amount of genetic material may be unchanged.

karotype: a gross chromosome analysis that is done by drawing blood, growing the cells in a culture, analyzing the white blood cells, photographing the chromosomes and then arranging the chromosomes in pairs for display and assessment.

keloid: excessive scar tissue formed during healing.

labial (adj.): relating to the lip; the outer part of the dental arch that touches the lip.

labial tubercle: the prominent projection on the inferior border, or free edge, of the midsection of the upper lip.

labioversion: when the upper incisors are displaced anteriorly, with overjet greater than 2 mm, causing the maxillary incisors to protrude out toward the lips.

labyrinthitis: inflammation of the labyrinth, which is sometimes accompanied by vertigo and deafness.

laminar airflow: airflow through the nasal cavity that is steady and smooth due to the lack of significant resistance.

laminography: use of a radiograph to measure distances and angles between particular landmarks.

language: refers to the meaning or message that's conveyed back and forth during communication.

laryngeal web: a congenital anomaly that consists of a band of tissue between the vocal folds, usually in the anterior portion of the larynx, and that can cause respiratory stridor.

laryngomalacia: abnormally soft cartilage in the epiglottis and aryepiglottic folds at birth, resulting in loud inspiratory stridor that is particularly pronounced when the infant cries or breathes deeply.

lateral cephalometric X-rays: still radiographs of the head taken in the sagittal plane.

lateral pharyngeal walls: the side walls of the throat.

lateral view: an X-ray view that shows the velum and posterior pharyngeal wall in a midsagittal plane; the orientation of the lateral view is as if we were able to look through the side of the head to view these structures from the side.

Latham appliance: a two-piece acrylic dental appliance that is used prior to the lip and alveolus repair to close the gap between the greater and lesser maxillary segments from a wide cleft of the primary palate.

Le Fort I osteotomy: a surgical cut in the bone that transversely separates the maxilla just above the base of the nose so that the maxilla and palate can be moved as a single unit.

Le Fort II osteotomy: a surgical cut in the bone that includes both the nasal pyramid and the alveolar arch.

Le Fort III osteotomy: a surgical cut in the bone that includes cheek bones, orbital rims, nasal pyramid, and alveolar arch.

lesser segment: palatal segment on the cleft side.

levator sling: the levator veli palatini muscles from each side interdigitate and blend together to form a muscle sling.

levator veli palatini: paired muscle that forms the main muscle mass of the velum, primarily responsible for velar elevation.

lingual: related to the tongue; the inner part of the upper and lower dental arch that is in contact with the tongue.

lingual frenulum: (pl. frenula) a narrow fold of mucous membrane that extends from the floor of the mouth to the midline of the under surface of the tongue; see *frenum* and *frenulum*.

lingual tonsils: a mass of lymphoid tissue located at the base of the tongue that extends to the epiglottis.

linguoversion: when the upper teeth are inside the lower teeth; also known as *anterior crossbite* or *underjet*.

lip adhesion: a simple, straight-line surgical procedure to temporarily repair a cleft lip; this procedure is performed so that the subsequent lip pressure will draw the segments together, making the final repair more successful.

lip pits: depressions in the bottom lip that are usually bilateral and are associated with Van der Woude syndrome with cleft palate.

lipodermoids: fatty tissue.

lobulated tongue: the tongue appears to have multiple lobes, with fissures between each lobe.

lower esophageal sphincter (LES): sphincter at the base of the esophagus that relaxes to allow a bolus to enter the stomach.

macro: large.

macroglossia: large tongue.

macrostomia: a large mouth opening, often due to failure of fusion between the maxillary and mandibular process of embryonic development of the face.

mala: (adj. malar) relating to the cheek or cheekbone (zygomatic bone).

malar hypoplasia: lack of cheekbone development.

malformation: defect in basic embryological plan due to chromosomal or genetic factors.

malleus (hammer): one of the ossicles in the middle ear; is firmly attached to the tympanic membrane and articulates with the incus.

malocclusion: improper dental or skeletal relationship of the maxillary and mandibular arches so that the arches do not close together normally.

mandibular hypoplasia: lack of mandibular development, causing a small, retrusive mandible; see *micrognathia* and *retrognathia*.

mastoid cavities: a section of the temporal bone that is porous and located just behind the ear.

mastoiditis: inflammation or infection in any part of the mastoid process.

maxillary hypoplasia: lack of development of the maxilla, causing midface retrusion or deficiency and concavity of the midface.

maxillary retrusion: characterized by a small upper jaw (maxilla) relative to the lower jaw (mandible); a common anomaly, especially in individuals with repaired cleft lip and palate secondary to the inherent deficiency in the maxilla due to the cleft and the possible restriction in maxillary growth with the surgical repair; also known as *midface deficiency*.

meatus: an opening, channel or passageway; usually the external opening of a canal; see *nasal meatus*.

median palatine raphe: the thin white line that can often be seen running longitudinally down the middle of the velum. This is an embryological suture line for the velum.

median palatine suture line: embryological suture line that begins at the incisive foramen and ends at the posterior nasal spine; separates the paired palatine processes of the maxilla and the horizontal plates of the palatine bones; also known as *intermaxillary palatine suture line*.

meiosis: a special process of cell division that results in gametes (spermatocytes or oocytes) with 23 chromosomes rather than the 46 that are found in somatic cells.

mesial (adj.): the direction toward the midline, following the curvature of the dental arch.

messenger RNA (mRNA): ribunucleic acid (RNA) that has had the introns removed and is transported from the nucleus to the cytoplasm to function as a template for protein synthesis.

metacentric: chromosomes with a centrally located centromere.

metopic: related to the forehead or anterior portion of the cranium.

micro: small.

microcephaly: small head circumference in comparison to age-matched peers.

microform cleft: see *form fruste.*

microglossia: small tongue.

micrognathia: a small or hypoplastic mandible; see *mandibular hypoplasia.*

micropenis: small penis.

microphthalmia: small eyes.

microstomia: a small mouth opening.

microtia: hypoplasia or absence of the external ear (pinna or auricle); often accompanied by aural atresia (a blind or absent external auditory meatus).

middle ear: a hollow space within the temporal bone.

middle ear effusion: collection of fluids within the middle ear space due to the eustachian tube dysfunction.

middorsum palatal stop: an abnormal articulation production that is often compensatory for anterior oral cavity crowding; produced as a stop consonant that is articulated with the middle of the dorsum against the middle of the hard palate; is usually substituted for the lingual-alveolar sounds (/t/ and /d/), for the velar sounds (/k/ and /g/), and in some cases, for sibilant sounds (/s/, /z/, /sh/, /ch/, and /j/); also called a *palatal dorsal production.*

midface deficiency: see *maxillary retrusion.*

midface retrusion: concavity of the midface due to maxillary hypoplasia.

mitosis: the process of separating duplicated chromosomes; the reconstitution of two cell nuclei.

mixed resonance: a combination of hypernasality, hyponasality, or cul-de-sac resonance during connected speech.

modified barium swallow (MBS): see *videofluoroscopic swallowing study (VSS).*

Moebius syndrome: involves specific cranial nerve damage with weakness affecting the oral and facial musculature.

molars: teeth that are designed for grinding; on each side of the maxillary and mandibular arch, there are the first molars (6-year molars), the second molars (12-year molars), and the third molars (wisdom teeth); upper molars have four cusps, two buccal and two palatal (or lingual) cusps, and lower molars have five cusps, three buccal and two lingual cusps.

mongoloid slant: upward slant of the eyes.

monosomy: absence of an entire chromosome of a pair of homologous chromosomes.

morphogenesis: the process of embryonic tissue formation.

mosaicism: an anomaly of chromosome division resulting in the presence of cells with two or more different genetic makeups, or a different number of chromosomes, in a single individual.

mucoid effusion: a thick, mucus-like fluid in the middle ear.

mucoperiosteum: tissue that consists of a mucous membrane and periosteum; covers the hard palate.

mucosa: see *mucous membrane.*

mucous membrane: (adj. mucosal) the lining tissue of the nasal cavity, oral cavity, and pharynx; consists of stratified squamous epithelium and lamina propria; also known as *mucosa.*

mucus: a clear, viscid secretion of the mucous membranes.

multidisciplinary team: a group of professionals from various disciplines who work independently in evaluating and treating patients with complex medical needs; members of this type of team have well-defined roles and cooperate with each other, but there is little communication and interaction among the team members.

multifactorial inheritance: a characteristic in the phenotype that is the result of a combination of many genes at different loci and/or factors from the environment; the combination of genes and other factors all have a small added effect to form the characteristic in the phenotype.

musculus uvulae: a paired muscle that creates a bulge on the posterior nasal surface of the velum during phonation; during contraction, this bulge provides additional bulk and stiffness to the nasal side of the velum and helps to fill in the area between the velum and posterior pharyngeal wall, contributing to a firm velopharyngeal seal.

mutation: a change in the sequence of base pairs in the DNA molecule that is reflected in subsequent divisions of the cell; a change in the chemistry of the gene that is reflected in the subsequent genotype and phenotype.

mutation: a change in the sequence of a molecule of DNA; mutation can be as small as a substitution of a single base pair or as large as the deletion of an entire chromosome.

myopia: nearsightedness.

myringotomy: a surgical puncture of the tympanic membrane so that fluid can be drained or suctioned out of the middle ear.

naris: (pl. nares) nostril.

nasal air emission: an inappropriate flow of the airstream through the nose during speech, causing distortion of the speech; usually caused by velopharyngeal dysfunction; also called *nasal escape.*

nasal airway resistance: attenuation of the nasal airflow due to any condition that obstructs or restricts the patency of the nasopharynx or nasal cavity.

nasal bridge: the bony structure that is located between the eyes and corresponds to the middle of the nasofrontal suture; also known as *nasion.*

nasal grimace: a muscle contraction during speech that is typically noted either above the nasal bridge (in the area between the eyes) or around the nares; occurs as an overflow muscle reaction when there is an attempt to achieve velopharyngeal closure; usually accompanied by nasal air emission.

nasal meatus: any of the three passages in the nasal cavity that lie directly under a nasal concha; see *meatus.*

nasal molding: a method of repositioning the nasal septum and ala in the infant prior to cleft lip repair; usually involves an intraoral/nasal appliance combined with taping.

nasal regurgitation: reflux of fluids into the nasopharynx and nasal cavity during drinking or vomiting.

nasal root: where the nose begins at the level of the eyes.

nasal rustle: a fricative sound that occurs as air pressure is forced through a partially opened velopharyngeal valve causing the airflow to become turbulent and resulting in bubbling of secretions above the opening; also called *nasal turbulence.*

nasal septum: a wall separating the nasal cavity into two halves; consists of the vomer bone, the perpendicular plate of the ethmoid, and the quadrangular cartilage and is covered with mucous membrane; see *septum.*

nasal sil: the base of the nostril opening.

nasal sniff: an uncommon compensatory articulation production that is produced by a forcible inspiration through the nose; usually substituted for sibilant sounds, particularly the /s/, and typically occurs in the final word position.

nasal snort: a burst of nasal air emission that is produced by a forcible emission of air pressure through the nares during consonant production, resulting in a noisy, sneezelike sound.

nasal turbulence: see *nasal rustle.*

nasalance score: represents the relative amount of nasal acoustic energy in the person's speech as determined by the Nasometer; the ratio of nasal acoustic energy over total (oral plus nasal) acoustic energy during speech as determined through the use of the Nasometer; the score represents the mean of the percentage points that are calculated for an entire speech passage.

nasalance distance: the range between the maximum and minimum nasalance.

nasalance ratio: the minumum nasalance divided by the maximum nasalance.

nasalization of oral phonemes: an obligatory error due to an open velopharyngeal valve.

nasendoscopy: see *nasopharyngoscopy.*

nasion: see *nasal bridge.*

nasogastric (NG) tube: a tube placed through the nose and down to the stomach and used for feeding.

nasogastric (ng) tube feeding: a method of feeding through the use of a tube that is placed in the nose and goes down to the stomach.

nasogram: a contour display on a computer screen that represents the nasalance results of the spoken passage on the Nasometer.

nasolabial fistula: a fistula in the alveolus (under the lip) that is often deliberately left by the surgeon during the initial repair to allow for maxillary growth. It is later closed by a bone graft. Often called *intentional fistula.*

Nasometer: a computer-based instrument (Kay Elemetrics, Inc., Pinehurst, NJ) that measures the relative amount of nasal acoustic energy in a patient's speech.

nasopharyngeal airway: a tube that used to improve the airway of infants, such as those with Pierre Robin sequence; the tube is placed in the nose of the infant in such a way that one end sticks out of the nose and the other end extends to below the region of tongue obstruction.

nasopharyngoscope: a type of endoscope that is used for examination of the pharynx, larynx, and velopharyngeal mechanism.

nasopharyngoscopy: a minimally invasive endoscopic procedure that allows visual observation and analysis of the velopharyngeal mechanism or larynx during speech through the use of a scope (nasopharyngoscope) that is inserted through the nose until it reaches the nasopharynx; can be used to evaluate velopharyngeal function, phonation, or swallowing; also called *nasendoscopy* or *videoendoscopy.*

nasopharynx: the part of the pharynx, or throat, that lies above the soft palate and just behind the nasal cavity.

nondisjunction: the failure of one or more chromosomes to separate in cell division.

nonpneumatic activities: as they relate to the velopharyngeal valve: swallowing, gagging, and vomiting.

nosocomial infections: infections that are acquired while in the hospital.

nucleotides: building blocks of DNA that consist of a 5-carbon sugar chemically bonded to a phosphate group and a nitrogenous base.

obligatory errors: speech characteristics that are the product of structural abnormality or dysfunction; includes hypernasality, nasal air emission, weak consonants, and short utterance length; also known as *passive speech characteristics* where the articulation placement (the function) is normal, but the abnormality of the structure causes distortion of speech.

oblique view: X-ray view that allows the examiner to see the lateral pharyngeal walls and velum during connected speech; used primarily if the base view cannot be obtained due to enlarged adenoids or the inability to hyperextend the neck.

obstructive sleep apnea (OSA): a period during sleep when the individual is exerting muscular forces to inspire, but is unsuccessful in moving air into the lungs due to a blockage in the pharynx; often caused by enlarged tonsils, enlarged adenoids, or pharyngeal hypotonia during sleep.

obturator: a generic term to describe a device that can be used to cover a hole; see *palatal obturator.*

occlusal cant: a sloping, transverse occlusal plane caused by impaired vertical maxillary growth on one side, which is compensated by vertical alveolar growth in the mandible on the same side; common in patients with unilateral cleft lip/palate and those with hemifacial microsomia.

occlusion: the relationship between the maxillary and mandibular teeth when the jaws are closed as when biting.

occult submucous cleft: a defect in the velum that is under the mucous membrane and not visible on the oral surface; this defect can usually be viewed on the nasal surface of the velum through nasopharyngoscopy.

ocular: related to the eyes.

oligogenic model: a variation of the multifactorial model of inheritance, where a trait may be determined by the interaction of multiple genes with little environmental influence; a small number of genes may contribute most of the risk.

omphalocele: where part of the intestines may be outside of the abdomen in the region of the umbilical cord.

open bite: occurs when one or more maxillary teeth fail to occlude with the opposing mandibular teeth; primarily affects the anterior dentition (anterior open bite) and less commonly the posterior dentition (lateral open bite).

ophtha: related to the eyes.

optic: related to the eyes.

oral frenulae: oral tissue webs.

oral manometer: an instrument that was used in the past to provide a gross measurement of airflow abilities during blowing or negative pressure during sucking; the patient was required to blow into a catheter or suck the catheter; this is no longer considered valid because information is now available about the physiological differences between blowing or sucking activities and speech.

oral resonance: the result of the sound energy vibrating (resonating) in the oral cavity during speech.

orbicularis oris: the muscle that encircles the mouth and serves to close the lips.

organ of corti: the part of the inner ear where the mechanical energy introduced into thecochlea is converted into electrical stimulation.

orogastric tube feeding: a method of feeding through the use of a tube that is placed in the mouth and goes down to the stomach.

oronasal fistula: see *palatal fistula*.

oropharyngeal isthmus: the opening from the oral cavity to the pharynx; bordered superiorly by the velum, laterally by the faucial pillars, and inferiorly by the base of the tongue.

oropharynx: the part of the pharynx, or throat, that lies below the soft palate at the level of the oral cavity or just posterior to the mouth.

orthodontist: the professional who is responsible for aligning misplaced teeth and correcting discrepancy in jaw size to improve the dental and facial aesthetics and the function of the dentition.

orthognathia: (adj. orthognathic) the study of the causes and the treatment of conditions related to malposition of the bones of the jaw.

orthognathic surgery: surgery that involves the bones of the upper jaw (the maxilla) and the lower jaw (the mandible).

Orticochea sphincteroplasty: see *sphincter pharyngoplasty*.

osseointegrated implants: implants that are inserted in the bone; used for retention of bridges and prosthetic devices.

ossicles: (adj. ossicular) three small bones in the middle ear that conduct sound energy from the tympanic membrane to the cochlea; include the malleus, incus, and stapes.

osteotomies: surgical cuts in a bone so that the bone can be placed in a more functional and appropriate position.

otic: relating to the ear (otitis, otolaryngologist, otorrhea, microtia, etc.).

otitis media: a bacterial infection and inflammation of the middle ear.

otitis media with effusion: an inflammation of the middle ear that is accompanied by a build-up of fluids.

otolaryngologist: the physician who is responsible for monitoring middle ear function and treating middle ear disease, assessing and treating anomalies and disease of the oral cavity, pharynx, nasal cavity, and upper airway and lower airway; also known as the *ear, nose and throat specialist (ENT)*.

otorrhea: a type of ear disease with discharge.

otoscope: an instrument used to visualize the tympanic membrane.

overbite: the vertical overlap of the upper and lower incisors; can be measured in millimeters but is often reported as a percentage of coverage of the lower incisors by the upper incisors; normal overbite is approximately 2 mm or about 25%; greater amounts are called either deep overbite, or *deep bite*.

overjet: the horizontal relationship between the upper and lower incisors; typically measured in millimeters from the labial surface of the lower incisor to the labial surface of the upper incisor with the teeth in occlusion; a normal amount of overjet is about 2 mm with upper incisors and lower incisors in light contact; excessive overjet is where the maxillary incisors are labioverted or stick out toward the lips.

overlay dentures: dentures that fit over the existing teeth and usually provide more vertical dimension.

palatal (adj.): the inner part of the upper and lower arch that is in proximity to the surface of the hard palate.

palatal fistula: a hole or opening in the palate that goes all the way through to the nasal cavity; may be the result of a breakdown of the area of a previously repaired cleft, the result of maxillary expansion, or even growth; also called *oronasal fistula.*

palatal lift: a prosthetic appliance that can be used to raise the velum for speech in cases where the velum is long enough to achieve velopharyngeal closure, but does not move well, often due to neurological impairment.

palatal obturator: a prosthetic appliance that can be used to cover an open palatal defect, such as an unrepaired cleft palate or a palatal fistula; this device can be used to improve an infant's ability to achieve compression of the nipple for suction or can be used to close a palatal defect for speech.

palatal orthopedics: a method used to align the alveolar segments in both unilateral and bilateral clefts of the palate prior to surgical correction; also known as *infant oral orthopedics.*

palatal section (of a prosthesis): the body portion of a prosthetic appliance that fits over the palate.

palatal vault: the rounded dome on the upper part of the oral cavity.

palatal-dorsal production: see *middorsum palatal stop.*

palate: the bony and muscular partition between the oral and nasal cavities.

palatine aponeurosis: a sheet of fibrous tissue located just below the nasal surface of the velum and extending about 1 cm posteriorly from its attachment on the posterior border of the hard palate; consists of periosteum, fibrous connective tissue, and fibers from the tensor veli palatini tendon; provides an anchoring point for the velopharyngeal muscles and adds stiffness to that portion of the velum; also called *velar aponeurosis.*

palatine processes: paired bones of the maxilla that are just behind the incisive suture lines and form the anterior three quarters of the maxilla.

palatine tonsils: masses of lymphoid tissue between the anterior and posterior faucial pillars on both sides of the oral cavity; also called simply the *tonsils.*

palatine torus: see *torus palatinus.*

palatoglossus: paired muscles that act antagonistically to the levator veli palatini to depress the velum or elevate the tongue; these muscles contribute to lowering the velum for the production of nasal speech sounds.

palatomaxillary suture line: see *transverse palatine suture line.*

palatopharyngeus: paired muscle of the pharynx; the horizontal fibers are thought to be associated with the sphincteric action of the velopharyngeal valve, assisting with velopharyngeal closure by pulling the lateral pharyngeal walls medially to narrow the pharynx.

palatoplasty: palate repair.

palpebra: (pl. palpebrae, adj. palpebral) eyelid.

palpebral fissures: opening between the eyelids.

panendoscope: an older illuminated instrument that included an optical tube that is placed in the mouth and turned upward for visualization of the velopharyngeal sphincter; no longer used.

parathyroid glands: glands responsible for making parathyroid hormone, which helps regulate calcium levels in the blood.

paresis: (adj. paretic) weakness of muscle movement; partial or incomplete paralysis.

partial trisomy: duplication of a piece of a chromosome rather than the entire chromosome so that there is a part of a chromosome with the pair.

Passavant's ridge: a shelflike ridge that projects from the posterior pharyngeal wall into the pharynx during speech; occurs as a result of contraction of specific fibers of the superior pharyngeal constrictor muscles; found in normal speakers and speakers with velopharyngeal dysfunction.

passive speech characteristics: see *obligatory errors.*

pedigree: pictorial representation of family members and their line of descent; used by geneticist to analyze inheritance, particularly for certain traits or anomalies.

penetrance: the frequency of the expression of a genotype in a phenotype; if the trait does not appear 100% of the time when the gene is present, then it is said to have reduced penetrance.

periosteum: a thick, fibrous membrane that covers the surface of bone.

peripheral sleep apnea: see *obstructive sleep apnea.*

perpendicular plate of the ethmoid: the bone that projects down to join the vomer and lies between the vomer and the quadrangular cartilage; forms part of the nasal septum.

pharyngeal affricate: a compensatory articulation production that is produced when the tongue is retracted so that the base of the tongue articulates against the pharyngeal wall; is the combination of either a pharyngeal plosive or a glottal stop and a pharyngeal fricative.

pharyngeal flap: a type of pharyngoplasty designed to be a passive soft tissue obturator of the middle of the velopharyngeal sphincter to improve or correct velopharyngeal function.

pharyngeal fricative: a compensatory articulation production that is produced when the tongue is retracted so that the base of the tongue approximates, but does not touch, the pharyngeal wall; a friction sound occurs as the air pressure is forced through the narrow opening that is created between the base of the tongue and pharyngeal wall.

pharyngeal plexus: a network of nerves that lies along the posterior wall of the pharynx and consists of the pharyngeal branches of the glossopharyngeal and vagus nerves, which provide motor innervation for the velar muscles that contribute to velopharyngeal closure.

pharyngeal plosive: a compensatory articulation production that is produced with the back of the tongue articulating against the pharyngeal wall; also called *pharyngeal stop.*

pharyngeal stop: see *pharyngeal plosive.*

pharyngeal tonsil: see *adenoid.*

pharyngeal wall augmentation: an implant that is surgically placed or injected in the posterior pharyngeal wall, or a rolled flap on the pharyngeal wall; placed in the area of the velopharyngeal opening to correct velopharyngeal dysfunction.

pharyngoplasty: a surgical procedure of the pharynx that is designed to correct velopharyngeal dysfunction.

pharynx: (adj. pharyngeal) the walls of the throat between the esophagus and nasal cavity.

phenotype: the manifestations of a genotype; range of characteristics associated with a genetic syndrome.

philtral ridges: the raised lines on either side of the philtrum, which are embryological suture lines that are formed as the segments of the upper lip fuse.

philtrum: (adj. philtral) a long dimple or indentation that courses from the columella down to the upper lip and is bordered by the philtral ridges on each side.

phonation: the sound generated by the vocal folds as they vibrate.

phoneme-specific nasal air emission (PSNAE): nasal air emission that is due to velopharyngeal mislearning rather than a structural or physiological cause; occurs due to the use of a posterior nasal fricative as a substitution for oral sounds; usually substituted for sibilant sounds, particularly s/z.

Pierre Robin sequence: a congenital condition that consists of micrognathia, glossoptosis, and cleft palate; there is often upper airway obstruction for several months after birth.

pinna: the delicate cartilaginous framework of the external ear; functions to direct sound energy into the external auditory canal; also known as the *auricle* or *concha*.

piriform aperture: literally means pear-shaped opening; the opening to the nostril or nasal cavity.

pyriform aperture stenosis: narrowing of the anterior nasal openings.

plagiocephaly: asymmetric or abnormal skull shape.

pleiotropy: the phenomenon where a single gene can affect multiple unrelated systems.

plosive sounds: pressure-sensitive consonants that require a build-up of intraoral pressure prior to a sudden release; include /p/, /b/, /t/, /d/, /k/, /g/.

pneumotachograph: an airflow device that consists of a flowmeter and a differential pressure transducer; one of the components of aerodynamic instrumentation to measure velopharyngeal orifice area or nasal resistance.

pneumatic activities: as they relate to the velopharyngeal valve: blowing, whistling, sucking, and speech.

polycythemia: an increase in the normal number of red blood cells.

polydactyly: extra fingers and/or toes.

polymorphism: variability in genes that contributes to the uniqueness of individuals.

polysomnography: a diagnostic test during which a number of physiologic variables are recorded during a sleep study.

posterior crossbite: involves any combination of teeth distal (posterior) to the canines where the maxillary teeth are inside the mandibular teeth; usually occurs because the maxilla is too narrow.

posterior nasal fricative: an abnormal articulation production that is produced with the velum somewhat down so that air pressure goes through a velopharyngeal opening, creating a friction sound with audible nasal air emission; typically used as a substitution for sibilant sounds, particularly s/z; associated with phoneme-specific nasal air emission (PSNAE).

posterior nasal spine: a protrusive projection in the middle of the posterior border of the hard palate.

posterior pharyngeal wall: back wall of the throat.

preauricular tags: projection of scalp and skin tags from the area of the ear to the cheek.

premaxilla: a triangular-shaped bone that is bordered on either side by the incisive suture lines; this bony segment normally contains the central and lateral maxillary incisors.

premolars: teeth that typically have two cusps, although they may sometimes have three.

pressure equalizing (PE) tubes: see *ventilation tubes*.

pressure-flow technique: procedure using aerodynamic instrumentation to evaluate the dynamics of the velopharyngeal mechanism during speech; also used to evaluate nasal respiration and to quantify upper airway obstruction through measurements of nasal airway resistance.

prevalence: in epidemiological terms, refers to a measure of existing cases of a disorder in a given population.

primary dentition: stage of dental development where there are 10 teeth in the upper arch, 10 teeth in the lower arch and usually spacing between all of the primary teeth.

primary palate: the lip and palate anterior to the incisive foramen; includes the lip and alveolus.

prognathia: (adj. prognathic) protrusive mandible caused by mandibular hyperplasia.

prognathism: having a large mandible.

prolabium: the tissue that normally makes up the central portion of the upper lip between the philtral columns but is isolated when there is a bilateral cleft lip.

proptosis: (adj. proptotic) protrusion of the eyeball.

prosthesis: (adj. prosthetic) a fabricated substitute for a body part that is missing or malformed; also called a *prosthetic device*.

prosthodontist: a dental professional who deals with the restoration of teeth and the development of appliances to replace or improve the appearance of oral and facial structures or to assist with feeding and velopharyngeal closure.

provisionally unique syndromes: patterns of multiple anomalies in what appears to be an underlying syndrome, although a diagnosis cannot be made because the pattern is not one that has been previously described or reported.

psychologist: the professional who assesses a patient's psychosocial needs, and assists the patient and family in dealing with the medical, social and emotional challenges that occur due to the patient's anomalies.

pterygoid process: a part of the sphenoid bone that contains the medial pterygoid plate, the lateral pterygoid plate, and the pterygoid hamulus, all of which provide attachments for muscles in the velopharyngeal complex.

purines: nitrogenous bases of nucleotides in a DNA molecule that consists of adenine and guanine.

ptosis: drooping of the eyelids.

purulent effusion: the fluid in the middle ear that is like pus.

pyrimidines: nitrogenous bases of nucleotides in a DNA molecule that consist of thymine and cytosine.

quad helix: a palatal expansion device that consists of bands on the most posterior molars, and frequently the primary canines, which are connected by a palatal spring that has two posterior and two anterior loops.

quadrangular cartilage: the cartilage that forms the anterior nasal septum and projects anteriorly to the columella.

radiography: the use of the roentgen rays (X-rays) to image internal body parts.

ramus: the upturned, perpendicular extremity of the mandible on both sides.

raphe: (pronounced *rayfay*) a line of union between two bilaterally symmetric structures; the palatine raphe is the midline of the mucosa of the hard palate that runs from the incisive papilla posteriorly over the entire length of the hard palate.

rapid palatal expander: a palatal expansion device that consists of two or four molar bands and a jackscrew connecting them in the middle of the palate; turning the screw creates the necessary force to widen the dental arches.

receptive language: the understanding of a message that is sent.

recessive inheritance: a trait that is expressed only in individuals who are homozygous for the gene involved in that they have inherited the same gene for the trait from both parents (e.g., blue eyes); when the same allele is needed from both parents for expression of a trait.

reduction therapy: a form of speech therapy where a prosthetic device is used to stimulate the movement of the velopharyngeal structures to avoid the need for surgery, or reduce the extent of the surgery needed.

replication: the process of making two identical DNA molecules from one, resulting in two double strands, each containing one original and one complementary newly synthesized strand of DNA.

resonance: the quality of the voice that results from the vibration of sound in the pharynx, oral cavity, and nasal cavity.

retrognathia: (adj. retrognathic) when one or both jaws is located posterior to its normal position; usually used in reference to a retrusive mandible; associated with micrognathia (mandibular hypoplasia).

reverse pull headgear: a device used to advance the maxilla and improve an anterior crossbite.

ribonucleic acid (RNA): a nucleic acid which is found in the nucleus and cytoplasm of all cells.

ribosomes: organelles within the cell that function in protein synthesis.

right sided aortic arch: abnormality where the aortic arch is on the right side rather than the left.

rhinomanometry: procedure for measuring nasal airway resistance; involves measurement of the pressure encountered by air passing through the nasal cavity.

rolled flap: a flap of tissue is surgically raised from the posterior pharyngeal wall and is rolled up on to itself to form a bulge on the posterior pharyngeal wall; used to fill in a velopharyngeal gap.

rotameter: used for the calibration of the pneumotachograph; uses a compressed air supply to provide a known rate of airflow.

rugae: folds, ridges, or creases in a structure; the transverse ridges in the mucosal covering of the hard palate.

rule of 10s: a guideline for the appropriate time for a cleft lip repair, which says that the infant must be at least 10 weeks of age, 10 pounds, and have a hemoglobin of 10 gm prior to the lip repair.

saccule: a sensory organ within the inner ear that provides a sensation of acceleration.

sagittal pattern: the least common pattern of velopharyngeal closure; the lateral pharyngeal walls move medially to meet in midline to effect closure; the velum may move to close against the lateral pharyngeal walls rather than against the posterior pharyngeal wall.

sagittal plane: the median, longitudinal plane of the body; a plane of view for X-ray procedures.

salpingopharyngeal folds: folds that originate from the torus tubarius at the opening to the eustachian tube on both sides of the pharynx and then course downward to the lateral pharyngeal wall; consist of glandular and connective tissue.

salpingopharyngeus: paired muscle that arises from the inferior border of the torus tubarius and courses vertically along the lateral pharyngeal wall and under the salpingopharyngeal fold; is not felt to have a significant role in achieving velopharyngeal closure given its size and location.

scaphocephaly: skull that is oblong from front to back; caused by premature closure of the sagittal suture.

secondary palate: structures that are posterior to the incisive foramen, including the hard palate (excluding the premaxilla) and the velum.

semicircular canals: the loop-shaped tubular parts of the inner ear that provide a sense of spatial orientation; the loops are oriented in three planes at right angles to each other.

sensitivity: the extent to which a test is able to correctly identify positive results; proportion of true positive results as intended to be revealed by a test.

sensorineural hearing loss: a type of hearing loss due to a problem with the creation of nerve impulses within the inner ear or the transmission of the nerve impulses through the brainstem to the auditory cortex.

septum: a thin wall separating two cavities; see *nasal septum.*

sequence: the occurrence of a pattern of multiple anomalies within an individual that arise from a single known or presumed prior anomaly or mechanical factor; where one anomaly leads to the development of the other anomalies as in Pierre Robin sequence.

serous effusion: fluid in the middle ear that consists of a very thin, watery liquid.

sex chromosomes: the 23rd pair of chromosomes (X and Y) that function in determining gender.

sialorrhea: drooling.

sibilant sounds: speech sounds that are produced by the friction of air pressure as it is emitted anteriorly through the incisors; includes /s/, /z/, /sh/, /ch/, /zh/, and /j/.

Simonart's band: a strand of soft tissue in the area of the cleft lip that is due to partial, yet incomplete, embryonic fusion of the upper lip.

single tooth crossbite: a crossbite that involves only one upper and one lower tooth.

sleep apnea: cessation of respiration during sleep due to upper respiratory obstruction or central (neurogenic) causes, or to a combination of both.

soft palate: see *velum.*

sometimes-but-not-always (SBNA): a term for an individual who demonstrates inconsistent velopharyngeal closure; the individual may be able to achieve total closure with effort, but has difficulty maintaining closure consistently and over a prolonged period of time.

somia: refers to body.

specificity: the extent to which a test correctly identifies true negative results; the proportion of individuals with negative test results for what the test is intended to reveal.

speech aid appliance: see *speech bulb obturator.*

speech bulb obturator: a prosthetic device that can be considered when the velum is too short to close completely against the posterior pharyngeal wall; this device consists of a retaining appliance and a bulb (usually of acrylic) that fills in the pharyngeal space for speech; also known as a *speech aid appliance.*

sphincter pharyngoplasty: a type of pharyngoplasty to create a dynamic sphincter that encircles the velopharyngeal port; also known as the *Orticochea sphincteroplasty.*

stapes: one of the ossicles in the middle ear; acts as a piston to create pressure waves within the fluid-filled cochlea.

stenosis: an abnormal narrowing or stricture of a canal (e.g., choanal stenosis, pharyngeal stenosis, or subglottic stenosis).

stertorous: a heavy snoring sound in respiration.

stoma: the surgical opening into the trachea through which the patient can breathe following a tracheostomy.

stomia: refers to the mouth.

stress: related to increased muscular effort and subglottic pressure during the production of a syllable; stressed syllables are produced with greater articulatory precision, are longer in duration, and are higher in pitch and intensity than unstressed syllables.

submetacentric: when the centromere of a chromosome is closer to one end than the other.

submucous cleft palate: a congenital defect that affects the underlying structures of the palate, while the structures on the oral surface are intact; can involve the muscles of the velum and also involve the bony structure of the hard palate.

succedaneous teeth: secondary or permanent teeth.

suckling: an early form of sucking characterized by extension-retraction movements of the tongue.

superior pharyngeal constrictor: paired muscle of the pharynx; the upper fibers are responsible for the medial displacement of the lateral pharyngeal walls to effectively narrow the velopharyngeal port.

supernumerary tooth: an extra tooth; usually erupts in the line of the cleft.

syndactyly: fusion or webbing of the digits (fingers and/or toes).

syndrome: a pattern of multiple anomalies or malformations that regularly occur together and are pathogenically related and, therefore, have a common known or suspected cause; craniofacial syndromes (involving the head and face) cause affected individuals to look alike, even when there is no family relationship (e.g., Down syndrome).

synostosis: abnormal fusion or premature fusion of the two or more normally separated bones; see *craniosynostosis.*

tailpiece (of a prosthetic device): the part of a palatal lift or speech bulb appliance that extends posteriorly to either raise the velum or close the nasopharynx behind the velum.

telecanthus: increased distance between the medial canthi of the eyelids.

temporomandibular joint: the joint of the mandible and temporal bone.

tensor veli palatini: paired muscles that are believed to be responsible for opening the eustachian tubes to enhance middle ear aeration and drainage.

teratogen: an external chemical or physical agent, such as cigarette smoke, drugs, viruses, or radiation, that can interfere with normal embryological development and result in congenital malformations.

tetralogy of Fallot: most common congenital heart defect; includes ventricular septal deviation (VSD), dextroposition (right-sided) aortic arch, right ventricular hypertrophy, and pulmonary stenosis; often associated with a syndrome.

thymus: the organ in the chest which is the source of T-lymphocytes.

TONAR: developed by Fletcher in 1970, this was the first instrument to measure nasal and oral acoustic energy during speech; predecessor to the Nasometer.

tongue-tie: see *ankyloglossia*.

tonsillectomy: surgical procedure to remove the tonsils; done to resolve recurrent infection or to eliminate oral cavity obstruction.

tonsils: see *faucial tonsils*.

torus palatinus: a normal variation, not an abnormality, that consists of a prominent longitudinal ridge, or exostosis, on the oral surface of the hard palate in the area of the median palatine suture line; found most often in Caucasians, particularly those of northern European descent, and reportedly common in the northern Native American and Eskimo populations.

torus tubarius: a ridge in the nasopharyngeal wall, posterior to the opening of the eustachian tube, caused by the projection of the cartilaginous portion of this tube.

Towne's view: a radiographic view that is sometimes used as an alternative to the base view because it also provides an en face orientation; it allows the examiner to look down into the port.

tracheoesophageal (TE) fistula: congenital opening between the trachea and the esophagus; causes aspiration during feeding.

tracheostomy: a surgical procedure that involves placement of a tube directly in the trachea; done to relieve upper airway obstruction, which can be life threatening.

transcription: the process of creating a strand of RNA that is complementary to a given strand of DNA.

transdisciplinary team: an interdisciplinary team where members understand the other disciplines and how they relate to the total care of the patient; this understanding of the various disciplines allows them to be able to see the "big picture" in the care of the patient.

transducers: as part of aerodynamic instrumentation, used to convert the detected air pressure or flow into electrical signals for further processing.

translocations: the result of a transfer of genetic material between two or more chromosomes; may not be associated with any abnormalities in the individual because the total amount of genetic material may be unchanged.

transverse palatine suture line: an embryological suture line that separates the paired palatine processes of the maxilla, which form the anterior three quarters of the maxilla, and the paired horizontal plates of the palatine bones; also known as the *palatomaxillary suture line*.

treating team: the team members provide a consultation regarding the total care of the patient and also offer treatment.

trigonocephaly: the top of the skull is triangular-shaped with a pointed forehead.

trisomy: a condition where there is an extra chromosome in an homologous pair of chromosomes; for example, trisomy 21 or Down syndrome in humans is a condition where the cell contains 47 rather than 46 chromosomes.

tubercle (of the lip): the somewhat prominent point at the inferior border of the midsection of the upper lip.

turbinates: bony structures in the nose that are covered with mucosa; the superior and middle turbinates are parts of the ethmoid bone and the inferior turbinate, which is the largest, is part of the sphenoid bone; see *concha*.

turbulent flow: airflow through the nasal cavity that is affected by obstacles, irregularities, and convolutions.

tympanic membrane: thin tissue that separates the outer ear from the middle ear; transmits sound energy through the ossicles to the inner ear; also called the *eardrum*.

underjet: a reversal of the normal incisor position, with the maxillary incisors linguoverted or facing inward toward the tongue; also called *linguoversion* or *anterior crossbite*.

Universal Blood and Body Fluid Precautions (UBBFP): guidelines for infection control that were developed by the Centers for Disease Control and Prevention (CDC) in Atlanta.

upper esophageal sphincter (UES): the upper end of the esophagus that normally is closed, but stretches open as the bolus travels through the hypopharynx and into the esophagus.

utricle: a sensory organ within the inner ear that provide a sensation of acceleration.

U-tube water manometer: a device that consists of a U-shaped glass tube partially filled with water and is used for the calibration of pressure transducers.

uvula: a teardrop-shaped structure that is typically long and slender and hangs freely from the back or free edge of the velum; it has no known function.

uvulopalatopharyngoplasty (UPPP): a surgical procedure for the treatment of the obstructive sleep apnea in adults; involves the excision of the remaining tonsil and resection of the free margin of the soft palate and uvula; the anterior and posterior tonsillar pillars are sewn together to open the oropharyngeal inlet.

Van der Woude syndrome: includes cleft palate and bilateral lip pits, which are small depressions in the bottom lip; has a 50% recurrence risk for future pregnancies.

variable expressivity: variability in the clinical presentation (phenotype) of patients with a particular genetic disorder; a gene can result in variations in the phenotype from a very pronounced effect in one individual to a barely noticeable effect in another.

velar aponeurosis: see *palatine aponeurosis*.

velar dimple: the area on the oral side of the velum where it bends during phonation or velopharyngeal closure; can be noted through an intraoral examination.

velar eminence: a bulge on the nasal surface of the velum during phonation which comes from the musculus uvulae muscles; can be seen through nasopharyngoscopy.

velar fricative: a compensatory articulation production that is produced with the back of the tongue in the same position as for the production of a /y/ sound so that a small space is created between the back of the tongue and the velum; a fricative sound is produced as air is forced through that small opening.

velar stretch: the process where the velum elongates as it elevates to achieve velopharyngeal closure.

veloadenoidal closure: the velum commonly closes against the adenoid during speech in children who have a prominent adenoid pad.

velopharyngeal dysfunction (VPD): one of the generic terms that is used to describe abnormal velopharyngeal function, regardless of the cause.

velopharyngeal inadequacy (VPI): one of the generic terms that is used to describe abnormal velopharyngeal function, regardless of the cause.

velopharyngeal incompetence (VPI): a neuromotor or physiological disorder that results in poor movement of the velopharyngeal structures.

velopharyngeal insufficiency (VPI): an anatomical or structural defect that precludes adequate velopharyngeal closure by causing the velum to be short relative to the posterior pharyngeal wall.

velopharyngeal mislearning: inadequate velopharyngeal closure due to faulty learning of appropriate articulation patterns.

velum: the part of the palate that is located in the back of the mouth and consists of muscles that are covered by the same mucous membrane as the hard palate; frequently referred to as the *soft palate.*

ventilation tubes: small tubes that are surgically inserted in the eardrum to provide an alternate route for air to enter the middle ear for ventilation if the eustachian tube is nonfunctional; also called *pressure equalizing (PE) tubes.*

ventral surface: the lower surface, as of the tongue.

ventricular septal defect (VSD): congenital discontinuity of the tissue that separates the lower chambers of the heart.

ventricular septum: the tissue that separates the two lower chambers of the heart.

verbal apraxia: see *apraxia (of speech).*

verbal language: meaning or message that is conveyed through speech.

vermilion: the red pigmented portion of the upper and lower lips.

video endoscopy: see *nasopharyngoscopy.*

videofluoroscopic speech study: an evaluation of the velopharyngeal mechanism and other oral and pharyngeal structures during speech using videofluoroscopy.

videofluoroscopic swallowing study (VSS): a radiographic procedure that allows an overall view of the oral, pharyngeal, and esophageal phases of swallowing as well as the interactions between the phases; also referred to as a *modified barium swallow (MBS).*

videofluoroscopy: a radiographic procedure used to examine deep structures of the body during movement; the images are recorded on a videotape.

vocal nodules: bilateral, circumscribed enlargements on the vocal folds that are the result of abuse, overuse, or misuse of the voice; commonly seen in patients with mild velopharyngeal dysfunction due to the strain in the vocal tract with attempts to achieve velopharyngeal closure; can also occur secondary to the use of compensatory articulation productions, particularly glottal stops.

vomer: a flat bone of trapezoidal shape that is positioned so that it is perpendicular to the palate; the inferior border meets the nasal surface of the maxilla in midline and forms the inferior and posterior portion of the nasal septum.

Waldeyer's ring: a complex of lymphoid tissue, including the adenoids, tonsils, and lingual tonsil, which encircles the pharynx and plays a role in the immune system.

W-arch: a variation of the quad helix palatal expansion device.

well-type manometer: similar to a U-tube water manometer but provides for the direct reading of applied pressures; has a calibrated reservoir filled with water or oil and is used for the calibration of pressure transducers.

white roll: the white border tissue that surrounds the red tissue, or vermilion, of the upper and lower lips.

Wilms tumor: a malignant tumor of the kidney; a risk for individuals with Beckwith-Wiedemann syndrome; a liver tumor called hepatoblastoma X-linked inheritance: an inherited trait from genes located on the X chromosome; the trait is usually more pronounced or is lethal in males because males have only one X chromosome as opposed to females who have two X chromosomes.

zona pellucida: a bluish area in the middle of the velum that is the result of abnormal insertion of the levator veli palatini muscles, effectively causing the velum to be thin and almost transparent in appearance.

zygoma: the bone of the skull that forms the prominence of the cheek and articulates with the frontal, sphenoid, temporal, and maxillary bones. It is also known as the *zygomatic bone* or *malar bone*.

INDEX

Page numbers with f indicate reference to a figure and those with t indicate a table